Medical Diagnosis and Therapy

CARDIAC ARREST DRUGS

DRUG	DOSAGE	SUPPLIED	COMMENT
Epinephrine	IV bolus 1 mg repeated q 3–5 min.* Tracheobronchial 10 ml (1:10,000)	10 ml (1 mg in 1:10,000 dilution)	Do not give with $NaHCO_3$ in same IV
Sodium Bicarbonate	IV bolus 1 mEq (mmol)/kg, usually 50 mEq (mmol) initially; then ½ initial dose q 10 to 15 min	50 ml of 8.4% = 50.0 mEq (mmol) 1 Amp = 44 mEq	Not used routinely. Recommended for trial after 7th shock, pH <7.1, or 10 min. in asystole
Atropine	In asystole 1 mg q 2–5 min (max of 3 mg, 0.04 mg/kg) Bradycardia 0.5 mg q 5 min to 2 mg	10ml = 1 mg 5 ml = 0.5 mg (UK, 1 ml amp = 0.6 mg or 1 mg)	
Lidocaine	75–100 mg IV bolus simultaneous infusion 2–3 mg/min	50 mg in 5 ml (1%) 100 mg in 10 ml (1%) 100 mg in 5 ml (2%)	
Bretylium Tosylate for VF	5 mg/kg IV bolus (undiluted). CPR, 1 min. If counter-shock fails, repeat 10 mg/kg (max 30 mg/kg)	500 mg in 10 ml amp (UK 50 mg/ml; 2 ml amp)	Hypotension Do not give epinephrine or norepinephrine simultaneously
Propranolol for VF	USA: 1 mg over 2–5 min (q 2–5 min to max 5/mg) UK: 1 mg over 2 min (q 2 min to max 5 mg)		Useful in recurrent VF if lidocaine fails
Metoprolol	5 mg IV over 5 min		
Calcium Chloride	2.5 to 5 ml 10% (5–7 mg/kg 250–500 mg) IV bolus, Repeat 10 ml IV in 5 min	10 ml 10% $CaCl_2$	*Not recommended* in cardiac arrest, except with hyperkalemia or post verapamil Do not give with $NaHCO_3$

q = every; *high doses may be tried (unproven) 2, 3, 5 mg, 3 min apart

Modified from: Khan, M. Gabriel: Cardiac Drug Therapy, 3rd Ed. London, W. B. Saunders, 1992

Medical Diagnosis and Therapy

M. Gabriel Khan

MB BCh (Hons), MD, FRCP (London), FRCP (C), FACP

Associate Professor of Medicine

University of Ottawa

Cardiologist, Ottawa General Hospital

Ottawa, Canada

Lea & Febiger

PHILADELPHIA · BALTIMORE · HONG KONG
LONDON · MUNICH · SYDNEY · TOKYO

A WAVERLY COMPANY

Lea & Febiger
Box 3024
200 Chester Field Parkway
Malvern, Pennsylvania 19355-9725 U.S.A.
(610) 251-2230

Executive Editor: R. Kenneth Bussy
Development Editor: Tanya Lazar
Project Editor: Raymond Lukens
Production Manager:
Samuel A. Rondinelli

Library of Congress Cataloging-in-Publication Data

Medical diagnosis and therapy / [edited by] M. Gabriel Khan.
p. cm.
Includes index.
ISBN 0-8121-1602-X
1. Internal medicine—Handbooks, manuals, etc. I. Khan M. I. Gabriel.
[DNLM: 1. Diagnosis. 2. Therapeutics. WB 141 M4892 1994]
RC55.M383 1994
616—dc20
DNLM/DLC
for Library of Congress 93-37038
CIP

NOTE: Although the author(s) and the publisher have taken reasonable steps to ensure the accuracy of the drug information included in this text before publication, drug information may change without notice and readers are advised to consult the manufacturer's packaging inserts before prescribing medications.

Reprints of chapter may be purchased from Lea & Febiger in quantities of 100 or more. Contact Sally Grande in the Sales Department.

PRINTED IN THE UNITED STATES OF AMERICA

PRINT NUMBER: 5 4 3 2

Preface

The aim of this book is to provide house staff, students, and clinicians with an accurate and up-to-date source of easily retrievable information on how to manage the medical diseases and conditions most frequently encountered in medical wards and emergency departments. The text provides practical advice that allows house staff to solve on-call problems in internal medicine; it presents a bedside approach with diagnostic hallmarks, advice on relevant investigations, and discussions of drug or interventional therapy.

It takes more than knowledge to write a medical bestseller or a text that is worthy of being in circulation for more than 50 years. In order to accomplish this objective, we strived to provide:

- accuracy;
- up-to-date information;
- depth of coverage in areas of internal medicine relevant to hospital practice;
- clarity of writing and emphasis on practical information; and
- succinctness.

The several areas of internal medicine are well represented by the 27 eminent clinical teachers who have had considerable practice on medical wards and are well-recognized authors in their fields. The cardiology section is largely derived from my recent book, *Cardiac and Pulmonary Management*, which has been described in the foreword by Dr. Henry J. L. Marriott as "a masterpiece . . . up-to-date, thorough, meticulously detailed and accurate." Dr. Eric J. Topol, Chairman, Department of Cardiology, The Cleveland Clinic Foundation, assisted with the chapter on Acute Myocardial Infarction. Dr. John G. Bartlett, Chief, Infectious Diseases, Johns Hopkins Hospital, has enhanced the work with his section on Infectious Diseases. Dr. Joseph P. Lynch, III and Galen B. Toews of the Pulmonary and Critical Care Division, University of Michigan Medical Center, have contributed comprehensive chapters on pneumonias and pulmonary infections. The text provides considerable coverage of endocrinology and rheumatology to fulfill the needs of students and house staff who often need to consult a pocket companion to resolve difficult but appealing endocrine and rheumatologic entities.

In-depth coverage of cardiology, rheumatology, endocrinology, gastroenterology, hematology, and pulmonary and infectious diseases was achieved by the omission of oncology, dermatology, and conditions that do not require hospitalization or emergency room management. Oncology is a specialized subject that requires complex management, including chemotherapeutic "cocktails" used in some hospitals, cities, or countries and not in others. Overdose/poisoning has not been included because management is usually efficiently administered by a poison control division that is readily accessible by phone in most cities.

Appropriate therapy and decision-making strategies require:

- accurate diagnosis;
- consideration of pathophysiology;
- knowledge of the action of pharmacologic agents and their correct indications; and
- advantages and disadvantages of interventional therapy.

These topics are sufficiently covered to allow the application of rational therapy. Carefully thought out, practical decision-making algorithms and numerous tables enhance the quality of the text.

The tersely written, bulleted style allows the text to accommodate a wealth of relevant clinical information on diagnosis and therapeutics that should appeal to students, house staff, internists, and all who render care to medical patients.

Finally I must express warm appreciation to R. Kenneth Bussy, Tanya Lazar, Nancy Roberson, CEO, Raymond Lukens and Sam Rondinelli of Lea & Febiger for their indispensable cooperation.

M. Gabriel Khan
Ottawa, Canada

Contributors

John G. Bartlett, MD
Professor of Medicine
Chief Infectious Diseases
Johns Hopkins Hospital
Baltimore, MD

Richard Beaser, MD
Consultant Endocrinologist
Diabetes Center
Joslin Clinic
Boston, MA

Sanjiv Chopra, MD
Associate Professor of Medicine
Harvard Medical School
Director, Clinical Hepatology
Beth Israel Hospital
Boston, MA

Diana S. Dark, MD
Associate Professor of Medicine
Division of Pulmonary and Critical Care Medicine
University of Kansas Medical Center
Kansas City, KS

John F. Goodwin, MD, FRCP(Lond), FACC
Professor Emeritus of Cardiology
Postgraduate Medical School
London, UK

Samuel L. Gross, MD
Professor and Division Chief
Hematology/Oncology
University of Florida
Gainesville, FL

Robyn L. Houlden, MD
Assistant Professor
Division of Endocrinology
Department of Medicine
Queen's University
Kingston, Canada

Shiv L. Jindal, MD
Associate Professor of Medicine
Nephrology Division
Ottawa Civic Hospital
Ottawa, Canada

F. Charles Jennette, MD
Professor of Medicine
Nephrologist
School of Medicine
University of North Carolina
Chapel Hill, NC

Gerald R. Kerby, MD
Professor of Medicine
Division of Pulmonary and Critical Care Medicine
University of Kansas Medical Center
Kansas City, KS

M. Gabriel Khan, MB BCh, MD, FRCP(Lond), FRCP(C), FACP
Associate Professor of Medicine
University of Ottawa
Consultant Cardiologist
Ottawa General Hospital
Ottawa, Canada

Richard Lechtenberg, MD
Clinical Professor of Neurosciences
University of Medicine and Dentistry of New Jersey
Newark, NJ

Richard W. Light, MD
Professor of Medicine
University of California at Irvine
Irvine, CA
Associate Chief of Staff for Research and Development
Veterans Administration Medical Center
Long Beach, CA

Joseph P. Lynch, III, MD
Associate Professor of Internal Medicine
Division of Pulmonary and Critical Care Medicine
University of Michigan Medical Center
Ann Arbor, MI

Paul L. Marino, MD, PhD, FCCM
Clinical Associate Professor
Department of Medicine and Surgery
University of Pennsylvania
School of Medicine and Surgery
Director of Critical Care
Presbyterian Medical Center of Philadelphia
Philadelphia, PA

Davendra Mehta, MD, MRCP (UK), PhD
Division of Cardiology
Mt. Sinai Medical Center
One Gustave L. Levy Place
New York, NY

David M. Nierman, MD, FRCP
Assistant Professor of Medicine
Associate Director, Medical ICU
The Mount Sinai Medical Center
New York, NY

Amy O'Brien-Ladner, MD
Assistant Professor of Medicine
Division of Pulmonary and Critical Care Medicine
University of Kansas Medical Center
Kansas City, KS

Lucy B. Palmer, MD
Assistant Professor
Department of Medicine
Pulmonary and Critical Care Division
State University of New York at Stony Brook
Stony Brook, NY

Susan K. Pingleton, MD
Professor of Medicine
Director Pulmonary and Critical Care Medicine
University of Kansas Medical Center
Kansas City, KS

Stuart Roath, MD, FRCP
Head, Department of Hematology
University of Southampton
Southampton General Hospital
Southampton, England

Sanjeev Saksena, MD, FACC
Clinical Associate, Professor of Medicine
UMDNJ–New Jersey Medical School
Newark, NJ
Director, Arrhythmia and Pacemaker Service
Eastern Heart Institute
Passaic, NJ

Robert P. Sheon, MD, FACP
Clinical Professor of Medicine
Medical College of Ohio
Senior Rheumatologist
Toledo Clinic
Toledo, OH

Galen B. Toews, MD
Professor of Internal Medicine
Chief, Division of Pulmonary and Critical Care Medicine
University of Michigan Medical Center
Ann Arbor, MI

Eric J. Topol, MD
Chairman, Department of Cardiology
Director, Center for Thrombosis and Vascular Biology
Professor of Medicine, Ohio State University
The Cleveland Clinic Foundation
9500 Euclid Avenue
Cleveland, OH

Irving Waxman, MD
Instructor in Medicine
Harvard Medical School
Co-Director, Pancreatico-Biliary Center
Beth Israel Hospital
Boston, MA

Lewis J. Wesselius, MD
Associate Professor of Medicine
Pulmonary and Critical Care Medicine
University of Kansas Medical Center
Kansas City, KS

Contents

Hypertension

1

M. Gabriel Khan

Hypertension is designated as mild, moderate, or severe based on the height of diastolic BP

- Mild: 90–104 mm Hg
- Moderate: 105–114 mm Hg
- Severe: ≥115 mm Hg

No guidelines yet exist for grading the severity of systolic hypertension based on the level of systolic BP. Nonetheless, systolic hypertension is as important as diastolic hypertension in the causation of cerebrovascular and cardiac morbidity and mortality.

Systolic BP constantly >140 mm Hg in patients < age 65 and ≥165 mm Hg in patients > age 65 is significant and requires aggressive control, especially in patients with CHD, CHF, cardiomegaly, renal dysfunction, diabetes, or a strong family history of cardiovascular events

- Guidelines for the management of isolated systolic hypertension in patients aged 65–85 have been clarified by the results of the SHEP. The SHEP indicates a threefold and twofold ↑ in the risk of stroke and CHD in elderly hypertensive patients with systolic BPs >180 mm Hg. The treated patients in the SHEP showed a 36% ↓ in risk of stroke ($p = 0.0003$), a 27% ↓ in CHD event rates, and a 54% ↓ in risk of LV failure
- The SHEP results indicate that it is advisable to treat all patients aged 65–85 who have isolated systolic hypertension constantly >180 mm Hg. In patients with systolic BP in the range 180–240 mm Hg, a 20% to max 25% ↓ in systolic pressure is recommended, based on the results of the SHEP
- The diagnosis of mild hypertension requires care to avoid unnecessary overtreatment with medications that have potential side effects; ≥3 readings in the hypertensive range obtained on separate days are necessary to confirm the diagnosis
- BP measured in the office tends to be > that observed in the patient's home or at work. In mild hypertension, it may be necessary to wait 6 months to establish the diagnosis before beginning drug therapy. In some individuals, ambulatory BP readings or estimations at work or during exercise stress testing may prove helpful.

PRIMARY (ESSENTIAL) HYPERTENSION

- In about 95% of hypertensive adults aged 20–65, no identifiable cause can be determined. Their hypertension should be defined as primary, idiopathic, or essential. In approximately 5% of cases, a secondary cause for hypertension is present. (Secondary hypertension will be considered in this chapter after discussion of primary hypertension.)
- Information obtained from the patient's history, physical examina-

tion, response to previous drug therapy, CBC, urinalysis, serum creatinine, blood urea or BUN, electrolytes, total and HDL-C, ECG, and chest x ray should give clues that might initiate further investigation to identify the presence of secondary hypertension. In patients with primary hypertension, data obtained from the evaluation serve as a baseline and may influence the selection of an appropriate antihypertensive drug.

Non-Drug Therapy

Non-drug therapy should be rigorously tried in all patients with mild hypertension prior to drug therapy

- Weight ↓ virtually always results in a lowering of BP; small group sessions organized by weight loss clinics have the greatest success
- Low Na diet. A 2-g Na diet is sufficient, and compliance is feasible. Table 1–1 lists foods with their comparative Na content
- Cessation of smoking
- Avoidance of alcohol or ↓ in alcohol intake
- Removal of stress and/or learning to deal with stress
- Relaxation and exercise

These measures may result in adequate control of hypertension in ≤40% of patients with mild hypertension.

The Joint National Committee on the Detection, Evaluation and Treatment of Hypertension recommends that patients with diastolic pressures of 90–94 mm Hg receive a non-drug therapy trial for about 6 months, followed by drug therapy if pressures remain elevated. Also, systolic hypertension requires aggressive control; the rationale for this recommendation has been discussed earlier.

Drug Therapy

- Strive for monotherapy in the treatment of systolic or diastolic hypertension whenever possible. The ideal choice is a drug that is effective for 24 h when given once daily and that produces few or no adverse effects
- The Joint National Committee recommends the use of a β blocker, small-dose diuretic, ACE inhibitor, or Ca antagonist as the initial drug for the treatment of mild to moderate (diastolic) hypertension. Both systolic and diastolic hypertension, however, require the same attention and measure of control, and identical recommendations apply
- One of the 4 drugs stipulated above is chosen based on characteristics of the individual—such as age, race, and concomitant disease—to manage systolic and/or diastolic hypertension. Each of the 4 classes of first-step drugs has unique pharmacologic properties that can be tailored to the hemodynamic, neurohormonal, and volume-related factors as well as the concomitant diseases that may exist in certain subsets of hypertensive patients
- Patients < age 70 respond best to β blockers or ACE inhibitors, but β blockers have the advantage of providing some cardioprotection depending on the β blocker used and the presence or absence of smoking (see Chap. 2). The "Quality of Life Study" indicated that ACE inhibitors are superior to propranolol
- Patients > age 70 and blacks with low-renin essential hypertension respond best to diuretics or Ca antagonists, but β blockers and ACE

Table 1–1
List of Foods with Comparative Sodium (Na) Content

FOOD	PORTION	MG SODIUM
Bouillon	1 cube	900
Bacon back	1 slice	500
Bacon side (fried crisp)	1 slice	75
Beef (lean, cooked)	3 oz (90 g)	60
Garlic salt	1 teaspoon (15 ml)	2000
Garlic powder	1 teaspoon	2
Ham cured	3 oz (90 g)	1000
Ham fresh cooked	3 oz	100
Ketchup	1 tablespoon	150
Milk pudding instant whole	1 cup (250 ml)	1000
Meat tenderized regular	1 teaspoon	2000
Meat tenderized low Na	1 teaspoon	2
Olive green	1	100
Pickle dill	Large (10 × 4½ cm)	1900
Peanuts dry roasted	1 cup	1000
Peanuts dry roasted (unsalted)	1 cup	10
Wieners	1 (50 g)	500
CANNED FOODS		
Carrots	4 oz	400
(Carrots raw)		40
Corn whole kernel	1 cup	400
(Corn frozen)	1 cup	10
Corn beef cooked	4 oz	1000
Crab	3 oz	900
Peas cooked green	1 cup	5
Shrimp	3 oz	2000
Salmon salt added	3 oz	500
Salmon no salt added	3 oz	50
Soups (majority)	1 cup (250 ml)	1000
Sauerkraut	1 cup (250 ml)	1800
SALAD DRESSING		
Blue cheese	15 ml	160
French regular	15 ml	200
Italian	15 ml	110
Oil and Vinegar	15 ml	1
Thousand Island	15 ml	90
FAST FOOD		
Chopped steak	one portion	1000
Fried chicken	3 piece dinner	2000
Fish & chips	one portion	1000
Hamburger	double	1000
Roast beef sandwich	one	1000
Pizza	one medium	1000

Normal diet contains 1000 to 3000 mg sodium.
Modified from: Khan, M. Gabriel: Heart Attacks, Hypertension & Heart Drugs. 2nd Ed. Toronto, McClelland-Bantam Inc., 1990.

inhibitors are effective in >50% of blacks and the elderly and may be suitable for use in these patients

- Ca antagonists are effective at all ages and in all grades of primary and secondary hypertension but provide less cardioprotection than β blockers or ACE inhibitor
- In females with a high risk for osteoporosis, diuretics are first choice as they are the only antihypertensive agents that ↑ bone mass. The SHEP has confirmed a salutary effect of low-dose diuretics with or without added β-blocker therapy on cardiovascular and cerebrovascular mortality in patients aged 65–86 who have isolated systolic hypertension
- In refractory smokers, hepatic-metabolized lipophilic β blockers such as propranolol are not advisable because their salutary effects are blunted, whereas timolol, acebutolol, and metoprolol retain protective effects

Table 1–2 summarizes individual patient characteristics and suggests a rational approach to the choice of an initial antihypertensive drug. Knowledge of the response and side effects of previous drug therapy aids in the selection of an appropriate drug. Figure 1–1 gives suggested steps in how to manage patients with mild and moderate hypertension. When combination drug therapy is necessary, rational therapy comprises the combination of 2 first-choice agents or a first choice combined with a second-choice agent, as indicated in Table 1–2. The following combina-

Table 1–2
Which Drug to Choose as Initial or Monotherapy for Mild Hypertension Based on Patient Characteristics

PATIENT TYPE	BETA BLOCKER	DIURETIC	ACE-I	C	CA	ALPHA1-BLOCKER	ALPHA1, BETA-BLOCKER
Age >70	2	1	2	4	1	4	4
Age <70, relatively healthy	1	2	2	4	3	4	4
Blacks	1	1	3	4	2	4	4
Any age group:							
Ischemic heart	1	3	3	4	2	RCI	4
LVH	1	3	1	3	2	RCI	4
Aneurysms	1	3	2	3	2	RCI	3
Cerebral ischemia	1	3	2	3	2	4	4
Heart failure	CI	1	1	RCI	RCI	4	CI
Diabetes:							
Insulin-dependent	RCI	3	1	3	1	3	3
Prone to hypoglycemia	CI	3	1	3	1	3	3
Mild hyperlipidemia	1	3	2	4	2	3	4
HDL < 35 mg%	1	4	1	4	1	3	4
Osteoporosis or women age >40	1	1*	2	4	2	4	4
Women < age 40	1	1	RCI†	4	RCI†	4	4
Chronic lung	CI	1	1	4	1	4	CI

ACE-1 = Angiotensin-converting enzyme inhibitor
C = Centrally acting adrenergic inhibitor
CA = Calcium antagonist
CI = Contraindicated
RCI = Relative contraindication
* = Increases bone mineral density
† = Risk during pregnancy
1 = first choice; 4 = poor choice
Modified from: Khan, M. Gabriel: Cardiac Drug Therapy. 3rd Ed. London, W.B. Saunders, 1992.

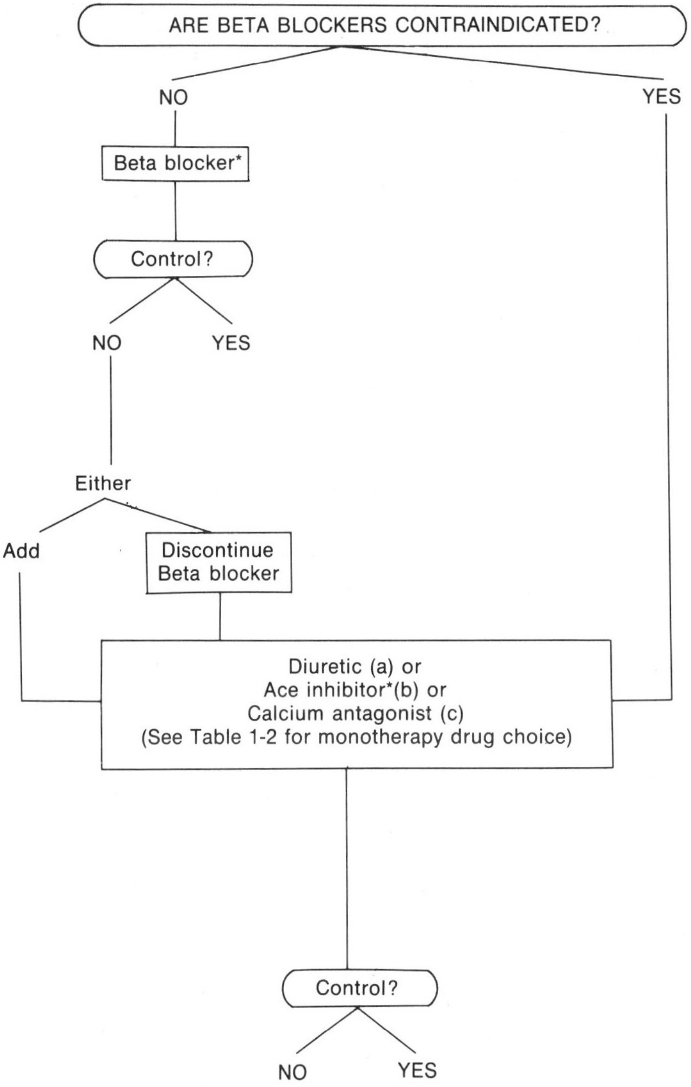

* Both cardioprotective

Figure 1–1. Steps in how to treat mild to moderate hypertension

tions are suggested, depending on patient characteristics listed in Table 1–2

- Age <70 or in the elderly: A β blocker plus a Ca antagonist (nifedipine extended release or amlodipine); a β blocker plus a small dose of a thiazide diuretic; or a β blocker plus an ACE inhibitor, although their effects are not always complimentary, the latter 2 agents are cardioprotective. If a diuretic agent is used and hypokalemia is observed, the thiazide should be switched to a K-sparing diuretic, preferably thiazide plus amiloride (Moduretic; Moduret); spironolactone should be avoided, and triamterene may cause renal calculi. Amiloride is the only diuretic agent that has salutary antiarrhythmic properties

- CHD: In patients with CHD or in those who are at high risk for CHD events, a β blocker plus amlodipine or nifedipine extended release is a natural choice. The reader is advised to consult Chapter 2 for the appropriate selection of a Ca antagonist. It must be emphasized that ACE inhibitors and alpha$_1$ blockers may cause a ↑ in angina and are relatively contraindicated in patients with CHD manifested by unstable angina
- Hypertension in a patient with significant hyperlipidemia presents a difficult decision-making scenario. Beta blockers cause about a 6% ↓ in HDL-C levels. Acebutolol, however, has been shown to cause no significant change in HDL-C levels in patients treated for >1 year (Chap. 9). These agents do not ↑ LDL-C. In addition, hypertensive patients who have hyperlipidemia are at high risk for CHD events, and β-blocking drugs afford cardioprotection, albeit modest. Thus, a logical therapeutic combination is acebutolol plus an ACE inhibitor or Ca antagonist, along with control of hyperlipidemia with diet and/or drug therapy where indicated. Although alpha$_1$ blockers do not cause lipid derangements, they may adversely affect the cardiovascular system and are thus graded a poor choice for most hypertensive scenarios. Figure 1–1 gives suggested steps in how to treat mild to moderate hypertension with monotherapy and appropriate combinations. Table 1–3 gives the dosage and Table 1–4 the more common adverse effects of antihypertensive drugs

BETA BLOCKERS

Beta blockers are considered first-choice therapy for the management of hypertension in several subsets of patients in whom no contraindications to β blockade exist (Table 1–2; Fig. 1–1).

Indications include

- Patients < age 70 in whom high renin essential hypertension is more prevalent than in the elderly. Beta blockers are indicated in elderly patients with hypertensive, hypertrophic "cardiomyopathy" with impaired ventricular relaxation because diuretics and ACE inhibitors are contraindicated in these patients
- Beta blockers are first choice in patients with CHD manifested by angina, silent ischemia, and following MI
- First choice in patients with arrhythmias
- Patients with LVH are at high risk for sudden death; β blockers are the only cardioactive agents that have been proven to prevent sudden cardiac death
- Patients with increased adrenergic activity, including the younger age group, who often have high plasma norepinephrine levels, and patients with hyperkinetic heart syndrome, alcohol withdrawal hypertension, or the hyperdynamic β-adrenergic circulatory state, with labile or elevated BP and palpitations
- Orthostatic hypertension, with an exaggerated ↑ in diastolic pressure on standing, usually indicates increased adrenergic tone; β blockers have a salutary effect in this subset
- Patients prone to postural hypotension may benefit since these agents, unlike all other antihypertensives, do not usually ↓ systemic vascular resistance

Table 1–3
Daily Dosage of Antihypertensive Drugs

	DOSE (MG)		
	INITIAL	USUAL MAINTENANCE	MAXIMUM*
ACE INHIBITORS†			
Captopril (Capoten)	12.5–25	50–100	150
Enalapril (Vasotec)	2.5–5	10–20	40
Lisinopril (Prinivil, Zestril)	2.5–5	10–20	40
Benazepril (Lotensin)	5	5–30	40
Fosinopril (Monopril) 10 mg	5–10	10–30	40
Perindopril	1–2	2–6	8
Quinapril (Accupril)	2.5–5	5–30	40
Ramipril (Altace)	1.25–2.5	2.5–5	20
ALPHA-ADRENERGIC BLOCKERS			
Prazosin (Minipress)	1 (0.5, UK)	5–15	20
Terazosin (Hytrin)	1	2–10	15
CALCIUM ANTAGONISTS			
Amlodipine (Norvasc)	2.5–5	5–10	10
Diltiazem‡ 60, 90, 120 mg	90	180–240	360
Cardizem CD	180	180–240	300
Cardizem SR 90, 120 mg	90	180–360	360
Adizem SR (UK) 120 mg	120	120–360	360
Nifedipine			
Nifedipine Extended Release:			
Adalat CC, Procardia XL, Adalat XL(C) 30, 60, 90 mg	30	60–90	120
Adalat PA 10 mg (C)	20–40	40–80	120
Adalat Retard 10 mg (UK)			
Adalat Retard 20 mg (UK)	20–40	60–80	80
Verapamil 80, 120 mg, 40, 80, 120, 160 mg (UK)	160	160–360	480
Calan SR 120, 180, 240 mg	120	120–360	480
Isoptin SR 120, 180, 240 mg	120	120–360	480
Verelan 120, 240 mg			
Nicardipine 20, 30 mg	40	40–60	90
Cardene			
Nitrendipine	5	5–20	40
Baypress			
Felodipine			
Plendil 5, 10 mg	5	5–10	15
Isradipine 2.5, 5 mg	2.5–5	5–10	30
DynaCirc			
CENTRAL ACTING			
Clonidine (Catapress)	0.1	0.2–0.8	1
Guanabenz (Wytensin)	4	8	16
Guanfacine (Tenex)	1	1	3
Methyldopa (Aldomet)	250–500	500–1000	1500
BETA BLOCKERS			
Acebutolol (Sectral, Monitan)	200–400	400–800	1000
Atenolol (Tenormin)	25–50	50–100	100
Labetalol (Trandate, Normodyne)	100–400	500–1000	1200

Table 1–3 (*Continued*)

	DOSE (MG)		
	INITIAL	USUAL MAINTENANCE	MAXIMUM*
Metoprolol (Toprol XL, Lopressor, Betaloc)	50	50–200	300
Nadolol (Corgard)	40–80	40–160	160
Penbutolol (Levatol)	20	20–40	80
Pindolol (Visken)	7.5–15	10–15	30
Proprandolol (Inderal)	40–120	160–240	240
Inderal LA	80	80–240	240
Sotalol (Sotacor, C, UK)	80	160	240
Timolol (Blocadren)	5–10	10–20	40
DIURETICS			
Bendroflumethiazide	2.5	2.5	5
Bendrofluazide (UK)	2.5	2.5–5	5
Benzthiazide	12.5	2.5	50
Chlorothiazide	125	250	500
Chlorthalidone	12.5	25	50
Hydrochlorothiazide	12.5–25	25–50	50
Hydroflumethiazide	12.5–25	25–50	50
Indapamide	2.5	2.5	2.5
Methylclothiazide	2.5	2.5	5
Metolazone	1.25	2.5	10
Polythiazide	2	2	4
Quinethazone	25	25	50
Trichlormethiazide	1	2	4
Bumetanide	0.5	1–5	10
Furosemide (Frusemide, UK)	40	40–160	240

* In clinical practice, a dose less than the manufacturer's maximum is advised and reduces the incidence of adverse effects.
† See Table 1–6
‡ Not appropriate for the elderly or those with renal or hepatic impairment (British National Formulary, 1992)
C = Canada
UK = United Kingdom
Note: All drugs are available in the United States, except where labeled "C" or "UK."

- First choice for patients with aneurysms
- In females > age 55, β blockers are a rational choice because the incidence of myocardial rupture is high in hypertensive women who sustain a first infarction. Beta blockers protect sufficiently from myocardial rupture to warrant their use in patients considered at risk. The combination of a β-blocking agent and a low-dose diuretic is advisable if prevention of osteoporosis also requires therapeutic consideration

There is still no clear consensus regarding the mechanisms by which β-blocking drugs cause a ↓ in BP. An interplay of mechanisms appears to be responsible. Negative chronotropic and inotropic effects lead to a ↓ in cardiac output and some ↓ in BP. Antagonism of sympathetically mediated renin release and ↓ in plasma renin have a role. Added mechanisms include CNS effects, ↓ in norepinephrine release, ↓ in plasma volume and venomotor tone, resetting of baroreceptor levels, and inhibition of the catecholamine pressor response to stress.

Dosage: See Table 1–3. (Individual β blockers are discussed in Chap. 2.) It is advisable to use a small dose initially, then titrate to a moderate dose that is within the "cardioprotective" range. If BP is not adequately controlled, it is advisable to add another agent rather than to use the manufacturer's suggested max dose. At very high doses of a β-blocking drug, cardioprotective properties are lost. A 20-mg daily dose of timolol produced significant ↓ in mortality in the Norwegian Post Myocardial Infarction Trial. In the BHAT, 160–240 mg propranolol achieved a ↓ in mortality; acebutolol (400 mg qd) has been shown to cause a 48% ↓ in cardiovascular mortality. The effect on mortality at lower doses is unknown, and animal experiments using larger doses indicate increased

Table 1–4
Adverse Effects of Antihypertensive Drugs

DRUG TYPE	ADVERSE EFFECTS
Beta Blockers	Bronchospasm, exacerbation heart failure, bradycardia, fatigue, dizziness, masking and worsening of hypoglycemia, rarely impotence, nightmares, depression
Thiazide Diuretics	Hypokalemia, hyponatremia, dehydration, postural hypotension, gout, glucose intolerance, impotence, muscle cramps, postural hypotension
Nifedipine Extended Release	Headache, flushing, edema, dizziness, jitteriness, heartburn
Verapamil and Diltiazem	Above, plus bradycardia, rarely sinus arrest, heart block, precipitation of heart failure, constipation, hepatic dysfunction
ACE Inhibitors	First-dose syncope, hypotension, angioneurotic edema, pruritic rash, cough, wheeze, hyperkalemia, worsening of renal failure, loss of taste, mouth ulcers, cerebral circulatory insufficiency, rare: neutropenia, agranulocytosis, proteinuria, membranous glomerulopathy, impotence, pemphigus, hepatitis, +ve ANA.
Centrally acting (methyldopa, clonidine, guanfacine, guanabenz)	Postural hypotension, drowsiness, dry mouth, parotitis, depression, lethargy, impotence, rebound hypertension
Alpha$_1$ blockers	First-dose syncope, postural hypotension, palpitations, precipitation of angina, impotence, retrograde ejaculation, progression of aneurysmal dilatation
Labetalol and other alpha$_1$-beta blockers	No first-dose syncope, otherwise similar to effects given under alpha$_1$ blockers and beta blockers plus +ve ANA, rare lupus-like syndrome, hepatic necrosis

mortality. Therefore, Table 1–3 gives 40 mg as the max dose for timolol and 240 mg for propranolol—not 80 mg and 480 mg, respectively, as quoted by other sources. In the management of hypertension, it is advisable not to exceed the 30-mg dose for timolol, 600 mg for acebutolol, 240 mg for propranolol, and 200 mg for metoprolol extended release.

Pharmacologic Features and Subtle Differences

- The usual classification into cardioselective and nonselective is an oversimplification (see Table 1–5). Atenolol and metoprolol are cardioselective β-adrenergic blockers. At high doses, however, these agents can produce bronchospasm, because a small quantity of β receptors is present in the lungs
- The lipophilic agents are metabolized in the liver and obtain high brain concentration, which may confer some adverse effects. Recent studies suggest that increased brain concentration and ↑ of central vagal tone may confer greater cardiac protection provided that salutary effects are not nullified by cigarette smoking. Abald et al. in a rabbit model showed that while both metoprolol (lipophilic) and atenolol (hydrophilic) caused equal β blockade, only metoprolol caused a ↓ in sudden cardiac death. Metoprolol, but not atenolol, caused a significant ↑ in RR interval variation that indicates a ↑ in parasympathetic tone. Only the β blockers with lipophilic properties—acebutolol, metoprolol, timolol and propranolol—in non-smokers have been shown in clinical trials to prevent sudden cardiac death. It is important for the physician to select an appropriate β blocker with the understanding that β blockers are not all alike
- Statements in editorials such as "beta blockers do not reduce cardiac mortality in hypertensives" must be considered erroneous because β blockers possess subtle differences that are clinically important. It is not surprising that cardiac mortality was not reduced by propranolol in smokers in the large hypertension clinical trials of the 1980s. Thus, meta-analyses do not reflect the max cardioprotective effects of β-blocking agents
- The protective cardiovascular effects of hepatic-metabolized β blockers such as propranolol, oxprenolol, and penbutolol are blunted by cigarette smoking.
- Only timolol, metoprolol, and acebutolol have been shown to be effective in preventing cardiac deaths in smokers and nonsmokers. Insisting that the patient stop smoking is important in preventing cardiovascular events and allows salutary effects of medication to emerge. However, patients who insist on smoking ↑ their risk of sudden death and other CHD events, and in this large group of patients, the choice of a β blocker is important

Beta blockers with more than moderate ISA are not recommended because they may blunt the cardioprotective lifesaving potential. Acebutolol has only mild ISA activity, however, and has been shown to ↓ cardiovascular mortality. Acebutolol is the β-blocking agent of choice in hypertensive patients with hyperlipidemia and/or if other β blockers cause symptomatic bradycardia (see Chap. 9).

Contraindications

- CHF
- Asthma, severe COPD, allergic rhinitis
- Severe PVD
- Heart block, sick sinus syndrome
- Diabetics prone to hypoglycemia—however, if β-blocker therapy is needed in patients with stable or mild diabetes, a cardioselective agent such as metoprolol is preferred.

Table 1–5
Pharmacologic Features of Beta Blockers

	ATENOLOL	ACEBUTOLOL	METOPROLOL	NADOLOL	PENBUTOLOL	PROPRANOLOL	PINDOLOL	TIMOLOL	SOTALOL	LABETALOL
Cardio selectivity β1	+ + +	+	+ + +	none	none	none	none	none	none	none
Intrinsic sympathomimetic activity (ISA) (partial agonist)	—	+	—	—	+	—	+ + +	—	—	+
Hydrophilic	+ + + +	+	—	+ + + +		—	+	+	+ + + +	
Lipophilic*	—	+ + +	+ + +	—	+ + + +	+ + + +	+ +	+ +	—	+ + +
Hepatic metabolized	—	+ + +	+ + + +	—	+ + +	+ + + +	+ +	+ +	—	+ +
Renal excretion	Yes	Partial	None	Yes	Partial	None	Partial	Partial	Yes	No
Alpha₁ blocker	—	—	—	—	—	—	—	—	—	—

\+ = mild
\+ + + + = maximum
* Increase concentration in brain

Adverse Effects: These include precipitation of CHF in patients with poor LV systolic function (EF<30%). Symptomatic bradycardia is bothersome in <10% of treated patients, bronchospasm may be precipitated in asthmatics and patients with COPD. Dizziness, weakness, fatigue, vivid dreams, rarely depression, and very rarely psychosis and loss of hearing may occur. Lipophilic β blockers (propranolol, oxprenolol, penbutolol) have a higher incidence of CNS adverse effects than hydrophilic agents (atenolol and nadolol). Impotence occurs in <2% of patients. Based on studies utilizing >39,000 patients, 0.4% reported impotence. The incidence is much < observed with the use of diuretics and is not > that reported for ACE inhibitors or Ca antagonists. Raynaud's phenomenon and worsening of intermittent claudication are bothersome features of β-blocker therapy. A few cases of exacerbation of psoriasis have been reported. Labetalol is a β blocker with alpha$_1$ blocking activity and has 2 major adverse effects not observed with pure β-blocking agents: Postural hypotension is not uncommon, and life-threatening hepatic necrosis has been observed.

Caution: Avoid abrupt cessation of β-blocker therapy in patients with CHD because angina may worsen. If necessary, discontinue β blockers gradually over 2–3 weeks and instruct the patient to refrain from moderate exertion. Rarely, rebound hypertension is precipitated.

Interactions

- With hepatic-metabolized β blockers are observed when drugs such as cimetidine or chlorpheniramine, which ↓ hepatic blood flow, are used concomitantly
- Hypertensive crisis can occur with cough and cold remedies containing phenylpropranolamine
- An increased risk for anaphylactoid reaction from contrast media and immunotherapy in patients on β blockers has been reported

DIURETICS

These economical, one-a-day drugs can be recommended as first line in selected patients. Table 1–2 indicates the rationale for the choice of diuretics in many subsets of hypertensives. The SHEP confirms the salutary effects of low-dose diuretic therapy. In the SHEP, chlorthalidone, 12.5–25 mg alone or in combination with atenolol, resulted in a significant ↓ in the risk of stroke, MI, and LVF. The exact mechanism of action by which diuretics produce a ↓ in BP is unknown. A ↓ in vascular volume, negative Na balance, and longterm arteriolar dilation occurs.

Indications: Small-dose diuretic therapy is particularly useful in the following categories of patients

- >age 65
- Blacks, who usually have low renin hypertension
- Concomitant CHF or renal dysfunction
- Particularly females > age 45, who may be at risk for osteoporosis. Diuretics are the only antihypertensive drugs that have been shown to ↑ bone mineral density and to ↓ the risk of hip fractures in both women and men
- As second-line agent to enhance the BP-lowering effect of β blockers, ACE inhibitors, vasodilators, and/or centrally acting drugs.

Disadvantages

- Hypokalemia occurs in <25% of patients treated with 25–50 mg of HCTZ or an equivalent dose of another thiazide daily. This occurrence is dose related. A 25- or 50-mg dose of HCTZ is expected to cause a ↓ in serum K of about 0.3–0.6 mEq/l, respectively, in susceptible individuals. Patients given a thiazide should be screened in 2 months and then q 6 months for hypokalemia. If hypokalemia develops, it is advisable to change to a K-sparing diuretic (Moduretic or Dyazide) after correction of the K deletion

- Patients who show hypokalemia despite K supplements or K-sparing diuretics are best treated by replacing the diuretic with an ACE inhibitor
- Diuretics have not been shown to consistently prevent the development of LVH or to produce regression
- Hypertensive patients treated with diuretics and followed for >14 years showed a major ↑ in the incidence of glucose intolerance; discontinuation of diuretics promptly reversed the hyperglycemic response. The mechanism for the development of diuretic-induced glucose intolerance appears to be the result of a suppressive effect of hypokalemia on insulin secretion. Shortterm studies have indicated that diuretics cause minor elevations in serum cholesterol and decreases in HDL. However, longterm trials with large numbers of patients, such as the Medical Research Council Hypertension Trial, showed no significant difference in serum cholesterol before and after 3 years of treatment with diuretics. Total cholesterol levels and HDL-C levels did not change after 4–5 years of therapy with chlorthalidone in the SHEP.

Dosage (See Table 1–3). *Adverse Effects:* Impotence, weakness, and fatigue; the incidence of impotence is > that observed with the use of β blockers. Hyponatremia may develop over a period of weeks or years in some susceptible individuals; electrolyte imbalance and hypomagnesemia; gout; rarely, thrombocytopenia, agranulocytosis, and pancreatitis. Thiazide appears in breast milk, crosses the placental barrier, and can cause decreased placental perfusion, fetal or neonatal thrombocytopenia, jaundice, and acute pancreatitis. Avoid during pregnancy and lactation.

Interactions occur with oral anticoagulants and steroids; a ↑ in serum lithium levels may occur; NSAIDs, including aspirin, interfere with the diuretic effect of furosemide.

Bendrofluazide (Aprinox, Berkozide, Centyl, Neo-NaClex, Urizide). *Supplied:* tablets; 2.5, 5 mg. *Dosage:* 2.5–5 mg qd

Hydrochlorothiazide (Hydrodiuril, Esidrix, Oretic, Hydrosaluric, Direma). *Supplied:* tablets; 25, 50, 100 mg. *Dosage:* Commence with 12.5 mg; then, if needed, usual maintenance 25 mg, max 50 mg once daily. Alternate-day therapy may suffice in some patients with mild hypertension.

POTASSIUM-SPARING DIURETICS

These agents are very useful in the management of hypertension; they also conserve magnesium. They are usually used in combination with other diuretics

- **Dyazide** (HCTZ 25 mg and triamterene 50 mg, a K-sparing diuretic)
- **Moduretic; Moduret** (UK and Canada) (HCTZ 50 mg and amiloride 5 mg, a K-sparing diuretic)
- **Moduret** 25 or **mini-Moduretic** (HCTZ 25 mg and amiloride 2.5 mg, UK and Europe) is a useful combination

Contraindications to the use of K-sparing diuretics include renal failure, concomitant use of ACE inhibitors and/or K supplements; with renal calculi avoid triamterene.

OTHER DIURETICS

Indapamide (Lozol; Lozide, Canada; Natrilix, UK). Indapamide is chemically related to chlorthalidone but has an added mild vasodilator effect, which is not related to diuretic action. The incidence of hypokalemia is similar to that of thiazides, but indapamide produced no disturbances in blood lipid, blood glucose, or insulin levels in hypertensive patients administered 2.5 mg qd for 1 year. Because approximately 60% of indapamide is excreted by the kidney, the drug should not be administered to patients with mild renal dysfunction. Dosing interval does not require adjustment, but periodic evaluation of serum K and creatinine is advised. Supplied: tablet; 2.5 mg. Dosage: 1 tablet each morning. A dose >2.5 mg qd is not advisable. In some patients with mild hypertension, alternate-day therapy may be effective.

Furosemide (Frusemide, UK). This powerful loop diuretic is less effective than thiazides in mild hypertension. However, thiazides, with the exception of metolazone, lose their natriuretic effect when the GFR falls below 25 ml/h while loop diuretics retain their effectiveness. Furosemide is therefore not advised for the treatment of hypertension except when there is concomitant CHF or severe renal dysfunction.

Timolide (timolol 20 mg and HCTZ 25 mg). Dosage: 1 tablet qd. The disadvantage of 2 tablets qd is excessive dose of thiazide.

Kalten (atenolol 50 mg, HCTZ 25 mg, and amiloride 2.5 mg). Kalten is available in Europe and has the advantage of being K-sparing. Dosage: 1 tablet qd.

ANGIOTENSIN-CONVERTING ENZYME INHIBITORS

These agents have provided a major advance in the management of hypertension. They are useful first-line agents (see Table 1–2). These inhibitors of ACE prevent the conversion of angiotensin I to the potent vasoconstrictor, angiotensin II. This action causes arteriolar dilation and a ↓ in total systemic vascular resistance as well as diminished sympathetic activity causing vasodilation (but HR does not ↑ as occurs with other vasodilators) and a ↓ in aldosterone secretion. The ↓ in aldosterone secretion causes both Na excretion and K retention. The pharmacologic profile of ACE inhibitors is given in Table 1–6; for dosages see Table 1–3.

Indications

- ACE inhibitors are most effective in patients with high renin hypertension and especially in Caucasians < age 65, but are effective in the elderly
- Hypertensives with LV dysfunction or CHF
- Diabetics with hypertension of all grades. Importantly, mild hypertension (systolic 140–160 mm Hg, diastolic 90–95 mm Hg) in diabetics must be aggressively treated, preferably with an ACE inhibitor
- Patients with renal dysfunction: ACE inhibitors appear to preserve nephron life (see contraindication solitary kidney and/or critical renal artery stenosis)

Table 1–6
The Pharmacologic Profile and Dosages of ACE Inhibitors

	CAPTOPRIL	ENALAPRIL	LISINOPRIL	RAMIPRIL
USA and Canada	Capoten	Vasotec	Prinivil, Zestril	Altace
UK	Capoten	Innovace	Carace, Zestril	Tritace
Europe	Lopril, Lopirin	Xanef, Renitec	Carace, Zestril	Tritace
Pro-drug	No	Yes	No	Partial
Action				
apparent (hours)	½	2–4	2–4	3–6
peak effect (hours)	1–2	5	4–8	3–6
duration (hours)	8–12	12–24	24–30	24–48
Half life (hours)	2–3	11	13	14–30
Metabolism	Partly hepatic	Hepatic	None	Partial
Elimination	Renal	Renal	Renal	Renal
SH group	Yes	No	No	No
Approved use USA**	Hypertension	Hypertension	Hypertension	Hypertension
Heart failure	Yes	Yes	No	No
Equivalent dose	100 mg	20 mg	20 mg	10 mg
Initial dose	12.5 mg	2.5 mg	2.5 mg	1.25–2.5 mg
Total daily dose				
hypertension	50–150 mg	5–40 mg	5–40 mg	2.5–20 mg
heart failure	25–100 mg	5–20 mg		
Dose frequency*	2–3 daily	1–2 daily	1 daily	1 daily
Supplied	12.5, 25, 50, 100 mg	2.5, 5, 10, 20 mg	5, 10, 20, 40 mg 2.5 UK; 5, 10, 20, 40 mg	1.25, 2.5, 5, 10 mg

* Increase dosing interval with renal failure
** Also approved for hypertension: Benazepril (Lotensin) Fosinopril (Monopril); Quinapril (Accupril): see Table 1–3 and text

Advantages

- ACE inhibitors are most effective in patients with high renin hypertension. They have been shown to cause regression and prevention of LV hypertrophy. Other vasodilators may not prevent the development of hypertrophy, presumably because they cause sympathetic stimulation that results in a ↑ in HR and increased myocardial O_2 requirement
- Unlike ACE inhibitors, other vasodilators (particularly $alpha_1$ blockers, hydralazine, and minoxidil) cause Na and water retention, and diuretics are usually required to achieve successful antihypertensive effects. The BP-lowering response to various doses of captopril flattens after about 75 mg or equivalent ACE inhibitor doses. A captopril dose >100 mg produces little further ↓ in BP. However, addition of a diuretic stimulates the renin angiotensin system and enhances the BP-lowering effect of ACE inhibitors. When diuretics are added, BP ↓ is similar in white and black hypertensive patients
- These agents have been shown to ↓ mortality in patients with NYHA Class II, III, and IV CHF, and they are first choice, along with diuretics, in the management of hypertensive patients who have CHF or LV systolic dysfunction (see Chap. 4). In addition, they blunt diuretic-induced hypokalemia
- ACE inhibitors do not alter lipid levels or cause glucose intolerance. Thus, they are advisable in patients with hyperlipidemia and/or diabetes mellitus or suspected insulin resistance. They ↓ diabetic proteinuria and appear to preserve nephron life in diabetics and in patients with renal failure
- Impotence, weakness, and lethargy observed with methyldopa and

diuretics are rarely observed with the use of ACE inhibitors, and quality of life is not adversely affected as may occur with several other antihypertensive agents

Contraindications

- Renal artery stenosis of a solitary kidney or severe bilateral renal artery stenosis
- Severe anemia
- Urticaria, angio-edema
- Aortic stenosis
- Hypertrophic and restrictive cardiomyopathy; hypertensive, hypertrophic "cardiomyopathy" of the elderly with impaired ventricular relaxation
- Severe carotid artery stenosis
- Hypertensive patients with concomitant unstable angina
- Uric acid renal calculi
- Pregnancy and breast feeding
- Porphyria
- Relative contraindications include patients with collagen vascular diseases or concomitant use of immunosuppressives, since neutropenia and rare agranulocytosis observed with ACE inhibitors appear to occur mainly in this subset of patients

Adverse Effects: Hyperkalemia in patients with renal failure, pruritus and rash in about 10% of patients, and loss of taste in approximately 7% of patients. A rare but important adverse effect is angioedema of the face, mouth, or larynx, which may occur in approximately 0.5% of treated patients and can be fatal. Rarely, mouth ulcers, neurologic dysfunction, GI disturbances, and proteinuria occurs in about 1% of patients with pre-existing renal disease. Neutropenia and agranulocytosis are rare and occur mainly in patients with serious intercurrent illness, particularly immunologic disturbances, altered immune response, or collagen vascular disease. Cough occurs in about 10% of treated patients, and wheezing, myalgia, muscle cramps, hair loss, impotence or decreased libido, hepatitis or occurrence of antinuclear antibodies, and phemphigus occasionally occur.

Interactions with lithium, allopurinol, acebutolol, hydralazine, NSAIDs, procainamide, pindolol, steroids, tocanide, immunosuppressives, and other drugs that alter immune response. Drugs that ↑ serum K levels have been emphasized.

Captopril (Capoten). *Supplied:* tablets; 12.5, 25, 50, 100 mg. *Dosage:* Commence with 12.5 mg bid, 1/2 h before meals; ↑ over days or weeks to 25–75 mg bid, which is the dose required by the majority of patients. The max suggested dose is 150 mg qd in severe hypertension. Serious side effects are more common in patients given a daily dose of ≥200 mg. Increase the dose interval in renal failure. Decrease the initial dose to 6.25 mg in the elderly or if a diuretic is used concomitantly.

Captopril 100 mg = approximately 20 mg enalapril, 20 mg lisinopril, 20 mg ramipril, 50 mg alecepril, 750 mg pentopril.

Enalapril (Vasotec; Innovace, UK). *Supplied:* tablets; 2.5, 5, 10, 20 mg. *Dosage:* 2.5–5 mg qd; ↑ over days to months to 10–30 mg qd in 1 or 2 divided doses with or without food. Max 40 mg qd or less often in renal failure. In the elderly or in patients receiving a diuretic, begin with a dose of 2.5 mg qd.

Cilazapril (Inhibace). *Supplied:* tablets; 1, 2.5, 5 mg. *Dosage:* 1–2.5 mg qd; Max 5 mg qd.

Lisinopril (Prinivil, Zestril). *Supplied:* tablets; 2.5 (UK), 5, 10, 20, 40. *Dosage:* 2.5 mg once daily; ↑ to 10–30 mg; max 40 mg qd or less often in renal failure. Discontinue diuretic for 2–3 days prior to commencing lisinopril and resume later if required.

Benazepril (Lotensin). *Supplied:* 5, 10, 20, 40 mg. *Dosage:* 5 mg; ↑ as needed to usual maintenance 5–30 mg; max suggested 40 mg. Commence with 2.5 mg in the elderly or if a diuretic is given concomitantly. Not affected by food or antacids or antibiotics; some hepatic elimination occurs.

Fosinopril (Monopril). *Supplied:* tablets; 10, 20 mg. *Dosage:* 5–10 mg once daily; ↑ slowly, if required, to 20 mg and with assessment of renal function; max 40 mg qd with or without food but avoid taking within 2 h of antacids. Initial dose 2.5 mg in the elderly or in patients receiving a diuretic. Fosinopril is the only phosphinic acid class of the ACE inhibitors; the carboxylic acid class includes benazepril, enalapril, lisinopril, quinapril, and ramipril; captopril is the only sulphydryl agent. Monopril has an advantage of compensatory hepatic elimination in patients with renal failure and minimizes accumulation in patients with renal insufficiency.

Perindopril (Conversyl, UK). *Supplied:* tablets 2 mg. *Dosage:* 2 mg qd; ↑ if required, after monitoring BP, to 4–8 mg qd. Discontinue diuretic 3 days prior and resume later, if needed.

Quinapril (Accupril; Accupro, UK). *Supplied:* tablets; 5 mg; 10, 20, 40 mg. *Dosage:* 5 mg once daily; usual maintenance 20–40 mg qd. Reduce the initial dose to 2.5 mg qd in the elderly, renal dysfunction, or with diuretic use. Interaction: tetracyclines.

Ramipril (Altace; Tritace, UK). *Supplied:* capsules; 1.25, 2.5, 5, 10 mg. *Dosage:* 1.25 mg once daily; ↑, if needed, to 2.5–5 mg and with assessment of renal function; max 20 mg qd.

Capozide. *Supplied:* Contains 15 mg captopril and 30 mg HCTZ; in the UK, 50 mg captopril and 25 mg HCTZ. Combinations should be used preferably only after BP is stabilized on 2 drugs given separately. *Dosage:* 1/2–1 tablet qd; max 2 tablets qd.

Vaseretic. *Supplied:* Contains 10 mg enalapril with 25 mg HCTZ. *Dosage:* 1/2–1 tablet qd; max 2 tablets qd.

CALCIUM ANTAGONISTS

The BP-lowering effects of Ca antagonists are due to peripheral arteriolar dilation. Normally, Ca enters the cells through slow Ca channels and binds to the regulatory protein troponin, removing the inhibitory action of tropomyosin, which in the presence of adenosine triphosphate, allows interaction between myosin and actin, resulting in contraction of the muscle cell. Ca antagonists inhibit Ca entry into cells by blocking voltage-dependent Ca channels, thereby inhibiting contractility of vascular smooth muscle and producing vasodilation.

Table 1–7 gives the pharmacologic and clinical effects of Ca antagonists. The dihydropyridine Ca antagonists amlodipine, nifedipine, felodipine, nicardipine, and nitrendipine are more potent vasodilators and more effective antihypertensive agents than verapamil; diltiazem has modest vasodilator properties, and high doses are usually required to achieve adequate lowering of BP. In addition, verapamil and diltiazem have added EP effects on the sinoatrial and A-V nodes and can produce

Table 1–7
Pharmacologic and Clinical Effects of Calcium Antagonists

	NIFEDIPINE	DILTIAZEM	VERAPAMIL
Decrease systemic vascular resistance	Marked	Mild	Moderate
Blood pressure	Marked reduction	Mild reduction	Moderate reduction
Coronary dilation	Mild	Mild	Mild
Cardiac output	Mild increase	No change	No change or mild decrease
Heart rate	No change or very slight increase	No change	Mild decrease
Negative inotropic	Very mild	Mild	Moderate
Sinus node depression	None	Moderate	Moderate
AV Conduction	No change	Mild reduction	Moderate reduction
Antihypertensive effect	Excellent	Mild	Good
Antianginal effect	Good	Good	Excellent
Precipitates heart failure	Rarely*	Yes, if EF <40%	Yes, if EF <40%**
Combination with beta blocker	Relatively safe	Caution	Relative contraindication†

* In patients with severe left ventricular dysfunction
** Contraindicated in all patients with left ventricular dysfunction
† May cause severe bradycardia, sinus arrest

bradycardia, sinus arrest, and A-V block in susceptible individuals with disease of the sinus and A-V nodes.

Advantages

- Ca antagonists do not usually ↓ the BP of normotensive individual; the higher the BP the greater the lowering effects on BP
- They can be used without a diuretic since they have a mild natriuretic effect; their effectiveness may or may not be enhanced by adding a diuretic
- Ca antagonists are useful in hypertensive patients with coexisting angina and PVD or when β blockers produce adverse effects or are contraindicated
- They do not cause abnormalities of lipid or glucose metabolism nor influence K and uric acid excretion and have advantages over diuretics in this subset of patients
- Nifedipine has shown modest but significant regression and inhibition of progression of atheromatous obstruction of coronary arteries in patients with coronary artery disease
- Most Ca antagonists prevent LVH and cause regression, although some reports show a lack of salutary effects
- Ca antagonists, particularly amlodipine and nifedipine extended release, cause no serious adverse effects, and their use requires virtually no laboratory monitoring when compared with diuretics and ACE inhibitors. Individual Ca antagonists have advantages that are important in terms of their adverse effects
- Amlodipine and nifedipine have less potential than verapamil and diltiazem to cause serious adverse effects. Amlodipine and nifedipine have no EP effects and, although uncommon, verapamil and diltiazem can produce bradycardia, sinus arrest, and A-V block in susceptible

individuals. Verapamil has significant negative inotropic activity and can precipitate CHF. Diltiazem has mild negative inotropic activity

- It is relatively safe to combine amlodipine or nifedipine extended release with a β blocker in the management of hypertension and when associated with angina. Verapamil must not be added to a β blocker, and diltiazem must be used with caution. Nifedipine does not alter digoxin levels; however, verapamil and diltiazem cause about a 47% ↑ in digoxin level and may rarely precipitate bradycardia and A-V block. Verapamil and diltiazem cannot be combined with amiodarone or quinidine, but nifedipine is not affected; nifedipine produces much less constipation than verapamil and has greater acceptance than verapamil in the elderly
- Other dihydropiridines are expected to show the same benefit as nifedipine but cause a higher incidence of minor adverse effects when compared with amlodipine or the extended-release nifedipine formulation

Ca antagonists have few disadvantages when compared with other antihypertensive agents.

Adverse Effects: The approved long-acting preparations for hypertension-amlodipine (Norvasc), nifedipine extended release (Procardia XL, Adalat XL, Adalat PA, Adalat Retard), diltiazem (Cardizem SR, Cardizem CD), and verapamil SR—produce pedal edema, mild facial flushing, dizziness, headaches, leg cramps, gastroesophageal reflux, and rarely sexual dysfunction in much the same frequency. Minor side effects include gingival hypertrophy, blurred vision, muscle cramps, and burning in the gums. Rare side effects include depression, psychosis, and worsening of renal failure. Diltiazem may cause mild elevation in liver function tests and rarely acute hepatic injury. The incidence of adverse reactions with Cardizem SR is reported as approximately 13% higher in the elderly and caution is necessary to titrate the dosage. Care is required in patients with severe hepatic dysfunction, and dosage, especially of diltiazem and verapamil, must be reduced to avoid toxicity. Ca antagonists should be avoided in pregnancy and by lactating mothers. Nifedipine has been used with salutary effects during the last trimester of pregnancy as shortterm therapy for the control of accelerated hypertension of pre-eclampsia. Further studies are required to document safety of longterm therapy.

Contraindications: Moderate or severe aortic stenosis. Diltiazem and verapamil are contraindicated with sick sinus syndrome, arrhythmia, bradycardia, heart block, LV dysfunction, or EF <40%.

Interactions: See Table 1–8.

Amlodipine (Norvasc). *Supplied:* tablets; 5, 10 mg. *Dosage:* 5 mg once daily; ↑ if needed to 10 mg. In the elderly, hepatic impairment or as added therapy initial dose 2.5 mg qd. Because amlodipine is extensively

Table 1–8
Calcium Antagonists—Drug Interactions

	DIGOXIN LEVEL	QUINIDINE	AMIODARONE	BETA BLOCKER
Nifedipine	No change	No change or ↓	No change	Safe
Diltiazem	40% ↑	↑	Sinus arrest	Caution*
Verapamil	50–75% ↑	↑	Contraindicated	Contraindicated*

* See text.

metabolized by the liver and half-life is 56 h in hepatic dysfunction, caution is necessary in these patients. Once-daily amlodipine provides gradual onset of action and steady plasma levels over 24 h with minimal peak-to-trough effects. This agent has been safely administered to patients with Class II-III CHF and may be used in hypertensives with mild or moderate LV dysfunction with close follow-up, especially if other agents are contraindicated. The drug has a role in hypertensives with concomitant angina and/or LV dysfunction. FDA-approved for both hypertension and angina.

Diltiazem (Cardizem, Cardizem SR, Cardizem CD, Anginyl, Adizem-SR, Britiazim, Calcicard, Herbesser, Tildiem, Tilazem). *Supplied:* tablets; 60, 90, 120 mg; Cardizem SR 90, 120 mg (UK, Adizem SR 120 mg); Cardizem CD 180, 240, 300 mg. *Dosage:* 60 mg bid; ↑ if needed to 240–360 mg qd. The SR preparation given bid has a side effect profile similar to nifedipine extended release. Cardizem CD 180–240 mg once daily, max 300 mg.

Nifedipine extended release (Adalat CC, Procardia XL or Adalat XL 30, 60, 90 mg; Adalat PA 10, 20 mg tablets; Adalat Retard 10, 20 mg). *Dosage:* Procardia XL or Adalat XL 30 mg once daily; ↑ if needed to 90 mg once daily. Adalat PA or Retard 10–40 mg bid (given with or after food); max 90 mg qd. For pharmacokinetics, see Chapter 2.

Nitrendipine (Baypress). *Supplied:* tablets; 10 mg. *Dosage:* 5–10 mg once or bid; ↑ as needed to 20 mg once or twice daily.

Nicardipine (Cardene). *Supplied:* capsules; 20, 30 mg. *Dosage:* 20 mg tid; max 30 mg tid.

Felodipine (Plendil, also Renedil in Canada). *Supplied:* tablets; 5, 10 mg. *Dosage:* 5 mg once daily; max 15 mg. In the elderly or in patients with liver dysfunction, BP should be carefully monitored because high plasma concentrations of felodipine may occur and caution is needed in dosing. The 5-mg dose should suffice in the elderly.

Isradipine (DynaCirc; Prescal, UK). *Supplied:* tablets; 2.5, 5 mg. *Dosage:* 1.25 mg; ↑ to 2.5 mg bid; maintenance 2.5–5 mg bid, max 10 mg bid. Elderly: 1.25–2.5 mg qd.

Verapamil (Isoptin, Calan, Cordilox. See Table 1–3). *Supplied:* tablets; 80, 120 mg; SR 120, 180, 240 mg. *Dosage:* 80 mg tid, increasing to 120–160 mg tid; preferably 120 mg SR once or twice daily. The max dose, 1-1/2 tablets of the 240-mg sustained release, should be used with caution; constipation may limit the dosage. Cautions: Combination with a β blocker may cause severe bradycardia or sinus arrest because of similar EP effects. Verapamil may produce bothersome constipation, especially in the elderly. Serum digoxin levels may be increased 50–75% by verapamil and about 45% by diltiazem. See Interactions Table 1–8.

VASODILATORS

$Alpha_1$ blockers and hydralazine have a small role in the management of hypertension not controlled by other agents or their combinations. The advent of ACE inhibitors have appropriately decreased the need for $alpha_1$ blockers.

Indications

- Advisable only when β blockers, diuretics, ACE inhibitors, or Ca antagonists are contraindicated or cause adverse effects

- Combination therapy with β blockers in selected patients

Disadvantages: $Alpha_1$ blockers cause a ↑ in HR and in peak velocity multiplied by HR. Thus, these agents ↑ cardiac work and are contraindicated in patients with CHD; also, they may ↑ the propensity to develop aneurysms. They cause a ↑ in circulating norepinephrine and activate the renin angiotensin system, causing Na and water retention; thus, diuretics are often required to potentiate their BP-lowering action. The combination with diuretics causes a further ↑ in cardiac ejection velocity. These agents do not consistently prevent LVH or cause regression. Because of these disadvantages, an alpha-blocking agent is considered a poor choice for initial or second-line therapy for mild or moderate hypertension and so indicated in Table 1–2.

Contraindications: Patients with aneurysms (undoubtedly, aneurysms may remain occult for several years); severe anemia; moderate or severe aortic stenosis; angina, including silent ischemia.

Dosage: See Table 1–2. *Adverse Effects:* Orthostatic hypotension, first-dose syncope, dizziness, impotence, retrograde ejaculation, confusion, rarely paranoid behavior, and psychosis.

Prazosin (Minipress). *Supplied:* capsules; 1, 2, 5 mg (Canada, UK). *Dosage:* Withhold diuretics 1–2 days. Give 0.5–1 mg test dose at bedtime, then 1 mg bid, increasing to 5 mg bid or tid.

As with the use of other vasodilators, after several months of therapy a diuretic may be required to prevent Na and water retention and to improve antihypertensive effects. At doses of prazosin >6 mg qd, the addition of a β blocker is often required to prevent a ↑ in HR and improve BP control.

Terazosin (Hytrin). *Supplied:* tablets; 1, 2, 5 mg. *Dosage:* 1 mg at bedtime; ↑ slowly if needed to 5 mg once daily; occasionally bid dosing is necessary. Maintenance 2–10 mg, max 15 mg qd. The drug has action and effects similar to prazosin, but a 12- to 24-hour duration of action and better bioavailability. Terazosin 5 mg = approximately 10 mg prazosin.

Hydralazine. *Supplied:* tablets; 10, 25, 50 mg. *Dosage:* 25–50 mg tid; max 200 mg qd. IV 10–20 mg/h, maintenance 5–10 mg/h.

CENTRALLY ACTING AGENTS

Commonly used centrally acting agents include methyldopa, guanabenz, guanfacine, and clonidine.

Indications: Patients who fail to respond to first-line drugs; in patients with severe or resistant hypertension combination with diuretics, Ca antagonists and/or ACE inhibitors.

Disadvantages: These drugs cause postural hypotension, rebound hypertension, and some sedation. Dry mouth is typical for clonidine, guanabenz, and guanfacine. Impotence and depression are not uncommon. Methyldopa is contraindicated in active liver disease. Hepatitis, fatal necrosis, and a rare myocarditis have been reported. Coombs' positive hemolytic anemia may occur with this agent.

Clonidine. *Supplied:* tablets; 0.1, 0.2 mg. *Dosage:* 0.1 mg at bedtime, then bid; maintenance 0.2–0.8 mg, max 1 mg qd.

Guanfacine. *Supplied:* tablets; 1 mg. *Dosage:* 1 mg at bedtime; ↑ to 2 mg over several weeks; 1 mg bid may be necessary with or without a diuretic. The max 3-mg dose commonly produces adverse effects.

Guanabenz. Supplied: tablets; 4, 8 mg. Dosage: 4 mg bid, max 10 mg qd.

Methyldopa. Supplied: tablets; 125, 250, 500 mg. Dosage: 250 mg bid; ↑ if needed to 500 mg bid or tid; max 2 g qd. IV 250 mg over 60 mins q 4–6 hr. Contraindications: active liver disease, depressive states, pheochromocytoma.

ACCELERATED, RESISTANT, OR MALIGNANT HYPERTENSION

In patients with moderate or severe essential or secondary hypertension treated with antihypertensive agents, acceleration and refractoriness of hypertension may occur because of

- Poor compliance
- Increased salt intake in salt-sensitive individuals
- Rebound from discontinuation of centrally acting drugs, clonidine, guanfacine, methyldopa, and, rarely, β blockers or Ca antagonists
- Drug Interactions: Phenylpropranolamine combined with β blockers. NSAIDs ↓ the natriuretic action of diuretics and the BP-lowering effect of ACE inhibitors and β blocker; acetylsalicylic acid or other NSAIDs may interfere with the diuretic effect of loop diuretics
- Renal failure: In this situation, thiazides are rendered ineffective and BP may ↑

Treated or untreated patients may present with severe hypertension that is difficult to control, including the rare presentation with malignant hypertension and diastolic BP >140 mm Hg with or without end-organ damage. The presence of papilledema is not essential for the diagnosis of malignant hypertension.

In about 15% of cases with severe resistant hypertension, a secondary cause is present. Renal artery stenosis is an important cause in both young and older patients. Atherosclerotic occlusion of the renal artery may suddenly worsen, thus causing accelerated hypertension.

Pheochromocytoma and other causes of secondary hypertension must be excluded. See Secondary Hypertension, later in chapter.

Therapy

In most cases of severe hypertension with diastolic BP >115 mm Hg, combination drug therapy is necessary. Renal failure causes resistance to thiazide diuretics, and high doses of furosemide combined with other agents may be required. Provided that CHF or other contraindications to β blockade are absent, β blockers are useful in most patients who have severe hypertension, regardless of the underlying cause. All antihypertensive agents, with the exception of β blockers, cause a ↓ in systemic vascular resistance and fortunately have different sites of action. Therefore, they may be combined in these difficult scenarios.

Additional drug therapy is selected to affect each regulatory system

- Loop diuretics to control renal and other volume-dependent hypertension
- ACE inhibitors or Ca antagonists, particularly nifedipine, to ↓ peripheral vascular resistance
- Centrally and peripherally acting drugs that interfere with alpha-

mediated vasoconstriction, e.g., methyldopa, clonidine, or guanfacine, and $alpha_1$ blockers prazosin or terazosin

If edema or severe renal failure is present, 160–320 mg furosemide may be required. If the diuretic and BP-lowering effects are inadequate, metolazone, 5–10 mg, added to furosemide or bumetanide often produces a salutary response. However, hypokalemia may ensue with this potent but useful diuretic combination.

SUGGESTED COMBINATION THERAPY

Combination 1. Beta blocker plus diuretic plus nifedipine at adequate doses; e.g., propranolol 240 mg plus furosemide and nifedipine extended release 90–120 mg qd (other Ca antagonists if adverse effects occur with nifedipine). Then, if needed, add centrally acting methyldopa or clonidine. Then, if needed, an $alpha_1$ blocker is cautiously added to maximize the vasodilator effect of nifedipine. *Caution:* The latter combination can cause severe hypotension.

Combination 2, where there is no suspicion of tight renal artery stenosis or a solitary kidney: ACE inhibitor plus diuretic plus a centrally acting agent. Then, if needed, add a β blocker plus or minus an $alpha_1$ blocker

- The dose of centrally acting agents and vasodilating alpha blockers may be increased if orthostatic hypertension is not controlled, and the dose of these agents should be decreased if orthostatic hypotension is present
- For hypertension resistant to combination drug therapy, as outlined, minoxidil 2.5–10 mg combined with diuretics and β blockade plus nifedipine may be considered, but baseline echocardiogram and ECG are advisable. The occurrence of serosanguinous pericardial effusion with tamponade is an undesirable effect of minoxidil therapy

Hypertension with diastolic BP >140 mm Hg without end-organ damage, classified as urgent hypertensive crisis, is not an indication for parenteral therapy. Oral medications, especially with oral nifedipine capsules, usually result in a sufficient ↓ in BP over 1–2 h, then further control is achieved over the following few days.

HYPERTENSIVE EMERGENCIES

Diastolic BP consistently >140 mm Hg with evidence of target organ damage—e.g., retinal hemorrhages, papilledema, acute pulmonary edema, decreased renal function, cerebrovascular accident, or hypertensive encephalopathy—requires immediate but carefully monitored, modest ↓ of BP. A 20–25% ↓ from baseline diastolic and/or systolic BP avoids relative hypotension and is sufficient to produce salutary effects.

Patients with consistently elevated diastolic BP >130 mm Hg in the absence of end-organ damage designated as having urgent hypertensive crisis are adequately managed with oral nifedipine in combination with other orally acting antihypertensive agents, as discussed earlier.

Table 1–9 gives guidelines and choice of drug therapy for the management of hypertensive emergencies associated with various conditions and complications

- Hypertensive emergencies are often associated with a malignant phase of essential hypertension, renal failure, cerebrovascular accidents, hypertensive encephalopathy, and rarely pheochromocytoma
- In dissecting aneurysm, BP may be markedly elevated or remain modestly elevated in the range of 160–190 mm Hg systolic, diastolic 90–100 mm Hg, and is considered a special hypertensive emergency, as BP must be promptly lowered within minutes. This is usually achieved by using nitroprusside; a β blocker is also necessary to ↓ the rate of rise of aortic pressure and to prevent further dissection
- In patients with cerebrovascular accident, caution is required because elevations in BP may fluctuate, being triggered by cerebral irritation, and it is essential to carefully monitor the BP for a few hours to confirm that the diastolic pressure is constantly elevated. The need for lowering the BP should be carefully considered and, if deemed necessary, the slow controlled titrated lowering of BP with the use of either nitroprusside or labetalol is used, depending on the cause of hypertension, underlying disease process, and complication. There is some evidence that nitroprusside increases intracranial pressure, but clinically the drug is effective
- Labetalol is a reasonable alternative, provided that precautions for the use of a β-blocking drug are enforced. Labetalol causes postural hypotension, and the patient must remain in bed. Also, the BP-lowering effect may occasionally last 1–12 h whereas the hypotensive effect of nitroprusside dissipates within minutes of cessation of the infusion
- Pulmonary edema due to severe hypertension can be controlled with oral nifedipine and furosemide. If myocardial ischemia is suspected, nifedipine is contraindicated and nitroglycerin IV infusion is advisable (see Table 2–9). The combination of IV nitroglycerin and furosemide should suffice, but if pressure remains markedly elevated, nitroprusside is indicated. Labetalol is contraindicated with CHF; captopril could be used in this situation
- Renal failure is usually associated with volume overload, and furosemide 80–160 mg IV should be administered. Oral nifedipine also has a role, and in this subset, sublingual nifedipine has been used widely and successfully. The oral preparation, however, lowers BP as quickly as sublingual administration and is the preferred route. Failure of nifedipine therapy should prompt the use of labetalol IV infusion as well as continuation of oral nifedipine capsules to wean the patient off labetalol as quickly as possible

Drug Therapy

Nitroprusside infusion reduces BP to any desired level in almost all patients and is the treatment of choice for most hypertensive emergencies that require the lowering of BP, except when nitroprusside is contraindicated. Caution is needed in patients with inadequate cerebral circulation (see Table 1–10). _Dosage:_ 50 mg sodium nitroprusside in 100 ml 5% dextrose water is a convenient solution for use with a nitroprusside infusion pump. See Table 1–10 for the appropriate rate of infusion based on the weight of the patient. Wrap the infusion bottle in aluminum foil or other opaque material to protect it from light. The solution must be used within 4 h. Start the infusion at 0.5 μg/kg/min and ↑ by 0.2 μg/kg/min q 5 mins until the desired BP is obtained. _Dosage Range:_

Table 1–9
Treatment of Hypertensive Emergencies Associated with Complications

AGENT	HEART FAILURE	ENCEPHALOPATHY	CEREBRAL HEMORRHAGE	OTHER CVA	RENAL FAILURE	PHEO	DISSECTING ANEURYSM	PRE-ECLAMPSIA
Nitroprusside	1	1	1	1	CI	2	1	CI
Nitroglycerin	1 or 2	—	—	—	—	—	—	—
Nifedipine	*2†	3*	CI	CI	1 or 2	3	CI	2 or 3+
Diazoxide	CI	2	CI	3	1	CI	CI	CI
Labetalol	CI	2 or 3	1* or 2	1* or 2	1 or 2	AT	2*	2 or 3+
Propranolol**	CI	4 or AT	4 or AT	4 or AT	2 or AT	AT***	1 AT	3 or AT
Trimethaphan	CI	—	—	—	—	—	2	CI
Hydralazine	CI	CI	4	4	2 or AT	CI	CI	1
Furosemide	AT always	4 or AT	—	—	AT always	CI	CI	CI
Methyldopa	4	4 or AT	4	4	3	CI	—	1 or 2
Captopril	1, 2 or AT	—	—	—	—	—	CI	CI
Phentolamine	—	—	—	—	—	1	—	CI

1 = first choice
2 & 3 = second or third choice
4 = rare use or if other drugs unavailable
AT = added therapy, provides reduction in dosages of combined drugs reduces adverse effects, ensures oral agent commenced early
CI = contraindicated
* = if nitroprusside unavailable, give oral 10 mg nifedipine capsule see dagger
** = or other beat blocker
*** = atenolol or other $beta_1$, selective drug used if severe tachyarrhythmia
— = not recommended
† = CI in myocardial ischemia
+ = Not approved by the FDA

Caution: The goal is to produce an immediate but only modest and preferably titrated reduction in blood pressure.

Table 1–10
Nitroprusside Infusion Pump Chart [Nitroprusside 50 mg (1 vial) in 100 ml (500 mg/l)]

	WEIGHT (kg)						
	40	50	60	70	80	90	100
Dosage (μg/kg/min)				Rate (ml/hr)			
0.2	1	1	1	2	2	2	2
0.5	2	3	4	4	5	5	6
0.8	4	5	6	7	8	9	10
1.0	5	6	7	8	10	11	12
1.2	6	7	9	10	12	13	14
1.5	7	9	11	13	14	16	18
1.8	9	11	13	15	17	19	22
2.0	10	12	14	17	19	22	24
2.2	11	13	16	18	21	24	26
2.5	12	15	18	21	24	27	30
2.8	13	17	20	23	27	30	34
3.0	14	18	22	25	29	32	36
3.2	15	19	23	27	31	35	38
3.5	17	21	25	29	34	38	42
3.8	18	23	27	32	36	41	46
4.0	19	24	29	34	38	43	48
4.5	22	27	32	38	43	49	54
5.0	24	30	36	42	48	54	60
6.0	29	36	43	50	58	65	72

The above rates apply only for a 500 mg/l concentration of nitroprusside. If a different concentration must be used, appropriate adjustments in rates should be made. Start at 0.2 μg/kg/min. Increase slowly. Average dose 3 μg/kg/min. Usual dose range 0.5–5.0 μg/kg/min.
From: Khan, M. Gabriel: Hypertension. *In* Cardiac Drug Therapy. 3rd Ed. London, W.B. Saunders, 1992.

0.5–6 μg/kg/min. It is important to begin oral antihypertensive agents as soon as possible so that the patient can be weaned off nitroprusside.

<u>Contraindications:</u> Pregnancy, severe anemia, and severe hepatic dysfunction because cyanide poisoning may occur; if renal disease is present and the use of nitroprusside is extended for >2 days, thiocyanate may accumulate.

Nifedipine administered as capsules is a most useful agent in the management of hypertensive emergencies and is of special value in patients with hypertensive encephalopathy and renal failure. Nifedipine is contraindicated in the management of cerebrovascular accidents, including hemorrhage, and in patients with myocardial ischemia because in these situations a slow, careful titration is needed to avoid a rapid ↓ in BP which may precipitate cerebral or myocardial ischemia.

<u>Dosage:</u> 10-mg capsule q 2–4 h for 4–8 doses, along with furosemide if volume hypertension or renal failure is present. The nifedipine dosage is structured qid. When BP is under control, a long-acting preparation, e.g., nifedipine extended release, Procardia XL, or Adalat XL 60–90 mg once daily is advisable for maintenance therapy

- An alternative initial schedule is the administration of sublingual nifedipine. A 10-mg capsule is perforated, squeezed, and the liquid kept sublingually for a few minutes. Alternatively, the patient is instructed to bite the capsule and then swallow it. This technique has been used extensively since 1982 with good results. Although sublingual nifedipine has gained widespread use, caution is needed because the route has not been approved by the FDA and is not warranted by the manufacturer. Sublingual nifedipine is safe in many situations, but occasionally cerebral infarction, myocardial ischemia, and MI have been precipitated. Importantly, nifedipine 10-mg capsule, used orally, causes BP lowering that is of the same magnitude and acts as rapidly as the sublingual approach. Thus, oral administration is the method of choice

Contraindications: Myocardial ischemia. Abrupt, uncontrolled ↓ in BP may lead to ischemia and infarction.

Labetalol. This alpha β blocker is indicated for the management of hypertensive emergencies caused by renal failure, clonidine withdrawal, and dissecting aneurysm, although in the latter situation a combination of nitroprusside and a β blocker is preferable. Dosage: IV infusion of 2 mg/min, 20–160 mg/h under close and continuous supervision. The patient must be recumbent during and for 4 h following the infusion. Hypotensive effects may last 1–12 h after cessation of the infusion. Alternatively, give bolus injections 20 mg over 1 min repeated after 5 min, if necessary, to a max of 200 mg. Excessive bradycardia can be controlled with IV atropine, 0.6–2 mg, in divided doses.

Diazoxide has been virtually replaced by nitroprusside, labetalol, and nifedipine. The drug is used when other medications are not available or when renal failure is present and there is concern for nitroprusside toxicity. The drug is of value in malignant hypertension and is used in hypertensive emergencies associated with renal failure and hypertensive encephalopathy.

Dosage: 150-mg IV bolus injected undiluted and within 30 seconds directly into a peripheral vein. The 300-mg dose is not recommended because it causes too great a ↓ in BP, is often unpredictable, and has caused cerebral and myocardial infarctions. Diazoxide has Na-retaining effects and must not be used in patients with CHF. Furosemide 40–80 mg IV should be given following a bolus of diazoxide. *Alternative Dosage Regimen:* A slow infusion of diazoxide 5 mg/kg, given at the rate of 15 mg/min over 20–30 min to a total dose of 300–450 mg, is safer than bolus therapy.

Contraindications: Cerebral hemorrhage, cerebrovascular accidents. Controlled BP ↓ is necessary in these situations when cerebral circulation is compromised.

Hydralazine. This vasodilator has a role when nitroprusside, nifedipine, and labetalol are not available. The drug is particularly useful for hypertensive emergencies associated with renal failure and in pregnancy. *Dosage:* A 10-mg test dose is followed in 30 min by IV infusion of 10–20 mg/h; maintenance dose is 5–10 mg/h. The addition of furosemide and a β blocker to hydralazine greatly enhances antihypertensive effects, and the latter agent prevents tachycardia.

Trimethaphan. This drug is indicated only for the management of dissecting aortic aneurysms when nitroprusside and labetalol are not available. *Dosage:* 50 mg trimethaphan in 500 ml 5% dextrose and water is given at 1–2 mg/min and increased, if needed, to 2–4 mg/min via an infusion pump. The head of the patient's bed should be elevated 45° to enhance the drug's orthostatic effect. An IV β blocker such as atenolol or propranolol is given to ↓ ejection velocity and pulsatile flow of blood, which may cause further dissection. For IV β blockers see Table 2–8.

Methyldopa is useful in hypertensive encephalopathy or renal failure. It is not the drug of choice in cerebrovascular accidents because of its sedative properties and slow onset of action, but is considered useful if other agents are not available and ↓ of BP is not required within the hour. Dosage: 250–500 mg IV q 4–6 h.

Nitroglycerin is useful in hypertensive states associated with myocardial ischemia, CHF, MI, and following CABS or other vascular reconstructive surgery and during cardiac catheterization. Dosage: See Infusion Pump Chart, Table 2–9.

HYPERTENSION IN PREGNANCY

- Hypertension in pregnancy is present if the BP taken ≥6 h apart is >140/90 mm Hg or if there is a ↑ above the baseline of 30 mm Hg systolic or 15 mm Hg diastolic. A mean arterial pressure >90 mm Hg (systolic pressure + twice the diastolic ÷ by 3) causes a twofold ↑ in perinatal mortality
- BP should be estimated with patient sitting or semi-reclined, because the BP may be lower in the recumbent position
- Beta blockers, methyldopa, and hydralazine have all been successfully used in the management of hypertension from the 16th week to delivery and for hypertensive complications during pregnancy. Reduced birth weight, neonatal bradycardia, and hypoglycemia have been reported with β blockers. However, recent results using β blockers have shown better control of BP and less effect on the fetus than observed with methyldopa or hydralazine
- A combination of pindolol and hydralazine has been used successfully in randomized studies. Atenolol 25–75 mg qd has had favorable short- and longterm comparison with methyldopa. Combination therapy lowers the dose of individual drugs and reduces adverse effects
- Caution is necessary to avoid using antihypertensive agents during the first and early half of the second trimester of pregnancy to prevent the rare possibility of inducing congenital malformations. Early pregnancy is fortunately associated with vasodilation, which protects from hypertension.

The antihypertensive agents methyldopa, β blockers, and hydralazine are considered relatively safe for chronic use from the 16th week to delivery. Agents suitable for shortterm use during the third trimester if no alternative exists include

- Thiazide diuretics at low dosages (see later discussion)
- Nifedipine 10–20 mg bid for hypertensive emergencies during the last trimester if other agents are not effective, are contraindicated, or cause serious adverse effects. Nifedipine should be avoided during labor because Ca antagonists may cause cessation of uterine contractions. Diltiazem and verapamil are contraindicated in pregnancy and during lactation. These agents must not be used concomitantly with magnesium sulfate because severe hypotension may occur

Drugs contraindicated: Nitroprusside (there is a risk of cyanide toxicity and fetal death) and ACE inhibitors (these agents may cause skull defects and oligohydramnios or may disturb fetal and neonatal renal function and BP control).

Atenolol. Dosage: 25 mg once daily; ↑ to 50 mg qd only after several determinations of BP, preferably made during 2 office or clinic visits. Maintenance ≤50 mg in the morning, 25 mg at night; max 50 mg bid. Longterm results are similar to those observed with methyldopa. Atenolol should not be used during lactation because the concentration in breast milk is high and adverse effects to infants have been reported.

Propranolol. Dosage: 20–40 mg tid; ↑ if needed to a max 80 mg bid. While the drug is well tried, atenolol is the preferred agent during pregnancy, propranolol is the only β blocker advised during lactation because concentration in breast milk is < that of other β blockers.

Labetalol. Dosage: 100–200 mg bid; max 800 mg qd is effective. The drug has been implicated in causing retroplacental hemorrhage. Postural hypotension, perioral numbness, itching of the scalp, positive ANA, and Lupus-like syndrome have been observed. Acute hepatic necrosis is a rare but life-threatening complication. Thus, labetalol must not be considered just another β-blocking drug.

Methyldopa. Dosage: 125–250 mg bid; ↑ the dose only after several reassessments over 2 or 3 visits; max suggested 500 mg bid.

In a study of 117 methyldopa-treated women, 1 (.9%) fetal death occurred and 9 (7.2%) fetal deaths occurred in the control group of 125 women. No significant differences were noted at 7-year follow-up of children born to women in both groups.

If BP control is urgently needed prior to delivery, methyldopa is preferred to β-adrenergic blockers. The addition of hydralazine may be required if methyldopa is not sufficiently effective.

Hydralazine (Apresoline). This pure arterial vasodilator may be used during the last trimester if BP is not adequately controlled with atenolol, pindolol, or methyldopa. The drug is teratogenic in animals. Hydralazine causes Na and water retention that requires the unwarranted use of a thiazide; sinus tachycardia may also be troublesome, necessitating β blockade. Fetal thrombocytopenia has been reported. This agent is best reserved for a short period of therapy, 1–2 weeks, in the last trimester, along with a small dose of methyldopa or atenolol. Dosage: IV: 5 mg bolus over 1–2 min, repeated in 20 min; then, if needed, infusion 5 mg to max of 15 mg/h, with constant fetal monitoring of HR and maternal BP. Oral: 25 mg tid for a few weeks.

Thiazide diuretics are relatively contraindicated since they ↓ placental blood flow, causing low birth weight. Thrombocytopenia, neonatal jaundice, and occasionally pancreatitis may occur. Preeclampsia is associated with reduced plasma volume. and thiazides are not recommended. Several studies have indicated freedom from serious adverse effects, but results are questioned and the use of thiazides remains restricted. Low-dose thiazide therapy may be considered in the third trimester if other agents are contraindicated or unavailable, particularly in the following category of patients: Those whose hypertension predated conception or manifested prior to midpregnancy; hypertension causing CHF associated with volume overload. Dosage: HCTZ 12.5, max 25 mg qd, or bendrofluazide 1.25–2.5 mg qd for a period of 1–6 weeks, when alternative therapy should be considered.

Hypertensive Crisis of Pregnancy

Severe hypertension of pregnancy, especially near term or during labor, associated with diastolic pressures >105 mm Hg may require urgent treatment with the following agents and/or combinations.

Hydralazine (Apresoline). *Dosage:* 5 mg IV over 10–20 min, then 5–10 mg q 20–30 mins, OR, after the first bolus, give by IV infusion 5 mg/h, ↑ to 10 mg, max 15 mg/h, with continuous evaluation of HR and BP and fetal monitoring; fetal distress may occur. In the UK, the drug is initially given by the above method or by IV infusion; 200–300 μg/min; maintenance usually 50–150 μg/min.

Methyldopa. *Dosage:* 500 mg orally causes BP ↓ within 6 h. IV 250–500 mg in 100 ml 5% dextrose in water, over 30 min to 1 h, q 6 h.

Labetalol. *Dosage:* IV bolus 10–60 mg q 20 min is effective and appears to cause less fetal distress than hydralazine. Practitioners should ascertain if labetalol is approved for IV use in their area of practice prior to use.

Magnesium sulfate is extremely useful in patients with pre-eclampsia to prevent convulsions. *Dosage:* 4 g diluted in 100–200 ml IV solution infused over 20 min, then 2 g/h with careful monitoring of BP and urinary output. The drug is continued during labor and for ≥24 h post partum. Combination therapy utilizing the vasodilator action of hydralazine, the central action of methyldopa, and enhancement by magnesium sulfate usually produces salutary effects with less adverse effects than observed with high doses of a single agent. Magnesium sulfate has only mild antihypertensive effects and is not considered an antihypertensive agent. The major benefit of this drug is to prevent seizures associated with pre-eclampsia. *Caution:* Magnesium sulfate must not be used concomitantly with nifedipine because severe hypotension may be precipitated; magnesium sulfate should be avoided in patients with renal failure.

SECONDARY HYPERTENSION

Causes of secondary hypertension and their approximate incidence include

- Renal parenchymal disease — 3%
- Renovascular disease — 1%
- Cushing's syndrome — 0.1%
- Pheochromocytoma — 0.1%
- Primary hyperaldosteronism — 0.1%
- Coarctation — 0.1%
- Estrogens — 0.4%
- Alcohol — ≥0.2%

Renal Parenchymal Disease

The history and physical and laboratory screening indicate the type and duration of the underlying disease. Screening includes assessment for

- Presence and type of urinary casts
- Degree of proteinuria and anemia
- Level of serum creatinine, urea or BUN, serum Ca, phosphate, and albumin

Common underlying diseases: Chronic glomerulonephritis, diabetic nephropathy, collagen vascular disease, polycystic kidney, chronic pyelonephritis, interstitial renal disease.

A ↑ in total peripheral resistance, hypervolemia, increased total body Na stores, and a high cardiac output contribute to the hypertension of renal failure.

THERAPY

Furosemide. As emphasized under the section on diuretics, above, thiazides lose their natriuretic effect in patients with GFR <25 ml/h or serum creatinine >2.3 mg/dl (203 μmol/l). Dosage: Furosemide 80–240 mg qd or bumetanide 5–10 mg qd may be expected to produce sufficient natriuresis, which is best reflected in the degree of weight loss. Rarely, ≤500 mg furosemide or 240 mg plus 5 mg metolazone may be required.

Beta Blockers. These agents combined with diuretics are effective in reducing BP in patients with chronic renal failure. Atenolol, nadolol, and sotalol are excreted by the kidney; their dosing interval should be increased, and the total daily dose may have to be reduced in chronic renal failure. Propranolol and metoprolol are actively metabolized, do not require dose adjustment, and are preferred for the management of hypertension with severe renal failure. Timolol and pindolol are partially excreted by the kidney but usually require little or no adjustment in dosage.

Calcium Antagonists. Nifedipine has had extensive trials and been proven effective in reducing total peripheral resistance, which is usually markedly increased in patients with chronic renal failure. Nifedipine and diltiazem are metabolized, and dosages may not require alteration. However, a few cases of patients with renal failure reportedly showed deterioration with nifedipine and diltiazem; recovery of function occurs upon discontinuing the Ca antagonist. Verapamil may accumulate with renal failure and is not advisable. Nifedipine has commonly replaced hydralazine in the combination β blocker plus diuretic plus vasodilator, but hydralazine may be added to the combination because the mechanism of vasodilation is different and the effect is additive.

Hydralazine. When Ca antagonists are contraindicated or produce adverse effects, hydralazine has a role in lowering total peripheral resistance and BP and has proven effective in patients with severe hypertension associated with renal failure. Dosage: 25–100 mg bid. The dosage interval for hydralazine should be increased with chronic renal failure, with creatinine clearance <25 ml/min.

Central Acting Agents. Methyldopa, clonidine, and guanfacine are useful in combination with furosemide and nifedipine or appropriate agents in managing resistant renal hypertension, including patients on dialysis. Dosing should be reduced to once daily, preferably at bedtime.

Renovascular Hypertension

Diagnostic considerations in renovascular hypertension include

- Age of onset (< age 30 or > age 50)
- Sudden onset of malignant, accelerated, or resistant hypertension accompanied by renal bruit
- Sharp rise in serum creatinine after the use of an ACE inhibitor, which is indicative of significant renal artery stenosis

In such circumstances, the incidence of significant renovascular hypertension is 20–33%. Increased diagnostic suspicion is obtained from observation of the IV pyelogram or renal scan. Where available, digital subtraction angiography is preferred to renal arteriography. A difference between the 2 renal veins from the abnormal and suppressed contralateral kidney, giving a renal vein renin ratio >1.5, strongly suggests significant renal artery stenosis, but results are often insufficient to justify the investigation.

Drug management includes the judicious use of combination therapy

- Beta blocker, thiazide (furosemide if renal failure is present), and amiloride if K conservation is necessary
- ACE inhibitors are contraindicated in patients with severe bilateral renal artery stenosis or stenosis of a solitary kidney since in these patients renal circulation is dependent on high levels of angiotensin II. Thus, a sharp ↓ in renal blood flow may occur, and renal failure may ensue with the loss of a solitary kidney
- Angioplasty and surgery are equally effective and superior to drug therapy in patients in whom renal artery stenosis is due to fibrous dysplasia and hypertension is present for <3 years with normal renal function. Angioplasty has a role in patients who are poor surgical candidates. Restenosis post angioplasty frequently occurs, but a second dilation may be rewarding. In patients with unilateral renal artery stenosis, elevation of serum creatinine indicates that nephrosclerosis is present in the contralateral kidney, and a salutary effect of angioplasty or revascularization is unlikely
- Surgery appears to be somewhat more effective than angioplasty for atherosclerotic renovascular disease. Either therapy is advisable for atherosclerotic occlusion in younger patients with unilateral renal artery disease, especially when hypertension is difficult to control with antihypertensive agents. A serum creatinine level >1.4 mg/dl (124 μmol/l) and the presence of CHD increases the surgical mortality rate

Pheochromocytoma

Less than 0.1% of patients with moderate to severe diastolic hypertension are expected to have a pheochromocytoma

- Approximately 10% of these tumors of the adrenal medulla are bilateral
- 10% are malignant
- 10% are outside the adrenals
- 10% are familial
- Patients with familial or bilateral pheochromocytomas may be part of the Type II Multiple Endocrine Neoplasia syndrome and should be screened for medullary carcinoma of the thyroid and hyperparathyroidism

DIAGNOSTIC HALLMARKS

- Severe headaches and profuse sweating
- Palpitations and tremor
- Pallor due to vasoconstriction
- Paroxysmal or diastolic hypertension; severe ↑ of BP with induction of anesthesia, surgery, or use of histamine, phenothiazines, or tricyclic antidepressants
- Postural hypotension
- Weight loss

The catecholamine metabolic pathway involves conversion of tyrosine to normetanephrine and metanephrine (see Fig. 1–2).

The following investigations are usually diagnostic

- Elevated 24-hour urine total metanephrine is the most reliable urinary screening test
- Free catecholamines and VMA are often elevated, but interference with urinary screening occurs with phenothiazines, chloral hydrate, and other drugs. Beta blockers, thiazides, Ca antagonists, and ACE inhibitors, however, cause no interference. A special diet and avoidance of several drugs for ≥3 days are necessary for accurate VMA results
- A ↑ in plasma catecholamines: An assessment is carried out with a heparin lock in an arm vein; the patient is sedated with 1 mg of sublingual lorazepam (Ativan) and is allowed to lie quietly for 20 min. Blood is then drawn for epinephrine and norepinephrine levels
- Elevated dopamine serum level is estimated on the same blood sample taken for epinephrine because dopamine may be the only chemical produced by some malignant pheochromocytomas. Plasma catecholamines may be mildly elevated with stress and essential hypertension, diuretics, prazosin, and other $alpha_1$ blockers, hydralazine, labetalol, and Ca antagonists. A CT scan may reveal a tumor. I^{131}MIBG enters chromaffin tissue and a MIBG scan helps identify extra adrenal tumors

THERAPY

Phentolamine (Regitine; Rogitine, Canada and UK). Hypertensive crisis may require the use of phentolamine prior to the administration of phenoxybenzamine. Dosage: An infusion of 10–20 μg/kg/min or 5–60 mg over 10–30 min at a rate of 0.1–2 mg/min. The drug has a rapid onset of action and lasts only 10–20 min. *Caution:* Deaths due to arrhythmia and acute MI have been reported, and β blockade may be required. If β blockers are used, care is required in patients who are considered at high risk for precipitation of CHF.

Nitroprusside. When used to ↓ BP during a crisis, nitroprusside is effective, but complicating tachyarrhythmias may cause problems with management, and β blockade should not be used without adequate alpha blockade. (See infusion Pump Chart, Table 1–10.)

Phenoxybenzamine (Dibenzyline). Oral therapy with this nonselective alpha blocker is commenced once the BP is under control or if the BP is not severely elevated after control with phentolamine or other agent. Dosage: 1–2 mg/kg qd in 2 or 3 divided doses, usually 10 mg q 8–12 h. Increase q 3 or 4 days by 10 mg to a max 50 mg tid. Phenoxybenzamine therapy is usually required for control of BP over a period of 1–2 weeks prior to surgery. The drug is contraindicated in CHF.

Nifedipine. This agent, used universally for the management of all grades of hypertension, may be used in the emergency setting, with temporary beneficial results expected in some patients. It may occasionally avoid the use of nitroprusside (see Table 1–9).

Patients with pheochromocytoma are hypovolemic, and alpha blockade causes vasodilation. Thus, a marked ↓ in BP may occur, causing severe postural hypotension. Increase in salt intake and vigorous saline infusion are usually required during the 1 to 2 weeks prior to surgery to prevent severe postural hypotension, but careful monitoring is required to prevent the precipitation of CHF. Postoperative hypotension may be avoided by discontinuing phenoxybenzamine several days prior to surgery.

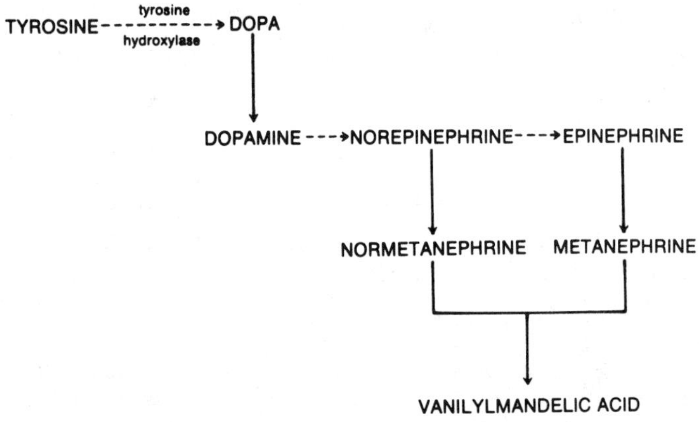

Figure 1–2. Catecholamine metabolic pathway

Beta Blocker. These agents must not be used prior to adequate alpha blockade because unopposed stimulation of alpha receptors can cause a severe ↑ in BP. Beta blockade may be required after 1 week of alpha blockage if catecholamine-induced arrhythmias require control. A $beta_1$ selective drug such as atenolol is preferable to propranolol.

Captopril has been successfully used to ↓ BP and ameliorate CHF in a patient with catecholamine-induced "cardiomyopathy" secondary to pheochromocytoma.

Metyrosine (Metirosine, UK) (alpha-methyl-L-tyrosine) (Demser). This agent is an inhibitor of tyrosine hydroxylase (see Fig. 1–2) and, hence, the synthesis of catecholamines. Metyrosine reduces catecholamine production by about 70% and has a role in the preoperative management of pheochromocytomas as an alternative to phenoxybenzamine. The drug is particularly useful for the management of inoperable tumors. *Dosage:* 250 mg qid; ↑ daily by 250 mg to reach a max of 4 g qd. *Adverse Effects:* Severe diarrhea, sedation, extra pyramidal symptoms, and hypersensitive reactions.

Surgery. A transabdominal incision is advisable to allow a search of all abdominal chromaffin tissue. Enflurane is considered the safest anesthetic agent as it does not stimulate catecholamine release or sensitize the myocardium to catecholamines. Management of fluid blood volumes necessitates the use of a Swan-Ganz catheter. Elevated BP is controlled with nitroprusside or nitroglycerin, especially in patients where the occurrence of CHF is predictable. Postoperative hypotension and CHF present a greater hazard with the use of alpha blockers and β blockade than with the use of nitroprusside or nitroglycerin.

A surgical cure is expected in 80% of patients. Approximately 10% of patients have a recurrence, and patients should be screened annually for 5 years. The 5-year survival is about 95% for patients with benign tumors and 45% for patients with malignant tumors.

Coarctation of the Aorta

Hypertension in the arms with weak, absent, or delayed femoral pulses is a hallmark. After the age of 10, chest x ray shows notching of the fourth to eighth ribs bilaterally or unilaterally and right sided if the coarctation is proximal to the left subclavian.

THERAPY

Drug therapy is often required in the adult prior to surgical correction. Coarctation of the aorta causes activation of the renin angiotensin aldosterone system; thus, ACE inhibitors are first-line agents. All patients should be screened for septal defects, polycystic kidneys, and berry aneurysms; the latter not uncommonly causes the patient's demise.

Surgical repair may not be curative. Postoperative hypertension may be a problem requiring antihypertensive therapy. Aortic dissection may occur distal or proximal to the site of surgical repair. Also, restenosis may require balloon angioplasty, and close follow-up is essential.

Two risk factors have been identified for premature death after surgery

- Age at the time of surgical correction: The younger the patient, the better the outcome
- Hypertension, both preoperative and postoperative, carries a guarded prognosis

Suggested Reading

Khan M Gabriel: Hypertension in Cardiac and Pulmonary Management. Philadelphia, Lea & Febiger, 1993.

SHEP Cooperative Study Group: Prevention of stroke by antihypertensive drug treatment in older persons with isolated systolic hypertension: Final results of the Systolic Hypertension in the Elderly Programs (SHEP). JAMA *265*:3255, 1991.

Joint National Committee on Detection, Evaluation and Treatment of High Blood Pressure. The 1992 Report of the Joint National Committee on Detection, Evaluation, and Treatment of High Blood Pressure (JNC-V). Arch Intern Med 153:154; 1993

Angina

2

M. Gabriel Khan

CLASSIFICATION

- *Stable angina:* No change in the past 60 days in frequency, duration, or precipitating causes. Pain duration <10 mins. In >90% of patients, stable angina is caused by a >70% obstruction in ≥1 coronary artery. In <10% of individuals, a lesser degree of atheromatous obstruction, coronary artery spasm, or small vessel disease is present

The Canadian cardiovascular classification grading of angina is widely used to differentiate mild, moderate, or severe stable angina

- Class 1 Angina: Pain is precipitated only by severe and usually prolonged exertion
- Class 2 Angina: Pain on moderate effort, e.g., precipitated by walking uphill or by walking briskly for >3 blocks on the level in the cold, against a wind, or provoked by emotional stress. There is "slight limitation of ordinary activity"
- Class 3 Angina: Marked limitation of ordinary activity; pain occurs on mild exertion, usually restricting daily chores. Unable to walk 2 blocks on the level at comfortable temperatures and at a normal pace
- Class 4 Angina: Chest discomfort on almost any physical activity, e.g., dressing, shaving, walking <100 feet indoors. Pain may be present at rest
- *Unstable angina:* Braunwald's classification of this heterogenous population of patients is given in Table 2–1.

STABLE ANGINA

Pathophysiology

Myocardial ischemia is a dynamic process. It is now clear that 3, not 2, determinants play a major role in the pathogenesis of myocardial ischemia, which may manifest as the chest pain of angina or remain painless as with silent ischemia.

The 3 determinants of myocardial ischemia are

- Concentric or eccentric coronary atheroma causing > about 70% stenosis; concentric plaques are observed mainly with stable angina and there is a tendency for them to be eccentric in patients with frequent rest pain and in those with unstable angina
- Increased myocardial O_2 demand
- Release of catecholamines occurring at the onset of angina and during the episode in the vast majority of patients with stable angina. Release

Table 2–1
Classification of Unstable Angina

	SEVERITY
Class I	New-onset, severe, or accelerated angina. Patients with angina of less than 2 months' duration, severe or occurring three or more times per day, or angina that is distinctly more frequent and precipitated by distinctly less exertion. No rest pain in the last 2 months.
Class II	Angina at rest. Subacute. Patients with one or more episodes of angina at rest during the preceding month but not within the preceding 48 hr.
Class III	Angina at rest. Acute. Patients with one or more episodes at rest within the preceding 48 hr.
	CLINICAL CIRCUMSTANCES
Class A	Secondary unstable angina. A clearly identified condition extrinsic to the coronary vascular bed that has intensified myocardial ischemia, e.g., anemia, infection, fever, hypotension, tachyarrhythmia, thyrotoxicosis, hypoxemia secondary to respiratory failure.
Class B	Primary unstable angina.
Class C	Postinfarction unstable angina (within 2 weeks of documented myocardial infarction).
	INTENSITY OF TREATMENT
1.	Absence of treatment or minimal treatment.
2.	Occurring in presence of standard therapy for chronic stable angina (conventional doses of oral beta blockers, nitrates, and calcium antagonists).
3.	Occurring despite maximally tolerated doses of all three categories of oral therapy, including intravenous nitroglycerin.

Modified from Braunwald E.: Unstable angina: A classification. Circulation *80*:410, 1989, by permission of the American Heart Association, Inc.

of catecholamines may actually initiate ischemia, which stimulates further catecholamine release, and a vicious circle perpetuates the O_2 lack (Fig. 2–1)

When angina is manifest, ≥1 coronary artery is expected to show a >70% stenosis on angiography. The obstructive plaque of atheroma is often focal and usually occurs in the proximal portion of a coronary artery; this combination of proximal and focal lesions dictates the success of angioplasty and bypass surgery. In <10% of individuals, and especially in diabetics, multifocal longer segmental or diffuse disease exists in the distal coronary tree

- Figure 2–2 shows coronary angiographic anatomy. An obstructive lesion in the LAD artery prior to the septal or first diagonal branch is considered proximal and highly significant because it can jeopardize >50% of the LV myocardium. LAD lesions after the first diagonal affect only about 20% of the myocardium. In approximately 85% and 15% of individuals, the right coronary or left circumflex artery supplies the posterior diaphragmatic portion of the interventricular septum and the diaphragmatic surface of the left ventricle, respectively, and is referred to as the dominant artery. The term "dominant" does

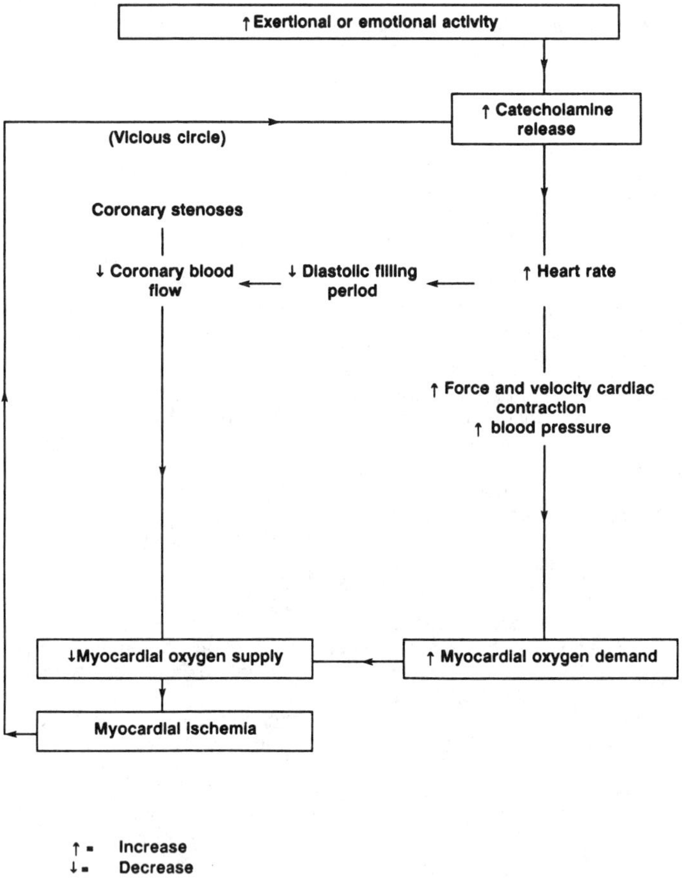

Figure 2–1. Pathophysiology of angina.

not imply a more important artery but does have some clinical bearing on decision making in the management of angina

- A 25% ↓ in the outer radius of a normal coronary artery results in about a 60% ↓ in a cross-sectional area. However, in an artery with 75% stenosis, a 10% ↓ in the outer radius would produce a complete occlusion
- During periods of exercise or exertion, catecholamine release causes a ↑ in HR, a ↑ in the velocity and force of myocardial contraction producing an elevation in BP, and a ↑ in myocardial O_2 demand. In the presence of significant coronary artery stenosis, an O_2 deficit may occur. Myocardial ischemia increases catecholamine release, resulting in an additional ↑ in HR and BP, with further O_2 lack, and the vicious circle ensues. Importantly, the coronaries fill during the diastolic period, which is shortened during tachycardia
- Pharmacologic agents that inhibit the initiation or interrupt the dynamic process described above provide rational therapy for myocardial ischemia. It is, therefore, not surprising that β-adrenergic blocking

drugs produce salutary effects in the majority of patients with stable angina and represent first-choice oral medications for the management of angina

- In contrast to the β-blocking drugs, dihydropyridine Ca antagonists, when used alone, tend to ↑ HR and, along with other Ca antagonists, do not inhibit the cardiovascular actions of catecholamines. Nitrates also ↑ HR
- An important consideration in relation to coronary artery spasm is that ischemia from this cause also triggers catecholamine release and worsening of angina. However, coronary artery spasm is a rare cause of myocardial ischemia manifest as stable angina

Diagnosis

- Diagnosis is based on a careful relevant history. The pain of angina is typically a retrosternal discomfort precipitated by a particular activity, especially walking quickly up an incline or against the wind. Pain or discomfort disappears within seconds to minutes of stopping the precipitating activity, in keeping with the concept of O_2 supply versus myocardial demand. Discomfort may start in the lower, middle, or upper substernal area, the lower jaw, or the arm. Typically, the discomfort is a tightness, constriction, squeezing, heaviness, pressure, strangulation, burning, nausea, or an indigestion-like feeling of gradual onset that disappears at rest, except with unstable anginal syndromes. Occasionally, the pain is described as sharp, and at times, discomfort is replaced by shortness of breath on exertion

CORONARY ANGIOGRAPHIC ANATOMY: REPRESENTATION IN STANDARD PROJECTIONS

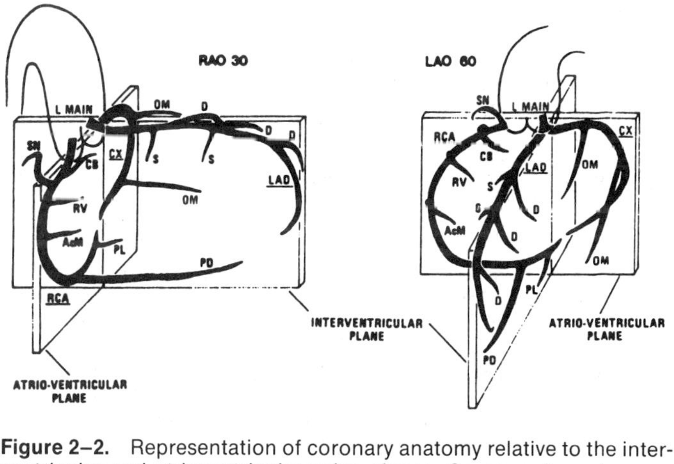

Figure 2–2. Representation of coronary anatomy relative to the interventricular and atrioventricular valve planes. Coronary branches are as indicated—L Main (left main), LAD (left anterior descending), D (diagonal), S (septal), CX (circumflex), OM (obtuse marginal), RCA (right coronary), CB (conus branch), SN (sinus node), RV (right ventricular), AcM (acute marginal), PD (posterior descending), PL (posterolateral left ventricular). From: Grossman W, Baim DS: Cardiac Catheterization, Angiography and Intervention. 4th Ed. Philadelphia, Lea & Febiger, 1992, p 200.

- The area of pain is usually at least the size of a clenched fist, often occupying most of the central chest area. The patient uses ≥2 fingers, the entire palm of the hand, or the fist to indicate the pain site. A pencil point area of pain is rarely caused by myocardial ischemia
- Relief of pain in an individual with stable angina always occurs within minutes of cessation of the precipitating exertional or emotional activity. Relief with sublingual nitroglycerin occurs within 1–2 mins

Investigative Evaluation

- Patients with the same clinical symptoms may have very different prognoses depending on coronary anatomy; 1-, 2-, or 3-vessel or left main stenoses; and on LV function
- The failure to predict outcomes based on the clinical presentation often necessitates evaluation with exercise stress testing and echocardiography. Thallium scintigraphy is required in some. It is necessary to evaluate the coronary reserve and degree of proximal stenosis. The goal of initial investigations is to stratify the risk so that those at higher risk can progress to angiography early
- Lipid levels: Total serum cholesterol and HDL are not affected by daily food intake. It is best to request their measurement with the patient in a nonfasting state at the same time as the office visit, as this routine saves patient's time and money. If the total cholesterol >240 mg/dl (6.2 mmol/l) then request total cholesterol, LDL, and triglycerides with the patient fasting 14 h (see Chap. 9)
- The Hb is necessary to exclude the rare occurrence of angina precipitated by anemia in patients with atheromatous coronary stenosis. Renal function, approximately assessed by the serum creatinine, is relevant to the choice and dosage of medications
- The ECG is expected to be normal in >70% of patients with stable angina, except in individuals with previous MI or concomitant hypertension. However, even a normal record makes a valuable baseline with which to compare future tracings
- Exercise stress testing is important in assessing the coronary reserve and in formulating strategies for other therapeutic interventions, especially in patients with Class 1 and 2 angina. It is also useful in assessing the effect of medical therapy. However, the test is not useful in evaluating atypical chest pain, especially in women. The test is

---

Figure 2–3. Nomogram of the Prognostic Relations Embodied in the Treadmill Score. Determination of prognosis proceeds in five steps. First, the observed amount of exercise-induced ST-segment deviation (the largest elevation or depression after resting changes have been subtracted) is marked on the line for ST-segment deviation during exercise. Second, the observed degree of angina during exercise is marked on the line for angina. Third, the marks for ST-segment deviation and degree of angina are connected with a straight edge. The point where this line intersects the ischemia-reading line is noted. Fourth, the total number of minutes of exercise in treadmill testing according to the Bruce protocol (or the equivalent in multiples of resting oxygen consumption [METs] from an alternative protocol) is marked on the exercise-duration line. Fifth, the mark for ischemia is connected with that for exercise duration. The point at which this line intersects the line for prognosis indicates the five-year survival rate and average annual mortality for patients with these characteristics.

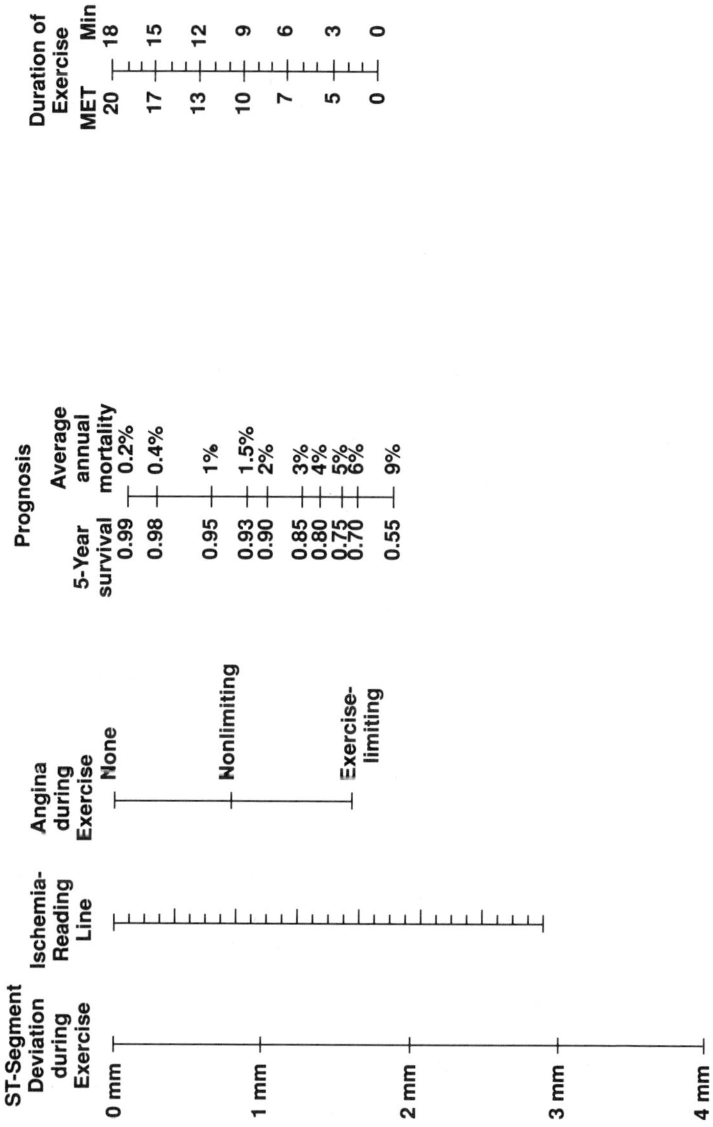
ST-Segment Deviation during Exercise
0 mm
1 mm
2 mm
3 mm
4 mm
Ischemia-Reading Line
Angina during Exercise
None
Nonlimiting
Exercise-limiting
Prognosis
5-Year survival
0.99
0.98
0.95
0.93
0.90
0.85
0.80
0.75
0.70
0.55
Average annual mortality
0.2%
0.4%
1%
1.5%
2%
3%
4%
5%
6%
9%
Duration of Exercise
MET
20
17
13
10
7
5
0
Min
18
15
12
9
6
3
0

contraindicated in patients with aortic stenosis, and obstructive cardiomyopathy

- Patients < age 60 with angina who can complete >6 mins of a Bruce protocol treadmill exercise test, achieving >85% of maximal HR without chest pain or ischemia changes, can usually be managed with medical therapy. Patients who can tolerate >9 mins of a Bruce protocol appear to have a good prognosis. In this subset, if medical therapy is judged by physician and patient to be yielding adequate control of symptoms, coronary angiography is usually not required. See nomogram of the prognostic relations embodied in the treadmill score, Figure 2–3
- A positive exercise stress test is indicated by ≥1 mm flat or down-sloping ST segment depression, 80 millisecond after the J point occurring in 3 consecutive beats. A strongly positive test is indicated by ST segment depression within the first 3 mins of exercise, down-sloping ST segment depression of ≥2 mm, persisting for >4 mins on cessation of exercise or occurring at low work load: HR <120/min, systolic pressure <130 mm Hg, i.e., a low rate pressure product. Patients in this category have a poor prognosis and are expected to have a large area of myocardium involved by the ischemic process. Patients with strongly positive tests, ischemia occurring prior to 6 mins, and/or hypotension during exercise have a high probability of having multivessel or left mainstem disease and are, therefore, at significant risk. Coronary angiography is warranted with consideration for coronary angioplasty or CABS in such patients
- Thallium 201 perfusing the myocardium is removed by myocardial cells. A positive test, a cold spot on the scan, absent thallium uptake with filling in later views, indicates ischemic myocardium. The test is generally performed in conjunction with an exercise test and is useful in patients with LV hypertrophy and atypical chest pain in which conventional exercise stress testing gives a high rate of false positives. The validity of the test depends on achieving a reasonably high rate pressure product during the preliminary stress period
- Thallium scintigraphy has several limitations. Proper methodology is necessary: Image artifacts are common and can lead to false positive interpretation; false positive results may occur because of overlying breast shadows, while right ventricular blood pool may attenuate inferoposterior myocardial activity; myocardial apical thinning causes a local ↓ in thallium activity that can be mistaken for ischemic disease; LBBB may produce a false positive scan. Most of these difficulties are of importance in relation to fixed defects, reversibility being a strong indicator of myocardium at risk. Negative scans may occur with significant lesions in the circumflex or diagonal branches of the LAD. Widespread disease with global ↓ in uptake will also, paradoxically, yield a negative result
- Dipyridamole or adenosine thallium scintigraphy is a useful investigation in patients with Class 2 angina with the absence of pain at rest who are unable to exercise because of arthritis or PVD. Patients with Class 3 angina require coronary angiographic assessment. Dipyridamole thallium scintigraphy is contraindicated in patients with unstable angina, post-infarction angina, and non Q wave infarction; within 3 months of infarction, these patients require coronary angiography. Also, dipyridamole scintigraphy is contraindicated in patients with asthma and COPD
- Echocardiography may be required in some patients to assess LV systolic function. Stress echocardiography has a role in selected patients
- *Coronary Angiography.* Indications include: Patients who require coronary angioplasty or CABS (see indications for these interventions);

ideally, all patients with angina in good general health and with absence of severe concomitant disease that would contraindicate CABS. Patients with painless ischemia have the same risks as patients with angina and must be evaluated and given consideration for angioplasty or CABS if severe obstructive disease is discovered

Therapy

General control of risk factors is the necessary first step: Weight ↓, cessation of smoking, removal or avoidance of stress, control of hypertension with suitable agents, maintenance of a serum cholesterol <200 mg/dl (5.2 mmol/l), LDL <160 mg/dl (4 mmol/l) (see Chap. 9).

Suggested steps in therapy for stable angina are given in Figure 2–4.

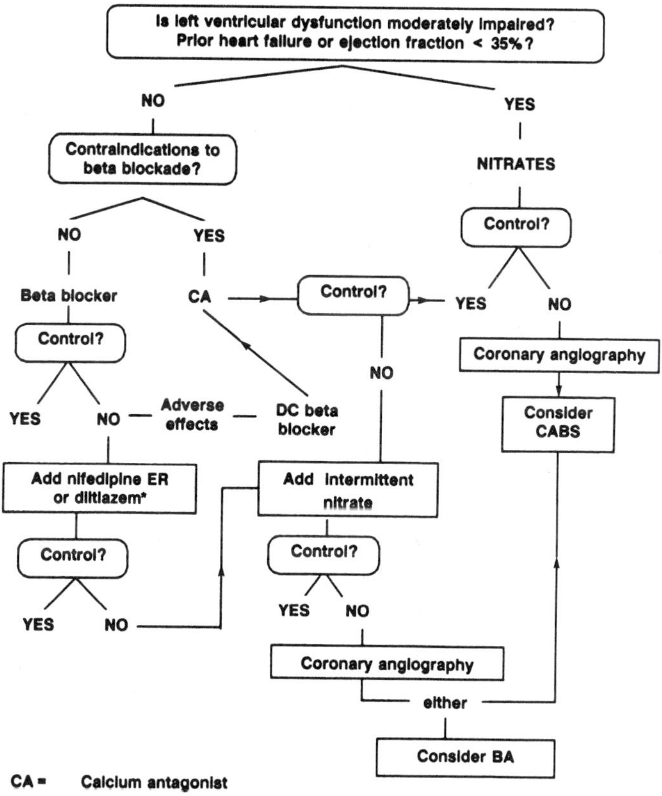

CA = Calcium antagonist
CABS = Coronary artery bypass surgery
DC = Discontinue
* Caution with beta blocker combination; avoid if ejection fraction <40%
BA = Balloon angioplasty
ER = Extended Release

Figure 2–4. Suggested steps in medical therapy for stable angina.

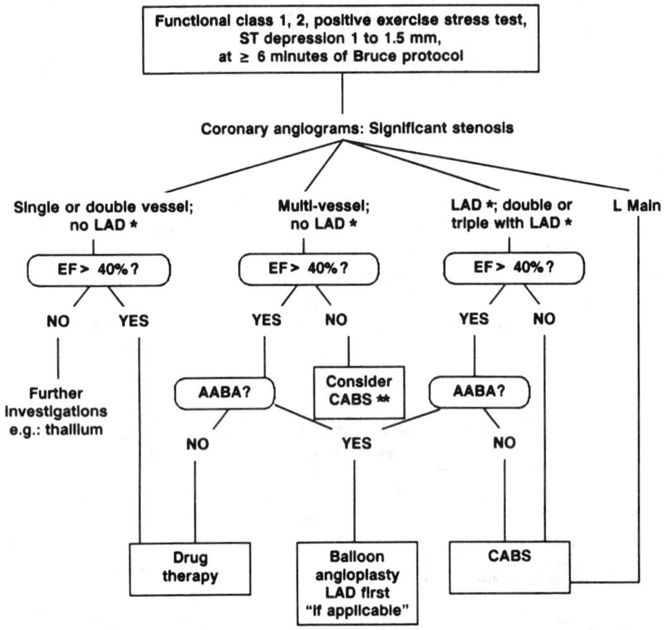

* LAD = Left anterior descending severe proximal stenosis
EF = Ejection fraction
AABA = Angiographically acceptable for balloon angioplasty
** CABS = Coronary artery bypass surgery

Figure 2–5. Decision-making in the management of angina (class 1, 2).

Figures 2–5 and 2–6 give decision-making steps in the management of varying grades of stable angina formulated on knowledge derived from

- The assessment of the patient according to the Canadian Cardiovascular Society functional or similar classification (or similar assessment of clinical severity of angina)
- The exercise stress test
- The anatomic site of atheromatous coronary obstruction, degree of stenosis as determined by coronary angiography, and number of involved vessels
- The presence or absence of lesions angiographically acceptable for balloon angioplasty (Type A) or probably acceptable lesions for balloon angioplasty
- Radionuclide or echocardiographic assessment of LV function. Patients with significant proximal coronary stenosis affecting 3 major vessels or 2 vessels including the LAD and moderate or severe LV dysfunction, EF <40% (>20%), show greater benefits from surgery as opposed to medical therapy; surgery is considered to have advantages over angioplasty in these patients. However, patients with severe LV dysfunction without reversible ischemia do not benefit from CABS

- The patient's age: Patients aged 35–60 are managed preferably by balloon angioplasty if the lesions are considered angiographically acceptable. Thus, surgery is deferred as long as possible to avoid the high risk of vein graft occlusion 10 years later (Table 2–2). The ACC/AHA Task Force Report (1991) strongly advises a left internal mammary artery anastomosis to the LAD. The artery remains attached at its origin from the left subclavian. This is the surgical procedure of choice for all patients, but especially for the relatively young; the 10-year occlusion rate is 5%, as opposed to 15% for internal mammary graft and 50% for vein graft (Table 2–2). Even so, internal mammary graft or anastomosis is deferred, if possible, by angioplasty in the younger patient

The algorithms in Figures 2–4, 2–5, and 2–6 give therapeutic guidelines and cannot include all clinical situations.

Although bypass surgery is superior to drug therapy when severe proximal stenosis of the LAD artery is present, there is no evidence

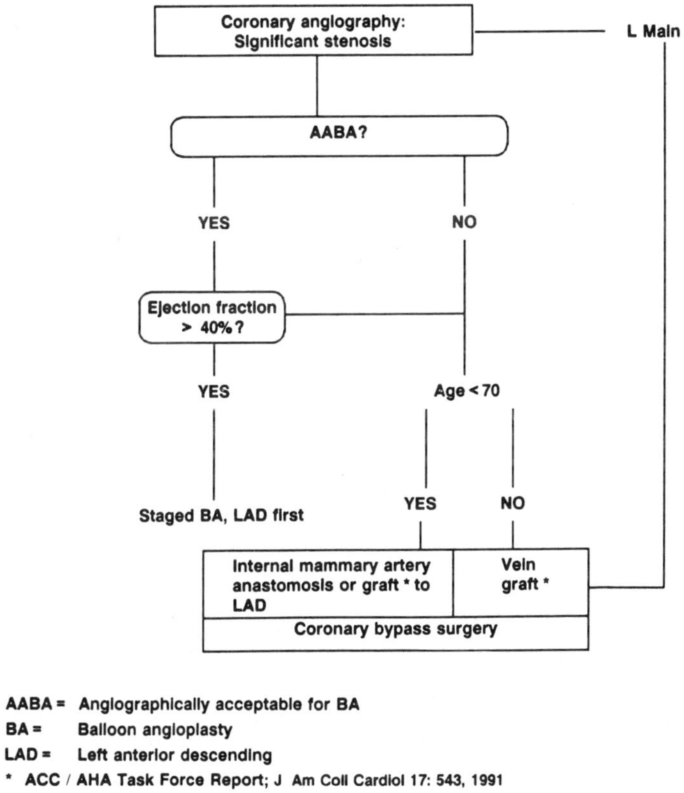

Figure 2–6. Decision-making in the management of severe angina (class 3, 4, or class 2 with a strongly positive exercise test).

Table 2–2
Results and Complications of Coronary Artery Bypass Surgery

OCCURRENCE	1 WEEK (%)	1 YEAR (%)	5 YEARS (%)	10 YEARS (%)	15 YEARS (%)
Survival	99	95	87	76	60**
Perioperative myocardial infarction (MI)	2–5				
MI fatal, nofatal			5	15	35
Reoperation for bleeding	1–4				
Occusion					
vein graft occlusion	6–10*	12–20*	20	40–50	60
vein graft to LAD				25–30	30–40**
vein graft to other vessels				30–50	60
internal mammary graft				10	
internal mammary anastomosis***				5**	
Symptomatic improvement	90	70			
Asymptomatic angina free	80		50		
Sudden cardiac death				5	10

* = Aspirin 1 hour postoperative = 1.6 and 5.8% (see Table 2–13)
** = ACC/AHA Task Force Report J Am Coll Cardiol, *17*:543, 1991
*** = Preferred technique
LAD = Left anterior descending

indicating that the procedure is superior to angioplasty in patients with good LV function (EF >50%) where the lesion is suitable for angioplasty. Therefore, young patients in this group with relatively good LV function, EF >40%, should be given a trial of angioplasty. Bypass is reserved for later use, utilizing left internal mammary artery anastomosis.

Patients suitable for medical management usually have the following characteristics

- Stable angina functional Class 1 to 2
- Good effort tolerance, negative or weakly positive treadmill exercise test, e.g., beyond 6 mins of the Bruce protocol. Patients who are unable to exercise because of intermittent claudication or arthritis cannot be graded as Class 1 and 2
- Good ventricular function, radionuclide EF, or estimate from echocardiogram >40%
- Absence of left main disease
- Presence of multi-vessel disease in the absence of severe proximal stenosis of the LAD (Fig. 2–5)
- Concomitant disease and contraindications to CABS
- Age >75 and not in good general health
- Lesions not ideal for intervention

Most patients with stable angina Class 1 and 2 are managed with sublingual nitroglycerin and a one-a-day β blocker. The rationale for a β-blocking drug as a first-choice oral agent is discussed shortly (Table 2–3).

Failure to achieve about a 75% symptomatic relief with an adequate dose of a β blocker (Table 2–4) might result in the addition of a second agent or the patient may learn to cope with mild angina that quickly disappears on cessation of a precipitating activity. Either a Ca antago-

Table 2–3
Beta Blocker: First-Line Oral Drug Treatment in Angina Pectoris

EFFECT ON	BETA BLOCKER	CALCIUM ANTAGONIST	ORAL NITRATE
Heart rate	↓	↑ ↓ —	↑
Diastolic filling of coronary arteries	↑	—	—
Blood pressure	↓ ↓	↓ ↓	—
Rate pressure product	↓	—*	—
Relief of angina	Yes	Yes	Variable
Blood flow (subendocardial ischemic area)†	↑	↓	Variable
First-line treatment for angina pectoris	Yes	No	No
Prevention of recurrent ventricular fibrillation	Proven	No	No
Prevention of cardiac death	Proven	No	No effect
Prevention of pain due to CAS	No	Yes	Variable
Prevention of death in patient with CAS	No	No	No

* RPP variable decrease on exercise, but not significant at rest or on maximal exercise
† Distal to organic obstruction
CAS = coronary artery spasm; ↑ = increase; ↓ = decrease; — = no change
From: Khan M. Gabriel: Beta-adrenoceptor blockers. *In* Cardiac Drug Therapy. 3rd Ed. London, W. B. Saunders, 1992.

nist or a nitrate is considered second choice (Fig. 2–4). If a β blocker is being used, then amlodipine or nifedipine extended release 30–90 mg qd is advisable. If a β blocker is contraindicated but verapamil is not, then verapamil should be used as the drug of first choice. The rationale for this approach is discussed under Ca antagonists and combination therapy. If a nitrate is selected as second line, a sustained release preparation is selected and given once daily or, at most, bid. Preparations and suggested timing of dosing of nitrates are shown in Table 2–5.

Table 2–4
Dosage of Beta Blockers for Angina

BETA BLOCKER	INITIAL DOSE* (mg daily)	MAINTENANCE (mg daily)
Atenolol (Tenormin)	25–50	50–100
Acebutolol (Sectral, Monitan)	100–400	400–1000
Metoprolol (Lopressor)	50–100	100–300
Toprol XL**	50–100	100–300
Nadolol** (Corgard)	40	40–160
Propranolol Inderal	80–120	80–240
Inderal LA**	80	120–240
Timolol (Blocadren)	10	10–30

* Elderly: halve initial dose
** Given once daily, all others preferably two divided doses to cover early morning catecholamine surge

Table 2–5
Oral and Transdermal Nitrate Preparations and Dosage

NITRATE	DOSAGE	
Isosorbide dinitrate (Isordil)	Initial Maintenance	15 mg at 700, 1200, 1700 hours 30 mg at 700, 1200, 1700 hours
Isosorbide dinitrate sustained release	Initial Maintenance	40 mg at 700 hours 40 mg at 700, 1400 hours
Isosorbide mononitrate (ISMO)	Initial Maintenance	10 mg at 700, 1400 hours 20 mg at 700, 1400 hours
Isosorbide mononitrate sustained release supplied as 20, 40, 50 or 60 mg	Initial Maintenance	20–30 mg at 700 hours 40–60 mg at 700 hours
Nitroglycerin (*oral* tabs) (glyceryltrinitrate oral tablets in UK)	Initial Maintenance	1.3 mg at 700, 1400 hours 2.6 mg at 700, 1400 hours
Nitroglycerin (*buccal* tablets)	Initial Maintenance	1 mg 1, 2, or 3 mg at 700, 1400 hours
Nitroglycerin (transdermal) (glyceryltrinitrate) Ointment (paste) 1 in. = approx. 16 mg	1–2 inches	700, 1400 hours
Phasic-release nitroglycerin patch: e.g., Transderm-nitro 0.4, 0.6 mg/hour	1 patch	700 Remove at 1900 hours

If symptoms remain bothersome, triple therapy with β blockers, Ca antagonists, and nitrates is warranted, but this action should prompt consideration for coronary angiography and interventional therapy.

BETA BLOCKERS

- Release of catecholamines plays a major role in the initiation and perpetuation of myocardial ischemia in patients with atheromatous coronary stenosis (Fig. 2–1). Beta blockers can inhibit the initiation of ischemia, interrupt the dynamic process, and provide rational and effective therapy as well as prolong life (Fig. 2–7)
- Beta blockers are competitive inhibitors of catecholamines (which they structurally resemble) at β-adrenergic receptors. Their action depends on the ratio of drug to catecholamine concentration at β adrenoceptor sites. Beta receptors are part of the adenyl cyclase system situated in the cell membrane. The ventricle contains β_1 and β_2 adrenergic receptors in the proportion 70:30. $Beta_2$ predominate in the lung. Adenylcyclase in the presence of the stimulatory form of the G protein converts adenosine triphosphate to cyclic adenosine monophosphate (cyclic AMP), the intracellular messenger of β stimulation

Beta blockade results in

- Decrease in HR. Cardiac work is reduced and the increased diastolic interval allows for improved diastolic coronary perfusion especially during exercise
- Decrease in velocity of cardiac contraction further reduces myocardial O_2 demand, which is particularly important during exertional activities
- Decrease in cardiac output results in a ↓ in systolic BP and causes a ↓ in the rate-pressure product and a ↓ in myocardial O_2 requirement

(Table 2–3). The salutary effects of β-adrenergic blockade are shown in Figure 2–7. These effects are not observed with other antianginal agents

- A ↓ in ejection velocity reduces hyperdynamic shearing forces imposed on the arterial wall; this might be important at the site of atheroma. Thus, it is possible that β blockers may ↓ the incidence of plaque rupture and thus protect from fatal or nonfatal MI. These agents ↓ the incidence of myocardial rupture
- Partial inhibition of exercise-related catecholamines that might initiate vasoconstriction in segments of coronary arteries where atheroma impairs the relaxing effect of the endothelium
- Increase in VF threshold and, thus, a ↓ in the incidence of VF, which may be responsible for the high mortality during the early hours of acute MI and also in VF occurring in other ischemic situations. Beta blockers are of proven value in the prevention of sudden death in the post-infarction patient
- A ↓ in early morning platelet aggregation and other salutary effects induced by a ↓ in catecholamine surges may eliminate the early morning peak of transient ischemic periods and ↓ the incidence of early morning mortality and sudden death from MI. Beta blockers have been shown to ↓ the incidence of sudden death in cardiac pa-

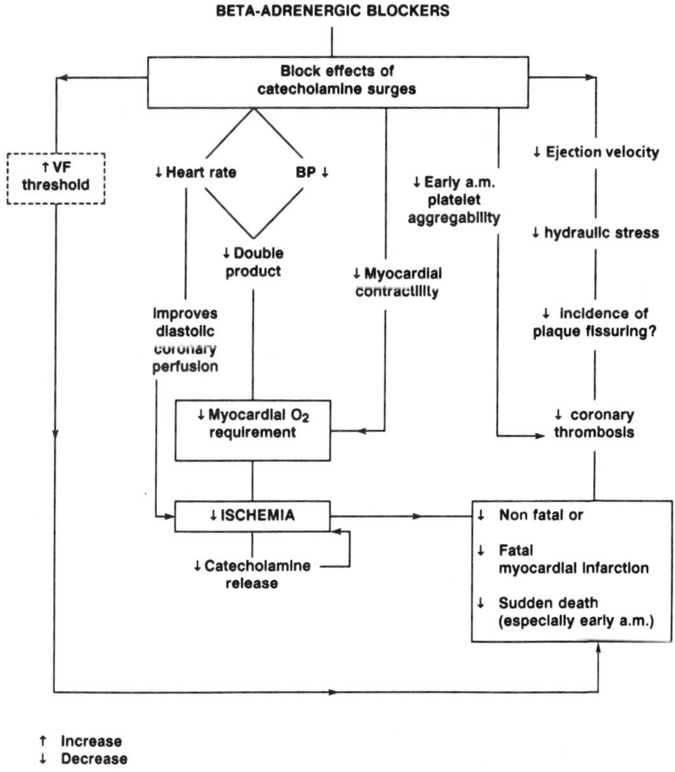

Figure 2–7. Salutary effects of beta-adrenergic blockade.

tients. This observation has not been documented for any other cardiac medication, including aspirin

- A ↓ in phase 4 diastolic depolarization is important in suppressing arrhythmias induced by catecholamines, which ↑ diastolic depolarization. This action is opposite to that of digoxin. Thus, β blockers are useful in the management of digoxin toxicity
- Decrease impulse traffic through the A-V node results in slowing of the ventricular response in AF or in the termination of PSVT
- Direct blood flow from the epicardial vessels to subendocardial ischemic areas. In contrast, dipyridamole, a vasodilator used in the management of angina in the early 1960s, is now used to dilate epicardial vessels and produce a "steal." Experimental evidence suggests that some Ca antagonists may also direct coronary blood flow from the subendocardium to dilated epicardial vessels. Nitrates appear to have an effect similar to Ca antagonists

The above-mentioned points have established β-blocking drugs as first-line oral agents in the management of stable angina and indicate the rationale for the algorithmic approach to drug therapy for stable angina given in Figure 2–4.

Dosages of available β blockers are given in Table 2–4. (For IV dosages see Table 2–7.)

Choice: Related to subtle differences

- Beta blockers with partial agonist activity, such as pindolol, should be avoided in patients with IHD since cardioprotection is not achieved. Acebutolol has only weak agonist activity and one study has shown a beneficial effect. Importantly, this agent does not adversely affect HDL-C as may occur with other β blockers (see Chap. 9)
- Do not use hepatic-metabolized β blockers, propranolol, or oxprenolol in smokers who won't quit, as the salutary effects of these agents are blunted by cigarette smoking (Chap. 1)
- Maximum protection appears to occur with proven agents: Timolol and metoprolol in smokers and in nonsmokers, propranolol in nonsmokers
- The subtle differences in β blockers may provide the solution for the apparent lack of protection of some β blockers. Lipophilic agents that achieve brain concentration may actuate more effective protection from the brain-heart interaction that appears to be involved in the genesis of sudden death in some subsets. This hypothesis must be tested in clinical trials, but predominantly hepatic-metabolized β blockers should not be given to smokers if all the benefits of β blockade are to be derived (see Chap. 1)

Cautions. Do not use in asthmatics, severe COPD or CHF (see Chap. 1 for adverse effects and Chap. 5 for use in CHF).

Atenolol (Tenormin) *Supplied:* tablets; 25, 50, 100 mg. *Dosage:* 25–50 mg for 1–4 weeks, then 50–100 mg once daily. Observations have confirmed that in some patients, a once daily dose of atenolol may not completely cover the 24-hour period and the patient may be at risk between 6 and 8 a.m. during the early morning period of catecholamine surge. Holter monitoring of patients has documented early morning ischemia in some patients administered atenolol once daily. Thus, it is advisable to give half the dose at 7 a.m. and half at bedtime. Elderly and nonwhite patients usually require a reduced dose to achieve β blockade. Reduce the dose and ↑ the dosing interval in renal failure.

Atenolol is a cardioselective agent. The pharmacologic properties of β blockers are given in Table 1–5.

Acebutolol (Monitan, Sectral) *Supplied:* 200, 400 mg. *Dosage:* 200 mg bid, to a max of 1,000 mg qd. Acebutolol is mildly cardioselective, possesses mild partial agonist activity, and causes no significant ↓ in HDL-C levels during longterm administration (see Chap. 9).

Nadolol (Corgard) *Supplied:* tablets; 40, 80, 120, 160 mg. *Dosage:* 40 mg once daily for 1–2 weeks, then maintenance 40–160 mg qd. Clinical practice has documented that the max dose of nadolol is much < that recommended by the manufacturer, and the above dosage is < that given in the package insert. The drug is nonselective and hydrophilic, has a prolonged action beyond 24 h, and covers the risk periods when given once daily. As with other β blockers, adverse effects occur beyond a certain dose range. The drug is eliminated by the kidney, and the dose must be decreased with renal dysfunction.

Metoprolol (Toprol XL, Lopressor, Betaloc) *Supplied:* tablets; 50, 100 mg (Toprol XL 50, 100, 200 mg; Betaloc-SA: 200 mg; Lopressor-SA: 200 mg). *Dosage:* Metoprolol 50–100 mg bid; max 300 mg qd. Metoprolol is a cardioselective β blocker, but this effect is maintained up to a dose of 200 mg qd. A metoprolol dose beyond this dosage or atenolol >50 mg qd can precipitate bronchospasm. However, when cardioselective drugs are given, bronchospasm is more easily reversed with albuterol (salbutamol) or other β agonists than when β_1 and β_2 nonselective β blockers are used. Toprol XL (metoprolol succinate) extended release tablets are effective when administered once daily, 100–300 mg qd.

Propranolol (Inderal; Angilol, Berkolol, UK) *Supplied:* tablets; 10, 40, 80, and 120 mg capsules; Inderal-LA (80, 120, 160 mg). *Dosage:* 20–40 mg tid for several weeks, ↑ if needed to 160–240 mg qd or Inderal-LA, 120–240 mg once daily. The drug is noncardioselective, lipophilic, and hepatic-metabolized.

Timolol (Blocadren; Betim, UK) *Supplied:* tablets; 5, 10 mg. Timolol is a noncardioselective β_1, β_2 adrenergic blocking agent that is partially lipophilic and hydrophilic. Thus, the drug causes fewer CNS side effects than metoprolol or propranolol. If vivid dreams occur with metoprolol or propranolol, a switch to timolol or nadolol is advisable. Because the drug is only partially metabolized in the liver, it is effective in smokers and nonsmokers. (See Beta Blocker, Subtle Differences, Chap. 1.). *Dosage:* 5 mg bid for 1–2 weeks, then 10–15 mg bid. This dose is much smaller than the max dose recommended by the manufacturer.

NITRATES

The action of nitrates is given in Figure 2–8.

The mononitrates are unaffected by the liver, whereas isosorbide dinitrate undergoes extensive hepatic metabolism. Mononitrates, on entering the walls of veins and arteries, combine with sulfhydryl groups with the formation of nitric oxide, which activates guanylate cyclase to produce cyclic guanosine monophosphate, which in turn brings about relaxation of vascular smooth muscle at the doses commonly used, with maximal dilation of veins and minimal dilation of arteries. The profound venous dilation causes ↓ in preload and, at high nitrate dosage, a modest ↓ in afterload occurs. Sulfhydryl groups become depleted by continued exposure to nitrates and tolerance develops with little or no resulting venous dilation. Thus, 24-hour therapy with nitrates is of no value to the patient. A minimum daily 10-hour nitrate-free interval is necessary for the intracellular regeneration of sulfhydryl groups and to maintain the effectiveness of the nitrate preparation.

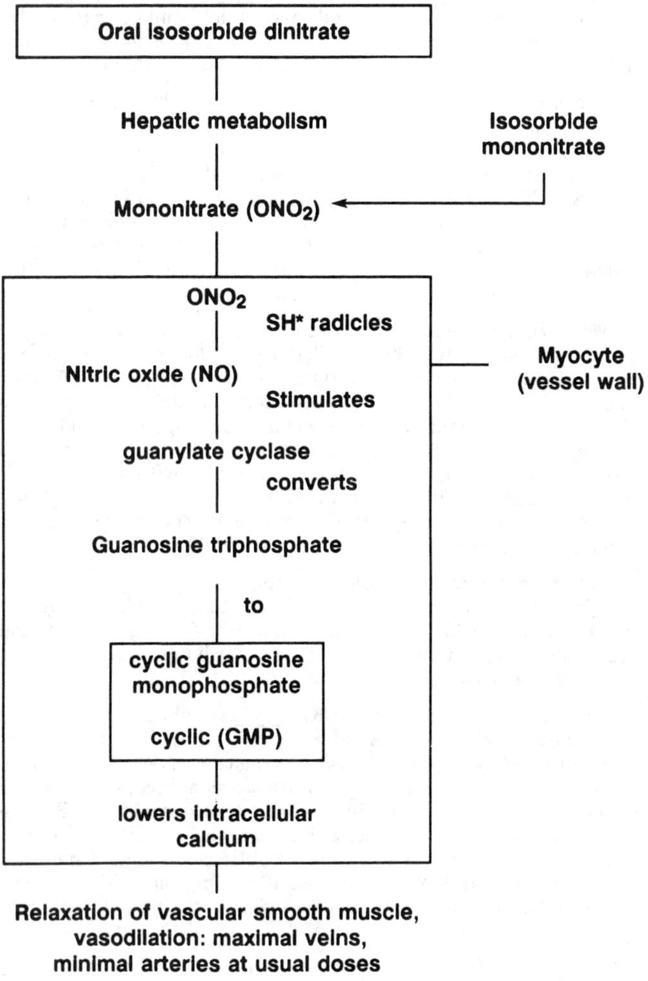

*SH = Sulfhydryl radicles required for formation of NO, oxidized by excess exposure to nitrates become depleted, leading to nitrate tolerance

Figure 2–8. Nitrates' mechanism of action.

Indications: Second-choice management of Class 2 and 3 stable angina; angina with concomitant LV dysfunction (shortness of breath and effort tolerance may be improved by nitrate therapy); angina with concomitant mild or moderate hypertension; combination therapy with β blockers or if β blockers are contraindicated combined with verapamil or diltiazem; pre- and postoperative management of the cardiac patient undergoing surgery; intraoperative hypertension.

Contraindications: HCM, constrictive pericarditis, or cardiac tamponade; hypovolemia; right ventricular infarction; severe uncontrolled glaucoma with very high nitrate dosing, especially IV nitrates.

Adverse Effects: Syncope, especially in the elderly, and an increased incidence with added ACE inhibitors, diuretics, alcohol, or alpha blockers. Tachycardia, mild palpitations, dizziness, and flushing commonly occur. Headaches are often bothersome; >25% of patients are intolerant and discontinue the drug. Indigestion and halitosis may occur. High-dose nitrates may cause a ↓ in arterial O_2 tension and are relatively contraindicated in severe COPD and hypoxemic situations. Methemoglobinemia has been noted with prolonged high dosage and withdrawal symptoms have been observed with high-dose, longterm use.

Interactions: Heparin resistance with high nitrate dosage. ACE inhibitors, alpha blockers, and diuretics also ↓ preload tachycardia may be increased when nitrates are used with dihydropyridine Ca antagonists.

Nitroglycerin. *Supplied:* sublingual tablets; 0.15, 0.3, and 0.6 mg (in the UK, glyceryl trinitrate: 300, 500, 600 μmg). spray; nitrolingual spray, 0.4 mg/metered dose, 200 doses/vial. *Dosage:* 0.3 mg is given if the systolic BP is <130 mm Hg, 0.6 mg if >130 mm Hg systolic. The patient should be instructed on how and when to use nitroglycerin

- Sit and put 1 tablet under the tongue or use the sublingual spray. Avoid taking the drug while standing except when accustomed to such usage. Nitroglycerin is less effective when used with the patient lying, since less pooling occurs in the limbs and the drug is thus less effective in relieving pain
- Take a nitroglycerin tablet before activities that are known to precipitate angina
- Take a second tablet if pain is not relieved in 2 mins. After taking the second nitroglycerin tablet, chew and swallow a junior aspirin (80 mg) or a regular 325 mg aspirin tablet. Aspirin is used here for its effect in preventing coronary thrombosis
- Go to the nearest emergency room if pain persists beyond 10 mins, using a third nitroglycerin during transport if marked weakness or faintlike feeling is not present
- Take nitroglycerin for acute shortness of breath but not if the symptoms are dizziness or palpitations in the absence of pain
- Keep nitroglycerin tablets in dark, light-protected bottles. If exposed to light, they may only last a few months
- Use 2 bottles, 1 for stock supply with the cotton wool within a well-stoppered bottle, kept in the refrigerator. This will last 1–2 years. The second bottle containing no cotton wool should contain a few month's supply and be refilled when needed

Dosage: Dosage of other nitrates is given in Table 2–5.

CALCIUM ANTAGONISTS

- Verapamil is the most potent antianginal Ca antagonist but is not the safest agent for general use. The pharmacologic and clinical effects of Ca antagonists are given in Table 1–7. Verapamil is more effective than diltiazem because of a more prominent negative inotropic effect; in addition, verapamil causes a greater ↓ in systemic vascular resistance. If β blockers are contraindicated, verapamil is a reasonable choice, provided that there are no contraindications to the use of this agent

- Dihydropyridines have no EP and minimal negative inotropic effects. The rapid-acting nifedipine capsule may cause a ↑ in HR and has been reported to ↑ anginal episodes. Undoubtedly, early studies were done using nifedipine capsules, which have a rapid onset of action and cause mild provocation of angina in some patients with stable angina. However, the administration of extended release formulations, e.g., Procardia XL (Adalat XL in Canada) or amlodipine (Norvasc) virtually abolishes this adverse effect and allows the drug to be used freely in all patients with stable angina who are unable to take a β-blocking drug. Dihydropyridines are a rational choice for use in conjunction with β blockers (see Table 2–7). Diltiazem and dihydropyridines have about equal antianginal effects

Calcium Antagonist Beta Blocker Combination. Verapamil should not be combined with a β blocker since there is a high incidence of bradyarrhythmias, including life-threatening sinus arrest and asystole; CHF may be precipitated. Diltiazem combined with a β blocker may cause sinus arrest or asystole. Although the occurrence is rare, caution is necessary and patients should be properly selected prior to prescribing this combination. Sinus bradycardia is not uncommon. Dihydropyridines can be safely combined with β blockers since they have no effect on the sinus or A-V nodes. Care is needed when dihydropyridines or diltiazem is added to β blockers in patients with LV dysfunction, since CHF can be precipitated.

Indications. Consider Ca antagonists as second line in the management of stable angina, Class 2 and 3, advisable only when β blockers are contraindicated or produce bothersome effects

Advantages. More effective than nitrates in the management of angina and do not carry the risk posed by a 10-hour drug-free interval. One-a-day preparation exists. These agents do not ↓ preload and are useful in angina patients with HCM, in which nitrates are relatively contraindicated. Angiographic studies, including the International Nifedipine Trial on Antiatherosclerotic Therapy (INTACT), have demonstrated that Ca antagonists appear to prevent progression of early atheromatous lesions and may cause some regression. Although the observed effect is quite modest, it could occasionally signify longterm gains for a wide range of patients with CHD. Ongoing studies will clarify this issue.

Disadvantages. Sinus node dysfunction, A-V block with verapamil or diltiazem. High incidence of constipation with verapamil. Ca antagonists do not significantly ↓ the incidence of fatal MI. Verapamil and diltiazem ↑ the risk of CHF in patients with LV dysfunction and should be avoided in this subset when the EF is <40%. Nifedipine may be given a trial in patients without overt CHF and EF >35% if a β blocker is contraindicated. Ca antagonists are commonly and inappropriately used in this large group of cardiac patients in whom β blockers, when used with due caution, are often effective, well tolerated, and likely to have salutary effects on prognosis. The Ca antagonists may, however, have to be used judiciously when β-blocking agents are ineffective or contraindicated. Dosages of Ca antagonists and the adverse effects of extended release Ca antagonists are shown in Tables 2–6 and 2–7. *Interactions:* Digoxin level is increased with verapamil, diltiazem, and nicardipine; Verapamil and diltiazem interact with β blockers, quinidine, disopyramide, amiodarone (Table 2–8).

Contraindications. Aortic stenosis; sick sinus syndrome and A-V block with verapamil and diltiazem; CHF or suspected LV dysfunction; MI with CHF (EF <40% for verapamil and diltiazem; EF <35% for nifedi-

Table 2–6
Dosages of Calcium Antagonists for Angina

PREPARATION	INITIAL	DOSAGE MAINTENANCE (daily mg)	MAXIMUM (daily mg)
Amlodipine (Norvasc)	5 mg/d	5–10	10
Nifedipine Extended Release Procardia XL; Adalat XL (C) 30, 60, 90 mg tabs	30 mg *once daily*	60–90	90
Adalat Retard 20 mg (UK)	20 mg BID	40–80	80
Diltiazem 60, 120 mg tabs (30, 60, C)	60 mg TID	180–240	360
Cardiazem 60, 90, 120 mg	60 mg TID	180–240	360
Cardiazem SR (C) 60, 90, 120 mg capsules Tildiem (UK) 60 mg Adizem SR (UK) 120 mg	60–90 mg BID	180–240	360
Verapamil 80, 120 mg tablets	80 mg TID	240–360	360

BID = twice daily
TID = three times daily d = daily
C = Canada

Table 2–7
IV Beta Blockers Dosage

DRUG	DOSAGE
Atenolol	2.5 mg rate 1 mg/min repeated if necessary at 5-minute intervals to a maximum of 10 mg
Atenolol (IV infusion)	150 μg/kg over 20 minutes repeated every 12 hours if required
Esmolol (infusion)	3–6 mg over 1 minute then 1 to 5 mg/minute, see text
Metoprolol	5 mg rate 1 mg/min repeated if necessary at 5-minute intervals to a maximum of 10–15 mg. Re-evaluate patient and ECG prior to each dose
Propranolol	1 mg rate of 0.5 mg/min repeated, if necessary, at 5-minute intervals to a maximum of 5–10 mg or 0.025–0.05 mg/kg over 15–30 minutes.

Caution: The systolic blood pressure should not be allowed to fall less than 100 mm Hg or a 10–15 mm fall from baseline, or up to 25 mm Hg in hypertensives.

Table 2–8
Nitroglycerin Infusion Pump Chart*

DOSE (μg/min)	INFUSION RATE (ml/h)
5	0.75
10	1.5
15	2.3
20	3
25	3.8
30	4.5
40	6
50	7.5
60	9
80	12
100	15
120	18
140	21
160	24
180	27
200	30
220	33
240	36
260	39
280	42
300	45
320	48
340	51
360	54
380	57
400	60

Commence dosing 5 to 10 μg/minute, increase by 5 μg/minute every 5 minutes until relief of chest pain. Decrease the rate if systolic blood pressure is <100 mm Hg or falls >20 mm Hg below the baseline systolic or diastolic blood pressure <65 mm Hg.

* 100 mg nitroglycerin in 250 ml 5% dextrose/water = 400 μg/ml

pine); presence of marked β blockade (avoid the use of verapamil or diltiazem); unstable angina (do not use nifedipine if a β blocker cannot be used).

Amlodipine (Norvasc) _Supplied:_ tablets; 5, 10 mg. _Dosage:_ Commence with 5 mg. Increase if needed over a 2- to 14-day period to 10 mg. Most patients will require 10 mg for anginal control. A max of 5 mg is suggested for the elderly or patients with hepatic impairment. No adjustment in initial dosing is required in patients with renal dysfunction. Of the available Ca antagonists, this agent has the least negative inotropic effects and can be used in patients with borderline LV dysfunction (EF 30–40%)

- Gradual rate of association and dissociation with receptor sites produces a gradual onset of action
- May bind to both dihydropyridine and nondihydropyridine sites

Once-daily dosing results in steady plasma levels for a full 24 h with negligible peak-to-trough effects and thus allows for early am ischemia protection.

- No significant effect on HR, cardiac conduction or digoxin levels
- Uncommon dose-related adverse effects (10 mg dose) include edema (10%), dizziness (3.4%), flushing (2.6%), palpitations (4.5%)

Nifedipine; Nifedipine Extended Release (Procardia XL; Adalat XL 30, 60, 90 mg in Canada; Adalat Retard 10, 20 in the UK). *Supplied:* See Table 2–6. *Dosage:* Nifedipine extended release, 30–60 mg qd, usual maintenance 60 mg qd, ↑ to 90 mg if required. As outlined in Chapter 1, an extended release preparation is preferred because the capsule formulation causes a quick release and a higher incidence of adverse effects. Pharmacokinetics: See Chapter 1.

Diltiazem. *Supplied:* tablets: Cardizem 60, 90, 120 mg (30 mg in Canada); Cardizem SR capsules 60, 90, 120 mg, Canada; Adizem SR 120 mg, Tildiem, UK; Anginyl, Dilzem, Herbesser, Tilazem, in other countries). *Dosage:* 60 mg tid or qid, ↑ slowly to 90 mg tid. The effective dose range is 240–360 mg qd. In the elderly or patients with renal dysfunction, give 30–60 mg bid. *Caution:* Caution is required to carefully select patients prior to giving a combination of diltiazem and a β blocker. The SR preparation appears to cause a higher incidence of adverse effects than the tablet formulation. Avoid in patients with LV dysfunction, EF <40%. Reduce dose in hepatic or renal dysfunction.

Verapamil. *Supplied:* tablets; 80, 120 mg (Cordilox 40, 80, 160 mg; Berkatens 40, 120, 160 mg available in the UK). *Dosage:* Initial, 80 mg bid; maintenance 80–120 mg tid. A higher dose is not advisable in angina. Reduce dose with hepatic dysfunction and renal failure. *Cautions.* Avoid in acute MI if bradycardia, A-V block, hypotension, LV failure, or LV dysfunction with an EF <40% is present. Not advisable in patients taking β blockers, except under close supervision in properly selected patients (see Contraindications of Calcium Antagonists and Chap. 1 for further details on individual Ca antagonists).

UNSTABLE ANGINA

Pathophysiology

In the majority of cases of unstable angina, atheromatous plaques are eccentric with irregular borders and a narrow neck on angiography. A ruptured or fissured plaque with overlying platelet thrombus is a common finding confirmed by several investigators during angioscopy. In addition, silent ischemia is frequently observed in patients with unstable angina, and prognosis is worse in this subset. See Classification Table 2–1.

Therapy

Figure 2–9 gives suggested steps in treating unstable angina

- Aspirin, 325 mg, chewed or swallowed for a rapid effect, then 160–325 mg coated aspirin is given qd

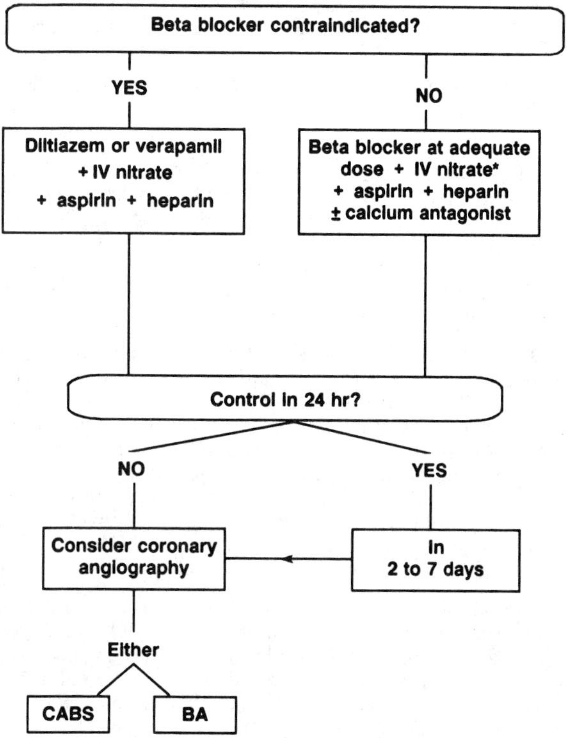

* = Oral if IV not available
CABS = Coronary artery bypass surgery
BA = Balloon angioplasty

Figure 2–9. Suggested steps in therapy for unstable angina.

- Heparin IV is commenced, 5,000 U and then continuous infusion (see later discussion and Chap. 11)
- Admission to a CCU: Monitor cardiac rhythm for 24–48 h, total CK and CK-MB q 4–6 h for 24 h, ECG q 6 h for 24–48 h to rule out acute MI
- Bedrest with bedside commode, fasting 8 h, allowed fluids only
- BP taken q 15–30 mins for a few hours, then q 1–2 h or as needed for 24–48 h and more often if IV nitroglycerin is used
- The patient is encouraged to report any recurrence of pain, however mild
- 5% dextrose in water to maintain IV line

- O_2 by nasal prongs 2–4 L/min
- Patients with Class A unstable angina: Diagnose and treat conditions that cause increases in myocardial O_2 demands (Table 2–1)
- Thrombolytic therapy does not improve morbidity or mortality and is not used routinely

Beta blockers. If not contraindicated, give propranolol 20 mg q 4 h or metoprolol 50 mg q 8 h, then metoprolol 100 mg q 12 h or equivalent dose of another β blocker. Hold dose if systolic BP is <100 mm Hg or if pulse is <50/min. If pain is present and unrelieved by nitroglycerin, the first dose of a β-blocking drug can be given IV. The IV dosage of β blockers is given in Table 2–7 and Table 3–4.

No cardioactive agent has been shown to ↓ cardiac mortality in unstable angina. This is not surprising since the dynamic obstruction cannot be ameliorated by a single agent. None the less, the role of a β-blocking agent and IV nitrate is most important and with concomitant aspirin and/or heparin often causes salutary effects for several weeks, during which time patients are selected for coronary angiography and interventional therapy.

Nitroglycerin. IV dosage is given in Table 2–8. Commence with 5–10 μmg/min, ↑ 5–10 μmg/min q 5 or 10 mins if needed to 100–200 μmg/min. Titrate to eliminate all episodes of chest pain and do not lower the systolic BP below 100 mm Hg. Dose to ↓ arterial pressure 10–15 mm Hg and ≤20 mm Hg in a hypertensive patient or ↓ mean arterial pressure by 10%. Although tolerance to IV nitroglycerin has been shown to occur after 24–48 h of infusion, concern should not be given to the development of tolerance in patients with unstable angina; the IV nitroglycerin dose is titrated upward. This administration is often successful in controlling pain, especially when time is allowed: 24–48 h to attain adequate therapeutic dosage of β blockers and/or Ca antagonists.

Calcium Antagonists. If a β blocker is used, diltiazem or nifedipine extended release are added. If a β-blocking drug is contraindicated, give diltiazem 30 mg q 6 h for 24 h, then 60 mg q 6 h, increasing if needed to 90 mg q 6 h. Caution is needed when the triple combination is used, since all 3 drugs (β blockers, nitrates, and Ca antagonists) can cause excessive ↓ in BP, which can worsen ischemia. Ca antagonists do not ↓ mortality in patients with unstable angina. Nifedipine or other dihydropyridines should not be used alone or in combination with nitrates in patients with unstable angina since mortality might be increased. Verapamil or diltiazem should not be given if sinus node disease, bradycardia, A-V block, CHF, or LV dysfunction is present.

Aspirin. Causes a 50% ↓ in mortality and reinfarction in patients with unstable angina. No trial is available to show its effectiveness with stable angina, although the Physicians' Study indicates a favorable trend, and many patients must be treated to observe a beneficial effect. However, patients with angina are at risk, and an 80-mg tablet or 160- to 325-mg enteric coated tablet qd or every second day is advisable if there are no contraindications. With unstable angina, the emergency use of aspirin 325 mg followed by shortterm heparin limited to 48 h, followed by enteric coated aspirin 160–325 mg qd is advisable.

Heparin IV is as effective as aspirin in decreasing mortality and reinfarction. Since aspirin, as opposed to heparin, carries a slightly greater risk of bleeding during bypass surgery, which may require transfusion, some units routinely use heparin in place of aspirin.

PRINZMETAL'S (VARIANT) ANGINA

CAS is a rare cause of angina in which spasm of the coronary artery occurs often without identifiable stimuli. However, in some patients, exposure to cold, smoking, emotional stress, aspirin ingestion, or cocaine usage may trigger coronary spasm. Discontinuation of nitrates or Ca antagonists may cause a worsening of spasm. Use of a β blocker in the absence of vasodilator drugs may allow alpha activity with resulting vasoconstriction to predominate. However, although β blockers may ↑ spasm, the risk of serious complications is likely to be small and is certainly not high enough to justify withholding this form of therapy from the great majority of patients with angina or even from those whose symptom pattern includes 1 or 2 atypical features, in case spasm is present.

All patients with variant angina should be considered for coronary angiography since a significant number of them have underlying obstructive atheromatous coronary disease with spasm at the site of the lesion.

The clinical hallmarks of Prinzmetal's angina are

- Pain, usually at rest, often during sleep, (between 3 a.m. and 7 a.m.) and described as chronic angina at rest as distinct from unstable angina occurring at rest
- ECG shows ST segment elevation during pain
- Worsening of angina during β-blocker use
- Variable threshold angina

Control is usually achieved with

- Nitroglycerin tablets sublingually
- Cessation of smoking
- Aspirin may precipitate spasm and should be avoided if spasm is proven to be the cause of symptoms
- For chronic management, nitrates at high dosage allowing a 10-hour nitrate-free interval to prevent tolerance; the full 24-hour period at risk may not be covered. Ca antagonists are preferred. Nifedipine, verapamil, or diltiazem are equally effective. For dosage, see Table 2–6. Occasionally, it is necessary to combine both a Ca antagonist and a nitrate
- If the patient is admitted to the hospital, commence IV nitroglycerin 5–20 μmg/min, see Table 2–8 (Nitroglycerin Infusion Pump Chart)
- IV heparin to prevent coronary thrombosis

SILENT ISCHEMIA

- Symptomless or painless myocardial ischemia is common in patients with CHD. More patients die without warning or with only minutes of warning pain than from stable or unstable angina
- The incidence of silent ischemia is high in patients with unstable angina. Holter monitoring following noncardiac surgery in patients with stable angina and in post-MI patients has documented a high incidence of silent ischemia within the second to fourth day following surgery
- Patients with evidence of silent ischemia should be maintained on a β blocker and aspirin and evaluated with exercise stress testing or noninvasive imaging technique such as thallium scintigraphy. Those

with strongly positive exercise tests should be submitted to coronary angiography for consideration of an appropriate revascularization procedure

- Drug treatment of patients with a diagnosis of silent ischemia should commence with enteric coated aspirin, 160–325 mg qd; β blockers are advisable to protect from death and infarction, although this therapy has not been proven in clinical trials in patients with silent ischemia. Nitrates and Ca antagonists do not offer this protection and β blockers must remain the mainstay of therapy

INTERVENTIONAL THERAPY FOR ANGINA

Interventional therapy in the form of coronary angioplasty or CABS should be strongly considered in virtually all patients with unstable angina and in those with bothersome angina and/or functional Class 2 and 3 stable angina as illustrated in the decision-making algorithms (Figs. 2–4, 2–5, and 2–6). In several categories of patients, interventional therapy has advantages over medical therapy in amelioration of angina, a return to a normal lifestyle, and prolongation of life.

Balloon Coronary Angioplasty

- Coronary angioplasty and CABS each have a definite role. It is advisable, however, to delay surgery for as long as possible in patients < age 65 because >10% of patients post bypass surgery require reoperation in 5 years and >50% of bypass grafts occlude after the tenth year. Moreover, longterm survival and symptomatic benefit following reoperation are far less favorable with a mortality rate >4%, as opposed to <1% with primary surgery
- Angioplasty can be successfully carried out only when acceptable angiographic lesions are documented (Table 2–9). More difficult lesions may be considered for dilation, but only if deemed necessary and carried out by a highly experienced team. Since many patients have lesions that are not suitable for angioplasty, bypass surgery is required for relief of symptoms and prolongation of life in some subsets. Coro-

Table 2–9
Angiographically Acceptable Coronary Balloon Angioplasty Lesions

Proximal 70–95% stenosis*
Not totally occluded
Concentric
Discrete <10 mm length
Readily accessible
Nonostial
Location in nonangulated segment <45 degrees
Nontortuous
No major branch involvement
Absence of thrombus
Little or no calcification

* >60%

Table 2–10
Complications and Outcome of Coronary Balloon Angioplasty

Death	<1%
Acute myocardial infarction	<2%
Emergency bypass surgery	<2%
Restensosis at 6 months	30%
Annual mortality rate	1%
Rate of nonfatal myocardial infarction	2%
5-year follow-up	
Symptomatic improvement	60%
No fatal or nonfatal myocardial infarction or coronary artery bypass surgery	80%

nary angioplasty, when successful, and bypass surgery in similar symptomatic patients with severe proximal single vessel disease appear to give equally excellent 10-year results: Mortality, 0.6% per year; MI rate <1%. However, patients with single vessel disease with 50–60% vessel diameter narrowing have a good outcome with medical therapy, mortality <1% per year. In this subset, angioplasty with its predisposition for restenosis is not advisable unless angina is not controlled with intensive medical therapy: Intolerance to drugs, a strongly positive exercise test, or if thallium scintigraphy reveals a large area of ischemic myocardium

- The goal of angioplasty is pain relief. In complicated cases with multivessel disease or difficult lesions, the decision is made on an individual basis. As a general rule, patients do not undergo coronary angioplasty unless they are potential candidates for surgery, since bypass surgery will be required in about 3–5%. The indications and contraindications listed are in keeping with the AHA guidelines; complications are given in Table 2–10

Indications. Patients with stable angina Class 2 and 3, Canadian Cardiovascular Society classification with good LV function, EF >40%, and acceptable angiographic lesions with symptoms. Inadequately controlled by intensive medical therapy or in patients who have bothersome adverse effects of medications. Proximal single vessel disease with a 70–95% stenosis. Proximal single vessel disease with >70% vessel diameter narrowing with a documented large area of viable myocardium involved, dominant artery, moderate or strongly positive exercise test, and symptoms uncontrolled with medical therapy. Patients with Class 1 angina with documented myocardial ischemia, a strongly positive exercise test, a large area of myocardium at risk, and documented 75–95% proximal single vessel disease should be considered for angioplasty.

Controversial indications include: Double vessel disease with angina Class 1, 2, 3 in control with medical therapy, acceptable angiographic lesions, not high-grade proximal LAD obstruction with stenosis of another artery especially in patients < age 60 with EF >40%; young patients with unstable angina with suitable angiographic lesions and EF >40%.

Contraindications include

- Bypass surgical team not available
- Left main >50% stenosis not protected by a patent bypass graft to the LAD or left circumflex
- Triple vessel disease in symptomatic patients with strongly positive stress test, large area of variable myocardium at risk, or EF <40%

- Double vessel disease with high grade lesion proximal LAD with obstruction of another artery in association with a strongly positive stress test with EF <40%
- Calcified lesion
- Presence of thrombus
- Lesion with 50–60% vessel narrowing, thallium scintigraphy indicates small area of myocardium involved
- Low expected success rate in view of angiographic features of the lesion: Eccentric, >2 cm long, excessive tortuosity of proximal segment, extremely angulated or sharp bend, total occlusion
- Angiographic features suggest <80% chance of successful angioplasty, with a probable high restenosis rate and a moderate risk of occlusion: Length 10–20 mm, eccentric, angulated segment >45°, moderate calcification or ostial location, total occluded artery marked tortuosity
- Angiographic features suggest <60% chance of successful dilation and a very high risk of acute closure: A diffuse lesion >20 mm in length, excessive tortuosity of the proximal segment, angulation >90°, complete occlusion

Restenosis. Success in angiographically acceptable lesions indicates a >20% ↑ in luminal diameter or a <50% residual stenosis. Approximately 90% of patients with proximal single vessel stenosis that is angiographically acceptable for dilation achieve successful angioplastic dilation, although nearly 25% require a second dilation, which is often successful.

Restenosis 3–6 months post coronary angioplasty occurs in approximately 30% of patients (Table 2–10). Fortunately, the second dilation is often successful. Prevention of restenosis presents a major challenge. The process is not significantly prevented by aspirin, dipyridamole, ticlopidine, or omega 3 fatty acids and several test medications.

Coronary Artery Bypass Surgery

The results and complications of CABS are given in Table 2–2. Overall mortality of CABS is about 1–2%, with 96% survival at 1 month and 95%, 87%, 76%, and 60% at 1, 5, 10, and 15 years, respectively.

Approximately 50% of saphenous vein grafts occlude by 10 years postoperative. This incidence is highest in patients with hypertension, hyperlipidemia, diabetes, and in persistent smokers. Some studies indicate 40% occlusion at 10 years and approximately 25–40% for LAD vein grafts. Use of the internal mammary artery as a graft results in <15% occlusion at 10 years.

The most important advance in ↓ of graft occlusion has resulted from the use of the left internal mammary artery. The artery is left attached to its origin from the left subclavian artery, mobilized, and anastomosed to the LAD artery. The 10-year occlusion rate is only 5% (Table 2–2).

CABS protects from sudden death, with only a 5 and 10% incidence at 10 and 15 years, an important indicator of the role of ischemia in promoting this tragic outcome.

Indications

- For relief of angina uncontrolled by intensive medical therapy, especially if symptoms intensely hinder the patient's lifestyle
- Intolerance to drugs in severely symptomatic patients
- Patients with significant obstructive lesions considered angiographically unacceptable for balloon angioplasty

To relieve symptoms and prolong life in

- Left main coronary stenosis with ≥50% ↓ in luminal diameter
- Proximal LAD ≥75% plus second vessel with >50% overall diameter ↓
- Strongly positive exercise test, large area of myocardium involved in the ischemic process
- EF <40% but >20% with 2 or 3 vessel disease
- Three vessel disease with EF <40% but higher than 20%. The internal mammary artery anastomosis to the LAD gives results superior to vein grafts and should be done in patients < age 65. Patients aged 70 and older should benefit sufficiently from a vein graft to the LAD artery if angioplasty is not feasible

CASE STUDY: DECISION MAKING IN MANAGING ANGINA

Case 1: A 46-year-old male with mild angina (Class 1 to 2), positive exercise test, 80–90% proximal stenosis of the LAD artery. Choice of therapy: Angioplasty preferred to surgery because of young age, and acceptable angiographic single vessel lesion (Fig. 2–5). If restenosis in 6 months, repeat angioplasty; if recurrent angina, proceed to CABS with left internal mammary artery to the LAD, advisable in younger patients.

Case 2: A 52-year-old female with angina Class 2, positive exercise test, 90% proximal LAD, 80% proximal right coronary artery dominant, EF >40%, anterior wall hypokinesia. Choice of therapy: No clear answers concerning angioplasty versus surgery. If staged angioplasty chosen because of young age, acceptable angiographic lesion, and EF >40%, proceed with dilation of LAD first (Fig. 2–5). CABS with internal mammary artery to LAD can be done later, if needed, or if angioplasty results in occlusion.

If EF is <35%, choose CABS with internal mammary artery to the LAD. Treat male and female the same.

Case 3: A similar scenario to Case 2 but the patient is older than 65 or EF is <40%, a vein graft should be used (Figs. 2–5 and 2–6).

Case 4: A 72-year-old female with a 90% proximal LAD, 80% proximal right, 70% circumflex, Class 2 or 3 angina, positive stress test, EF between 30 and 40%. Choice of therapy: CABS using vein graft (Fig. 2–6).

Case 5: An 80-year-old patient in good health, an active golfer, with Class 3 angina that has been poorly controlled with intensive medical therapy. The EF is >40%; a proximal LAD artery 90% occluded. Choice of therapy: If the lesion is angiographically acceptable, angioplasty is advisable.

Suggested Reading

Khan, M Gabriel: Angina. *In* Cardiac and Pulmonary Management. Philadelphia, Lea & Febiger, 1993.

Rutherford JD, Braunwald E: Chronic ischemic heart disease. *In* Heart Disease. 4th ed. Philadelphia, W. B. Saunders, 1992.

Acute Myocardial Infarction

3

M. Gabriel Khan and Eric J. Topol

PATHOPHYSIOLOGIC IMPLICATIONS

- An acute MI is nearly always caused by occlusion of a coronary artery by thrombus overlying a fissured or ruptured atheromatous plaque. The ruptured plaque, by direct release of tissue factor and exposure of the subintima, is highly thrombogenic. Exposed collagen provokes platelet aggregation. Coronary angiography performed during the early hours of infarction has confirmed the presence of total occlusion of the infarct-related artery in over 90% of patients. It is not surprising that aspirin, through inhibition of platelet aggregation, reduces the incidence of coronary thrombosis and is especially useful in prevention of the progression of unstable angina to thrombosis and MI. Aspirin is particularly useful when given at the onset of chest pain produced by infarction. Aspirin, however, does not block all pathways that relate to platelet aggregation. In addition, aspirin does not ↓ the incidence of sudden death in patients with acute MI
- The increased morning incidence of acute MI documented in several studies of the diurnal variation of infarction is related to the early morning catecholamine surges, which induce platelet aggregation, and a ↑ in BP and hydraulic stress, which may lead to plaque rupture (See Fig. 2–7). Beta-adrenergic blockers have been shown to ↓ the early morning peak incidence of acute infarction and sudden death
- Unfortunately, when an atheromatous plaque ruptures, the thrombogenic effect of plaque contents cannot be completely nullified by the inhibition of all aspects of platelet aggregation, and chemical agents that can arrest the effects of these thrombogenic substances deserve intensive study. Agents such as hirudin, hirulog, and agatroban, direct antagonists of thrombin, have been shown to be superior to heparin in preventing coronary thrombosis in experimental models. Preliminary studies in patients suggest that direct thrombin inhibitors administered with aspirin is effective in the prevention of coronary thrombosis and requires testing in clinical trials. These studies may pave the way to further research that may uncover newer types of antithrombotic agents, more specific and superior to the coumarins, in preventing coronary thrombosis. The combination of a thrombin inhibitor, therefore, with aspirin may cause a significant ↑ in survival of patients with CHD, and large-scale clinical trials are in progress
- Coronary artery spasm appears to play a lesser role in the pathogenesis of coronary occlusion leading to infarction. Evidence of coronary vasoconstriction was found when angioscopy was performed shortly after infarction, and intermittent occlusion, presumably on a vasomotor basis, has been apparent in some cases. Vasoconstriction appears

to be a secondary factor, however, and since sudden plaque rupture is now proven to be the initiating event causing coronary thrombosis, the mechanisms underlying plaque rupture and its prevention deserve intensive study to no lesser degree than the important aspect of prevention of atheroma formation

- Use of a β-blocking agent may inhibit plaque rupture perhaps by its ability to ↓ cardiac ejection velocity. This action reduces hydraulic stress on the arterial wall that might be critical at the arterial site where the atheromatous plaque is predisposed to rupture (See Fig. 3–7). Recent experimental data suggest that hypolipidemic agents, antioxidants such as vitamin E or probucol, and ACE inhibitors, all have the capacity to ↓ plaque growth and perhaps rupture
- Occlusion of a coronary artery leads, in about 20 mins, to death of cells in areas of severely ischemic tissue, which will usually become necrotic over 4–6 h. Since early and late mortality are directly related to the size of the infarct, limitation of infarct size (or even prevention of necrosis) by means of thrombolytic therapy initiated at the earliest possible moment, is of the utmost importance
- The ischemic zone surrounding the necrotic tissue provides EP inhomogeneity that predisposes the occurrence of lethal arrhythmias. These arrhythmias are most common during the early hours after onset and contribute to one of the major mechanisms of sudden death

Extensive myocardial necrosis is the major determinant of CHF; papillary, septal, and freewall rupture; and cardiogenic shock, in which >35% of the myocardium is usually infarcted. The most effective means of reducing the extent of myocardial necrosis is the administration of thrombolytic therapy, aspirin, and a β-blocking agent as soon as possible after the onset of symptoms of coronary thrombosis.

DIAGNOSIS

Chest Pain

- Usually lasts >20 mins and often persists for several hours. However, the pain of infarction can last for only 15 mins and, occasionally, fatal infarction is ushered in by only a few minutes of severe pain or even unheralded cardiac arrest. Infarction may be silent, particularly in diabetic patients and in the elderly
- Typically retrosternal and across the chest
- Variations of a crushing, vise-like, heavy weight on the chest, pressure, tightness, strangling, aching
- At times, only a discomfort with an oppression and burning or indigestion-like feeling
- May radiate to the throat, jaws, neck, shoulders, arms, scapulae, or the epigastrium. At times, pain is centered at any one of these areas, e.g., the left wrist or shoulder, without radiation
- Usually builds up over minutes or hours, as opposed to aortic dissection, in which pain has an abrupt onset like a gunshot

Associated symptoms and factors include

- Diaphoresis, cold clammy skin, apprehension
- Shortness of breath, nausea, vomiting, dizziness
- Presyncope and rarely syncope may occur due to bradyarrhythmias, especially in inferior MI

- Occasionally, no pain. A marked ↓ in BP with associated symptoms, along with ECG findings, should suffice in making the diagnosis
- Painless infarcts (in about 10% of patients), especially in diabetics or the elderly. In these patients, associated symptoms are often prominent and serve as clues to diagnosis
- Over 50% of patients have a history of angina or prior infarction
- Approximately 33% of patients with acute infarction have no major risk factors: Death of a parent or sibling < age 55, hypercholesterolemia, cigarette smoking, hypertension, or diabetes. Absence of these factors should not influence the diagnosis

Physical Signs

- Patient appears apprehensive, anxious, cold, clammy
- Area of chest pain may be indicated with a clenched fist
- Tachycardia 100–120/min. A ↑ in BP due to increased sympathetic tone is observed in slightly >1/2 of patients with anterior infarction
- Bradycardia <60 beats/min and a ↓ in BP in about 2/3 of inferior infarcts; many of these patients become hypotensive, sometimes profoundly
- S4 gallop is common; S3 and S4 if in CHF or cardiogenic shock
- Murmur of MR due to papillary muscle dysfunction
- Crepitations, more prominent over the lower third of the lung fields, may be present
- Elevated jugular venous pressure due to left and right CHF or a very high venous pressure in the presence of right ventricular infarction or cardiac tamponade
- Frequently, there are no abnormal physical signs, and this finding in a patient with suggestive symptoms should not ↓ the level of suspicion that the patient may have an MI

Although sophisticated tests evolved in the 1980s to improve diagnostic accuracy, they are of limited value in the era of thrombolysis. Thus, a relevant history and correct interpretation of the ECG are of paramount importance in the implementation of early thrombolytic therapy, which will be of greatest benefit if given very early after symptom onset (<60 min).

Electrocardiogram

DIAGNOSTIC FEATURES OF ST SEGMENT ELEVATION ACUTE MI

- ST segment elevation of ≥1 mm in ≥2 limb leads or
- At least 2 mm ST elevation in ≥2 precordial leads

The above criteria, which have been used in most clinical trials of thrombolytic therapy, have become internationally standard and are considered diagnostic in patients with symptoms suggestive of acute MI. Where symptoms are not typical, the response to nitroglycerin is ascertained. Also, minimal ST segment elevation in black patients must be reassessed to exclude the occasional normal variant. There is clear recognition that Q waves may evolve early or late and cannot be relied upon for early diagnosis. Thus, the terms "transmural" and "nontransmural" have been abandoned and Q wave or non Q wave infarction cannot be categorized in the early phase. The best differentiating feature is ST segment elevation, which is present in 95% of patients with acute coronary thrombotic occlusion.

In addition, later ECG signs of infarction include

- Diminution of R waves (poor R wave progression)
- Evolving Q waves
- The simultaneous presence of reciprocal ST segment depression is important to confirm the electrocardiographic diagnosis
- Patients who are developing non Q wave infarction often manifest ST depression, or T-wave change

If the first ECG is not diagnostic of acute injury/infarction, but the patient is strongly suspected of having an acute coronary syndrome, the ECG is repeated q 30 mins until diagnostic changes are observed or until the CK and/or CK-MB results are reported. If the ECG is equivocal and there is a strong clinical impression that acute MI is present, valuable confirmatory information may be obtained from an echocardiogram.

Because the initial abnormality may not be fully diagnostic in up to 40% of cases, it is imperative to correlate the findings with accurate historical details. In patients with chest pain, new or presumably new Q waves in 2 leads with ST elevation are diagnostic in over 85% of cases

- Q waves are fully developed in 4–12 h and may manifest as early as 2 h from onset of chest discomfort or associated symptoms
- Evolutionary ST-T changes occur during 12–24 h but may be delayed up to 30 h
- Inferior MI ST elevation in lead 2, 3 and AVF with evolving Q waves and reciprocal depression in V_1-V_3. The latter depression may be due to reciprocal changes, but there is evidence to suggest that in some patients it is due to LAD disease. The evolutionary changes in repolarization that occur with inferior infarction evolve more rapidly than with anterior infarcts
- Tachycardia may ↑ ischemic injury, causing elevation of the ST segment that must be differentiated from extension of infarction or pericarditis. Importantly, reciprocal depression does not occur in pericarditis

NONDIAGNOSTIC ECG

Acute MI may be present with ECG changes that are nonspecific in 10–20% of cases and may result from

- Slow evolution of ECG changes. The tracing may remain normal for several hours
- Old infarction masking the ECG effect of a new infarct
- Inferior MI associated with left anterior hemiblock in which R waves are expected to be small in leads 2, 3, AVF
- LBBB
- Apical infarction
- Posterolateral infarction is not usually associated with ST elevation or Q waves

ST elevation of infarction must be distinguished from the following

- Acute pericarditis where the ST segment elevation is not confined to leads referrable to an anatomic segmental blood supply. Thus, elevation in lead 1 is accompanied by elevation in leads 2, 3, AVF; the ST elevation is concave, as opposed to convex, upward with an injury current of infarction; and reciprocal depression is absent (see Chap. 13)

- Early repolarization changes may mimic infarction but are often observed mainly in leads V5 and V6 with a subtle "fish hook" configuration. This feature is common in blacks
- LV aneurysm, in which there may be permanent ST elevation

ECG AND LOCATION OF INFARCTION SITES

- Anteroseptal: ST elevation V_1, V_2, V_3
- Anterior: ST segment elevation V_2-V_4
- Extensive anterior: V_1-V_6, 1 AVL
- Anterolateral: V_4-V_6, 1 AVL
- Inferior: 2, 3, AVF
- Posterior infarction: Tall R waves V_1, V_2, upright T waves occasionally ST depression V_1-V_2 and often inferior or inferolateral infarct signs
- Right ventricular infarction: ST segment elevation V_2, V_4R, often associated with inferior infarction

ECG AND SIZE OF INFARCTION

The extent of ST segment elevation gives clues to infarct size, but the correlation is not close. The site of infarction influences mortality but is not as paramount as the size of infarction, which can be reasonably ascertained from the number of leads showing ST elevation, as follows

- Small MI: 2 or 3 leads
- Moderate: 4 or 5 leads
- Large: 6 or 7 leads
- Extensive: 8 or 9 leads

Echocardiography in Acute Myocardial Infarction

Echocardiography is not required routinely in an uncomplicated MI, especially where the history and ECG are typical or with non Q wave infarction.

Indications

- Patients with cardiogenic shock often require assessment to determine the presence of mechanical complications: Septal rupture, severe MR, myocardial rupture, and tamponade. Color Doppler can provide quick results and, with the unconscious patient, a TEE is helpful and accurate
- To distinguish acute severe MR from papillary muscle rupture
- In patients with new LBBB with typical chest pain and history suggestive of acute infarction, echocardiography can assist with the diagnosis
- Patients with an atypical ECG pattern and clinical features of MI
- Suspected right ventricular infarction with high jugular venous pressure to assess right ventricular involvement and differentiate pericardial tamponade causing a high venous pressure
- To identify high-risk patients with multivessel disease. The contralateral remote zone should be hyperkinetic, but if it is not, this usually indicates significant noninfarct vessel atherosclerotic disease
- In patients with moderate CHF not clearing after $\geq$2 doses of furosemide, echocardiographic assessment of LV systolic function is useful prior to β-blocker therapy. Although radionuclide ventriculography gives a more accurate assessment of the EF, the estimate obtained from echocardiography is usually adequate to assist with the evaluation of outcomes and therapy

PUBLIC EDUCATION AND PHYSICIAN INTERACTION

It is estimated that in areas where thrombolytic therapy is available, 20–30% of patients with acute MI in North America and about 40% in the UK receive such treatment

- Thrombolytic therapy has proven valuable and reduces mortality and morbidity. Timing of treatment, however, is of great importance, and until recently it was uncertain as to the outer time boundary of therapy from symptom onset. In the recently completed Late Assessment of Thrombolytic Efficacy (LATE) double-blind placebo controlled trial of 5,700 patients treated between 6 and 24 h of symptoms, patients receiving tPA within 12 hours had a 27% ↓ of mortality compared with placebo. These data extend the time window of 0–6 h, established by GISSI-1 and ISSI-2, to 12 h
- The first hour of symptoms represents a huge opportunity for benefit for thrombolytic therapy. In the recent MITI trial, patients treated in the first 60 min had mortality reduced from 10% to 2%, and 40% of these patients had no infarct on thallium scintigraphy. In the GISSI-1 and ISIS-2 trials, ↓ in mortality was >50% compared with controls treated in the first hours. Unfortunately, <3% of patients actually received therapy in this time frame. The average delay in hospital admissions of 80–90 min largely accounts for the problem, is inexcusable, and should be reduced to <15 min
- Benefit is observed up to 12 h
- A major undertaking is the education of patients and the community at large about the importance of minimizing delays between the onset of symptoms of suspected heart attack and attention in the emergency room of the nearest hospital
- It is not easy to motivate healthy individuals, and efforts to educate the public in this area of their care have not been sufficiently fruitful. Leaflets and health booklets appear to have little impact. A concerted effort must be made by physicians' groups in individual communities in conjunction with audiovisual programs for the public. In addition, hospitals must adopt policies to enforce rapid triage in the emergency room; physicians must be encouraged to institute thrombolytic therapy within a few minutes of the patient's arrival

Delays to Be Avoided

- Reaching the emergency room >6 h after onset of symptoms: Patient and public education should address this issue
- Slow emergency room triage: Patients with chest pain should be allowed quick passage, not exceeding a 1-min delay at the so-called "triage area," to an area of the emergency room delineated for the rapid assessment of MI
- Waiting for attending physician
- Emergency room physician delay: The emergency room physician must be well trained to deal with patients who have chest pain. This physician must be allowed to give IV thrombolytic therapy (SK, TPA, or APSAC) to all those who qualify according to an approved, well-outlined hospital emergency room protocol for IV use of thrombolytic agents. The protocol should clearly show the indications and contraindications to IV thrombolysis, but should be simplified. The only well-documented contraindications are active bleeding, stroke, major

trauma or surgery in the past 6 months, and uncontrolled hypertension
- Waiting for CCU beds: Transfer is advisable after commencement of thrombolysis and initial hemodynamic stability is achieved. Thus, emergency rooms must be equipped to administer all functions that are available in the CCU
- Waiting 1–2 h for CK, CK-MB enzyme results: The CK is not usually sufficiently elevated within the first 4 h to establish the diagnosis of infarction and can be used only after the fact. The object is to ↓ or, in some cases, prevent enzyme release by rapid reperfusion of ischemic myocardium

RISK STRATIFICATION

On admission, risk stratification (see Table 3–3) assists in decision making, especially when relative contraindications to thrombolytic therapy are present. Characteristics of patients with acute MI who, on admission, have a high risk of death or complications include

- Large infarcts usually associated with moderate to severe CHF, pulmonary edema, with crackles observed over >1/3 of the lower lung field
- An EF <35%
- Cardiogenic shock indicating a large infarct or mechanical complication and high mortality
- Over age 75: The 1-year mortality >30% versus <10% in patients < age 70
- New LBBB
- New RBBB with LV failure
- Previous MI and recent infarction with CHF

Patients with cardiogenic shock and other selected high-risk individuals should be considered for transfer to an interventional cardiac catheterization laboratory for emergency angiography and possible infarct vessel angioplasty.

THERAPY

- Immediate relief of pain is of paramount importance since pain enhances autonomic disturbances that may precipitate sudden death. All patients should take or be given noncoated aspirin, 162–325 mg, immediately and then enteric coated, 160–325 qd. This dosage proved very effective in ISIS-2 (Table 3–2) and ISIS-3; a 325-mg dose was used successfully in GISSI-2 (Table 3–1). An initial large dose of 325 mg is strongly recommended because a lower dose may still leave substantial thromboxane activity at this crucial period and may take a few days before achieving >95% of inhibition of platelet activity. Beta blockers are administered without delay if there are no contraindications, and thrombolytic therapy is commenced in properly selected patients. These treatment modalities will be discussed in this chapter.

Table 3–1
Timing of Thrombolytic Therapy and Lives Saved by GISSI-1 and ISIS-2

	GISSI-1*		ISSI-2**	
	CONTROL	SK TREATED	CONTROL	SK & ASPIRIN TREATED
	5,860	5,852	8,595	8,592
Mortality:	13%	10.7%	11.8%	9.1%
Mortality reduction:	17.7%	Lives saved 130/5852 2/100 treated	22.9%	Lives saved 233/8595 3/100 treated
	Hours	Lives saved		Lives saved
	≤3	3/100		4/100
	3–6	2/100		2.6/100
	6–9	1/123		
	6–24	—		1/100

SK = Streptokinase
* = Modified from: Lancet, *1*:397, 1986
** = Modified from: Lancet, *2*:350, 1988

The reader is advised to consult Chapter 4 for a discussion of angioplasty and the management of complications of acute MI

- In all patients with uncomplicated infarction, treated with thrombolytic agents, a delayed strategy of coronary angiography or "watchful waiting" (with no angiogram unless angina or a positive functional test) is pursued. A conservative strategy has evolved based on the result of the TIMI-2 trial
- Patients for whom thrombolytic therapy is contraindicated should be considered for primary (direct) angioplasty of the infarct vessel if they can be transferred quickly (<90 min) to a facility with skilled operators and personnel to perform coronary intervention

Table 3–2
ISIS-2: Effects of Aspirin and Streptokinase Given Within 4 Hours and Within 24 Hours of Onset of Myocardial Infarction

	PLACEBO (I)	SK	ASPIRIN	SK + ASPIRIN	PLACEBO (I) + TABLETS	NEITHER
35-day vascular mortality; therapy within 4 hours	12.3%	8.2%	8.9%	6.4%	13.1%	
Within 24 hours	12% 1029/8595	9.2% 791/8592	9.4% 804/8587	8% 343/4292	11.8% 1016/8600	13.3% 568/4300

I = infusion
SK = streptokinase
Modified from: Lancet, *2*:350, 1988.
* Odds of death, 53% SD 8 Reduction; 2 $p < 0.00001$

Emergency Management

PAIN RELIEF

- Morphine: 4 mg IV over 1 min, repeated if necessary at a dose of 2–5 mg q 5–30 mins as needed at the rate of 1 mg/min
- A β blocker, preferably given IV for 2 doses then orally (see Table 3–4), if there is no contraindication. Beta blockade has been shown to abolish and may prevent recurrence of chest pain and decreases the need for morphine or nitroglycerin
- Nitroglycerin is usually given sublingually for 2 doses. Recurrence of chest discomfort after adequate administration of morphine and a β blocker should prompt the use of IV nitroglycerin (see Pump Infusion, Table 2–8)

CONTROL OF EARLY LIFE-THREATENING ARRHYTHMIAS

Lives can be saved by

- Prompt defibrillation or conversion of VT by medical teams or paramedics
- Lidocaine (lignocaine) IV: Effective for the control of VT, but its prophylactic use is *not* recommended (discussed later in this chapter)
- Beta blockers: May be required as therapy independent of pain control to abolish ventricular arrhythmias or to prevent their occurrence, especially if these arrhythmias are catecholamine-induced. These agents ↓ the incidence of VF; they should not be given with hypotension, bradycardia, or signs of CHF

TREATMENT OF AUTONOMIC DISTURBANCES

- Monitoring of the cardiac rhythm is routine practice
- Autonomic disturbances are triggered by ischemic tissue as well as pain and may result in sinus tachycardia and tachyarrhythmias that are associated with inappropriate catecholamine release, thereby intensifying ischemia, which further increases release of catecholamines. Alternatively, bradycardia may occur and the associated hypotension may enlarge the infarct. This vicious cycle results in a ↑ in infarct size, which can culminate in progressive CHF and shock
- Autonomic disturbances may be abolished by morphine and β blockade
- Symptomatic bradycardias with pulse rates <40/min are controlled with the judicious use of atropine (0.4–0.6 mg) IV given slowly q 5–10 mins as needed, to a max of 2 mg. *Caution:* Do not ↑ the HR beyond 60/min. Too rapid administration of atropine may result in sinus tachycardia in some patients and, rarely, VF may be precipitated

ANCILLARY THERAPY

- Oxygen 2–3 L/min via nasal prongs is given during the first few hours until assessment is completed, then O_2 is continued if the patient is short of breath, tachypneic, or if there is proven hypoxemia. Pulmonary edema causes hypoxemia, but ventilation perfusion mismatch plays a role. Cessation of O_2 administration indicates to the patient that some improvement is occurring and helps to allay anxiety

- Diet: Fluids only for 8–12 h until it is established that the infarction is uncomplicated, then light diet as tolerated with no added salt until the patient is discharged from the CCU
- A stool softener is routinely prescribed, e.g., docusate (100–200 mg) bid
- Bedrest and bedside commode for 24 h, then washroom privileges and ambulation
- Anticoagulants, for tPA, IV heparin 5,000 U/bolus, with thrombolytic therapy, 1,000 U/h, with careful adjustment of PTT between 60 to 85 sec (or 2.5 × control)
- Mild sedation: Oxazepam (15 mg) or a similar agent at bedtime; some patients may require twice daily dosing
- Psychologic management is discussed in Chapter 4

RECOMMENDATIONS FOR BALLOON FLOTATION RIGHT HEART CATHETER

Hemodynamic monitoring is required only when information is not available clinically and is needed to assess the degree of cardiac decompensation or to guide the administration of pharmacologic agents.

Indications include

- Cardiogenic shock or signs of systemic hypoperfusion
- Severe CHF
- Suspected mechanical complications: Ventricular septal or papillary muscle rupture, suspected severe MR, pericardial tamponade
- Diagnosis of right ventricular infarction when there is also a degree of LV failure
- Progressive or unexplained hypotension failing to respond to fluid administration in patients without pulmonary congestion

REDUCTION OF INFARCT SIZE AND MORTALITY; ACHIEVING INFARCT VESSEL PATENCY

- Infarct-related vessel patency is best achieved with early thrombolysis using IV SK, TPA, or APSAC. See discussion under Thrombolytic Therapy
- Aspirin, 162–325 mg, enteric coated, is administered qd. Aspirin administered at the onset of symptoms added to IV SK was shown in ISIS-2 to cause a significant improvement in survival (see Table 3–2). In this trial, aspirin reduced death by about 25% and the incidence of reinfarction by 50%. Also, aspirin is necessary following thrombolytic therapy to prevent reocclusion of the infarct-related vessel
- Beta blockade given at the earliest opportunity reduces infarct size and mortality. A β-blocking agent is advocated by the ACC/AHA Task Force and the early use of these agents for the management of acute MI has now been appropriately adopted worldwide. The above guidelines applied to patients with ST elevation (probable evolution to Q wave infarct) and ST depression (probable evolution to non Q wave infarct) are given in Figures 3–1 and 3–2
- Patients with large anterior infarcts considered high risk (Table 3–3), and in whom thrombolytic therapy is contraindicated or ischemia persists, should be considered for urgent coronary angiography and angioplasty if a highly skilled team is available (Fig. 3–1)

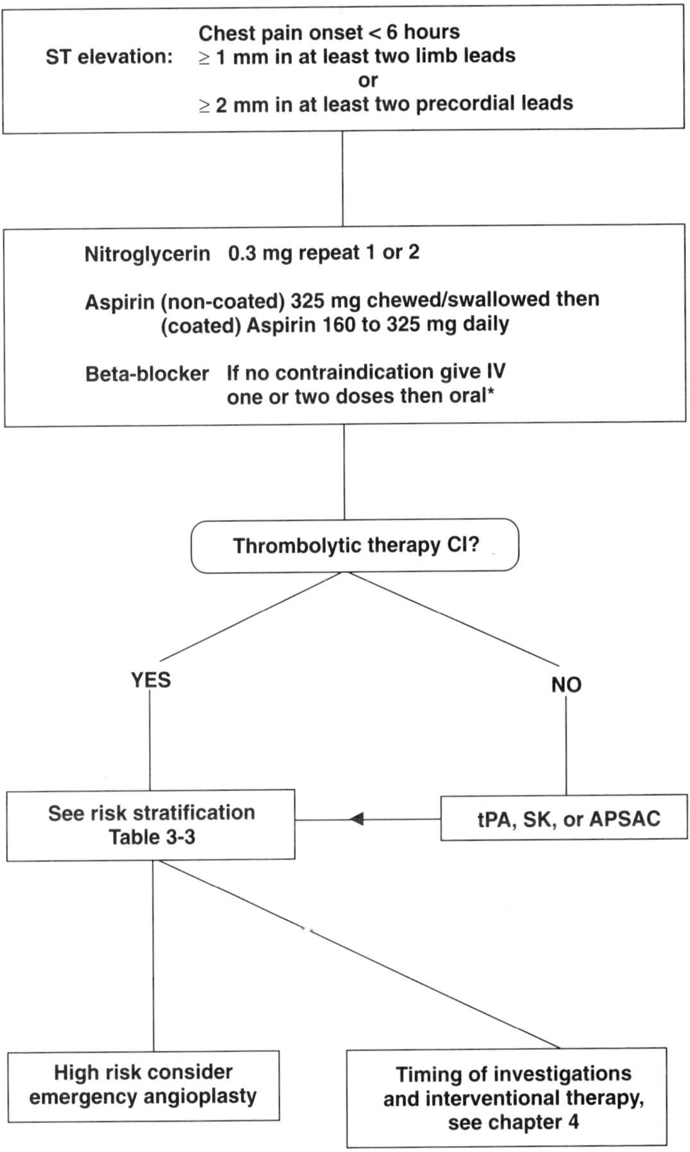

Figure 3–1. Management of acute myocardial infarction: ECG ST elevation (probable evolution of Q wave infarct). * = see Table 3–4; CI = contraindicated; tPA = tissue plasminogen activator; SK = streptokinase.

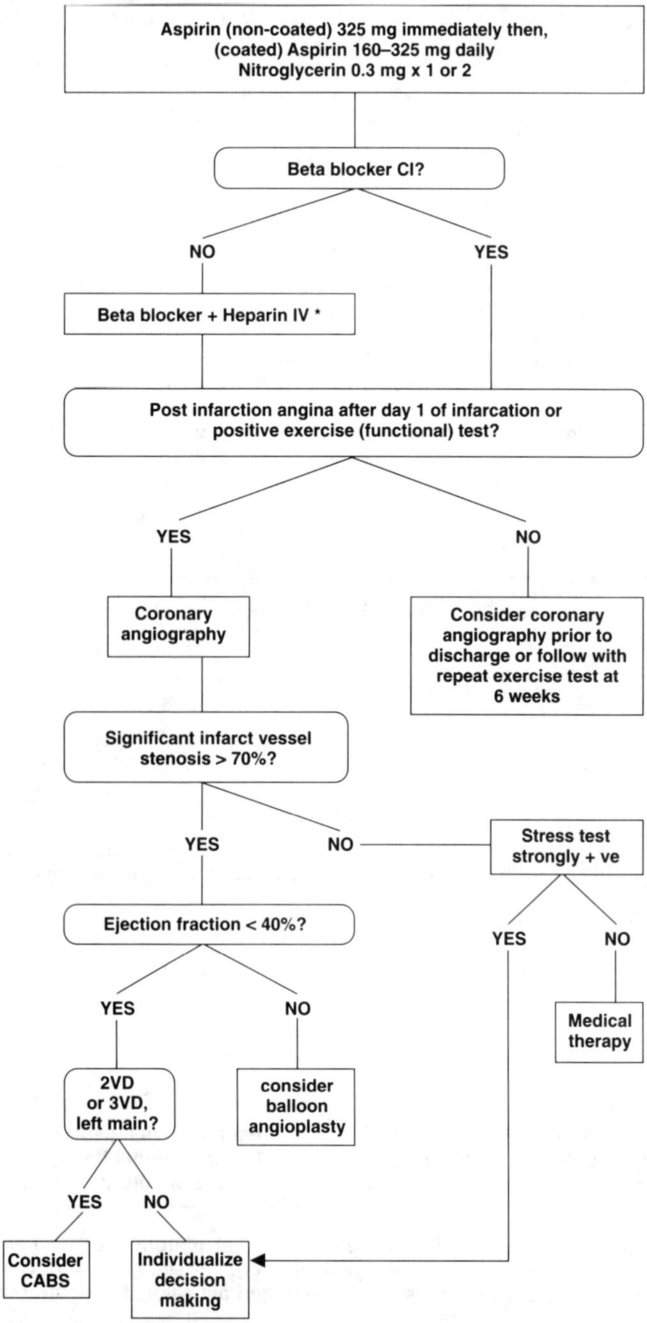

Figure 3–2. Algorithm** for the management of acute myocardial infarction: ECG ST depression (probable evolution to non Q infarct).
* TIMI-3 No benefit of thrombolytic agents
** Algorithms do not cover all scenarios
CABS = Coronary artery bypass surgery
VD = Vessel disease.

Table 3–3
Acute Myocardial Infarction In-Hospital Mortality Risk Stratification

PARAMETERS	*APPROXIMATE MORTALITY %
Average	13
Age	
75–85	24
65–74	15
50–65	9
<50	<7
Cardiogenic shock	80
Large anterior** infarcts associated with	
a) Severe heart failure pulmonary edema	>30
b) Previous infarct and heart failure ejection fraction <30%	>25
c) Q wave anterior infarct heart rate >100/min blood pressure <110 mm Hg	>20
New left bundle branch block proven infarction	>20
Q wave anterior infarct uncomplicated	12
Q wave inferior	3
Non Q wave infarction	3
Q wave and age <55 uncomplicated	7
Non Q wave age <55	1

* Recent pooled trial results
** Anterior, anterolateral

Thrombolytic Therapy

Reduction in major events and mortality is achieved by thrombolytic therapy instituted within 12 h of onset of symptoms.

Pooled mortality results of recent trials in over 42,000 patients randomized 21,034 to thrombolytic therapy, 20,979 to placebo, were 10% in the treated group and 11.7% in the control group. These percentages account for 350 lives saved. The treatment of 21,000 patients saved 2 lives in 100 patients < age 60 treated within 6 h from onset of symptoms, 7 lives in patients 60–69 years old, and 8 lives in those > age 70. Thus, the 70- to 75-year-old patients derived the greatest absolute benefits from thrombolytic therapy.

There is currently no ideal thrombolytic agent. From GISSI-2 and ISIS-3 the 3 approved agents—SK, TPA, and anistreplase (APSAC)—are equally effective.

Tables 3–1, 3–2, 3–5, and 3–6 give relevant results of GISSI-1, ISIS-2, GISSI-2, and ISIS-3.

Thus, until recently no evidence of any real difference in 5-week mortality between SK and TPA or APSAC has been observed despite randomization of over 60,000 patients in ISIS-3 and GISSI-2. Assessment of global and regional LV function 3 weeks after a first infarction indicates similar effects for SK and tPA. It is important to note that tPA must be used in conjunction with IV heparin to achieve excellent late patency rates and avoid reocclusion.

The choice of thrombolytic therapy remains controversial owing to the high cost of TPA and APSAC and the increased incidence of stroke (4/thousand patients treated) for these 2 agents. (See Fig. 3–3.) However,

Table 3–4
Dosage of Beta Blockers in Acute Myocardial Infarction*

IV*	ORAL DOSAGE 1ST 7 DAYS	1 WEEK TO 2 YEARS
Atenolol (IV 5 mg over 5 min, 10 min later 5 mg over 5 min)	10 min after last IV dose give 50 mg oral/daily	50 mg daily
Metoprolol (IV 5 mg at a rate of 1 mg/min 5 min later 2nd 5 mg bolus 5 min later 3rd 5 mg bolus)	8 hours after IV 25 to 50 50 mg twice daily	50 to 100 mg twice daily
Propranolol (IV not approved for MI in USA)	20 mg three times daily	80 mg long-acting, increasing to 160 mg once daily; maximum 240 mg daily
Timolol	5 mg twice daily	10 mg twice daily

* Contraindications: bronchial asthma, severe heart failure, systolic BP <100 mm Hg, 2nd- or 3rd-degree AV block

** Halt IV if the following events develop: heart rate <50/minute, 2nd- or 3rd-degree AV block, PR >0.24, systolic BP <95 mm Hg, marked shortness of breath, wheezes, or crackles >⅓ of the lung fields, or pulmonary capillary wedge pressure >22 mm Hg, if this parameter is being monitored.

the results of the GUSTO study provided some solution to the controversies and defined the role of IV heparin. The net clinical benefit of the aggressive thrombolytic regimens, of front-loaded tPA which open the infarct vessel faster than previous strategies used along with carefully titrated IV heparin in GUSTO, a 41,021-patient trial in 15 countries and 1,100 hospitals demonstrated a 14% mortality reduction compared with streptokinase or combined TPA and streptokinase published in September 1993. It was shown that a small ↑ in hemorrhagic stroke for these aggressive regimens will be acceptable for the trade-off of a more extensive "net" mortality ↓.

Table 3–5
Timing of Thrombolytic Therapy on Events, Mortality and Effect of Heparin* in GISSI-2

HOURS		tPA	SK	HEPARAIN SQ	NO HEPARIN
≤3	Events →	973/4449 21.9%	962/4481 21.5%		
3–6	Events →	454/1729 26.3%	430/1711 25.1%		
	Deaths →	556/6182 9%	536/6199 8.6%	518/6175 8.3%	574/6206 9.3%

Modified from: Lancet, *336*:65, 1990

* Subcutaneous

** Death plus heart failure beyond 4 days, plus extensive left ventricular damage in the absence of heart failure; treatment <3 hours, maximum benefit

Table 3–6
Effects of Allocated Treatment on Deaths in Days 0–35 Among (i) All Patients and (ii) Patients Presenting Within 0–6 H With ST Elevation

	FIBRINOLYTIC COMPARISONS			Difference %SK–%tPA		Difference %SK–%APSAC	
	SK	tPA	APSAC				
(i) All patients	13 780	13 746	13 773	%	SD	%	SD
Any	1455 (10.6%)	1418 (10.3%)	1448 (10.5%)	0.24	0.37	0.05	0.37
(*a*) Timing							
Day 0–1	699 (5.1%)	649 (4.7%)	700 (5.1%)	0.35	0.26	−0.01	0.26
Day 2–7	357 (2.6%)	415 (3.0%)	378 (2.7%)	−0.43	0.20*	−0.15	0.19
Day 8–35	399 (2.9%)	3544 (2.6%)	370 (2.7%)	0.32	0.20	0.21	0.20
(*b*) Antithrombotic allocation							
Aspirin plus sc heparin	726 (10.5%)	684 (10.0%)	722 (10.5%)	0.58	0.52	0.06	0.52
Aspirin alone	729 (10.6%)	734 (10.7%)	726 (10.6%)	−0.09	0.53	0.03	0.52
(ii) 0–6 h, ST elevation	8643	8571	8622	%	SD	%	SD
Any	861 (10.0%)	822 (9.6%)	855 (9.9%)	0.37	0.45	0.05	0.46
(*a*) Timing							
Day 0–1	421 (4.9%)	389 (4.5%)	408 (4.7%)	0.33	0.32	0.14	0.33
Day 2–7	201 (2.3%)	236 (2.8%)	218 (2.5%)	−0.43	0.24	−0.20	0.23
Day 8–35	239 (2.8%)	197 (2.3%)	229 (2.7%)	0.47	0.24	0.11	0.25
(*b*) Antithrombotic allocation							
Aspirin plus sc heparin	425 (9.8%)	389 (9.1%)	427 (9.9%)	0.69	0.63	−0.13	0.64
Aspirin alone	436 (10.2%)	433 (10.1%)	428 (9.9%)	0.05	0.65	0.22	0.65

* $2p < 0.05$.
From: ISIS-3: A randomized comparison of streptokinase vs. tissue plasminogen activator vs. anistreplase and of aspirin plus heparin vs. aspirin alone among 41,299 cases of suspected acute myocardial infarction. Lancet, *339*:759, 1992.

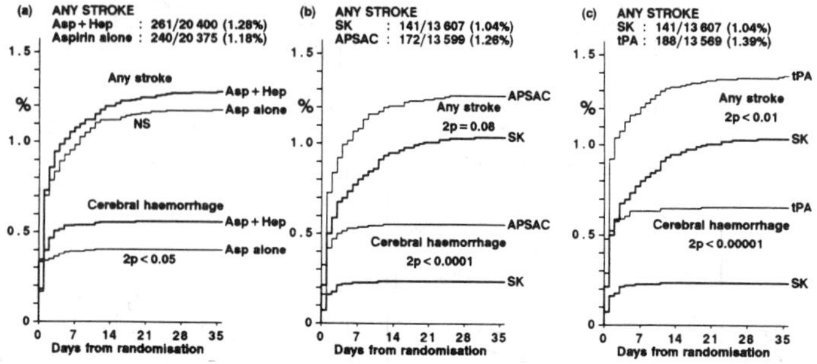

Figure 3–3. Cumulative percentage with any stroke (upper lines) and with (definite or probable) cerebral hemorrhage in hospital up to day 35 or prior discharge. (a) All patients allocated aspirin plus heparin (thicker line) vs. all allocated aspirin alone; (b) all patients allocated streptokinase (SK) (thicker line) vs. all allocated APSAC; (c) all patients allocated SK vs. all allocated tPA. From: ISIS-3: A randomized comparison of streptokinase vs. tissue plasminogen activator vs. anistreplase and of aspirin plus heparin vs. aspirin alone among 41,299 cases of suspected acute myocardial infarction. Lancet, *339*:757, 1992.

INDICATIONS FOR THROMBOLYTIC THERAPY

Guidelines for the administration of thrombolytic therapy are shown in Figure 3–4

- Patients ≤75 years old, seen within 6 h of onset of symptoms with clinical and ECG diagnoses consistent with acute MI (with ≥2 mm ST elevation in ≥1 precordial leads or ≥1 mm ST elevation in ≥2 limb leads) are candidates for thrombolytic therapy

Probable indications include

- Patients > age 75 in good general health should *not* be excluded if seen within 6 h of pain onset where the impending infarction is large or extensive and there is no contraindication to thrombolytic therapy. ISIS-3 indicated that patients > age 75 showed the greatest benefits. However, thrombolytic therapy should be used with great caution in patients > age 80 because most studies indicate increased risk of major bleeding in this subset of patients. In 1 study, SK caused a twofold increased risk of major hemorrhage that resulted in a mortality of 17% in patients > age 75 and 1% in those < age 75. It must be reemphasized that IV heparin and a thrombolytic agent in patients over age 80 should be used with caution until further large, randomized studies show proven benefit at low risk in these patients. When thrombolytic therapy is considered necessary in healthy patients over age 75 with large infarcts seen within 6 h, the combination of aspirin and the cautious use of SK is advisable, preferably without heparin use
- Patients with new LBBB seen within 6 h of onset of chest pain. This subset represents a high-risk group and was shown to benefit in the ISIS-3 study
- Patients with new RBBB, proven acute infarction, associated with CHF
- Patients seen within 12 h from onset of symptoms with evidence of ongoing ischemia: Pain still present or stuttering episodes in the presence of continuing elevation of ST segments and CK and CK-MB ele-

vation. Caution is required in patients seen after 12 h because late reperfusion appears to ↑ the risk of myocardial rupture and it is necessary to weigh the risks involved

Absolute contraindications include

- Active internal bleeding within the prior weeks
- Suspected aortic dissection
- Recent head injury or cerebral neoplasm
- Recent trauma, major surgery within 6 weeks
- Recent prolonged or clearly traumatic CPR
- History of cerebrovascular accident known to be hemorrhagic
- Cerebrovascular accident within 6 months
- Severe hypertension, uncontrolled BP >200/110 mm Hg

Relative contraindications include

- Known bleeding diathesis or current use of anticoagulants
- Active peptic ulcer without bleeding; patient on medications

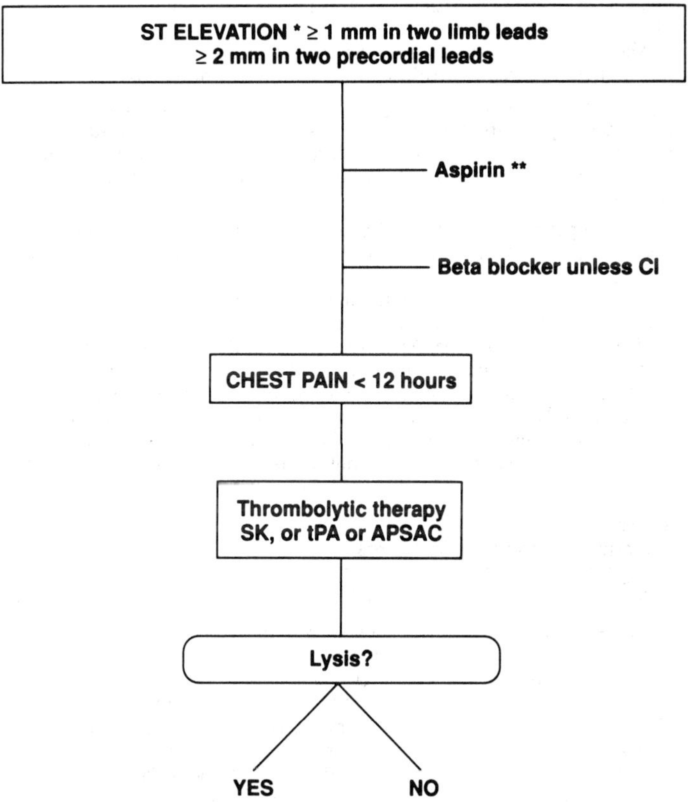

Figure 3–4. Guidelines for thrombolytic therapy.
* Probable Q wave infarct
** Aspirin (non-enteric coated) 160–325 mg, chewed/swallowed plus beta blocker IV or oral (see Table 3–4)
CI = contraindicated.

- History of severe hypertension under drug treatment; systolic >180 mm Hg, diastolic >110 mm Hg
- Significant liver dysfunction or esophageal varices
- Underlying malignancy
- Elderly patients who are confused, lethargic, or agitated

Complications of thrombolytic therapy include

- Bleeding, especially in patients requiring invasive procedures. Intracranial bleeding reportedly occurs in 0.3–1.4% and is more common in patients > age 70
- Rarely myocardial and splenic rupture, cholesterol embolization
- Hypotension and allergic reaction occur in approximately 5–10% with SK or anistreplase

Streptokinase (Streptase, Kabikinase) Action: SK combines with plasminogen to form plasminogen activator complex. The complex converts free plasminogen to plasmin, which causes fibrinogenolysis and independent lysis of fibrin. SK also causes activation of fibrin-bound plasminogen; thus, 2 independent actions occur. The activator complex has a half-life of about 85 mins. The extensive coagulation defect begins rapidly after administration, remains intense for about 4–8 h, and dwindles over the following 36–48 h.

About 65% coronary reperfusion rate is observed when 1.5 million U of the drug are given within 3 h of onset of symptoms of infarction.

Dosage: See Table 3–7. Adverse Effects: Allergic reactions are seen in about 2% of patients. Edema, bronchospasm, angioneurotic edema, anaphylaxis reported in 0.1–0.5% with apparently no fatalities. Hypotension occurs in 6–8% of patients but usually is responsive to fluid administration.

Anistreplase (Eminase). APSAC is a 1:1 molecular combination of plasminogen and SK with a catalytic center protected by a chemical group.

Anistreplase is activated in the bloodstream; de-acylation to the active complex begins immediately and continues at a constant rate with a half-life of about 90 mins. An advantage over SK is the ease of administration by slow IV bolus. The drug produces about a 60% patency rate in about 40 mins with persistence of activity for 4–6 h. This agent is approximately as effective as SK or conventional dosing tPA in achieving vessel patency and this effect is enhanced by routine aspirin use. Concomitant heparin therapy is not advisable. Dosage: See Table 3–7.

Table 3–7
Dosage of Thrombolytic Agents

DRUG	DOSAGE
Streptokinase	1.5 million U in 100 ml 0.9% saline IV infusion over 30 to 60 minutes
Anistreplase (APSAC)	30 U in 5 ml sterile water or saline by slow IV bolus over 2 to 5 minutes
tPA (alteplase) (Manufacturer's dosage; product monograph 1990 to 1992)	6–10 mg IV bolus over 1–2 minutes then 50 mg IV infusion over 1 hour, 20 mg IV infusion over 2nd hour, 20 mg IV infusion over 3rd hour; 100 mg total dose
tPA Front-loaded (Author's recommendation)	15 mg bolus 0.75 mg/kg over 30 minutes (not >50 mg) 0.50 mg/kg over 60 minutes (not >35 mg) Total dose ≤100 mg

Tissue Plasminogen Activator (tPA; Activase) Tissue type plasminogen activator is the physiologic activator of plasminogen but has a higher affinity for fibrin-bound plasminogen. However, tPA's specificity for fibrin-bound plasminogen is relative and dose dependent. Activation of free plasminogen occurs with increasing dosage and blood levels of tPA. Thus, bleeding complications are similar to SK.

Because tPA therapy results in a significantly faster-achieved higher vessel patency rate (85% at 90 min) than SK, and tPA was used in ISIS-3 without the necessary combination with IV heparin for 6 days, further randomized studies using different heparin regimens are in progress. The net clinical outcome (total death plus stroke) in ISIS-3 was similar (11.1%) in the SK versus the tPA treated group. As outlined earlier, the GUSTO trial showed accelerated TPA led to a significant 14% mortality reduction compared with streptokinase. The preferred dose of tPA is a 15 mg bolus, 50 mg over 30 min, and the remaining 35 mg over the next 30 min. Plasma clearance is decreased with hepatic dysfunction and the drug is not advisable in patients who have hepatic disease. Dosage: See Table 3–7. *Adverse Effects.* These are essentially the same as listed under SK, except that allergic reactions do not occur and hypotension from the drug per se is quite unusual. Hypotension with all thrombolytics can occur as a result of the Bezold-Jarisch reflex.

Beta-Blocker Therapy

Acute coronary occlusion producing anteroseptal or anterior MI is often associated with sinus tachycardia. Necrotic tissue is surrounded for a time by a zone of severe myocardial ischemia and injury that causes pain. Both ischemia and pain initiate catecholamine release, and the vicious circle is perpetuated. During the early phase of infarction, the amount of myocardial damage is not fixed and a dynamic process is usually in evolution.

Beta blockers have a proven beneficial effect when relieving pain, ischemia, and injury current during the early phase of acute MI. Decreased mortality, modest ↓ in infarct size, and ↓ in the reinfarction rates have been documented in patients given IV β blockers, followed by oral therapy from day 1 and for 30–90 days, as well as up to 2 years post infarction. The early ↓ in mortality and infarction rates have been modest, but sufficiently significant to warrant early β-blocker therapy for all patients with anterior or anteroseptal infarcts, especially in those with sinus tachycardia, provided that the systolic BP is >100 mm Hg and there is no contraindication to β blockade. If adverse effects are feared, esmolol IV is advisable since its action dissipates in about 10 mins. However, in the United States, presently only metoprolol is approved for IV use during acute MI. Dosage: See Table 3–4.

The merits of β-adrenergic blockade in ischemic syndromes are given in Figure 2–7

- Decrease in HR prolongs the diastolic interval during which coronary perfusion normally occurs. Thus, a ↑ in blood flow may ensue to ischemic areas of myocardium. Necrotic tissue is not capable of salvage, but the area subject to infarction may remain ischemic for several hours, and increased perfusion to ischemic areas may limit the ultimate size of infarction
- Sinus tachycardia causes increased O_2 demand and can shift the balance in ischemic tissue toward necrosis; sinus tachycardia decreases VF threshold. Beta blockers relieve sinus tachycardia and associated hypertension and ↑ VF threshold; some trials showed ↓ in the incidence of VF

- Beta blockers ↓ phase 4 depolarization and thus suppress arrhythmias that may arise in ischemic tissue, especially when initiated by catecholamines
- Decrease in myocardial contractility decreases O_2 requirement
- Decrease in stress on infarcting tissue by the remaining myocardium appears to be responsible for the modest but important ↓ in the incidence of early myocardial rupture due to acute infarction
- In patients given thrombolytics, there is currently no confirmation of experimental findings that viability of ischemic myocardium is prolonged. However, β blockers have been shown to ↓ the incidence of post-thrombolytic ischemic events in patients
- Where there is some residual patency of the infarcted-related artery, β blockers do exert a strong anti-ischemic effect and will ↓ infarct size; in this group of patients, perhaps equivalent to non Q wave infarction, β blockers have been demonstrated to have a major impact on pain and serious events

Clinical trials have not adequately tested the use of β blockers during the first 3 h of onset of symptoms. The MIAMI trial is often quoted as showing a lack of effectiveness of early β-blocker use in reducing mortality. However, the mean treatment time was 11 h. In ISIS-1, 80% of patients were treated up to 8 h and <30% within 4 h of onset, resulting in a 15% ↓ in cardiovascular mortality with significant prevention of early myocardial rupture. Beta blockers were given to 720 patients at about 3–4 h after onset of symptoms in TIMI 2-B and resulted in a 47% ↓ in the incidence of reinfarction in 6 days; also, the incidence of recurrent chest pain was significantly decreased. However, a ↓ in mortality and myocardial rupture was not observed in TIMI 2, probably due to the small number of patients studied, resulting in a type II error. Pooled trial results with the use of β blockade covering mainly 4–6 h from onset of symptoms indicate a 23% ↓ in mortality occurring on day 1, then no significant ↓ during the next few weeks.

The ACC/AHA Task Force recommends β-blocker IV therapy given at the same time as aspirin, as soon as the diagnosis of acute MI is entertained. This is especially important in patients with anteroseptal and anterior MI with a HR >100 and/or systolic BP >110 mm Hg, where no contraindication to β blockade exists. In this subset, β blockers should be given in the emergency room at the same time as aspirin and sublingual nitroglycerin. No harm can ensue if the patient is not later selected for thrombolytic therapy. The concomitant use with a thrombolytic agent has been documented in TIMI 2-B and other trials as safe and worthwhile. Beta blocker therapy from day 7 for 2 years is expected to save 3 lives annually per 100 treated (see Chap. 4).

Early IV followed by oral β-blocker therapy should be strongly considered for all patients presenting with definite or probable acute infarction, in whom contraindications do not exist.

These agents are particularly strongly indicated in the following situations

- Sinus tachycardia unassociated with hypotension or clinically apparent CHF
- Rapid ventricular response to AF or flutter
- Administration of thrombolytic agents: To prevent arrhythmias and/or ischemia and improve survival
- Recurrent ischemic pain
- Moderate impairment of LV function with frequent or complex ventricular ectopy after the first week post infarction

Nitroglycerin. In patients with anterior infarction, there is evidence to suggest that IV nitroglycerin causes a slight ↓ in mortality. The

ACC/AHA Task Force considers the data inadequate to recommend the routine use of IV nitroglycerin in patients with uncomplicated acute MI.

IV nitroglycerin is not recommended in patients with uncomplicated MI. Cutaneous preparations have a role in some patients without hypotension for the relief of chest discomfort. *Indications* include

- Relief of chest pain unresponsive to morphine and β blockers
- Stuttering pattern of pain indicating continued ischemia
- Moderate to severe CHF or pulmonary edema complicating acute MI and PCWP >20 mm Hg

Contraindications include

- Hypovolemia
- Inferior infarction. Nitroglycerin is used cautiously only when needed to manage post-infarction angina and/or pulmonary edema, since hypotension may be precipitated
- Right ventricular infarction
- Cardiac tamponade
- Significant hypoxemia. IV nitroglycerin may accentuate hypoxemia by increasing ventilation perfusion mismatch

Adverse Effects. These include worsening of hypoxemia and severe hypotension that may ↑ ischemia. Preload ↓ may cause hypotension. Rarely, nitrates precipitate bradycardia and hypotension responsive to atropine. Oral, cutaneous, and other nitrates, including interaction with heparin, are discussed further in Chapter 2. *Dosage:* See Infusion Pump Chart, Figure 2–9. Commence with a 5 μmg bolus injection then ↑ the dose by 5–10 μmg/min q 5 or 10 mins to abolish chest pain and/or to achieve a mean arterial pressure ↓ of 10% and a maximal ↓ of 20% in hypertensive patients. The systolic BP must not be allowed to fall under 95 mm Hg or diastolic <60 mm Hg. HR should be maintained <110/min. Nitrate tolerance develops after about 48 h use of IV nitroglycerin, but in unstable patients, the dose is titrated up as required rather than leaving a nitrate-free interval.

Lidocaine (Lignocaine, UK). In the first 24–48 h, VPCs and short runs of VT bear little relation to the occurrence of VF. R on T are an exception but usually appear <2 mins before VF. Lidocaine is far from completely effective in preventing VF, and inexperienced staff are often tempted quite unnecessarily to push the dose to toxic levels to "control" VPCs, which are, in the main, quite harmless.

Probable indications include

- Frequent VPCs, causing hemodynamic disturbance in the absence of bradycardia where atropine is advisable
- Sustained VT (see Fig. 6–4)
- Following VT occurring in the first 24 h of infarction, lidocaine is given for 48 h
- Post VF or for repetitive VF

Recent trials and meta-analysis suggest that prophylactic lidocaine may actually ↑ mortality because of its ability to cause asystole.

Contraindications include: Sinoatrial dysfunction, which may precipitate sinus arrest; A-V block, all grades, which can cause asystole; patients recovering from asystole; idioventricular rhythm; severe CHF; porphyria. Relative contraindications include sinus bradycardia.

The prophylactic use of lidocaine in acute MI remains controversial in the United States and its widespread use has been greatly curtailed. The drug is associated with a ↑ in the occurrence of asystole. In the early hours of infarction, VF occurs in approximately 5% of patients and many patients must be treated to prevent some episodes of VF. A meta-

Table 3–8
Lidocaine (Lignocaine) Dosage

	NORMAL DOSAGE E.G.: 60–90 KG PATIENT	HALVE DOSE: ELDERLY, CHF, SHOCK, HEPATIC DYSFUNCTION, CIMETIDINE, SOME BETA BLOCKERS, HALOTHANE
1st IV Bolus	1.5 mg/kg	0.75 mg/kg
usually	100 mg	50 mg
2nd Bolus	0.75 mg/kg	0.5 mg/kg
usually	50 mg	25 to 30 mg
Concomitant infusion	2 to 4 mg/min (50 μg/kg/min)	1 to 2 mg/minute (20 μg/kg/min)

Therapeutic level 1.5 to 5 μg/ml, 1.5 to 5 mg/L, 6 to 26 μmol/L
Seizures: levels >6 mg/L
* Hepatic metabolized beta blockers: propranolol, metoprolol

analysis of 14 randomized trials indicated that lidocaine reduced the incidence of VF 33% without a ↓ in mortality. In areas where facilities for monitoring cardiac rhythm and/or for defibrillation are lacking or inadequate, the drug has a role. In heavily monitored units, lidocaine is unnecessary, and the cost is not justified. *Dosage:* bolus IV 1.0–1.5 mg/kg, 75–100 mg over 5 mins, during which time a continuous infusion of 2 mg/min for a 70- to 80-kg patient < age 70 is commenced (see Table 3–8). An additional bolus of 50% of the original amount given 10 mins after the first bolus prevents a dip in plasma level below the therapeutic range, which commonly occurs 20–60 mins after starting the infusion. In the elderly, bolus 0.75 mg/kg, then if needed, 25–30 mg IV bolus. Do not allow a time lapse of minutes between the bolus and commencement of the infusion, as inadequate blood levels may ensue. Halve the dose in patients with CHF, shock, hepatic dysfunction, or concomitant use of a hepatic-metabolized β blocker or cimetidine (see Table 3–9).

If frequent multiform ventricular ectopy persists, resulting in hemodynamic disturbance, an additional bolus, 0.5–1 mg/kg, is given q 10 mins for 2 or 3 doses if deemed necessary, and the infusion rate is increased to 3 mg/min. Reevaluate the clinical situation, including serum K, magnesium, presence of bradycardia or sinus tachycardia, and contraindications, and factors that ↑ lidocaine toxicity prior to increasing the rate to a max 4 mg/min for a patient <200 lbs (90 kg). *Adverse Effects*. The incidence of asystole appears to be increased by lidocaine use. Confusion,

Table 3–9
Warnings to Avoid Lidocaine (Lignocaine) Toxicity

1. Reduce bolus dose and infusion rate in the elderly (over age 70)
2. Determine the dose utilizing lean body weight
3. Decrease the dose in heart failure, hypotension, cardiogenic shock
4. Decrease dosage with hepatic dysfunction or concomitant use of cimetidine, propranolol, or drugs that decrease hepatic blood flow or metabolism
5. Previous seizure activity or central nervous system disease
6. Determine blood levels if infusion rates are high (≥4 mg/ml/min) or neurologic adverse effects

seizures, drowsiness, dizziness, lip or tongue numbness, slurred speech, muscle twitching, double vision, tremor, altered consciousness, respiratory depression or arrest, complete heart block in patients with impaired A-V conduction, hypotension due to peripheral vasodilation.

Calcium Antagonists

In a very small study of 288 post-infarction patients treated with diltiazem, 11 patients died, as opposed to 9 patients in the placebo group; diltiazem decreased infarction rates at 2 weeks. This small, shortterm study has been used to advance the claim that diltiazem is the drug of choice in the management of non Q wave infarction. Physicians have extended the drug's use to other ischemic syndromes with the hope that the drug will prevent reinfarction, but without bearing in mind that the drug does not significantly ↓ the cardiac death rate.

A second large, well-run study of 2,466 post-infarction patients treated with diltiazem showed a ↑ in total mortality due to diltiazem in patients with LV dysfunction. Thus, diltiazem is not recommended in acute MI, Q wave or non Q wave, if signs of LV dysfunction are present or if the EF is <40% (Fig. 3–2). There was a trend in favor of a ↓ in total events (death and/or reinfarction) in the small number of patients with non Q wave infarction treated for 1 year with diltiazem, but the evidence from this overall negative study is not sound enough to recommend diltiazem to all patients with non Q wave infarction. In the absence of ongoing chest pain, diltiazem has an uncertain role in the management of non Q wave infarction in patients with good LV function, who are unable to take a β-blocking drug and in whom further interventional therapy in the form of angioplasty or bypass surgery is contraindicated because of underlying ill health or age (see Chap. 4).

It is clear that Ca antagonists have no role in the routine management of acute MI. Meta-analysis indicates that this group of drugs does not significantly ↓ infarct size, infarction rates, or mortality in patients with acute MI. Nifedipine used without a β-blocking drug in patients with unstable angina may ↑ chest pain and shows no beneficial trend in mortality. Dihydropyridines should be avoided in patients with acute MI since they may ↑ HR and vasodilation may cause a ↓ in BP. Also, Ca antagonists may ↓ BP during the early hours of infarction. A ↓ in BP may contraindicate the use of lifesaving medications: β blockers, thrombolytic agents, IV nitroglycerin, and/or ACE inhibitors.

Verapamil should not be used in patients with acute MI because of its negative inotropic effect and strong propensity to precipitate CHF, sinus arrest, or asystole. The drug is advisable in selected patients with SVT or AF with an uncontrolled ventricular response after a trial of β blockers or digoxin in the absence of CHF.

Diltiazem is not indicated in acute MI since it increases mortality in patients who manifest LV dysfunction or in those with an EF <40%. Ca antagonists are not advisable in patients with acute MI and concomitant, severe COPD since these agents may ↑ hypoxemia.

Suggested Reading

The GUSTO Investigators. An international randomized trial comparing four thrombolytic strategies for acute myocardial infarction. N Engl J Med, *329*:673–682, 1993

ISIS-3 (Third International Study of Infarct Survival) Collaborative

Group: A randomised comparison of streptokinase vs. tissue plasminogen activator vs. anistreplase and of aspirin plus heparin vs. aspirin alone among 41,299 cases of suspected acute myocardial infarction. Lancet *339*:953, 1992

Khan, M Gabriel: Acute myocardial infarction. *In* Cardiac and Pulmonary Management. Philadelphia, Lea & Febiger, 1993

MacIsaac AE, Thomas JD, Topol EJ: Toward the Quiescent Coronary Plaque. J Am Coll Cardiol *22*:1228, 1993

Complications of Myocardial Infarction and Post-Infarction Care

4

M. Gabriel Khan

Knowledge of the probable outcome after MI is important in formulating an appropriate plan of management, as with Q wave versus non Q wave infarction. Acute MI in-hospital mortality is about 12–14% (Table 4–1). However, several characteristics alter the in-hospital and post-discharge mortality

- Age >70
- Prior MI, angina, or CHF is associated with a twofold or more ↑ in mortality
- Uncomplicated Q wave infarct with the absence of even mild CHF has a 7–8% mortality
- Non Q infarcts, in contrast to Q wave infarction, have a lower in-hospital mortality (about 2%) but a threefold higher incidence of reinfarction within the following 3 months, and angina occurs in 33–66% of patients during the first year post discharge
- On admission to the hospital, 40–50% of patients with Q wave infarction have mild to moderate CHF and the presence of this complication carries a twofold early mortality. Table 4–2 gives comparison outcomes in acute Q wave and non Q wave infarction. Overall, increasing age beyond 70 and the degree of CHF or ↓ in EF that relates to the size of infarction are the most telling predictors. Thus, frank pulmonary edema during day 1 and 2 prior to discharge or an EF <30% is most unfavorable
- Recurrence of ischemic symptoms after day 1 represents an unstable state and carries a high mortality if not appropriately managed

The complications of MI determine prognosis. The outcome can be improved, however, by appropriate pharmacologic therapy and by angioplasty in properly selected patients. The complications of acute MI are listed in Table 4–3.

HEART FAILURE POST INFARCTION

Mild interstitial edema occurs in >40% of patients with acute MI and responds to bed rest, O_2, morphine, and judicious use of furosemide.

Furosemide. This agent is the most frequently used diuretic because it causes venous pooling and has a rapid diuretic effect. <u>Dosage:</u> 20–40 mg IV repeated with care to avoid K depletion suffices in the majority of patients. In those who were receiving diuretics prior to infarction, magnesium depletion must be assessed and corrected.

Diuretic therapy improves symptoms, but excessive volume depletion

Table 4–1
Acute Myocardial Infarction: Mortality Risk Stratification

		APPROXIMATE %		
PARAMETERS	IN HOSPITAL	1 YEAR	3 YEAR	5 YEAR
Overall mortality	12–14	10–15		33*
Uncomplicated				
Anterior infarction	12	15	33	
Inferior infarction	3	5	12	
Complicated				
Anterior infarction				
Moderate heart failure	30	50	60	
Cardiogenic shock	80			
Ejection fraction				
<30%	30	50	60	
30–40%	15	25		
40–50%	5	15		
>50%	3			
Previous infarct	25	30	50	
Post-infarction Angina (Day 2 to 10)	20	20		
Anterior infarct				
Age >70	25			
Age <50	7			

* Unchanged 1960 to 1969, 1970 to 1979; (1980–1990 not available)

Table 4–2
Comparison of Outcomes in Acute Q Wave and Non Q Wave Infarction

	APPROXIMATE %	
PARAMETERS	Q WAVE	NON Q WAVE
Incidence prehospital	>90	<10
Mortality prehospital	Very high	Low
Incidence in hospital	80	20†
In hospital mortality		
All patients	12 (18)	6 (9)
First infarction	10 (15)	3 (5)
Incidence of moderate/severe heart failure	>20	<1*
Incidence of arrhythmias	High	Low
Incidence of post-infarction angina (12 months)	<40	>60
Reinfarction <3 months	6	10; 16**

* Except if previous Q wave infarction
** Pooled data prior to the use of aspirin, beta blockers, and diltiazem
† 10% in GISSI-2
( ) Pooled data, 1962 to 1988, prior to thrombolytic therapy and general use of aspirin and beta blockers.

Table 4–3
Complications of Myocardial Infarction

1. Heart Failure
2. Cardiogenic Shock
3. Recurrent Ischemia
   (a) Angina
   (b) Reinfarction
4. Early Mechanical Complications
   (a) Freewall rupture
   (b) Interventricular septal rupture
   (c) Mitral regurgitation
5. Late Mechanical Complications
   (a) Aneurysm
6. Electrical
   (a) Ventricular fibrillation
   (b) Ventricular tachycardia other tachyarrhythmias
   (c) Bradyarrhythmias, complete heart block
7. Left Ventricular Thrombus/Embolism
8. Psychologic

stimulates the renin angiotensin system and may paradoxically ↑ myocardial wall stress. It is advisable, therefore, to use a small dose of diuretic along with an ACE inhibitor if larger doses of a diuretic are considered necessary in the management of CHF caused by LV dysfunction.

Morphine. Dosage: 4–8 mg IV at a rate of 1 mg/min. Repeat, if necessary, at a dose of 2–4 mg/min. It is important to allay anxiety. Patients at this stage may not complain bitterly of chest pain, but mild discomfort increases apprehension, which must be avoided. Morphine produces venous dilation and thus reduces preload. In addition, the drug has a modest but important effect on elevating VF threshold. Morphine should be avoided in patients with right ventricular infarction since all drugs that ↓ preload are contraindicated in this setting.

Patients with Mild CHF

About 25% of acute MI patients admitted are in this category and have about a 10% mortality. They do not require hemodynamic monitoring if they respond over a few hours to appropriate doses of furosemide and morphine. Some of these patients may require low-dose IV dobutamine via a peripheral vein, according to clinical status, before resorting to Swan-Ganz catheterization. In this subset of patients, if there is evidence of hypoperfusion with oliguria and/or a ↓ in systolic BP <100 mm Hg or a ↓ >30 mm from baseline, hemodynamic monitoring is necessary to guide pharmacologic intervention.

Patients with Severe CHF

The prompt insertion of a balloon flotation catheter with intensive hemodynamic monitoring is usually required. The choice of a pharmacologic agent based on hemodynamic parameters is indicated in Table 4–4. Figure 4–1 gives an algorithmic approach to management. Severe CHF, pulmonary edema with PCWP >22 mg Hg, and a low cardiac index <2.2 L/min/m^2 carries an in-hospital mortality of about 30%. Large doses of pharmacologic agents and combination therapy are usually required

Table 4–4
Choice of Pharmacologic Agents in Patients with Acute Myocardial Infarction Based on Hemodynamic Parameters

DRUG EFFECT	FUROSEMIDE	IV NITRATES	DOBUTAMINE	DOPAMINE	NITROPRUSSIDE	ACE INHIBITORS
Preload	↓	↓	—	↑	↓	↓
Afterload	—	minimal ↓	minimal ↓	↑	↓	↓
Sinus tachycardia	No	Yes	minimal	Yes	Yes	No, minimal
Parameters						
Moderate heart failure PCWP ≥20 >24	Yes	Yes	Yes, if BP >70	Yes, if BP <70 and oliguria (on dobutamine)	BP >110 and >6h* post infarction	Oral maintenance weaning nitroprusside
Severe heart failure PCWP >24 Cardiac index >2.5 L/min/m²	Yes	Yes if BP >95	Yes if BP >70	Yes if BP <70‡	CI <6h	Yes
Cardiogenic shock if BP <95 PCWP >18 Cardiac Index <2.5 L/min/m²	CI	CI	Yes IABP	Yes	CI	RCI**
Right ventricular infarction JVP ↑	CI	CI	Useful with titrated volume infusion	Relative CI ↑ PA pressure	CI	CI

Yes = useful; ↓ = decrease; — = no change; ↑ = increase; BP = systolic blood pressure mm Hg; * = Coronary steal during ischemic phase of infarction; ** = See text; PCWP = Pulmonary capillary wedge pressure; IABP = Intra-aortic balloon pump; RCI = Relative contraindication; CI = Contraindication; ‡ = Dopamine, dobutamine combination

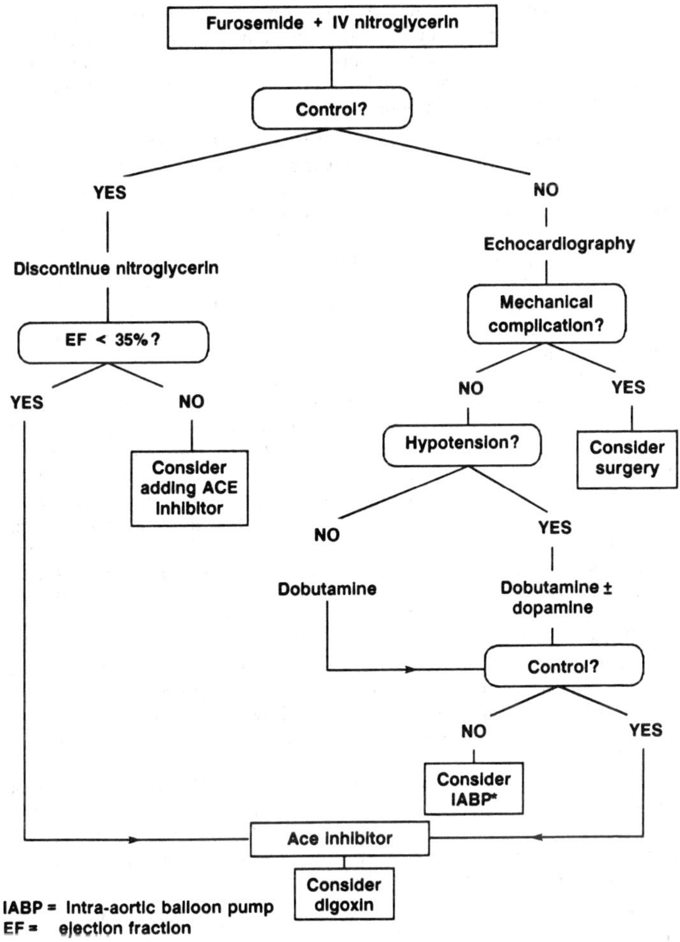

Figure 4–1. Management of moderate to severe heart failure: acute myocardial infarction in sinus rhythm

- Furosemide IV ≥80 mg, in repeated doses if pulmonary edema is present with the wedge pressure >24 mm Hg. The subsequent development of hypotension following an IV bolus of furosemide should alert the physician to the possibility of hypovolemia secondary to the diuretic or to the presence of right ventricular infarction. Care is required in some patients with severe CHF and concomitant cardiogenic shock to maintain a wedge pressure as high as 24 mm Hg provided that fulminant pulmonary edema is absent
- IV nitroglycerin is commenced if the systolic BP is >100 mm Hg, PCWP is >20, and right atrial pressure is increased in the absence of right ventricular infarction. Titrate the dose to attain an optimal wedge pressure of 14–18 mm Hg without causing a ↓ in systolic BP below 95 mm Hg or 10% from baseline (Table 2–8)

- A ↓ in BP is best managed with the use of dobutamine in combination with nitroglycerin. Other inotropes carry no advantages over dobutamine; if severe hypotension is present, dopamine is added, but amrinone or milrinone IV may be given a trial if severe hypotension is not present (see Cardiogenic Shock)

Digoxin may ↑ O_2 demand, but in this situation with known high mortality, there is little reason to withhold digoxin. The area of infarction is a necrotic zone and there is no evidence to support the notion that digoxin increases infarct size. Improvement in cardiac function and hemodynamics may have a salutary effect on the peripheral ischemic zone. The concern of increasing infarct size is irrelevant if severe CHF persists on the second day post infarction in the absence of recurrent chest pain or ECG signs of worsening ischemia. Digoxin is usually not advisable within the first 12 h of infarction, when the risk of ischemia and arrhythmia is at its highest.

If the echocardiogram shows no mechanical defect or tamponade, digoxin is advisable for the management of severe CHF or pulmonary edema. Also, when the patient is weaned off dobutamine, the action of digoxin is manifest. Patients with severe CHF often require digoxin along with ACE inhibitors on discharge (Fig. 4–1). Although the effect of digoxin on longterm survival post MI remains controversial, the risk of precipitating an arrhythmia with digoxin is low, as long as the serum K is maintained in the normal range. In patients who have been previously treated with diuretics, magnesium depletion may be a problem, and this should be addressed. <u>*Dosage:*</u> Digoxin IV is not normally required, except where AF with a fast ventricular response requires control. With sinus rhythm and severe CHF, give orally 0.5 mg immediately, then 0.25 mg at bedtime in patients < age 70 with normal renal function and in the absence of conditions in which there is an increased sensitivity to digoxin (see Table 5–3). Follow with 0.25 mg qd. In patients > age 70 and those with slight elevation of serum creatinine, 1.3–2.3 mg/dl (115–203 μmul/l), the maintenance dose should be reduced to 0.125 mg qd after the second day (see Chap. 5). Digoxin is particularly useful in post-infarction patients who have systolic BP ≤100 mm Hg. In these patients, nitrates or ACE inhibitors may further ↓ systolic BP and preload, causing decreased coronary and cerebral perfusion that may induce ischemia or presyncope.

ACE Inhibitors. In accordance with the SOLVD and SAVE trials, ACE inhibitors have appropriately assumed a major role in the acute and chronic management of patients with post-infarction CHF. These agents produce symptomatic improvement and also prevent the recurrence of CHF in patients with poor systolic function and an EF <40%. They cause a modest ↓ in mortality in patients with CHF with chronic IHD when used in conjunction with digoxin and diuretics (see Chap. 5).

The renin angiotensin system is activated during the early hours of MI and appears to be an important compensatory mechanism that serves to maintain BP. The arterial vasoconstrictor effect of angiotensin II causes an unnecessarily greater ↑ in afterload and ventricular wall stress, which initiates and perpetuates ventricular enlargement and an associated change in geometry with consequent further LV dysfunction. ACE inhibitors have been shown to attenuate these processes. Their effect on post-infarction ventricular remodeling provides salutary effects, even in the absence of CHF, and may result in the ↓ of cardiac mortality among patients with LV dysfunction.

ACE inhibitors are indicated during recovery from acute MI if mild CHF persists beyond day 3 and if not completely controlled with furosemide, morphine, and nitrates. ACE inhibitors should be given to virtually all patients who have severe CHF or pulmonary edema. ACE inhibitors must be used with caution, however, in patients who develop post-infarction angina or other manifestations of worsening ischemia because coronary artery perfusion beyond a critical stenosis may be reduced by these and other vasodilators.

Captopril. Dosage: 6.25 mg test dose or 3 mg if the BP is marginal. If there is no ↓ in BP and the systolic BP remains >110 mm Hg, give 6.25 mg tid. The dose may be slowly increased over the next week to 12.5 mg bid or tid. The majority of post-infarct patients require 25–75 mg of captopril or the equivalent dose of enalapril to achieve beneficial effects without adverse side effects of hypotension and presyncope, which are easily precipitated by the addition of nitroglycerin or oral nitrates. The benefits of afterload ↓ must be weighed against the risk of too dramatic a ↓ in BP and preload with consequent deleterious effects on coronary perfusion. Importantly, diastolic dysfunction is a feature of large infarcts and right ventricular infarction. In these settings, ACE inhibitors, nitrates, or other preload-reducing agents do not improve ventricular function and may be hazardous, especially in patients with right ventricular infarction. The dosage for enalapril is given in Chapter 5. Contraindications and interactions of ACE inhibitors are discussed in Chapter 1.

Intubation. Patients who manifest florid pulmonary edema and respond poorly to furosemide and IV nitroglycerin, with an arterial PO_2 <50 or PCO_2 >50 mm Hg, require mechanical ventilation and PEEP in addition to the other measures described. Caution: PEEP may ↓ cardiac output and precipitate hypotension.

CARDIOGENIC SHOCK

There are 2 hemodynamic subsets of pump failure and patients may move from one subset to another.

The clinical spectrum of pump failure and shock embraces

- Poor peripheral perfusion with cold cyanotic extremities
- Obtundation
- Oliguria
- Weak pulse
- Cuff systolic BP range
  Subset I—>100 mm Hg, LV filling pressure >15 mm Hg, CI <2.5 L/min/m^2
  Subset II—<90 mm Hg
- Patients with systolic pressures between 90 and 100 mm Hg may move toward Subset I or Subset II and close hemodynamic monitoring is necessary
- Symptoms and signs of LV failure

Salient therapeutic measures include

- Define LV filling pressure to exclude volume depletion
- If the LV filling pressure is <15 mm Hg, give a rapid IV fluid challenge over a very short period to ↑ the filling pressure to the range 18–23 mm Hg. A prolonged infusion must be avoided, as it can worsen pulmonary congestion without increasing LV filling pressure appreciably

If volume depletion and preload-reducing factors are excluded, management must rapidly progress to

- Stabilization of BP with dobutamine 2–10 μg/kg/min and/or dopamine 3–15 μg/kg/min (see Fig. 4–2, infusion pump charts, and Tables 4–5 and 4–6). Failure to stabilize the patient should prompt consideration of IABP and urgent coronary angiograms with a view to coronary angioplasty. This procedure has been shown to improve survival in patients with cardiogenic shock
- In patients with mechanical complications, relieving the load on the LV with afterload-reducing agents but without decreasing BP and perfusion to vital areas

Nitroglycerin has advantages over nitroprusside during the early hours of infarction since, at this stage, ischemia is often present. The drug is reserved for selected cases where continued ischemia is suspected of causing progression of infarction or LV dysfunction.

The drug reduces preload, which may be beneficial in some patients with severe pulmonary congestion but in whom BP is reasonably well maintained. However, patients with pump failure and severe shock may have deleterious effects from too great a ↓ in preload. Higher doses also ↓ afterload. Thus, careful hemodynamic monitoring is essential when using pharmacologic agents that alter both preload and afterload. _Dosage:_ Commence with 5 μg/min via pump-controlled infusion (see Nitroglycerin Infusion Pump Chart, Table 2–18). Increase by 5 μg/min q 10 mins. Do not allow a ↓ in systolic BP >10 mm Hg. The systolic BP should not ↓ to <90 mm Hg. If nitroglycerin alone causes improvement in the pump failure/shock syndrome, achieving an acceptable ↑ in cardiac output, continue the infusion for 24–48 h. During this period, therapy with an ACE inhibitor is introduced. If hypotension persists or worsens and preload is high, ↓ the nitroglycerin infusion and add dobutamine 2–5 μg/kg/min (Table 4–5). If the preload is low or BP decreases more precipitously, dopamine should replace dobutamine.

Dobutamine. _Dosage:_ 2–10.0 μg/kg/min, titrated to achieve a desired inotropic effect directed by several measurements of CO, A-V O_2 content difference, urine output and mentation (see Infusion Pump Chart, Table 4–5). Dobutamine should not be used alone in the severely hypotensive patient. Usually, if a dose >4–6 μg/kg/min is required and unacceptable hypotension exists, dopamine infusion is commenced at 5 μg/kg/min and dobutamine 4–6 μg/kg/min titrated up to a suggested max of 10 μg/kg/min of each agent. Occasionally, dobutamine titrated to a max of 20 μg/kg/min is necessary, especially if LV filling pressure exceeds 24 mm Hg, a situation in which dopamine is relatively contraindicated. Thus, if the systolic BP is <70 mm Hg and PCWP is >24 mm Hg, a combination of dobutamine and norepinephrine is indicated.

Dopamine. _Dosage:_ 2.5–10 μg/kg/min via a central line (see Infusion Pump Chart, Table 4–6). Dopamine at a dose of 0.5–4 μg/kg/min causes cardiac β stimulation and also stimulates renal dopaminergic receptors producing renal arteriolar dilation and a ↑ in urinary output. A dose of 4–6 μg/kg/min is initially advised if severe hypotension is present. At doses >4 μg/kg/min, beneficial renal effects are lost, and mainly alpha-adrenergic vasoconstriction occurs with minimal β stimulation that causes a ↑ in HR, CO, and BP. A dose >5 μg/kg/min is often required to raise systemic BP in severely hypotensive patients. In patients with cardiogenic shock, a dose >15 μg/kg/min without added dobutamine is seldom advisable, because at this dose, only marked alpha vasoconstriction occurs. It must be emphasized that while the combination

Table 4–5
Dobutamine Infustion Pump Chart (dobutamine 2 amps (500 mg) in 500 ml (1000 μg/ml))

WEIGHT (kg)	40	45	50	55	60	65	70	75	80	85	90	95	100	105
DOSAGE (μg/kg/min)							RATE (ml/hr)							
1.0	2	3	3	3	4	4	4	5	5	5	5	6	6	6
1.5	4	4	5	5	5	6	6	7	7	8	8	9	9	9
2.0	5	5	6	7	7	8	8	9	10	10	11	11	12	13
2.5	6	7	8	8	9	10	11	11	12	13	14	14	15	16
3.0	7	8	9	10	11	12	13	14	14	15	16	17	18	19
3.5	8	9	11	12	13	14	15	16	17	18	19	20	21	22
4.0	10	11	12	13	14	16	17	18	19	20	22	23	24	25
4.5	11	12	14	15	16	18	19	20	22	23	24	26	27	28
5.0	12	14	15	17	18	20	21	23	24	26	27	29	30	32
5.5	13	15	17	18	20	21	23	25	26	28	30	31	33	35
6.0	14	16	18	20	22	23	25	27	29	31	32	34	36	38
7.0	17	19	21	23	25	27	29	32	34	36	38	40	42	44
8.0	19	22	24	26	29	31	34	36	38	41	43	46	48	50
9.0	22	24	27	30	32	35	38	41	43	46	49	51	54	57
10.0	24	27	30	33	36	39	42	45	48	51	54	57	60	63
12.5	30	34	38	41	45	49	53	56	60	64	68	71	75	79
15.0	36	41	45	50	54	59	63	69	72	77	81	86	90	95
20.0	48	54	60	66	72	78	84	90	96	102	108	114	120	126

The above rates apply only for 1000 mg/l concentration of dobutamine. If a diff. rent concentration must be used, appropriate adjustments in rates should be made. Usual dose range 2.5–10 μg/kg/min.
From: Khan M Gabriel: Cardiac Drug Therapy. 3rd Ed. London, W.B. Saunders, 1992.

Table 4–6
Dopamine Infusion Chart
Dopamine (800 mg) in 500 ml 5% Dextrose/water
Use chart for: pump (ml/hour) *or*
microdrip (drops/minute)

Example: 60 kg patient at 4.0 μg/kg/minute
—pump—set pump at 9 ml/hour
—microdrip—run solution at 9 drops/minute

WEIGHT (kg)	40	50	60	70	80	90	100
DOSAGE (μg/kg/min)			RATE: ml/hour (pump)				
1.0	1.5	1.9	2.3	2.6	3	3.4	3.8
2.0	3	3.8	4.5	5.3	6	6.8	7.5
3.0	4.5	5.6	6.8	7.9	9	10.1	11.3
4.0	6	7.5	9	10.5	12	13.5	15
5.0	7.5	9.4	11.3	13.1	15	16.9	18.8
6.0	9	11.3	13.5	15.8	18	20.3	22.5
7.0	10.5	13.1	15.8	18.4	21	23.6	26.3
8.0	12	15	18	21	24	27	30
9.0	13.5	16.9	20.3	23.6	27	30.4	33.8
10.0	15	18.8	22.5	26.3	30	33.8	37.5
12.0	18	22.5	27	31.5	36	40.5	45
15.0	22.5	28.1	33.8	39.4	45	50.6	56.3
20.0	30	37.5	45	52.5	60	67.5	75

of dopamine (6–10 μg/kg/min) and dobutamine (2–10 μg/kg/min) has several merits, dosages of either drug >10 μg/kg/min have major disadvantages. If >15 μg/kg/min is required and the systolic or diastolic BP remains very low, with a PCWP >24 mm Hg, dopamine should be discontinued and norepinephrine infusion 2–10 μg/min should be tried in combination with dobutamine. Provided that filling pressures are adequate (>18 mm Hg), failure of dopamine 15 μg/kg/min to raise systolic pressure to >80 mm Hg, or diastolic >60 mm Hg, or both necessitates the addition of norepinephrine; max suggested dose is 20 μg/kg/min. The IABP is preferred if the decision is made to proceed with interventional therapy.

Nitroprusside. The drug is a powerful afterload-reducing agent and has a role, especially when the systolic BP is in the range of 100–120 mm Hg, in the presence of pump failure/shock syndrome. The drug can replace nitroglycerin in patients presenting with pump failure/shock syndrome after 8 h of infarction if ischemia is not present and afterload ↓ is considered necessary. The drug may cause a coronary steal and may have a deleterious effect when administered within 8 h of onset of chest pain. *Dosage:* Commence with 0.4 μg/kg/min with close monitoring of arterial pressure, ↑ the infusion given by infusion pump, and titrate the dosage in increments of 0.2 μg/kg/min q 2–5 mins (Table 1–10). A dose of ≤3 μg/kg/min should suffice to achieve salutary hemodynamic effects. (See Chap. 1 for further details.)

RIGHT VENTRICULAR INFARCTION

Right ventricular infarction is usually associated with inferoposterior infarction and, where present, frequently causes right-sided pump failure/shock. Approximately 25% of patients with inferior infarction show varying degrees of right ventricular infarction, but only those with a large affected area develop the characteristic signs. The diagnostic hallmarks of right ventricular infarction are given in Table 4–7.

Patients with extensive right ventricular infarction are very sensitive to volume depletion, and titrated volume infusion should be tried. The right ventricle is unable to deliver adequately the venous return to the left ventricle, however, and the reduced LV preload results in decreased systemic output. Thus, volume infusion is often partially or even completely ineffective but must be tried judiciously

Table 4–7
Right Ventricular Infarction

1. High jugular venous pressure with clear lung fields (exclude tamponade)
2. Kussmaul's sign present >90%
3. a) ECG evidence of inferoposterior infarct
   b) ST segment depresion V_1, V_2, or elevation in V_4 R
4. PCWP normal
5. Right atrial and right ventricular pressure >10 mm Hg
6. *Ratio right atrial to PCWP >0.8

* Present in <33% of patients
PCWP = Pulmonary capillary wedge pressure

- Dobutamine infusion should be commenced at 2 μg/kg/min and increased to a max of 10 μg/kg/min if needed (Table 4–5)
- Failure to respond to volume replacement and dobutamine is a strong indication for the use of IABP
- Sublingual or IV nitroglycerin is contraindicated in patients with right ventricular infarction since ↓ in preload must be avoided
- Nitroprusside, as well as diuretics and ACE inhibitors, ↓ preload and are not recommended
- Dopamine increases pulmonary vascular resistance and may ↑ right ventricular pump failure. Dobutamine is thus superior to dopamine in patients with right ventricular infarction, although the hypotensive effect may limit the dose that can be tolerated

POST-INFARCTION ANGINA

Definite post-infarction angina occurring after day 1 to discharge associated with ECG changes and correctly interpreted as due to worsening ischemia is an indication for coronary angiography with consideration of CABS or angioplasty. Careful selection of patients for this investigation, based on a diagnosis formulated by an experienced cardiologist or team, is essential to avoid a reflex angiographic rush to see the lesion.

Consider and exclude

- Pericarditis
- Esophagogastric origin of pain due to stress ulceration, esophagitis, and the effects of aspirin in individuals with sensitive stomachs
- Some patients with a stuttering pattern of pain due to ischemia or reinfarction respond readily to β-adrenergic blockers and/or IV nitroglycerin. In patients categorized at high risk for surgery, administration of tPA should be considered (see Chap. 3, thrombolytic therapy)

In the TIMI Phase 2 Trial, the incidence of coronary angiography for presumed post-infarction ischemia in tertiary and community hospitals was 48%, versus 32% that resulted in a greater frequency of angioplasty and bypass surgery, with no difference observed in end points of reinfarction or death at 40 days and 1 year. The results of TIMI 2 indicate that the conservative strategy adopted in the community hospitals using thrombolysis during the early hours of acute MI resulted in a significantly lower number of invasive procedures being done than in the tertiary care setting, with no apparent deleterious consequences.

The surgical mortality and survival of patients with post-infarction angina with an EF >50% are as good as those observed with elective surgery. When the EF is <35% and perhaps as low as 25%, CABS is preferred over angioplasty if the ischemic syndrome persists and lesions of the left main, triple vessel or double vessel, with proximal LAD are observed on angiography.

EARLY VENTRICULAR ARRHYTHMIAS

The mechanism of early infarction arrhythmias includes

- Disturbances of impulse generation/enhanced automaticity
- Disturbances of impulse conduction/reentry, focal conduction slowing

- Increased sympathetic and parasympathetic tone is a commonly prominent feature that influences the above underlying mechanisms

Precipitating factors are

- Ischemia with associated tissue acidosis and local ↑ in extracellular K concentration
- Catecholamine release: May induce arrhythmia as well as ↑ ischemia. Arrhythmias worsen ischemia and vice versa. Thus, a dynamic interplay perpetuates ventricular arrhythmias that may terminate in VF
- Hypokalemia from prior use of diuretics or induced by verapamil
- Hypomagnesemia due to diuretic use
- Hypoxemia
- Respiratory or metabolic acidosis or alkalosis
- Severe CHF probably related to extensive infarction

Ventricular Premature Contraction

VPCs occurring during the first 6 h of infarction and requiring therapy are managed with lidocaine (see Chap. 6).

During the later hospital phase, frequent VPCs (>10/h multifocal beats or couplets) may ↑ risk, but there is only limited evidence that antiarrhythmic therapy, other than β-blocking agents, prolongs life in these patients. The CAST indicated a ↑ in mortality among these patients with the use of flecainide and encainide. Patients with this category of arrhythmia should be given a β-adrenergic blocking agent such as metoprolol or timolol (propranolol in non-smokers) if there is no contraindication to the use of this class of drug. A study has shown improved survival among high-risk patients treated with amiodarone, but this finding requires confirmation (see Chap. 6).

Sustained Ventricular Tachycardia

- VT asymptomatic or mild symptoms with the pulse present occurring during the first 24 h of MI (rare at this time): Give lidocaine (lignocaine) IV 100 mg bolus. IV lidocaine infusion 2–3 mg/min is given for a time after conversion without waiting for recurrence (Fig. 6–4). If the drug is ineffective and the patient is hemodynamically stable, give procainamide IV 100 mg bolus at the rate of 20 mg/min and then 10 mg/min; max 24 mg/min not to exceed 1 g during the first hour. Procainamide has a negative inotropic effect and is not recommended for patients who manifest CHF or with EF <40%. The drug is, therefore, reserved for patients who fail to respond to lidocaine or who have recurrent VT but who remain hemodynamically stable
- The cardioverter should be prepared and connected to the patient while drug therapy is in progress
- Failure to control with lidocaine or procainamide requires synchronized cardioversion (see Fig. 6–4)
- Any breakthrough should be treated by adding a β blocker (if not already being administered) and, if needed, IV amiodarone 300 mg in 20 mins, preferably via a central vein followed by 50 mg/h for 6–12 h, then 30 mg/h if stable (see Chap. 6). IV amiodarone may cause hypotension and caution is required. With the availability of IV amiodarone, which is effective and has good tolerability, the use of bretylium has appropriately dwindled. If amiodarone IV is not available and VT or VF recurs, give bretylium, 5 mg/kg undiluted, rapidly as an IV bolus. Electrical defibrillation is then carried out. If VF persists,

bretylium dosage is increased to 10 mg/kg and repeated, if needed. *Caution:* IV bretylium has not been shown to be superior to lidocaine. Bretylium causes severe hypotension, and epinephrine or norepinephrine must not be used concomitantly. Most early ventricular arrhythmias settle down, and lidocaine is stopped after about 24 h
- VT no pulse present or hemodynamically unstable: Chest pain, shortness of breath, clouding of consciousness or obtundation, treat as VF (Fig. 6–4)

Supraventricular Arrhythmias

AF in acute MI is often precipitated by

- Large infarction of the atrium
- Chronic atrial enlargement
- CHF with atrial dilation
- Acute mitral regurgitation
- Increase catecholamines
- Acute pericarditis
- Hypoxemia
- Inferior infarction more commonly than anterior infarction, with occlusion of the right coronary or circumflex artery

Acute AF occurs within the first few hours of infarction in approximately 3% of patients and is often of short duration, lasting <2, 4, and 24 h in 50, 75, and 95% of patients, respectively.

AF is observed during the first few days of infarction in ≤15% of patients, and in 10% the onset is prior to infarction.

Management of AF depends on the hemodynamic and pro-ischemic effect of a rapid or uncontrolled ventricular response

- Hemodynamic compromise requires immediate electrocardioversion
- Asymptomatic patients or patients with CHF with a moderate ventricular response and normal BP should be slowly digitalized
- Digoxin may not reach peak effect for 8–24 h depending on the dosing schedule, but a rapid-acting drug is not essential. Importantly, the other available agents are hazardous in this setting
- Patients not in prominent CHF with systolic BP >110 mm Hg and rates of 120–150/min can be managed with a β-blocking drug. A fast rate of 140–160/min not causing hemodynamic compromise should respond to metoprolol or ultra-short-acting esmolol (see Table 3–4 for dosage)

The Ca antagonist verapamil slows the ventricular response, but the negative inotropic effect is more prominent than that of titrated small doses of esmolol or metoprolol and is not advisable in acute infarction unless the use of a β blocker is absolutely contraindicated by severe asthma.

Bradyarrhythmias

Early-occurring sinus bradycardia, symptomatic or associated with hypotension usually with rates <45/min, should be managed with atropine. Similarly, 2nd° or 3rd° A-V block occurring during the first few hours after onset of MI often responds to this agent. Patients with asystole should be given atropine.

Atropine. *Dosage:* 0.4–0.6 mg IV repeated if needed q 5 or 10 mins to a max of 2 mg. *Caution:* Rapid injection or too large a dose may cause unwanted sinus tachycardia and rarely VF. Dosage for asystole: 1 mg IV repeated in 2–5 mins during which CPR should continue. Total dose: 2.5 mg over 30 mins. In the latter situation, a large dose given promptly is essential, without concern for tachycardia causing increased myocardial O_2 demand. See Chapter 6.

Recommendations for Temporary Pacemaker Post Infarction

Indications include

- Asystolic episodes
- Complete heart block, unless escape rhythm is present >60/min and hemodynamics are good
- RBBB with left anterior or left posterior hemiblock or LBBB developing during acute infarction can be managed with external pacer with chest pads on standby
- Mobitz Type 2 2nd° A-V block
- Mobitz Type 1 2nd° A-V block with hypotension or CHF (see Chap. 7 for further details)

Pacemaker electrode insertion is not indicated in

- 1st° A-V block
- Mobitz Type 1 2nd° A-V block with normal hemodynamics
- Accelerated idioventricular rhythm with A-V dissociation
- Bundle branch block known prior to the acute infarction

LATE VENTRICULAR ARRHYTHMIAS

It is advisable to obtain Holter recordings for all patients at 1–3 weeks post MI to assist in assessing the risk profile, especially if the EF is <40%. A 24- or 48-hour Holter study is indicated if the patient complains of palpitations, presyncope, syncope, or other symptoms. Holter monitoring is advisable in patients to document the presence of significant arrhythmia requiring consideration of drug therapy.

Late-occurring sustained VT is very ominous. Sustained VT or complex ventricular ectopy occurring during the weeks following infarction greatly increases the risk of sudden death. These potentially lethal arrhythmias require antifibrillary therapy.

Currently, it is not known what pharmacologic agent is best for post-MI patients at highest risk. Beta-adrenergic blockers are the only antiarrhythmic agents that have been proven to prevent cardiac death or sudden death. However, there is evidence from one study that amiodarone may improve survival rates.

The BASIS investigated the effects of prophylactic antiarrhythmic therapy in patients with asymptomatic complex ventricular arrhythmias post infarction. Low-dose amiodarone, 200 mg qd, was given over 1 year. Cumulative mortality rates were 13% in the control group, 5% in the amiodarone-treated group ($p < 0.05$), and 10% in the individually treated patients who were administered mexiletine, quinidine, propafenone, sotalol, disopyramide, or flecainide. (Treatment failures were given amiodarone.) Arrhythmic events were also reduced in the amiodarone group. In contrast with the beneficial effects of β-blocking agents and possibly for amiodarone, other antiarrhythmic agents have been shown to ↑ mortality. Flecanide and encainide caused a ↑ in cardiac mortality observed in the CAST.

The management of patients with late nonsustained VT, at least in short runs, or complex ventricular arrhythmias is presently unsatisfactory. Suggestive steps include

- If a β-blocking drug is being administered as routine β-blocker post-MI prophylaxis, the dose should be increased: e.g., 100 mg metoprolol, 160 mg propranolol, 20 mg timolol, and 50 mg atenolol qd should be increased to 300, 240, 30, or 150 mg qd, respectively. A change from one of the aforementioned β-blocking agents to sotalol, 240–480 mg qd, may be effective and should be given a trial
- If β blockers are ineffective, poorly tolerated, or are contraindicated because of asthma or very poor LV function, many cardiologists will go to amiodarone, oral or IV as appropriate, as the next choice because of the high frequency of failure with other drugs
- The third choice is mexiletine, which has a low proarrhythmic effect and a minimal negative inotropic action. The drug is, however, poorly effective

Amiodarone and other antiarrhythmic agents are used only under close supervision by using repeated Holter monitoring, and the usual precautions are observed when prescribing amiodarone (see Chap. 6). The combination of amiodarone and a β-blocking agent (except sotalol) has a role in patients with lethal arrhythmias, as discussed in Chapter 6. Failure of this trial therapy should prompt consideration of selecting alternative treatment

- A combination of antiarrhythmic agents guided by EP testing, although the recommendation of antiarrhythmic therapy has several limitations
- Rare surgical excision of focus
- Catheter ablative techniques
- An implantable cardioverter-defibrillator, which has antibradycardia pacing and algorithms for pace termination of VT (Chapter 7)

MECHANICAL COMPLICATIONS

Mechanical complications should be strongly suspected in patients who develop sudden hemodynamic deterioration especially from the second post-infarct day onward with no new ECG changes occurring. The incidence and associated mortality of these complications are given in Table 4–8.

Severe Acute Mitral Regurgitation. A transient mitral regurgitant murmur is often present with acute MI caused by papillary muscle dysfunction. Severe acute MR is uncommon, however, occurring in <3% of patients with acute MI, and is usually due to

- Papillary muscle rupture: Partial rupture of the tip or rarely the trunk
- Rupture of the chordae tendineae
- Strongly suspect severe MR in the presence of acute inferior infarction on the second to fifth days in patients with pulmonary edema and/or hemodynamic deterioration developing out of proportion to the ECG changes. An EF in the normal range is typical of regurgitant flow. The posterior papillary muscle is most commonly affected with infero-posterior infarction

Table 4–8
Acute Myocardial Infarction-Mechanical Complications Incidence, Timing and Mortality

	% OF TOTAL ACUTE INFARCTS	INCIDENCE & TIMING	% OF TOTAL RUPTURE	% OF TOTAL IN-HOSPITAL MORTALITY	TYPE OF INFARCT
Cardiac rupture	3–10	Up to 50%; 2–3 days Up to 40%; day 1		20	
Free wall	2–8	10%; days 4–7 25%; day 1	85	15	
Papillary muscle rupture	1	75%; 3–5 days 25%; day 1–2 or 6–10	5	5	Commonly infero-posterior
Ventricular septal rupture	1–3	75%; 3–5 days 25%; 1–2 or 6–14	10	1–4	60% anterior 40% inferior
Severe mitral regurgitation	2%	1–5 days			
LV aneurysm	10–15	3 months			90% anterior 10% inferior

Echocardiography with continuous wave Doppler flow study has an important role

- If the Doppler flow study is in keeping with severe MR, proceed with catheterization. Large V waves on pulmonary capillary wedge and severe MR are observed on left ventriculography
- Patients with severe acute MR due to papillary muscle or chordal rupture require surgery. IABP provides support if needed during catheterization and to the operating room
- Patients with papillary muscle dysfunction and severe MR who are not hypotensive are managed with afterload-reducing agents. IV nitroglycerin has a role in relieving ischemia as well as reducing preload and causes minimal afterload ↓. Dobutamine and the use of IABP may be necessary to support BP where needed while considering interventional therapy

Ventricular Septal Rupture occurs in 1–3% of patients with acute MI

- Echocardiography should confirm the diagnosis, and right-sided catheterization with oximetry should show an O_2 step-up in the right ventricle
- The degree of hemodynamic compromise and the general health and age of the patient dictate the urgency and selection of pharmacologic and interventional therapies. Patients often come through angioplasty without problems on the IABP. Mortality exceeds 80% with medical therapy

- Surgery should not be delayed for some weeks, as was formerly recommended, in patients in whom the IABP produces some stability. This improvement is usually temporary, and although surgical mortality is high, repair of the lesion that is causing hemodynamic compromise gives the only hope of survival. Some centers use intraoperative angiography or angioscopy to define coronary occlusions for added management with CABS

Pericarditis. Approximately 40% of fatal MI show acute fibrinous pericarditis. The incidence of clinical pericarditis ranges from 5 to 25%. Pericarditis usually manifests during the second and fifth day post infarction, localized in the area overlying the infarct, but may diffusely involve the pericardial sac. Approximately 50% are symptomatic

- Discontinue heparin if pericarditis is proven
- Treatment is indicated for pain even when no friction rub is present
- Aspirin in full doses, 650 mg tid, is useful; NSAIDs should be avoided because indomethacin and similar agents may cause vasoconstriction and alter myocardial healing and appear to ↑ the incidence of myocardial rupture. Also, these agents cause retention of Na and water
- Pericarditis presenting between 2 and 6 months of infarction occurs in <0.1% of patients. Fever, increased sedimentation rate, and increased titer of heart reactive antibodies may be present; NSAIDs are best avoided because they cause vasoconstriction and ↑ stress on the myocardium
- Late pericarditis is treated with aspirin. Failure to respond or relapses should be managed with a short course of prednisone with aspirin overlapping ≥2 weeks before prednisone is withdrawn

PREDISCHARGE EXERCISE TEST

The ACC/AHA Task Force Report 1990 states that the best time to obtain the exercise test depends on patient characteristics, physician preference, departmental policies, and local laboratory expertise. The report adds that maximal exercise testing at 3 weeks post-infarction is a cost-effective alternative to submaximal predischarge testing on days 7–14 and can be used for evaluation of functional capacity as well as prognostication. Timing and relevance of post-infarction exercise stress testing is given in Table 4–9.

The Task Force emphasizes that a 10- to 14-day predischarge test does not allow for the early sixth- to seventh-day discharge of patients with uncomplicated infarction. The report appropriately states that the safety of predischarge submaximal testing is less well established and only evaluates functional capacity in properly selected patients. Testing at 3 weeks has proven to be safe, and the 10- to 14-day delay caused in patients with uncomplicated infarction appears to be associated with rare instances of intercurrent death or reinfarction. In one study of 1,000 patients, using 3-week testing, 0.5% sustained a cardiac event: Reinfarction occurred in 5 patients and cardiac death in 2 between the tenth day and 3 weeks. However, treadmill-induced deaths, although rare, tend to occur prior to 14 days post infarction. The results of a 3-week test can be correlated with that of several well documented studies

- Patients who complete ≥6 METs (1 MET equals the amount of O_2 used at rest) and experience no ECG ischemic changes have a <3% 1-year mortality

Table 4–9
Timing and Relevance of Post-Infarction Exercise Stress Testing

PARAMETERS	6–7 DAYS	10–14 DAYS	3 WEEKS
Function test	Yes	Yes	Yes
Prolongs hospital stay >7 days	No	Yes	Not applicable
Requires very careful selection of patients	Yes	Yes	Not as stringent
Safety established	No	Somewhat	Yes
Standard for comparison	Not well established	Not well established	Yes
Confusion in interpretation	Yes	Yes	Little
Cost	High, 2 tests required*	2 tests required	Acceptable
Mainly low-risk group tested	Yes	Yes	Can test all grades if needed
Prognostic value	No (Probable in some)	No (Probable in some)	Yes: Attain ≥6 METS <3% 1-year mortality Attain ≤4 METS >12% 1 year mortality

* Predischarge and at 6 weeks

- Inability to complete a treadmill workload of 4 METs is associated with a sixfold ↑ in the risk of death or nonfatal reinfarction in the subsequent year
- Patients who fail to achieve peak systolic BP >110 mm Hg, increased systolic pressure >10 mm Hg from baseline, have a poor prognosis
- Patients who develop ≥2 mm ST segment depression persisting for >2 mins at a HR of <120/min, have poor coronary reserve and should be considered for urgent interventional therapy

These conclusions are applicable to tests performed at 3 or 6 weeks but are of limited relevance to submaximal tests performed at 6–14 days post infarction.

DISCHARGE MEDICATIONS

Beta Blockers. If β blockers were commenced during the early hours of MI and no adverse effects were apparent, the β blockers should be continued. If not given at that time, β blockers should be administered prior to discharge and maintained for ≥2 years. Studies indicate that this approach is highly beneficial and cost effective.

Clinical trials indicate an impressive 33% ↓ in mortality due to β-blocker therapy. Mortality ↓ with propranolol is significantly less than that observed with timolol in smokers. As emphasized in Chapter 2, the efficacy of hepatic-metabolized β blockers is blunted by cigarette smoking. It is necessary to prescribe metoprolol or timolol to refractory smokers.

If there is no contraindication to β blockade, virtually all post-MI patients should receive timolol, 10 mg bid, or acebutolol, 200 mg bid, or metoprolol, 100 mg bid. Propranolol, 180–240 mg qd, is advisable only in nonsmokers. The ACC/AHA Task Force recommends that treatment begin within the first few days of infarction and continue for ≥2 years in virtually all patients if there are no contraindications to β blockers.

It is estimated that 70% of post-infarction patients are suitable for β-blocker therapy. Up to 20% of post-infarction patients are unable to receive β blockers because of contraindications, and a further 10% have relative contraindications.

Contraindications to longterm β-adrenergic blockade include severe LV failure, systolic BP <100 mm Hg, heart rate <60/min, type I, II, or III A-V block, and asthma or severe COPD.

Some cardiologists do not prescribe β blockers to so-called "low-risk" patients. However, risks are not accurately assured by stress testing. Because β blockers are capable of producing about a 28% ↓ in reinfarction rates, up to a 67% ↓ in sudden death, and a 33% ↓ in mortality, it is advisable to prescribe these medications to virtually all patients who can tolerate the effects at the relatively low dosage indicated above. Acebutolol, metoprolol, and timolol, are better tolerated than propranolol and are preferred. If mild adverse effects occur, the drug dosage should be decreased slightly or a switch should be made to another β-blocking agent. Subtle but important differences of various β blockers are discussed in Chapters 1 and 2. Patients should be encouraged to persist with therapy except when adverse effects are bothersome.

Protective effects of β-adrenergic blockade appear to relate to their ability to actuate

- A ↓ in early morning sudden cardiac death (see Fig. 2–7 and Table 4–10)
- A ↓ in the incidence of early myocardial freewall rupture
- A ↓ in lethal arrhythmias, yet causing only a modest suppression of VPCs
- A ↑ in VF threshold and a ↓ in the incidence of VF
- Proven ↓ in the incidence of fatal and nonfatal MI rates, possibly by decreasing hydraulic stress at the site of atheroma, thus preventing plaque fissuring and subsequent thrombosis. The action of β blockers to attenuate the hemodynamic effects of catecholamine surges may protect a vulnerable atheromatous plaque from rupture and consequent coronary thrombosis that leads to fatal MI, sudden death, or nonfatal MI
- Prevention of early morning platelet aggregation induced by catecholamines and decreased early morning peak incidence of acute MI and sudden death (Table 4–10)
- Decreased renin activity. This may have salutary effects on ventricular remodeling. Decreased aneurysmal expansion may occur

Table 4–10
Beta Blocker Reduction of Early Morning Sudden Cardiac Death

SUDDEN DEATHS	CONTROL	PROPRANOLOL	DECREASE
Total	78	60	23%*
5 to 8 a.m.	6	0	
5 to 11 a.m.	25	11	56%
11 to 4 a.m.	33	31	Similar

* Timolol: 67% reduction in sudden death
Modified from: Beta-Blocker Heart Attack Study Data. Am J. Cardiol, *63*:1518, 1989.

Table 4–11
Aspirin Reduction of Early Morning Myocardial Infarction But Not Sudden Death*

	ASPIRIN	PLACEBO	p VALUE
Fatal MI	10	26	0.007
Nonfatal MI	129	213	0.0001
Sudden death	22	12	0.08
Other coronary heart diease	24	25	
Stroke death	9	6	
Total cardiovascular death	81	83	
Total death	271	227	0.64

* 22,071 physicians aged 50–80: 325 mg aspirin alternate day over 5 years
Modified from: The Physicians' Health Study. NB Engl J Med, *321*:129, 1989.

In the United States, β-blocker usage in the post-infarction patient can prevent >15,000 deaths in the first year and up to 60,000 deaths over 5 years in patients at medium or high risk. The effectiveness of β blockers in the low-risk post-infarction population is modest but worthwhile because it is occasionally difficult to correctly assign risks based on prognostic parameters including post-discharge exercise stress testing. In addition, β-blocking agents prevent sudden cardiac death, and it must be emphasized that aspirin does not prevent sudden cardiac death. Adverse effects and dosage of β blockers are given in Chapter 2.

Acetyl Salicylic Acid (Aspirin). Dosage: Initial dose, regular aspirin 325 mg then enteric coated aspirin, 160–325 mg once daily.

Indications include unstable angina, stable angina, onset of acute MI, post-MI prophylaxis, prevention of fatal or non-fatal strokes in patients with cerebral TIAs or post stroke, post CABS to prevent graft occlusion, and lone AF in patients < age 70

Aspirin irreversibly acetylates the platelet enzyme cyclooxygenase, thus preventing platelets from forming the powerful aggregating agent thromboxane A2, resulting in a ↓ in platelet aggregation. One dose of 80 mg of aspirin inhibits cyclooxygenase for the 1-week life span of the circulating platelets. This action abolishes platelet aggregation that would occur in response to stimuli such as collagen, arachidonate, and second-phase aggregation by ADP and epinephrine. Aspirin, unfortunately, reduces the formation of the potent vasodilator prostacyclin, and the smallest possible dose is advisable, 80–160 mg qd, so as not to inhibit prostacyclin. Further studies will clarify the dose range. Currently, a dose of 160–325 mg qd is widely used in post-MI patients. Aspirin causes a ↓ in the early morning incidence of acute MI but does not prevent sudden death (Table 4–11). The incidence of GI bleeding is shown in Table 4–12.

Table 4–12
Gastrointestinal Bleed in the Physicians Study (22,071 Physicians)

	ASPIRIN	PLACEBO	p VALUE
Upper gastrointestinal	38	28	
Melena	364	246	0.00001
Transfusion	48	28	

Modified from: The Physicians' Health Study. N Engl J Med, *321*:129, 1989.

ACE Inhibitors. Some degree of ventricular enlargement is detectable in >40% of patients with Q wave transmural anterolateral infarction and is observed as early as 1 or 2 weeks after the event. Physical slippage and reorientation of myocyte bundles in the infarcted area occur, causing thinning and expansion. The left ventricle appears to undergo a variable amount of dilation with some hypertrophy of the non-infarcted area.

Stimulation of the renin angiotensin system plays an important role in augmenting diastolic and systolic wall stresses, producing further LV enlargement. The structural changes in the left ventricle, termed remodeling, appear to have some detrimental effects that may later ↑ the incidence of CHF.

Fortunately, ACE inhibitors favorably influence remodeling and improve EF; their use should be considered in post-infarct patients with anterior infarction in the absence of CHF but with EF <35%. The SAVE Study of 2,231 patients randomized to captopril or placebo 3–16 days post MI and with EF <40% showed a 17% ↓ in mortality and a 36% ↓ in risk of development of CHF in patients treated with captopril 6.25 mg tid, titrated to a max of 150 mg qd. It is advisable to treat patients with anterior infarction, EF <40% 3 days post MI with captopril 6.25 mg tid, increasing when stable to 100 mg qd.

Cholesterol-Lowering Agents. Serum cholesterol and HDL-C should be evaluated within a few days of admission to the hospital. These measurements can be done in a nonfasting state. If the serum cholesterol in patients < age 70 is >240 mg/dl (6.2 mmol/l), the test should be repeated and decisions should be made based on the degree of elevations (see Chap. 9). In the Framingham post-MI study, patients with cholesterol levels >7.11 mmol/l (274 mg/dl) proved to be at an increased risk for reinfarction and cardiac mortality compared with patients who had cholesterol levels <5.2 mmol/l (200 mg/dl). An increased risk was not observed in patients with cholesterol levels of 5–7 mmol/l (193–270 mg/dl).

In-hospital diet should reflect the dietary advice given to the patient. Instructions on the value and use of a low saturated-fat diet with a ↑ in polyunsaturated fatty acids, as outlined in the AHA guidelines or similar instructions, are appropriate for all patients. See Chapter 9, hyperlipidemias.

Suggested Reading

Khan M Gabriel: Complications of Myocardial Infarction and Post-Infarction Care. *In* Cardiac and Pulmonary Management. Philadelphia, Lea & Febiger, 1993.

Heart Failure

5

M. Gabriel Khan

The term "heart failure" (HF) is preferred to "congestive heart failure" (CHF) because manifestations of congestion may be absent at rest in some patients with moderate or severe LV dysfunction. Indeed, there may be no clinical manifestations of forward or backward failure at rest.

The management of HF requires the application of 5 basic principles to actuate a salutary effect

- Ensure a correct diagnosis, excluding mimics of HF
- Determine the underlying heart disease, if possible, and treat
- Define precipitating factors, because HF can be a result of underlying disease and is often precipitated by conditions that can be prevented or easily corrected
- Understand the pathophysiology of HF
- Know the actions of the pharmacologic agents and their appropriate indications

DIAGNOSTIC HALLMARKS

Symptoms. Dyspnea, orthopnea, PND, weakness, fatigue, edema, and a ↑ in abdominal girth are common complaints.

Physical Signs. Signs of LV failure include

- Crepitations (crackles) over the lower lung fields. Many patients are treated for HF based on the presence of crepitations. HF may be present without pulmonary crepitations, and crepitations may be present in the absence of HF. Crepitations that fail to clear on coughing may be due to atelectasis, fibrosis and restrictive lung disease, pneumonia, pneumocystis infection, lymphangitic carcinomatosis, and other causes of noncardiogenic pulmonary edema
- S_3 gallop or summation gallop (S_3 and S_4). An S_3 gallop may elude auscultation in patients with CHD, although a corresponding movement associated with rapid diastolic filling may be visible on careful inspection of the precordium. An S_3 or summation gallop is virtually always present in patients with DCM, even in the absence of HF

Signs of right ventricular failure include

- A ↑ in jugular venous pressure >2 cm above the sternal angle. The most common cause of right ventricular failure is left HF, and signs of this should be sought
- A prominent V wave of tricuspid regurgitation or an A wave of atrial hypertrophy
- A positive hepatojugular reflux usually indicates a right atrial pressure >9 mm Hg and a PCWP >15 mm Hg where right HF is secondary to left HF

- Bilateral leg or sacral edema. Edema may be absent with severe HF, and when present, edema is often assumed to be due to HF. If a diagnosis of HF is not confirmed by other findings and a basic cause for HF is not present, consider the edema to be due to stasis, venous insufficiency, or DVT, of lymphangitic origin, or induced by drugs such as NSAIDs or Ca antagonists

Chest X Ray. Look for

- Constriction of lower lobe vessels with dilation of those in the upper lobes. This sign is observed with pulmonary venous hypertension in LV failure, mitral stenosis, severe COPD, or x ray taken in the recumbent position
- Interstitial pulmonary edema: Pulmonary clouding, perihilar haze, Kerley B or A lines caused by edema and thickening of interlobular septa. Kerley B lines usually are localized to the periphery of the lower zones and appear as horizontal lines 1–3 cm in length and no wider than 0.1–0.2 cm. They occur transiently when pulmonary venous pressure exceeds about 22 mm Hg. A lines are less common, reflect thickened intercommunicating lymphatics, and appear as thin nonbranching lines, several inches in length, extending from the hilar region. The transient appearance of A and B lines is caused by LV failure and may persist if the lymphatic channels are obstructed by tumor, choked by dust particles in pneumoconiosis, or thickened by fibrosing alveolitis or hemochromatosis. They may be caused by viral infections or drug hypersensitivity
- Pleural effusions: Subpleural or free pleural, blunting of the costophenic angle, the right usually greater than the left
- Alveolar pulmonary edema, a butterfly pattern, may be unilateral
- Interlobar fissure thickening due to accumulation of fluid, seen best on the lateral film
- Dilatation of the central right and left pulmonary arteries
- Cardiomegaly

The heart size may be normal on chest x-ray, in many instances, with HF present due to

- Acute MI in patients with CHD. Cardiac dilation may not take place in a transverse direction and patients with ≥1 old infarcts may present with HF and a normal heart size on chest radiograph. Hypokinetic, dyskinetic areas may be observed on inspection or palpitation of the chest wall and are readily observed on echocardiography
- Mitral stenosis
- Aortic stenosis in some patients
- HF due to predominant diastolic dysfunction
- Cor pulmonale

The following radiologic mimics of HF should be excluded

- Lung infection, including all causes of ARDS
- Allergic pulmonary edema (heroin, nitrofurantoin)
- Lymphangitic carcinomatosis
- Uremia
- Increased CSF pressure
- High altitude pulmonary edema
- Alveolar proteinosis

ECG. Scrutinize the ECG for

- Acute or old infarctions
- Recent ischemia (assess by serial ECGs)
- LV aneurysm: ST segment elevation in 2 contiguous leads present >3 months post infarction

- Bradyarrhythmias or tachyarrhythmias, particularly AF with a fast ventricular response
- Left or right ventricular hypertrophy
- Left atrial enlargement, which is an early sign of altered LV compliance from LV hypertrophy and a common feature of MR and/or mitral stenosis

Echocardiography provides many diagnostic aids

- Decreased systolic function: An EF <35% is often seen in patients with moderate HF. The EF may not be decreased in patients with HF caused by MR or VSD and in patients with ventricular diastolic dysfunction. The radionuclide evaluation of EF is more accurate than that of echocardiography, but the latter is superior in detecting the presence and significance of valvular lesions and specific chamber enlargement
- Ventricular wall motion abnormalities, global hypokinesia, and chamber enlargement
- An approximate assessment of PA pressure is extremely useful
- Valvular abnormalities: Reasonably accurate assessment of the severity of MR and obstructive lesions can be ascertained by continuous wave Doppler (see Chap. 12)
- Exclude cardiac tamponade
- Assess pericardial effusion and pericardial calcification
- Diastolic dysfunction abnormalities
- Assess LVH, left atrial enlargement, and right ventricular hypertrophy
- The diagnosis of hypertrophic, dilated, or RCM

ASSESS FOR UNDERLYING CAUSE OF HEART FAILURE

A complete cure may be a rare reward if a surgically correctable lesion is uncovered

- Left atrial myxoma
- Significant MR: May be missed because of the presence of a poorly audible murmur due to low cardiac output, thick chest wall, or COPD
- ASD
- A-V fistula
- Constrictive pericarditis
- Cardiac tamponade: May simulate HF and must be excluded because usual HF medications, diuretics, ACE inhibitors, or nitrates can cause marked hemodynamic deterioration in patients with tamponade
- Pulmonary edema or HF is not a complete diagnosis. The basic cause must be stated as part of the diagnosis and an associated precipitant must be defined, if present

It is necessary to make a systematic search for the following basic causes of heart disease

- Myocardial damage: CHD and its complications, myocarditis; cardiomyopathy
- Ventricular overload: *Pressure overload:* Systemic hypertension, coarctation of the aorta, aortic stenosis, pulmonary hypertension. *Volume overload:* MR, aortic regurgitation, VSD, ASD, patent ductus arteriosus

- Restriction and obstruction of ventricular filling: Right ventricular infarction; constrictive pericarditis; cardiac tamponade (although not truly HF); restrictive cardiomyopathies (see Chap. 14); SHMDs (see Chap. 14); hypertensive, hypertrophic "cardiomyopathy" of the elderly; mitral stenosis and atrial myxoma
- Others: Cor pulmonale, thyrotoxicosis, high output failure: A-V fistula, peripartum cardiomyopathy, and beri-beri

SEARCH FOR PRECIPITATING FACTORS

- Reduction or discontinuation of medications, salt binge, increased physical and mental stress
- Increased cardiac work: Increasing hypertension (systemic or pulmonary), arrhythmias, pulmonary embolism, infections, increased activities, physical and emotional stress
- Progression or complications of the underlying disease: Acute MI, LV aneurysm, valvular heart disease with progression of stenosis or regurgitation
- Several drugs may precipitate HF: Alcohol, NSAIDs, β blockers, corticosteroids, disopyramide, procainamide, propafenone and other antiarrhythmics, Ca antagonists, Adriamycin, daunorubicin, mithramycin. Excessive alcohol intake can significantly ↓ LV contractility

PATHOPHYSIOLOGIC IMPLICATIONS

In most patients with HF, cardiac output is reduced due to poor LV systolic function. However, LV systolic function may be relatively normal in some patients with valvular regurgitant lesions, hypertensive heart disease, and RCM, in which diastolic dysfunction plays a major role in causing HF (Fig. 5–1).

HF is a syndrome identified by well-defined symptoms, signs, and/or hemodynamic findings caused by an abnormality of cardiac function that results in a relative ↓ in cardiac output and compensatory renal and neurohormonal adjustments (Fig. 5–1).

Cardiac output is the product of stroke volume and HR. Stroke volume is modulated by

- Preload
- Myocardial contractility
- Afterload

Preload is the extent of fiber stretch during diastole and is clinically represented by the end diastolic volume. The LV end diastolic or filling pressure is closely related, although in a nonlinear fashion, to end diastolic volume, and is an indication of LV preload. In the absence of obstruction to blood flow through the pulmonary veins and into the ventricle, the LV end diastolic pressure is in turn reflected by the PCWP or PA end diastolic pressure.

Decrease preload and diastolic dysfunction: The affected ventricle may contract well if adequately filled but may relax poorly, resulting in a diastolic dysfunction that is more prominent than the commonly occurring systolic dysfunction.

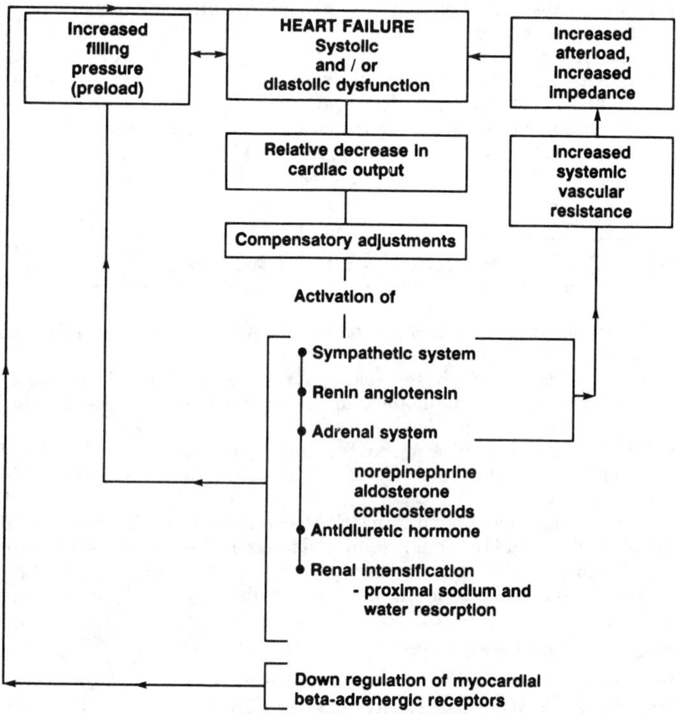

Figure 5–1. Pathophysiology of heart failure.

A ↑ in ventricular diastolic stiffness impedes diastolic stretch and causes failure to adequately fill the ventricle. Conditions that alter ventricular compliance, causing diastolic dysfunction, a ↓ in preload, and thus, a ↓ in cardiac output, include: MI (although systolic dysfunction is the main abnormality); cardiac tamponade; constrictive pericarditis; hypertensive heart disease; RCM; DCM; SHMD, e.g., amyloid; the aging heart; and hypertensive, hypertrophic "cardiomyopathy" of the elderly. Approximately 15% of patients with HF have mainly diastolic dysfunction with relatively preserved EF. Over 70% of patients with HF have systolic dysfunction and about 15% have both systolic and diastolic dysfunction.

In patients with predominant diastolic dysfunction, the heart size and EF are often normal. The heart fills less and empties less, and the percent ejected may be relatively normal, but the stroke and cardiac index are decreased. Since a ↓ in preload exists in the above conditions, the use of preload-reducing agents is relatively contraindicated. Hemodynamic and clinical deterioration may ensue with the use of diuretics, nitrates, ACE inhibitors, nitroprusside, or prazosin.

Afterload is represented by LV wall end systolic stress, which must be overcome to allow ejection of blood from the ventricle. A ↑ in afterload signifies a ↑ in myocardial O_2 demand.

Afterload is determined by: The radius of the ventricle (A), LV end systolic pressure (B), and arteriolar resistance or impedance (C). Afterload is highly dependent on A and B. In turn, B is dependent on cardiac index and C. A ↓ in systolic vascular resistance or a ↓ in BP is not identical with a ↓ in afterload. Also, a ↓ in systemic vascular resistance is not synonymous with a ↓ in arterial BP, as a compensatory ↑ in cardiac output occurs to maintain BP. The peripheral systolic pressure may be maintained because of colliding reflected pressure waves, despite a ↓ in central systolic BP.

Conditions causing a ↑ in afterload include: Aortic stenosis, pulmonary stenosis, coarctation, hypertension, and all causes of HF because of activation of the renin angiotensin and sympathoadrenal system.

LV dysfunction and HF due to systolic dysfunction improve with therapy directed at

- A ↓ in afterload, which improves ventricular emptying at a lowered demand for O_2
- A judicious ↓ in preload, in order to ↓ symptoms caused by pulmonary congestion but without bringing about an unwanted ↓ in cardiac output or a marked stimulation of the renin angiotensin system

Myocardial Contractility. A ↓ in myocardial contractility or systolic dysfunction is commonly caused by CHD, especially in patients with large areas of infarction. Rarely, DCM and myocarditis are implicated; and with late-stage volume overload due to valvular regurgitant lesions, myocardial damage occurs, culminating in pump failure.

COMPENSATORY ADJUSTMENTS IN HEART FAILURE

The body responds to the abnormality of cardiac function and a relative ↓ in cardiac output by bringing several homeostatic mechanisms into action (Fig. 5–1). This situation is similar to the body's reaction to severe bleeding over several hours, but the results are, of course, less than completely appropriate in HF

- The activation of the sympathetic system causes a ↑ in HR, force, and velocity of myocardial contraction in order to ↑ stroke volume and cardiac output. A ↑ in systemic vascular resistance occurs in order to maintain BP. The body's homeostatic response (indicated in Fig. 5–1) is appropriate but often not sufficient to compensate for the ↓ in cardiac index and increased filling pressures. It is, in fact, counterproductive in some ways. Also, sympathetic stimulation causes Na and water retention and a ↑ in venous tone in order to ↑ filling pressure that enhances preload, provided that there is no restriction to ventricular filling
- The renin angiotensin system is stimulated. Patients with mild HF show little or no evidence of stimulation of the renin angiotensin system. Stimulation of the system is observed in response to treatment with diuretics and is seen in untreated patients with more severe degrees of HF. The secretion of renin causes angiotensin I to be converted by ACE to the vasoconstrictor angiotensin II. This action occurs in the circulation and in the tissues

Angiotensin II supports systemic BP and cerebral, renal, and coronary perfusion through

- Arteriolar vasoconstriction and a ↑ in systemic vascular resistance
- Stimulation of central and peripheral effects of the sympathetic system
- Marked resorption of Na and water in the proximal nephron
- Enhanced aldosterone secretion, which brings about Na and water retention in the renal tubules, distal to the macula densa. Since the distal tubules only handle about 2% of the nephron's Na load, this latter contribution is small, compared to proximal Na resorption, but is a final tuning of Na balance
- Stimulating thirst and vasopressin release, thereby increasing total body water

Renal blood flow is preserved by selective vasoconstriction of postglomerular efferent arterioles. The adjustments, however, made to maintain BP and cerebral, coronary, and renal perfusion, cause a marked ↑ in afterload, which unnecessarily increases cardiac work and myocardial O_2 demand. Thus, HF increases.

NONSPECIFIC THERAPY

- Bedrest is necessary for patients with NYHA Class IV or acute HF requiring admission to the hospital. Most patients are able to walk to the bathroom, with assistance, but some may require a bedside commode for the first 24 h. It is important to quickly ambulate in order to avoid deep vein thrombosis and pulmonary embolism
- Heparin, 5,000 U q 12 h, is advisable until the patient is mobilized
- In patients ill enough to be admitted to the hospital and suspected of having hypoxemia because of a history of orthopnea, PND, and symptoms of pulmonary congestion or when hypoxemia is proven by ABG analysis, O_2 is given for 12–24 h. ABG analysis is not necessary in the majority of patients with HF. Oxygen, 2–3 l/min, by nasal prongs is usually adequate
- Overweight patients with HF benefit from weight ↓. The physician must have a basic understanding of salt intake to confidently advise the patient. Booklets prepared by the AHA and other organizations should be made available to the patient. Patients must recognize that salt added to meals at the table is only a minor part of the daily salt consumption and that increased salt in the diet can precipitate HF and an expensive admission to hospital. Table 1–1 lists a few commonly used foods and their Na content (see Chap. 1)

WHICH DRUG OR DRUG COMBINATION TO CHOOSE

In clinical practice, an appropriate drug or combination for patients with HF due to ventricular systolic dysfunction requires consideration of the patient's functional class. It is appropriate to utilize the NYHA functional class since several major clinical trials have incorporated this parameter in study design.

NYHA Functional Class

- Class I: Asymptomatic on ordinary physical activity associated with maximal oxygen consumption >20 ml/kg/min

- Class II: Symptomatic on ordinary physical activity with max VO_2 of 16–20 ml/kg/min
- Class III: Symptomatic on < ordinary physical activity with max VO_2 of 10–15 ml/kg/min
- Class IV: Symptomatic at rest or on any activity with max VO_2 of <10 ml/kg/min

Drug Therapy, NYHA Class IV Heart Failure

CONSENSUS studied only NYHA Class IV HF patients. In 253 randomized patients, the 6-month mortality was 44% in patients treated with diuretics and a digoxin combination and 26% in patients given enalapril in addition ($p < 0.002$). Forty-two percent of the group treated with added ACE inhibitors showed an improvement in functional class, compared with 22% in the control group ($p = 0.001$). A significant ↓ in mortality attributable to ACE inhibitor therapy was observed mainly during the first 6 months

- The current recommendation to treat NYHA Class IV HF patients with diuretics, digoxin, and an ACE inhibitor for life is appropriate, given the short life expectancy of Class IV patients, and is, of course, supported by the obvious symptomatic benefit, improved survival, and ↓ in sudden death that results from therapy

Drug Therapy, NYHA Class II and III Heart Failure

- Clinical trials have confirmed that monotherapy with diuretics, digoxin, or ACE inhibitors is not satisfactory for NYHA Class II patients in sinus rhythm who have an EF <35% and who have had overt HF
- Sufficient data strongly indicate that these patients should be managed with triple therapy: Diuretic, digoxin, and ACE inhibitor. This combination has been shown in both the SOLVD and VHeFT-II to improve survival, and in the SOLVD, significant ↓ in hospitalization for recurrent HF was achieved
- In the few patients in whom ACE inhibitors are contraindicated or cause adverse effects, the diuretic digoxin combination should suffice
- If angina or active ischemia is documented, the combination of diuretic, digoxin, and nitrate is preferable because ACE inhibitor therapy has been shown to cause a ↑ in angina in these patients
- When exercise performance is not improved by diuretic, digoxin, and ACE inhibitor therapy, the dose of ACE inhibitor should be halved and intermittent oral nitrate should be administered. Caution is necessary with this combination because a sharp ↓ in preload may result in syncope or presyncope

Studies that support or are relevant to the above recommendations include

- The CONSENSUS study has shown that triple therapy is lifesaving in Class IV patients, as discussed earlier
- SOLVD studied HF patients who had EFs ≤35%; 1,284 patients who had overt HF with EF <35% were randomly selected to receive enalapril 2.5–20 mg plus conventional therapy, and 1,285 patients were randomly assigned to a control group to receive conventional therapy. Approximately 30% of the study group were in NYHA Class III. At an average follow-up of 41 months, in Class III patients, there were 182 (47%) deaths in the enalapril group and 201 (51%) deaths in the placebo group. Total mortality in the enalapril group was 452 (35%)

Table 5–1
Effect of Treatment on Mortality and Hospitalization for Congestive Heart Failure, and Proportion of Patients Taking Angiotensin-Converting–Enzyme Inhibitors after Various Periods*

	MORTALITY			DEATH OR HOSPITALIZATION FOR HEART FAILURE			PROPORTION TAKING INHIBITORS†	
MONTHS-OF FOLLOW-UP	PLACEBO	ENALAPRIL	RISK REDUCTION (95% CI)	PLACEBO	ENALAPRIL	RISK REDUCTION (95% CI)	PLACEBO	ENALAPRIL
	number		*percent*	*number*		*percent*	*percent*	
3	69	47	33 (2–53)	164	92	46 (30–57)	6	92
6	126	91	29 (8–46)	259	150	45 (33–55)	10	88
12	201	159	23 (5–37)	401	262	40 (30–48)	12	86
24	344	277	23 (10–34)	559	434	30 (21–38)	20	83
36	450	396	16 (4–27)	680	555	28 (19–35)	23	82
48	504	443	17 (5–27)	731	607	27 (18–34)	30	83
Overall‡	510	452	16 (5–26)	736	613	26 (18–34)	—	—
	Z = 2.69; p = 0.0036			Z = 5.65; p < 0.0001				

* The 95% confidence intervals (CI) correspond to a two-sided p value of <0.05 or a one-sided p value of <0.025. Risk reductions were calculated by the log-rank test from the data available at each specific time.

† Values shown for 3 and 6 months were based on data obtained after the visits at 4 and 8 months, respectively. The inhibitors were angiotensin-converting–enzyme inhibitors.

‡ The total number of deaths were 518 and 458 when deaths after January 31, 1991, but before the patients' last visits, were included. See notes to Table 2.

From: The SOLVD Investigators: Effect of enalapril on survival in patients with reduced left ventricular ejection fractions and congestive heart failure. N Engl J Med, *325*:297, 1991.

Table 5–2
Captopril-Digoxin Multicenter Research Group Study*

PARAMETERS	DIURETIC	DIURETIC + DIGOXIN	DIURETIC + ACE INHIBITOR
Increase in EF	0.9%	4.4%	1.8%
Exercise time (seconds)	40	55	77
Recurrence of heart failure (not due to myocardial infarction)	20%	10%	10%

* 300 patients; New York Heart Association Class II and III heart failure
% = Approximate percentage
(Data obtained from JAMA *259*:1988)

versus 510 (39.7%) in the placebo arm, a 16% risk ↓ (p = 0.0036). Enalapril therapy resulted in a significant ↓ in hospitalizations; overall, 971 patients in the placebo group required hospitalization versus 683 patients in the enalapril group. Mortality ↓ was highest at 24 months of therapy, when the risk ↓ was 23% (Table 5–1). Although Class III patients did not achieve major mortality ↓, hospitalizations were decreased. In SOLVD, enalapril therapy resulted in a significant ↓ in mortality in NYHA Class II patients, who comprised 56.7% of the study group. There were 219 (30%) deaths in the enalapril group and 254 (35%) in the placebo group

- VHeFT-II randomized 804 Class II and III HF patients who had EF <0.45 (mean at baseline = 0.29). Enalapril (10–20 mg) added to standard therapy diuretic-digoxin was compared to ISDN-hydralazine added to standard therapy. Enalapril therapy resulted, at the end of 2-year follow-up, in a significant ↓ in mortality (18% versus 25% [p = 0.016] in the ISDN-hydralazine arm). The incidence of sudden death was reduced mainly in Class II patients. Only ISDN-hydralazine therapy, however, resulted in an increased body VO_2 at peak exercise. The venodilator effect of ISDN is more potent than enalapril at the dose administered. This may have contributed to the ISDN-hydralazine improvement in exercise performance since hydralazine therapy alone does not improve this parameter
- The Captopril-Digoxin MRG study compared the effects of placebo, digoxin, or captopril added to maintenance diuretic therapy at 6 months in 300 Class II and III HF patients, LV EF mean of 25%. Results are listed in Table 5–2. Digoxin significantly increased EF, compared to diuretics alone or a diuretic-captopril combination

Drug Therapy, NYHA Class I Heart Failure

Patients with mild LV systolic dysfunction who are asymptomatic generally do not require treatment with a diuretic, digoxin, or ACE inhibitor. The role of ACE inhibitors in Class I patients was evaluated in the SAVE Following MI Study. More than 20,000 patients within 3–16 days of MI, with an average EF of 31% by radionuclide ventriculography or without overt HF or post-infarction angina, were randomized and followed for 2 years. The SAVE data showed a 17% ↓ in risk of death compared with the control group (p = 0.020). Fewer patients in the captopril-treated group required hospitalization for the occurrence of HF (see Chap. 4). The SOLVD prevention arm showed that enalapril administered to patients without overt HF and an EF <35% caused a 37% reduced risk of developing HF and hospitalizations; but no significant changes in mortality or infarction rates were observed.

Diuretics

The main action of diuretics is to ↓ preload. Although this effect does not improve cardiac output or survival, diuretics are still first-line agents in the management of HF because they ameliorate bothersome, congestive symptoms and prevent costly hospitalization. As discussed earlier, they can be used alone as first-line therapy in patients with NYHA Class II HF with mild systolic dysfunction, especially when HF is precipitated by a reversible cause such as pneumonia, infection, arrhythmia, or NSAIDs. These patients are often controlled with a diuretic only and maintained without ACE inhibitor or digoxin therapy. Further reasons for the choice of diuretics in various grades of HF are given under the previous section regarding which drugs to choose.

Furosemide. _Action:_ Furosemide inhibits Na and chloride reabsorption from the ascending limb of the loop of Henle, with weak effects in the proximal tubule, which excretes the drug. IV furosemide has a venodilator effect; thus, preload ↓ occurs within minutes and relief of symptoms may occur before the appearance of increased urinary flow. The potency of action allows furosemide and other loop diuretics to retain beneficial effects in renal failure patients with GFRs as low as 10 ml/min. Thus, in patients with elevated serum creatinine, >2.3 mg/dl (203 μmol/l), furosemide retains activity, whereas thiazides, except metolazone, are not effective. _Supplied:_ tablets; 20, 40, 80, 500 mg ampules available in 10 mg/ml, 20 mg/2 ml, 40 mg/4 ml, and 250 mg/25 ml. _Dosage:_ IV 20–80 mg given as a slow IV bolus, 20 mg/min. _Caution:_ If renal failure is present, do not exceed 4 mg/min to prevent ototoxicity.

For acute HF of mild to moderate severity in patients with acute MI, small doses are advisable (20–40 mg IV repeated 1–2 h after careful assessment) in order not to ↓ cardiac output or produce further stimulation of the renin angiotensin system. For acute HF in patients with known NYHA Class III or IV, large doses may be required, depending on the extent of pulmonary congestion and the degree of respiratory distress (80 mg IV followed by 80–120 mg in 2–4 h and repeated q 8 or 12 h as needed; maintenance 40–120 mg once daily). Larger dosages may be required if urinary output is poor or if chronic renal failure is present (with serum creatinine >2.3 mg/dl, 203 μmol/l) or if severe pulmonary congestion with respiratory distress persists (with a JVP >5 cm), having excluded cardiac tamponade or mimics of HF. See earlier discussion on this topic.

Maintenance dose should be given before 9 a.m. qd. Split doses are rarely needed at 7 a.m. and 3 p.m. The afternoon dose should not be given later than 3 p.m. in order not to disturb the patient's sleep. It is preferable to give 160 mg once daily rather than 80 mg bid since the tubules may be resistant to the 80-mg dose in patients with severe HF. Doses >160 mg are preferably divided into 120 mg in the morning and 80 mg in the afternoon. Patients with Class IV ventricles and graded as NYHA Class IV require ≥120 mg in 1 day, alternating with 80 mg the next day to achieve adequate control.

Always maintain the serum K >4 mEq (mmol)/l. Patients who require large doses of furosemide >80 mg qd benefit from ACE inhibitor therapy, which normalizes serum K. When the combination is used, K supplements or K-sparing diuretics should not be given, except with carefully monitored serum K levels. Also, salt substitutes contain K and can cause hyperkalemia. Periodic measurements of serum K are advisable for all patients taking daily diuretics.

Adverse Effects: Hypokalemia, hypersensitivity in patients allergic to sulfur compounds, very rarely leukopenia, thrombocytopenia, precipitation of gout, hypocalcemia, hypomagnesemia. *Drug Interactions:* Cephalosporin or aminoglycoside antibiotics may show increased nephrotoxicity in patients with renal dysfunction when given large doses of loop diuretics. An increased reabsorption of lithium may occur, resulting in lithium toxicity; with chloral hydrate, hot flushes, sweating, and tachycardia may occur; NSAIDs antagonize the action of loop diuretics as well as thiazides; the effect of tubocurarine is increased.

Ethacrynic Acid. *Supplied:* tablets; 50 mg vials; 50 mg. *Dosage:* oral 50–150 mg qd, IV 50 mg diluted with 50 ml of 5% dextrose in water given slowly.

Ethacrynic acid is recommended when there is failure to respond to large doses of furosemide or when sulfonamide sensitivity exists. The drug causes slightly more chloride loss than furosemide and has slightly more adverse effects. However, uric acid elevation appears to occur less frequently than with thiazides or furosemide. Warfarin's anticoagulant effect is increased by ethacrynic acid.

Bumetanide. *Supplied:* tablets; 0.5, 1, and 5 mg ampules; 2, 4, 10 ml (500 μg/ml). *Dosage:* oral 0.5–1 mg qd, ↑ if needed to 2–5 mg qd. In patients with renal failure, ≥5 mg may be required. IV 1–2 mg repeated in 30 mins to 1 h if needed.

The drug has similar actions to furosemide but is reported to cause less magnesium loss (1 mg bumetanide is equivalent to 40 mg furosemide). The drug is more nephrotoxic than furosemide, and its use should be avoided with cephalosporins and aminoglycosides.

Thiazide Diuretics

Thiazide diuretics are advisable mainly in patients with NYHA Class II HF. However, hypokalemia occurs in up to 30% of patients and as many as 50% with chlorthalidone. Also, hypomagnesemia often occurs and goes undetected. K-sparing diuretics retain K and magnesium, and are useful in patients with mild HF (NYHA Class II). The patient may benefit from a K-sparing diuretic given 3–4 days per week only. See Chapter 1 for products and dosage.

Metolazone. *Supplied:* tablets; 2.5, 5, 10 mg. *Dosage:* 2.5–5 mg once daily; max 10 mg (rarely indicated). This thiazide diuretic has a unique property of retaining effectiveness when other thiazides become ineffective with GFR <30 ml/min. The combination of metolazone and furosemide is very useful in patients with refractory HF who fail to respond to large doses of furosemide or ethacrynic acid. In one reported study, in 15 of 17 patients with severe failure refractory to loop diuretics, digoxin, and ACE inhibitors, substantial improvement occurred, allowing discharge from the hospital. This potent combination is useful, but hypokalemia is often pronounced. Intermittent therapy (metolazone twice weekly) may help avoid this effect. In this situation, however, combination with an ACE inhibitor or K supplement often becomes necessary.

Digoxin (Lanoxin)

After >200 years of use and controversies in the 1970s regarding its efficacy and role, digoxin has been fully restored as the only oral positive inotropic agent available that significantly improves symptoms, signs, EF, and other hemodynamic parameters in patients with all grades of acute, recurrent, or chronic HF, with salutary effects occurring when combined with a diuretic and/or ACE inhibitor.

Clinicians who have used this drug for >30 years in patients with ventricular systolic dysfunction (NYHA Class III and IV HF) recognize the effectiveness of the drug when combined with diuretics and have documented the recurrence of HF when digoxin is discontinued. An S3 or summation gallop present during several days of treatment with diuretics and ACE inhibitors disappears within days of digitalization. Also, objective hemodynamic data are now available that clearly indicate the drug's salutary effects.

Digoxin has been shown to further improve cardiac function in patients with abnormal hemodynamic variables when stabilized on diuretics and ACE inhibitors.

Contraindications: Patients with sick sinus syndrome or A-V block of all grades.

Cautions: Many physicians avoid the use of digoxin in the first 24 h of MI, except in the management of patients with AF with hemodynamic compromise, in whom electrical cardioversion is preferred. The drug can be used judiciously in smaller initial doses within the first 24 h of infarction if moderate to severe HF is unimproved with the use of furosemide and nitrates and/or if dobutamine is not available.

Indications: HF associated with AF; patients in sinus rhythm (severe HF due to systolic dysfunction, particularly patients with NYHA Class III or IV, regardless of the presence of an S3 gallop. In these patients, the drug is combined with diuretics and ACE inhibitors); as part of triple therapy in patients with NYHA Class II HF and EF <35%; as the second-line agent for management of NYHA Class II HF patients with EF >35% in combination with diuretics (salutary effects are equal to those of ACE inhibitors combined with diuretics); where ACE inhibitors are contraindicated because of hypotension, renal failure, or bothersome adverse effects; patients with angina or NYHA Class II, III, or IV HF requiring furosemide dosage >40 mg qd (studies indicate that ACE inhibitors may worsen angina and are relatively contraindicated in these patients); the drug can be used, if indicated, in pregnancy and during breastfeeding.

Action: Inotropic effect: Digoxin increases the force and velocity of myocardial contraction and improves the EF. It combines with and partially inhibits the Na pump, the enzyme Na, and K-activated adenosine triphosphatase (Na K ATPase) located in the sarcolemmal membrane of the myocardial cell and increases the availability of intracellular Ca to contractile elements, resulting in enhanced myocardial contractility. This effect causes the Frank-Starling function curve to move upward and to the left.

Increase of vagal activity and a modest ↓ in sympathetic activity slow conduction velocity in the A-V node. This action is important in slowing the ventricular response in AF and the termination of PSVT. Mild slowing of the sinus rate occurs due to the mild ↓ in sympathetic activity

Increase in Phase 4 diastolic depolarization increases the activity of ectopic pacemakers

Pharmacokinetics: About 66% of the oral tablet dose is absorbed mainly in the stomach and the upper small bowel. Following absorption, the drug is widely distributed, but binding to skeletal muscle is particularly important because a low muscle mass in the elderly calls for a smaller loading dose. The mean serum half-life is approximately 36 h. It is advisable to wait until equilibration is reached to obtain a digoxin level that represents myocardial concentration. After IV and oral dosing, wait ≥3 h and 6 h, respectively, before obtaining a serum digoxin assay.

Dosing at bedtime is advisable so that an assay during a morning assignment would be appropriate.

Bioavailability is reduced as a result of decreased absorption due to: Malabsorption syndrome; colestipol, cholestyramine, Metamucil (or similar agents); antacids, metoclopramide, phenytoin, phenobarbital.

Absorption is enhanced by Lomotil and decreased intestinal motility.

An increased serum digoxin level may result from antibiotics, especially Neomycin, and some broad-spectrum antibiotics that may eliminate Eubacterium lentum, which partially metabolizes digoxin to inactive dihydrodigoxine and may thus cause increased digoxin absorption. However, this effect occurs in <10% of patients. Digoxin levels are also increased by quinidine, some Ca antagonists, and amiodarone.

Excretion is by the kidneys. Thus, undetected or unnoticed renal insufficiency is the commonest cause of digoxin toxicity.

After 1 mg oral dosing, peak onset of action occurs in 1–6 h, with serum levels usually >1 μg/ml; max inotropic action is observed in 4–6 h.

<u>Dosage:</u> 0.5–1 mg over 24 h prescribed as follows

- Orally: 0.5 mg immediately, 0.25 mg q 12 h for 2 doses, followed by an appropriate maintenance dose depending on age, renal function, and presence or absence of conditions that ↑ sensitivity to the drug (Table 5–2). If such conditions are present, halve the initial dose (or 0.25 mg bid) for 2 days, followed by maintenance dosage depending on age or renal function. In the UK, the British National Formulary recommendation is 0.125–0.25 mg bid for about 1 week and then once daily, having regard to renal function. However, 0.5 mg qd for 1 week may cause toxicity if an unsuspected ↓ in creatinine clearance is present, especially in the elderly, or if sensitivity exists. Also, in patients < age 70 with normal renal function, the initial 0.25 mg daily dose may not achieve adequate levels or salutary effects for several weeks
- Rapid oral method for AF with a ventricular response: 110–140/min in patients with HF not receiving digoxin. <u>Caution:</u> The patient is reassessed prior to each dose and the order for the drug is then written: 0.5 mg immediately, 0.25 mg q 4 or 6 h for 3 doses, followed by maintenance
- IV therapy for AF with a fast ventricular response >150/min where urgent digitalization is required in the absence of definite daily digoxin use in the previous week and the exclusion of sick sinus syndrome: 0.5 mg IV slowly over 10 mins with ECG monitoring, reassess before each dose, 0.25 mg over 10 mins q 2–4 h for 2 or 3 doses, followed by maintenance. It is often necessary to give 1.25–1.5 mg over 12 h to obtain satisfactory control of the ventricular response. Occasionally, higher doses are necessary to achieve a ventricular response <110/min, followed by maintenance dose. Alternatively, verapamil or a β blocker administered orally may be added to control a fast ventricular rate

Alternatively, it is recommended (in the UK) that digoxin be given by IV infusion (0.75–1 mg in 50 ml) over ≥2 h when rapid control of AF is required.

Suggested maintenance dosage with normal serum creatinine

- Age <70 (0.25 mg qd preferably at bedtime)
- Age >70 (0.125 mg at bedtime)

In patients with AF requiring further control of ventricular response, a 0.125-mg daily dose in addition to the maintenance dose indicated is often necessary. A 0.1875-mg tablet is available in some countries and is a convenient once-daily dose.

If renal failure is present, obtain a direct measurement of the creatinine clearance or determine the clearance by utilizing the lean body weight, age, sex, and serum creatinine.

Caution: Digoxin toxicity may occur in patients with known or unsuspected renal dysfunction, and especially in the elderly, in whom creatinine clearance is frequently reduced in the presence of a normal serum creatinine. In patients < age 70 with serum creatinine of 1.3–2.3 mg/dl (115–203 μmol/l), give 0.125 mg on alternate days and assess digoxin levels in about 10 days. In patients over age 70 with abnormal serum creatinine >2.3 mg/dl (203 μmol/l), it is advisable to avoid digoxin use because toxicity is a major concern. In this situation, treatment with diuretics and vasodilators is indicated and digoxin is relatively contraindicated. If needed, digitoxin can be used.

DIGOXIN TOXICITY

A ↓ in the incidence of definite or serious digitalis intoxication has materialized because of physician awareness of the pharmacokinetics: Absorption, binding, distribution, and excretion of the drug. In particular, the hazard in patients with renal dysfunction, including elderly patients with unsuspected impaired renal function with a normal serum creatinine, has sharply curtailed digitalis toxicity.

A lean skeletal mass, especially in the elderly, carries 2 important connotations

- Digoxin binds to skeletal muscle; thus, in individuals with lean, skeletal mass, more digoxin is available in the serum for myocardial binding. Therefore, there is a higher probability of toxicity in patients with lean skeletal mass, especially if renal dysfunction inhibits elimination of the drug
- Low skeletal muscle mass in the elderly reflects a lowered serum creatinine that leads the physician to believe that renal function is normal, when creatinine clearance may be reduced by ≥50%

Reduction of the maintenance dose in patients with conditions that ↑ sensitivity to digoxin (Table 5–3) and the appropriate use of digoxin serum assay are important precautionary measures. Conditions that ↑ or ↓ the bioavailability of digoxin, particularly drugs that cause interactions, are listed in Table 5–4.

Symptoms and signs of digitalis intoxication include

- GI: Nausea, anorexia, vomiting, diarrhea, abdominal pain, weight loss

Table 5–3
Conditions in Which There is an Increased Sensitivity to Digoxin and Conservative Dosing is Recommended

1. Elderly patients (age >70)	8. Hypercalcemia
2. Hypokalemia	9. Hypocalcemia
3. Hyperkalemia	10. Myocarditis
4. Hypoxemia	11. Low skeletal mass
5. Acidosis	12. Hypothyroidism
6. Acute myocardial infarction	13. Amyloidosis
7. Hypomagnesemia	

From: Khan, M Gabriel: Cardiac Drug Therapy, 3rd Ed. London, W.B. Saunders, 1992

TABLE 5–4
Digoxin Interactions

Increase serum levels
- Quinidine displaces digoxin at binding sites, decreases renal elimination
- Verapamil, diltiazem, nicardipine, felodipine, amiodarone, propafenone
  - ACE inhibitiors may decrease renal elimination
- NSAIDs decrease renal elimination
  - Lomotil, probanthine, decrease intestinal motility
- Erythromycin, tetracycline eliminate eubacterium lentum
- Spironolactone, digoxin assays falsely elevated
- Electrophysiologic interactions may occur with amiodarone, diltiazem, verapamil

Decrease serum levels or bioavailability
- Antacids, metoclopramide, cholestyramine, colestipol
- Metamucil, neomycin, phenytoin, phenobarbital, salicylazosulfapyridine

- CNS: Visual hallucinations; blue, green, or yellow vision; blurring of vision and scotomas; dizziness, headaches, restlessness, insomnia, and rarely mental confusion and psychosis
- Cardiac: There is a spectrum from occurrence of arrhythmia in digoxin free state, through latent arrhythmia precipitated by digoxin, to arrhythmia directly secondary to digoxin. First°, 2nd° or 3rd° A-V block; sinus pause >2 seconds; PAT with block (ventricular rate is often 90–120/min; the P waves may be buried in the T waves); accelerated junctional rhythm; VPBs, bigeminal or multifocal; VT; and rarely VF. Table 5–5 shows the incidence of arrhythmias caused by digoxin toxicity. In addition, deterioration in HF may be due to digoxin toxicity

No single serum digoxin concentration drawn at the appropriate time interval, >6 h after oral dosing, can indicate toxicity reliably, but the

Table 5–5
Major Manifestations of Digoxin Toxicity

	%
A. Non-life-threatening arrhythmias	
Multifocal VPCs	30
1° AV Block	15
Supraventricular tachycardia	25
B. Life-threatening arrhythmias	
3° AV Block	25
2° AV Block	15
Ventricular tachycardia	20
Ventricular fibrillation	10
Asystole	8
C. Noncardiac	
Nausea & vomiting	50
Hyperkalemia*	25

* Due to renal failure and/or inhibition of the sodium pump

likelihood increases progressively through the range 1.5–3 ng/ml or μg/l (1.2–3.5 nmol/l). Concentrations >3 ng/ml must be avoided. Levels <1.5 ng/ml drawn at the appropriate time are rarely associated with toxicity, except in patients with myocardial sensitivity as listed in Table 5–3. Digoxin toxicity in the patient with the absence of the conditions listed and a level <1 ng/ml is so rare as to exclude the diagnosis. Reviews indicate that digoxin-intoxicated patients have a mean serum digoxin level of 3.3 ng/ml.

MANAGEMENT OF DIGOXIN TOXICITY

- Discontinue digoxin
- Replace K if hypokalemia is present. Hold diuretics until serum K is in the normal range
- Clarify conditions that ↑ sensitivity to digoxin (Table 5–3). Toxicity is likely to be present if suggestive symptoms are manifest and if there is a precipitating cause for renal impairment or if the serum creatinine is elevated
- Assess digoxin level
- Assess ECG signs: Digitalis effect does not mean toxicity. (See brady-arrhythmias and tachyarrhythmias as listed under Adverse Effects)

Drug therapy is indicated for: Arrhythmias causing a threat to life, hemodynamic deterioration, or worsening of HF (the incidence of digoxin-induced arrhythmias is given in Table 5–5)

Bradyarrhythmias. Sinus bradycardia, 2nd° A-V block, and sino-atrial dysfunction are managed with atropine 0.4, 0.5, or 0.6 mg IV q 5 mins to max of 2 mg. Failure to respond to atropine or the presence of 3rd° A-V block is an indication for digoxin-specific Fab antibody fragments or temporary pacing (see Chap. 7). KCl is relatively contraindicated with bradyarrhythmias as K and digoxin synergistically depress conduction and may precipitate a higher degree of A-V block. If the serum K is in the range of 3.0–3.8 mEq (mmol)/l, K should be given IV at a rate <10 mEq (mmol)/h; a serum K <3 mEq/l may require an infusion rate >10 mEq (mmol)/h, and continuous monitoring of the cardiac rhythm is necessary

Tachyarrhythmias. VT, multifocal VPCs, or atrial tachycardia with block in the presence of hypokalemia. Potassium chloride. IV 40–60 mEq(mmol) in 1 liter of 0.9% or half normal saline over 4 h, except in patients with renal insufficiency or in patients with A-V block, because a ↑ in K may ↑ the degree of A-V block. KCl is diluted in 5% dextrose in water if HF is present. Magnesium sulfate may be of value in suppressing some cases of VT by blocking Ca currents that are involved in after depolarization. Lidocaine. Considered the drug of choice for control of ventricular arrhythmias secondary to digoxin intoxication after the correction of hypokalemia. The short duration of action and relatively low toxicity and availability are major advantages. <u>Dosage:</u> 1.5 mg/kg, 50–100 mg with a simultaneous infusion of 1–3 mg/min and repeat bolus in 10 mins. If lidocaine fails to control the tachyarrhythmia and if there are no contraindications, a β-blocking drug may be tried cautiously (see Tables 3–8 and 3–9 for IV dosage)

DIGOXIN-SPECIFIC FAB ANTIBODY FRAGMENTS

The treatment of digitalis toxicity has been revolutionized since the value of digoxin-specific Fab fragments was proven. The digoxin-specific antibodies bind to digoxin and accelerate digoxin removal from cellular membranes. Because the digoxin is bound, it is rendered inactive. The entire body load of digoxin is bound and pulled back into the blood stream; thus, the serum digoxin level may be high, but the bound level is inactive. Fab fragments are excreted by the kidneys with a half-life of 16–20 h.

A treatment response is observed within 20 mins and by 60 mins, >75% of patients show a salutary response. Most patients show complete recovery within 4 h. Approximately 3% of patients have a recurrence of toxicity within 7 days, especially patients receiving < the estimated adequate dose of Fab. Patients with severe digoxin toxicity may have hyperkalemia due to renal failure and/or inhibition of the Na pump.

Digitalis-induced hyperkalemia suggests imminent cardiac arrest. If serum K >5 mEq/l (mmol/l), digoxin-immune Fab is immediately indicated.

In patients with life-threatening tachyarrhythmias or bradyarrhythmias, the early use of digoxin-specific antibody is strongly recommended; pacing can be avoided. Supplied: (Digibind) powder for preparation of infusion; vial, 40 mg. Dosage: 2–3 vials, 80–120 mg; an estimated adequate dose is calculated using the patient's body weight and serum digoxin level if toxicity is due to therapy or based on the amount ingested for patients with overdose. (See product monograph.) Adverse Effects: These are uncommon. Hypokalemia is observed in <5% of patients and allergic reaction occurs in <1%. Caution: Rapid onset of hypokalemia should be anticipated following reversal of toxicity by Fab fragments. IV KCl should be given as needed to avoid hypokalemia.

ACE Inhibitors

When HF occurs, sensors in the heart, the aortic arch, and arterioles of the juxtaglomerular apparatus actuate a host of neurohormonal responses that are necessary for the perfusion of vital tissues, especially of the brain, heart, and kidneys. These responses, initiated by sympathoadrenal activation and enhanced by stimulation of the renin angiotensin system, result in marked vasoconstriction, which increases systemic vascular resistance in order to maintain central BP. Unfortunately, a ↑ in systemic vascular resistance increases afterload and contractile myocyte energy costs (Fig. 5–1).

ACE inhibitors prevent formation of the vasoconstrictor angiotensin II and, at the appropriate dose, provide sufficient vasodilation to bring about a ↓ in afterload and a ↓ in systolic ventricular workload. Thus, ACE inhibitors play a major role in drug therapy of HF (NYHA Class II, III, and IV). Although these agents have greatly improved the management and survival of HF patients, they do not replace loop diuretics and are used in combination with a diuretic, with or without added digoxin therapy; see earlier discussion of drug therapy, NYHA class II, III, and IV HF.

Captopril and enalapril are approved for the management of HF in the United States; in the UK and Europe, lisinopril, perindopril, quinapril, and ramipril are available. The dosages, pharmacologic profile of ACE inhibitors, and their adverse effects are given in Tables 1–2 and 1–3 and discussed in Chapter 1.

Captopril (Capoten). Supplied: tablets; 12.5, 25, 50, and 100 mg. Dosage: 6.25-mg test dose (a 3-mg test dose is administered to the elderly or patients considered at risk for hypotension). Observation is necessary for the next 2–4 h; BP should be taken q 15–30 mins for 1, 2, or 3 h post dosing. If there is no occurrence of hypotension or presyncope, give 6.25 mg bid for the first day, ↑ to 12.5 mg bid for 1–2 days, and then over days to weeks, ↑ to the usual maintenance dose of 37.5–50 mg qd (max of 75 mg qd). A dose >75 mg provides little added benefit. Marked lowering of the diastolic BP may occur with doses >50 mg qd, causing a ↓ in coronary perfusion that may worsen angina or silent ischemia. Caution is necessary to avoid hypotension and syncope.

It is often necessary to discontinue diuretics or halve the dose to allow the introduction of an ACE inhibitor at an appropriate dose. When the patient is stabilized on captopril (25–37.5 mg qd), the dose of loop diuretics can be increased as required to relieve congestion and shortness of breath. In renal failure, the dose interval is increased according to the creatinine clearance, so that a once-daily dose should suffice for a patient who has a 50% ↓ in creatinine clearance or a serum creatinine at the upper limit of normal or at max 2.3 mg/dl (203 μmol/l). The serum creatinine is an approximation of renal function, and caution is necessary in patients with renal failure.

Enalapril (Vasotec; Vasotec or Innovace, UK). _Supplied:_ tablets; 5, 10, 20 mg. _Dosage:_ 2.5 mg orally and observe for 2–6 h. If there is no hypotension, give 2.5 mg bid for a few days, and ↑ slowly over days or weeks to 5 mg to a max of 10 mg bid. If HF is refractory, systolic pressure exceeds 120 mm Hg and active ischemia is not present; a max dose of 20 mg in the morning and 10 mg at night may be tried cautiously. In patients with severe HF, the dose can be increased more rapidly when under supervision with careful monitoring of BP to avoid hypotension. As with captopril, the dose is often given once daily in patients with very mild renal dysfunction or in patients > age 70. It is advisable to ↓ the dose of loop diuretics prior to giving the first dose of enalapril, as with other ACE inhibitors.

An initial effect of hypotension is usually observed within 1–2 h after administration of captopril and within 2-1/2 to 5 h with enalapril. Withdrawal of diuretics does not always prevent marked hypotension or syncope, and caution is required at all times with the initiation of ACE inhibitor therapy.

Interaction: Important interaction occurs with NSAIDs. Aspirin has been shown to nullify the salutary hemodynamic effects of enalapril and a similar interaction is expected with other ACE inhibitors.

PULMONARY EDEMA

Cardiogenic causes include

- Pulmonary edema, commonly accompanied by left-sided HF, which may result from or be precipitated by complications of CHD, AF with uncontrolled ventricular response, other tachyarrhythmias, hypertension, MR or aortic valve disease, and DCM
- Mitral stenosis and, rarely, left atrial myxoma

Noncardiogenic causes include

- ARDS due to pneumonias, severe trauma, toxins, allergens, smoke inhalation, gastric aspiration, hemorrhagic pancreatitis (see Chap. 28)
- Drugs, narcotic overdose, severe hypoalbuminemia, uremia, and neurogenic causes. Lymphangitic carcinomatosis may mimic LV failure

Therapy for Cardiogenic Pulmonary Edema

- O_2 must be given at high concentrations to maintain an adequate PaO_2
- Furosemide (80–120 mg IV) usually produces an effect in 10 mins due to the drug's venodilator action, which produces a ↓ in preload followed in 30 mins to 1 h by diuresis that lasts for about 2 h. If the response is not adequate, a further dose of 40–120 mg IV is given, provided that hypotension is not present. A higher dose is usually required if severe renal failure is present
- Morphine remains an extremely useful drug to allay anxiety and relieve discomfort. Also, the drug causes pooling of blood in the periphery. Morphine is advisable, provided that severe respiratory insufficiency or untreated severe hypothyroidism is absent. Dosage: 3–5 mg IV at a rate of 1 mg/min. Repeat as needed at 15- to 30-minute intervals to a total dose of 10–15 mg/h
- Treat underlying problems such as severe hypertension: Give captopril or nitroprusside (see Nitroprusside Infusion Pump Chart, Table 1–10)
- Manage cardiac arrhythmias and administer digoxin to ↓ the ventricular response in AF
- Nitroglycerin: If the systolic BP is >100 but <120 mm Hg, give 0.3 mg sublingually; give 0.6 mg for systolic pressure >120 mm Hg. The application of a transdermal preparation, e.g., 1- to 1.5-inch nitropaste, or patch formulation is useful following the sublingual dose. However, transdermal application produces variable absorption and must not be relied upon within the first hour. Both sublingual and transdermal preparations should be avoided if the systolic pressure is <100 mm Hg. In severe cases, IV nitroglycerin is recommended (see Infusion Pump Chart, Table 2–8, Chap. 2)
- Nitroprusside is indicated if pulmonary edema is due to severe hypertension or mechanical complications of acute MI (see Infusion Pump Chart, Table 1–10)
- Aminophylline should not be used routinely. It has a role if bronchospasm and/or diaphragmatic fatigue are present. The drug increases the diuretic effect of furosemide and has mild anti-ischemic effects. Dosage: 2–4 mg/kg IV over 20 mins, then infusion 0.3–0.5 mg/kg/h. The smaller dose is used in the elderly or in patients with hepatic dysfunction (see Tables 16–5 and 16–6)
- Rotating venous tourniquets can be temporarily beneficial in patients with severe pulmonary edema unresponsive to standard therapy listed above. Tourniquets should be placed several inches distal to the groin and shoulders, and only 3 of the 4 tourniquets should be inflated at one time, to approximately 10 mm Hg below the diastolic pressure; one should be released q 15–20 mins
- Dobutamine is indicated if the above measures fail to control pulmonary edema in the presence of mild hypotension and severe LV systolic dysfunction; dobutamine is superior to amrinone IV. If respiratory failure complicates pulmonary edema, dopamine should be avoided because this agent may cause constriction of pulmonary veins, which results in a ↑ in pulmonary capillary hydrostatic pressure and lung fluid accumulation. Dosage: 2.5–7.5 μg/kg/min (see Infusion Pump Chart, Table 4–5)
- Digoxin: See earlier sections of this chapter. Digoxin is required if AF or flutter with a rapid ventricular rate is present; slower rates (100–120/min) may require slowing in patients with severe mitral stenosis

- Endotracheal intubation and mechanical ventilation may be required for patients with respiratory failure: If PaO_2 cannot be maintained at or near 60 mm Hg despite 100% O_2 at 20 liters/min or if there is progressive hypercapnia. Identify and treat precipitating factors, especially acute MI, arrhythmias, and infection

Non-cardiogenic pulmonary edema is discussed in Chapter 20.

Suggested Reading

Khan M Gabriel: Heart failure. *In* Cardiac and Pulmonary Management. Philadelphia, Lea & Febiger, 1993.

Pfeffer MA, Braunwald E, Moye LA, et al.: Effect of captopril on mortality and morbidity in patients with left ventricular dysfunction after myocardial infarction: results of the Survival and Ventricular Enlargement Trial. New Engl J Med *325*: 669, 1992.

SOLVD Investigators: Effect of enalapril on survival in patients with reduced ventricular ejection fractions and congestive heart failure. New Engl J Med *325*: 293, 1991.

SOLVD Investigators. Effect of enalapril on mortality and the development of heart failure in symptomatic patients with reduced left ventricular ejection fractions. New Engl J Med *327*: 685, 1992.

Uretsky BF, Young JB, Shahidi FE, et al: Randomized Study Assessing the Effect of Digoxin Withdrawal in Patients With Mild to Moderate Chronic Congestive Heart Failure: Results of the PROVED Trial. J Am Coll Cardiol *22*: 955, 1993.

Arrhythmias

6

M. Gabriel Khan

Accurate diagnosis—in particular, differentiation of VT and SVT is essential for appropriate management. The ECG diagnostic points for tachyarrhythmias are shown in Tables 6–1 and 6–2 and Figure 6–1

- Divide into narrow QRS or wide QRS
- Determine whether the rhythm is regular or irregular

The treatment of underlying conditions may cause amelioration and/or prevention of arrhythmia recurrence. The severity of the underlying diseases, particularly the degree of LV dysfunction, may dictate the choice of antiarrhythmic agent and the outcome. The prognosis of ventricular arrhythmias is closely linked to the degree of LV dysfunction. Echocardiographic EF is more cost effective than radionuclide because structural abnormalities including left atrial enlargement may be detected

- EF >50% carries a good prognosis
- EF 40–50% is commonly associated with benign arrhythmias and a fair prognosis
- EF 25–39% is often associated with potentially lethal arrhythmias
- EF <25% indicates a poor prognosis

Adverse effects of drug therapy are related to the degree of LV dysfunction. Drugs that may be used in patients with an EF<30% and other scenarios are given in Table 6–3.

The emergency management of arrhythmias calls for a quick assessment of

- The hemodynamic status: Is the BP<90 mm Hg and are there signs of peripheral hypoperfusion?
- The symptomatic status: Chest pain, shortness of breath, presyncope, syncope, or clouding of consciousness
- Cardiac decompensation: Signs of CHF

An essential step is to rapidly define the clinical setting and correct a precipitating cause in order to obviate the need for antiarrhythmic therapy or to appraise and prevent deleterious proarrhythmic effects of these agents.

Precipitating factors and/or clinical setting include

- Ischemia: As with acute MI or acute myocardial ischemia
- Those characterized by myocardial reperfusion: Post-thrombolytic therapy in acute MI, balloon deflation during coronary angioplasty, release of coronary artery spasm
- Hypotension
- Sick sinus syndrome or A-V block
- CHF
- Hypokalemia, hypomagnesemia, hyperkalemia
- Alkalemia, e.g., may develop rapidly in ventilated patients

Table 6–1
Differential Diagnosis of Narrow QRS Tachycardia

REGULAR	IRREGULAR
1. AVNRT Rate = 140–220 P waves usually buried and not apparent in the QRS or less commonly retrograde P barely visible in terminal QRS or very early ST segment, inverted in II, III AVF	1. Atrial fibrillation R–R intervals completely irregular Absent P waves
2. WPW with AV reentry, negative P wave Lead I suggest left-sided bypass tract Marked alternation in QRS amplitude highly suspect WPW	2. Atrial flutter: AR >250 Variable AV conduction
3. PAT with block, AR 150–200 VR usually <140 P wave often buried in T Isoelectric intervals between P waves	3. Multifocal atrial tachycardia (MAT) Three different P wave morphologies in any lead, variable P–P, PR, RR intervals Atrial rate = 100–200/minute R–R intervals completely irregular; may progress to AF
4. Sinoatrial trachycardia Average rate = 140/minute Sinus P waves present: Upright P waves in the ST segment	
5. Atrial flutter AR = 250–350 often 300/minute VR often 150–160/minute Conduction ratio often 2:1 Sawtooth pattern leads II, AVF Sharp-pointed "P" waves in V_1	
6. Ectopic atrial tachycardia	

AVNRT = AV nodal reentrant tachycardia
AR = atrial rate
VR = ventricular rate
AF = atrial fibrillation
VR = 240–300 suggests WPW

- Acidemia
- Hypoxemia
- Pulmonary disease, cor pulmonale, atelectasis, pneumothorax, and carcinoma of lungs. May precipitate atrial flutter or AF
- Infection
- Fluctuations in autonomic tone
- Acute blood loss
- Thyrotoxicosis
- Digoxin toxicity
- Proarrhythmic effects of antiarrhythmic drugs: Quinidine and other Class IA drugs may cause torsades de pointes, also caused by Class III agents (sotalol and rarely by amiodarone). More typical monomorphic VT and other lethal arrhythmias may be initiated by antiarrhythmic drugs
- Non-antiarrhythmics: β agonist, theophylline, terfenadine, and astemizole, especially in combination with erythromycin or ketoconazole
- Ruptured esophagus: May initiate atrial flutter or AF

Table 6–2
Wide QRS Tachycardia

REGULAR	IRREGULAR
1. Ventricular tachycardia Hallmarks a. Absence of an RS complex in all precordial leads b. QRS duration: R to S interval >100 msec* in one precorded lead RBBB QRS >140 msec* LBBB QRS >160 msec* c.† AV dissociation (cannon waves in neck) excludes atrial but not nodal tachycardia Suggested Features: d. Positive concordance (except WPW type A) e. Left axis −90 to +180 (−60 to −90 suggest VT) f. QS or rS in V_6 (R to S, ratio <1) or net negative QRS in V_6 g. V_1 "Left rabbit ear" taller than the right: slurred downslope of S wave in V_1 strongly suggests VT 2. SVT with known Right or LBBB 3. SVT with aberrant conduction: visible on aberrant atrial ectopic: small normal q: qRs in V_6 4. Atrial flutter: with wide QRS‡ with WPW§ (rare) 5. WPW anterograde through bypass tract§ (resembles VT)	1. Atrial fibrillation and WPW rate (200–300/min with aberrancy§) 2. AF and prior intraventricular conduction defect on recent ECG

* milliseconds
† AV block or dissociation excludes bypass tract
‡ AF treated with Class IC or IA agents may induce this arrhythmia
§ RR <205 milliseconds suggests WPW, treat as VT

Table 6–3
Ejection Fraction May Dictate Choice of Antiarrhythmic Agent

GROUP I	GROUP II	GROUP III
Ejection fraction (EF) <30% only safe agents* Amiodarone Mexiletine Quinidine Beta blockers†	EF >30% Beta blockers and agents used for Group 1*	EF >40% Agents given under Group I, II plus Class IA, IB Propafenone‡ Flecainide‡ Verapamil Diltiazem

* All other agents: hazard of precipitating heart failure
† Used judiciously in properly selected patients, absence of overt heart failure, EF down to 25%
‡ Limited indications (see text)

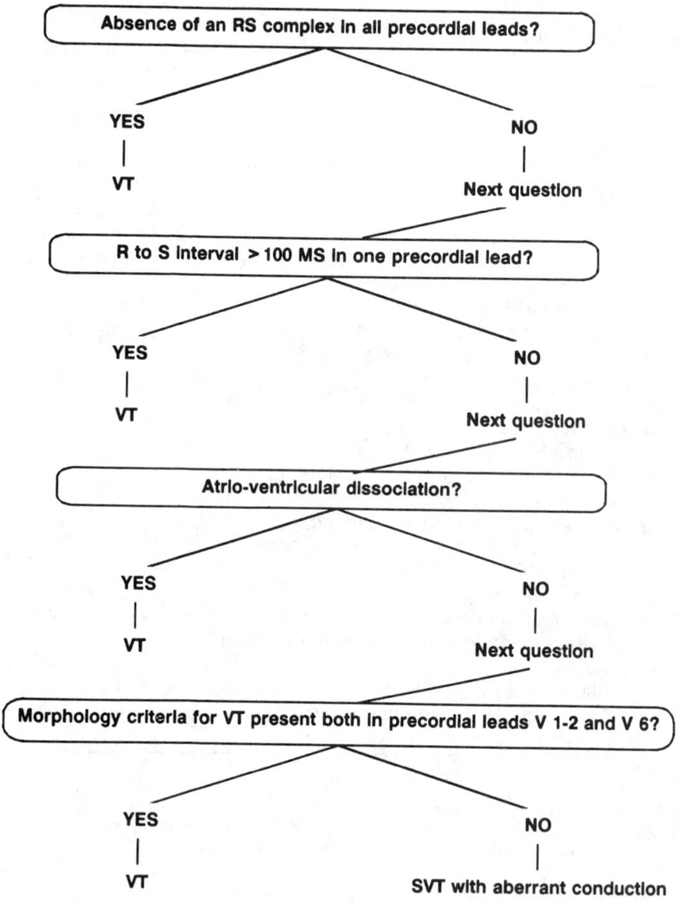

Figure 6–1. Algorithm for diagnosis of a tachycardia with a widened QRS complex. From: Brugada P, et al.: A new approach to the differential diagnosis of a regular tachycardia with a wide QRS complex. Circulation, *83*:1651, 1991.

SUPRAVENTRICULAR ARRHYTHMIAS

A-V Nodal Reentrant Tachycardia

PSVT in patients < age 35 usually occurs in an otherwise normal heart and has a good prognosis. However, AVNRT is not uncommon with organic heart disease caused by coronary, rheumatic, or other valvular heart disease, and rarely can be life threatening. The onset and termination are abrupt; HR varies from 140–220/min, with a regular rhythm (Table 6–1).

TREATMENT

Carotid sinus massage, patient rhythm monitored

- Response is either reversion to sinus rhythm or no effect at all, in contrast to atrial flutter, where slowing of HR virtually always occurs
- Not recommended in the elderly or in patients with known or highly suspected carotid disease, ischemia, or digitalis toxicity
- With the patient supine (head slightly hyperextended, turned a little toward the opposite side), locate the right carotid sinus at the angle of the jaw. Apply firm pressure in a circular or massage fashion for 2–6 sec, using the first and second fingers. It is necessary to monitor the cardiac rhythm and gauge exactly when to stop massage because asystole, although rare, can occur. If unsuccessful, after an interval of 2 min to allow acetylcholine to be manufactured in the A-V node, massage the left carotid sinus. If asystole occurs during the procedure, ask the patient to cough and/or give the patient ≥1 light chest thumps, which usually reverses transient asystole
- *Caution:* Never massage for >10 seconds.

Verapamil. *Caution:* Verapamil IV is contraindicated in patients with severe hypotension, CHF, LV dysfunction, cardiomegaly, acute MI, sick sinus syndrome (Fig. 6–2), suspected digitalis toxicity and concurrent use of β blockers, disopyramide, or amiodarone; do not use in wide QRS tachycardia, antidromic WPW, or if the refractory period of the accessory pathway is <270 millisec.

Dosage: Verapamil (5 mg IV) is given slowly over 1–2 min. Use 2.5 mg initially if LV function is believed to be slightly impaired. Resistance or recurrence of arrhythmia without a marked ↓ in BP should be treated with an additional 2.5- to 5-mg dose 10 min after the first dose. Occasionally an IV infusion is used, 1 mg/min to a total of 10 mg or 5–10 mg over 1 h; 100 mg in 24 h. Mild hypotension is not a contraindication, and further hypotension can be partially avoided by the administration of CaCl: 10 ml of a 10% solution over 5–10 min; calcium gluconate is an alternative; for sinus arrest or A-V block give CaCl and atropine 0.5 mg IV.

Adenosine (Adenocard). This ultra short acting agent has decreased the need for IV verapamil (Table 6–4), digoxin, or β blockers in the acute management of PSVT (Fig. 6–2).

Dosage Using a Peripheral Vein: 6 mg by rapid IV bolus injection over 2 sec rapidly flushed into a peripheral vein; if given via an IV line, the drug should be given as proximal as possible and followed by a rapid saline flush. Termination of arrhythmia is expected in <1 min, and the action of the drug lasts for <30 sec after injection. A second bolus injection of 12 mg is repeated 2 min after the first if the arrhythmia persists or recurs. The 12-mg dose may be repeated in 2–5 min, if required, and may be given via a larger vein than used in prior IV injection. Further recurrence of the arrhythmia calls for alternative therapy. In 10–30% of cases, arrhythmia recurs within minutes of the first injection of adenosine. A smaller dose is required if the drug is given through a central vein. A dose of 6 mg administered through a central vein in the same patient may have a potent effect, whereas a 12-mg dose may be ineffective when administered through a small peripheral vein. The drug should be used cautiously in patients with right to left shunting and must not be administered into the distal port of a balloon flotation catheter.

Table 6–4
Adenosine Versus Verapamil for the Management of Paroxysmal Supraventricular Tachycardias

PARAMETERS	FIRST CHOICE	SECOND CHOICE
Uncomplicated cases ventricular rate <220/min	Verapamil	Adenosine
Hypotension		
mild	Adenosine	Verapamil after pretreatment with calcium chloride or gluconate
moderate/severe	Adenosine	Verapamil CI
Left ventricular dysfunction heart failure cardiomegaly	Adenosine	Verapamil CI
Suspect pre-excitation (AVRT)	Adenosine	Verapamil CI
Wide QRS		
? aberrancy	Adenosine	Verapamil CI
Ectopic or multifocal atrial tachycardia	Verapamil	Adenosine ineffective

CI = contraindicated
R = relative
HF = heart failure

Action

- The drug has a depressant effect on the SA node and slows impulse conduction through the A-V node. These effects appear to be mediated at the cellular level by an increase in K and a decrease in Ca conductance. These EP effects are not antagonized by atropine
- After IV quick bolus injection, adenosine has a rapid onset of action within 5–30 sec and converts ≤90% of PSVTs to sinus rhythm
- The drug has a very short half-life (<2 sec) because it is avidly taken up and metabolized by adenosine deaminase in endothelial and red blood cells

Indications

- Termination of AVNRT and A-V reentrant reciprocating tachycardia. The drug causes termination of these arrhythmias in >90% of cases. It is the agent of first choice for these arrhythmias in patients with hypotension (Fig. 6-2) or other situations where rapid conversion to sinus rhythm is needed or as an alternative to electrical cardioversion
- In patients with PSVT that fails to terminate with a 10-mg dose of verapamil, or when contraindications or relative contraindications to verapamil exist
- The drug has advantages over verapamil in patients with A-V reentrant tachycardia utilizing an accessory pathway in the reentry circuit; adenosine may unmask latent pre-excitation when sinus rhythm is restored and can only produce very transient episodes of rapid pre-excited arrhythmia, as opposed to verapamil, which is contraindicated in these situations. Thus, adenosine is much safer than verapamil for use in patients with WPW or suspected WPW arrhythmias
- Adenosine, in decreasing A-V conduction, unmasks atrial flutter and assists with diagnosis
- Adenosine also has a role in patients with suspected SVT or wide

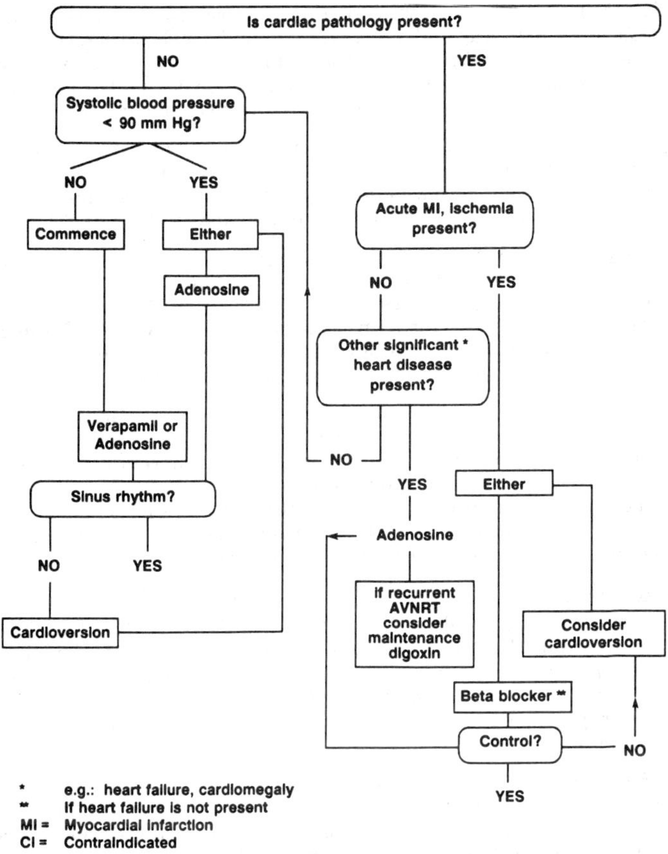

Figure 6–2. Suggested steps in how to treat AV nodal reentrant tachycardia (AVNRT). From: Khan M. Gabriel: Management of cardiac arrhythmias. *In* Cardiac Drug Therapy. 3rd Ed. London, W.B. Saunders, 1992.

complex tachycardia of uncertain type. In patients with misdiagnosed VT, verapamil may precipitate CHF and other life-threatening complications. Adenosine, in this situation, causes reversion if the rhythm is due to A-V nodal reentry, and its effect on VT is transient and not detrimental because of its ultrashort half-life

- Adenosine appears to have an important role and is relatively safe in infants with rapid PSVT with hemodynamic compromise, because repeat electrical cardioversion with 20 J can cause deleterious effects on the myocardium at this age. Adenosine pediatric dosage: 50 μg/kg; increase at 50 μg/kg increments if needed to 150 μg/kg (not included in the drug's product monograph but appears to be relatively safe at this dose range).

Adenosine indications may be limited by cost; adenosine is 60 times more expensive than verapamil. A multicenter study indicated that a 12-mg dose is usually required to achieve about a 90% success in conversion of the arrhythmia to sinus rhythm at a cost of $30 compared with a $.50 for 10 mg verapamil. Also, there is a high incidence of recurrence of the arrhythmia within minutes of the first successful conversion. The incidence varies from 10 to 33% a second injection is usually successful. Adenosine is not effective in ectopic atrial tachycardia and MAT.

Contraindications: 2nd° or 3rd° A-V block, except in patients with a functioning pacemaker; sinus node disease; known hypersensitivity to adenosine; asthma; chronic pulmonary disease with theophylline usage; unstable angina; acute MI (not given in the product monograph)

Adverse Effects: Minor adverse effects occur in 30–60% of patients. It is wise to advise the patient that minor transient adverse effects may occur, lasting 1/2–1 min. These effects include: facial flushing, dyspnea, chest pain or pressure, mild bronchospasm in patients with COPD, and, less commonly: nausea, vomiting, headache, transient hypotension, and sinus pauses with ventricular standstill of several seconds.

Caution: Safety in patients with myocardial ischemic syndromes is not established. A dose of 12 mg may be ineffective if given through a small peripheral vein, but 6 mg given through a central vein may have a potent effect. Do not administer the 12-mg dose through a central vein or porthole of a balloon flotation catheter. Avoid the use of adenosine in the presence of a prolonged QT interval because induced bradycardia may promote the precipitation of torsades de pointes.

Interactions

- Dipyridamole markedly enhances the sinoatrial and A-V nodal effects of adenosine. Dipyridamole decreases cellular uptake of adenosine, thereby inhibiting its metabolism. This interaction may be important in patients being given oral dipyridamole
- Aminophylline, caffeine, and other methyl xanthines completely antagonize adenosine.

Esmolol has an ultra-short action that confers major advantages over propranolol, atenolol, and metoprolol. The onset of action is rapid. The drug is quickly metabolized by esterases of red blood cells and has a half-life of 9 min that is unaffected by renal failure, CHF, or hepatic dysfunction. The drug is cardioselective and has the same contraindications as other β-blocking agents. Esmolol has a role in the management of uncomplicated cases of SVT not terminated by adenosine and where adenosine or verapamil are contraindicated, especially during acute MI or other ischemic syndromes.

Dosage: Initial loading infusion of 3–40 mg (usually 6 mg), IV infusion over 1 min (30 to max 500 μg/kg given over 1 min), and then maintenance infusion 1–5 mg/min (max 50 μg/kg/min). *Adverse Effects:* Mild transient hypotension occurs in <25% of patients, more commonly in those with systolic BP <100 mm Hg, and improvement occurs within minutes of discontinuing the IV infusion.

Propranolol. *Dosage:* 1 mg IV given over 2 min, repeated q 5 min to a max of 5 mg.

Metoprolol. *Dosage:* 5 mg IV bolus over 3 min; then, if required after 5 min, an additional bolus is given and repeated if needed 5–10 min later.

Phenylephrine has a role only in young patients with a normal heart when the BP is <90 mm Hg, when adenosine is not available, or when cardioversion is felt to be unnecessary. This alpha agonist increases BP, and vagal activity results in sinus rhythm. *Dosage:* 0.1 mg diluted with

5 ml or 5% dextrose IV bolus over 2 min; the BP is measured at 30-sec intervals and must not be allowed to exceed 140 mm Hg. Allow 1–3 min after each bolus for the BP to return to baseline value before giving an additional bolus. Max dose 0.5 mg. If this fails to produce sinus rhythm but stabilization of BP is achieved, verapamil can be given.

Digoxin is preferred if there are signs of CHF, hypotension, or severe cardiomegaly, or signs and symptoms of a sick heart. However, digoxin takes >2 h to have an effect and is not recommended where rapid restoration of sinus rhythm is required. *Dosage:* In the absence of digoxin use during the previous week, 0.5 mg IV by infusion over 10 min, followed in 30 min with 0.25 mg, then po 0.25 mg once daily, (see page 123).

DC Cardioversion may be necessary for patients who are hemodynamically unstable and should be used prior to drug therapy, or if such therapy appears unsuccessful.

Chronic maintenance for bothersome, frequently recurring SVT usually requires digoxin or a β blocker and occasionally a combination of both drugs. Verapamil 120 mg taken at the onset of SVT has a role in aborting attacks within 1-2 h and prevents ER visits.

Paroxysmal Atrial Tachycardia with Block

- The arrhythmia is usually due to digoxin toxicity. Atrial rate <200 excludes atrial flutter (see Table 6-1). If the HR is 90–120/min with a normal serum K, no treatment is usually required
- If the serum K is <3.5 mEq/l and a high degree of A-V block is absent, give KCI IV (60 mEq) in 1 L normal saline over 5 h

Multifocal Atrial Tachycardia

- MAT is usually seen in patients with COPD, hypoxemia, and theophylline toxicity. Treat the underlying cause
- If tachycardia is symptomatic or causes cardiac embarrassment, give verapamil 2.5–5 mg IV repeated in 30 min. IV verapamil is usually successful, and it should be followed by 80 mg 3 or 4 times daily until the underlying problem resolves. Often the arrhythmia causes no hemodynamic disturbances, especially at rates of 100–130/min and requires no drug therapy, or the initial dose of verapamil can be given orally
- Magnesium has a direct effect on K channels, increases intracellular K, and is effective in some patients
- A β blocker is more effective than verapamil, but caution is needed in patients with COPD. Metoprolol IV or oral may be given a trial if asthma or severe COPD are not present

Atrial Flutter

- Atrial flutter is usually due to underlying pathology, in particular CHD, MI, hypoxemia due to pulmonary embolism, pneumothorax, and COPD; also mitral valve disease and thyrotoxicosis. Removal of the underlying causes may be followed by spontaneous reversion to sinus rhythm
- Atrial flutter is easily converted to sinus rhythm by synchronized DC shock 25–50 J. This should be carried out if the patient is hemodynam-

ically compromised, a ventricular response is >200/min, or the patient is known or suspected to have WPW
- Patients with ventricular response <200/min: propranolol or other β blockers may be used to slow the ventricular response
- Digoxin converts atrial flutter to AF and slows the ventricular response
- Verapamil reduces the ventricular response and may occasionally cause conversion to sinus rhythm. Verapamil, digoxin, and β blockers are contraindicated in patients with WPW presenting with atrial flutter or AF. In this setting, verapamil or digoxin may precipitate VF
- Atrial pacing is effective in terminating atrial flutter

Atrial Fibrillation

- Diagnosis is readily made from the ECG. Causes of AF include rheumatic and other valvular heart disease, CHD, hypertension, cardiomyopathies, cor pulmonale, pulmonary embolism, thyrotoxicosis, sick sinus syndrome producing tachy and brady arrhythmias, WPW syndrome, alcohol abuse, post thoracotomy, esophago-jejunostomy, ruptured esophagus, carbon monoxide poisoning, and idiopathic
- Investigations should include echocardiogram to confirm underlying causes and evaluate left atrial size and presence of thrombus.

Digoxin is used in the majority of patients to control the ventricular response, except with HR >240/min, likely due to WPW. Symptomatic patients ventricular rate 150–220/min; give digoxin IV 0.5 mg slowly followed by 0.25 mg IV q 2 h to control the ventricular response. A total dose of 1 mg is usually necessary if the patient has not taken digoxin in the past 2 weeks. For patients who have taken digoxin recently, a dose of 0.125 IV should be tried followed by a further 0.125 mg 2 h later, if needed, followed by maintenance doses of 0.125–0.25 mg. qd. The serum K must be maintained above 4 mEq (mmol)/l.

Diltiazem IV slows the ventricular response, has less negative inotropic effect than verapamil, and can be given as a continuous infusion up to 24 h in patients in whom digoxin maintenance is not considered essential. Diltiazem should not be administered in patients with suspected LV dysfunction or known to have EF <40%.

Patients with recent onset of AF should be anticoagulated. Conversion to sinus rhythm may be achieved in some patients if it is felt desirable: conversion may be achieved after full digitalization and control of ventricular response by adding quinidine 200–300 mg q 6 h, or, if ventricular function is unimpaired, disopyramide may be used instead of quinidine. Conversion to sinus rhythm is achieved in about 50% of patients. DC conversion should be utilized in individuals with suspected WPW or HR >240, or unstable patients and acute MI with hemodynamic compromise. DC conversion is also deemed necessary in patients with severe aortic stenosis, obstructive cardiomyopathy, and right ventricular infarction in whom atrial transport function is of great importance. Patients with chronic AF benefit from slowing the ventricular response with digitalis, and those who have a fast ventricular response on exercise gain further benefit with the addition of small doses of a β blocker or oral verapamil.

Synchronized DC cardioversion is usually

<u>Contraindicated</u> in

- AF duration >1 year because sinus rhythm is usually not maintained.
- Cardioversion is often not considered worthwhile with chronic AF

since <40% of patients remain in sinus rhythm 1 year post conversion. Other reasons for not electing to convert include the course of anticoagulation 1–2 weeks prior and 3–4 weeks post. Embolization occurs in about 2% of patients as well as transient post-conversion arrhythmias. DC conversion is not advisable in patients with suspected digitalis toxicity because of the risk of precipitating VF. Patients with sick sinus syndrome may develop prolonged post-conversion arrhythmias. In patients with left atrial size >5 cm, sinus rhythm is usually not maintained. However, a clinical study indicates that left atrial size >5 cm is not a major determinant of failure to maintain sinus rhythm post conversion. Amiodarone has been shown to cause reversion and maintenance of sinus rhythm for ≤6 months in ≤60% of patients with atrial size <6 cm. For DC conversion, anticoagulants are not generally used if AF is 24 h duration. If AF is >24 h and conversion is necessary, oral anticoagulants are given. Digoxin is maintained for the period before conversion and is interrupted 24–48 h prior. Quinidine or disopyramide is given immediately after conversion and continued so as to increase the chance of perpetuating sinus rhythm, but this therapy is not of proven value. Light anesthesia, IV diazepam, or thiopental with a standby anesthesiologist is necessary

- Role of anticoagulants: Patients with recent onset and paroxysmal AF should be anticoagulated if there is no contraindication so as to prevent embolization. Risk of embolization is about 20% higher in patients with rheumatic heart disease and congestive cardiomyopathy, thus anticoagulation is strongly recommended. Patients with atrial flutter, however, do not require anticoagulants for conversion or for chronic use because embolization is not a complication.

Flecainide (Tambocor) IV is more effective than a combination of digoxin and quinidine in converting AF to sinus rhythm. The drug is effective mainly in patients with AF of recent onset (<6 weeks) or in patients with small atria (<4 cm). _Dosage:_ IV bolus 2 mg/kg over 10 min followed by oral treatment 200–300 mg qd. Flecainide given orally is useful in preventing recurrence of paroxysmal AF. Average oral dose 300 mg qd, max 400 mg. The drug is contraindicated in patients with CHF, poor ventricular function, and/or conduction defects. The manufacturers no longer recommend the drug for benign or potentially lethal arrhythmias. The CAST initiated this recommendation.

Wolff-Parkinson-White Syndrome

ECG changes are not always typical and depend on the distance between the SA node and the accessory pathway, and the resulting conducting times: intra-atrial, A-V node-His, bundle branch, and accessory pathway. Thus, when A-V nodal conduction is slowed, ECG features are more prominent and less apparent during exercise or when the accessory pathway is distant from the SA node.

ECG hallmarks include

- A PR interval <0.12 sec is observed in ≤80% of cases. In approximately 20% of patients, the PR interval is 0.12 sec or slightly longer, especially with advancing age
- A QRS ≥0.12 sec is not necessary for the diagnosis; in about 20% of cases, the QRS duration is <0.11 sec
- A delta wave is not always present
- Occasionally, a pseudo-infarction pattern "Q in leads 2, 3 or AVF" is present
- R wave as the sole or main deflection in V_1, V_2 referred to as Type A WPW suggests localization of the bypass tract in the left ventricle

- Type A pattern and a negative delta wave in leads 2, 3 and AVF; consider posteroseptal bypass tract
- Type A and isoelectric or negative delta in one of the following leads: 1, AVL, V_5, V_6; consider a left lateral bypass tract
- A negative P wave in lead 1 during tachycardia suggests a left-sided bypass tract
- In so-called Type B WPW, an S or QS is the dominant deflection in V_1, V_2, and may be mistaken for incomplete LBBB or voltage criteria for LVH. Type B pattern is more commonly seen with right-sided bypass tracts. The terms Type A and Type B are no longer considered important hallmarks, but they are ingrained in history and may serve to remind the physician of certain scenarios, e.g., tall R in V_1 is not always due to right ventricular hypertrophy or true posterior MI, but may be due to pre-excitation; also, Type B is present in ≤25% of cases of Ebstein's anomaly
- AF occurs in 15–39% of cases; if the refractory period is very short, a very fast ventricular response (240–300) may occur and precipitate VF. Rarely, atrial flutter is manifest (Table 6-5)
- Very rarely a wide QRS regular tachycardia may be caused by multiple mechanisms, including the antidromic form of tachycardia
- A clearly observed retrograde P wave in the ST segment suggests WPW tachyarrhythmia, whereas in AVNRT the P wave is usually lost in the QRS complex and is rarely seen in the ST segment
- The presence of alternation in QRS amplitude during tachycardia suggests the participation of a bypass tract
- Rate-related LBBB: Consider WPW

Also, patients can have ≥2 pathways with reciprocation, using them and not the A-V node, or may have AVNRT with conduction to the ventricles by the bypass tract.

The most common orthodromic arrhythmia in WPW syndrome is a circus movement in which the reentrant circuit uses the A-V node in the anterograde direction and the accessory pathway in the retrograde direction and is a reciprocating tachycardia. This situation is present in >85% of WPW arrhythmias. Rarely, a spontaneous change occurs in some patients from orthodromic to the rare antidromic tachycardia.

Antidromic tachycardia is an uncommon but clinically important form of tachyarrhythmia that occurs in 7–15% of patients with WPW; >66% have multiple bypass tracts. In antidromic WPW, the tachycardia uses the accessory pathway in the anterograde direction and the A-V node in the retrograde direction, resulting in rapid tachycardia.

Dizziness and syncope occur in >66% of patients with antidromic tachycardia and in <10% of patients with orthodromic tachycardia. Antidromic tachycardia may present as AF with rapid ventricular rates,

Table 6–5
Types and Approximate Incidence of Tachyarrhythmias in WPW Syndrome

TACHYCARDIA	APPROXIMATE %
1. AVRT	60
2. Atrial fibrillation	15–39
3. Atrial flutter	1
4. Regular wide complex QRS indistinguishable from VT (Atrial flutter or BBB during AVRT)	1
5. Ventricular flutter VF	3

RR <205 msec with a wide QRS complex. Table 6-5 gives types of tachyarrhythmias observed with WPW and their approximate incidence.

Associated diseases and mimicry include

- An increased incidence of WPW in patients with hypertrophic cardiomyopathy; echocardiographic assessment is advisable in all patients with WPW
- Approximately 25% of Ebstein abnormalities have Type B ECG pattern
- Q waves in 2 of the 3 inferior leads 2, 3 and AVF may be incorrectly diagnosed as inferior infarction
- Absence of R in V_1, and initial Q in V_2, simulate anteroseptal infarction
- Tall R waves in V_1 may incorrectly suggest right ventricular hypertrophy or true posterior infarction
- High QRS voltage may incorrectly suggest LVH
- Type B or Type A ECG pattern can be mistaken for incomplete LBBB or RBBB, respectively.

Therapy

- Emergency room management of AVRT previously in patients with WPW: Adenosine rapid bolus injection as indicated in the section, Management of AVNRT (see page 135)
- Patients with rapid ventricular response >240/min should be managed with IV procainamide. (*Caution:* Avoid in patients with hypertrophic cardiomyopathy.) In tachycardia, which could be pre-excited (e.g., AF or flutter), procainamide ≤10 mg/kg IV over 30 min, max 1 g in 1 hour, is reasonably safe provided that the patient is not hypotensive and does not become so. Failure to convert the arrhythmia or hemodynamic deterioration is an indication for prompt electrical conversion
- Amiodarone has a role in the prevention of paroxysmal AF with rapid rates. Failure to respond is an indication for EP studies with a view to ablative therapy.

MANAGEMENT OF VENTRICULAR PREMATURE BEATS AND VENTRICULAR TACHYCARDIA

- Guidelines for the management of benign, potentially lethal, and lethal arrhythmias are given in Table 6-6. An algorithm for the management of sustained VT is given in Figure 6-3
- The selection of an antiarrhythmic agent is often dictated by the efficacy, proarrhythmic effect, and propensity to cause serious adverse effect, especially CHF (Table 6-7)
- **Dosage** of antiarrhythmic drugs is given in Table 6–8
- Patients with benign arrhythmias require drug therapy only if symptoms are very bothersome. A β blocker should be given a 3-month trial. Benign arrhythmias may disappear or wax and wane; prolonged therapy may not be justified. Propafenone is of some value but is contraindicated with bundle branch block and significant COPD. Although rare, agranulocytosis has been reported
- In patients with potentially lethal arrhythmias but with EF 25–30%, only 3 agents can be considered: amiodarone, mexiletine, and quinidine (Table 6-8). They have only a mild negative inotropic effect. Encainide can precipitate CHF, and the manufacturer's caution must be

Table 6–6
Guidelines for the Management of Ventricular Arrhythmias

BENIGN ARRHYTHMIAS	POTENTIALLY* LETHAL	LETHAL (MALIGNANT ARRHYTHMIAS)
Normal heart: VPCs, couplets, Bigeminy ↓ No treatment reassurance If symptoms very bothersome or VT normal heart ↓ Beta blocker and reassurance; consider Mexiletine 2nd choice	Abnormal heart e.g., post myocardial infarction: Frequent VPCs multifocal, Nonsustained VT ↓ EF >30%; No overt CHF ↓ Beta blocker† ↓ Not controlled and symptomatic ↓ Mexiletine (unproven to improve survival) ↓ Not controlled ↓ Consider ↓ Amiodarone‡	a. Cardiovascular collapse b. Post cardiac arrest (VF) ↓ EP Studies: In approximately 25% of cases, can initiate and suppress with drug or combination and improve outcome ↓ In majority EF <30% trial sotalol† or Amiodarone or Amiodarone + beta blocker§ or Multiprogrammable implantable pacemaker-cardioverter-defibrillator, especially if EF ≤25% (see Chapter 7) or ablative treatment c. Torsades de pointes (see text)

* Only beta blockers significantly prolong life; amiodarone appears to do so only in the absence of heart failure
† Used judiciously, EF down to 25% (see text)
‡ Flecainide, moricizine, and propafenone not recommended for benign or potentially lethal arrhythmias.
§ Not sotalol

observed; the drug is also markedly proarrhythmic. The result of the CAST indicates that flecainide, encainide, and moricizine are contraindicated in benign or potentially lethal arrhythmias; *encainide is not approved for general use.*

Classification of Antiarrhythmics

A knowledge of the EP classification of antiarrhythmics is useful in understanding arrhythmia suppression, drug combinations, and proarrhythmic and some adverse effects. Class 1 drugs inhibit influx of Na into the cardiac myocyte (Fig. 6–4, Table 6–9). Class 1A (quinidine, disopyramide, and procainamide) slow phase zero and prolong the duration of the action potential. Class 1B (lidocaine, mexiletine, and tocanide) have relatively no effect on phase zero. Class 1C (flecainide, encainide, and propafenone) slow phase zero but have little or no effect on action potential duration. Class 2 comprises β-blockers. Class 3 comprises amiodarone, bretylium, and sotalol.

Antiarrhythmic Agents

Lidocaine (Lignocaine, UK) is used in the presence of acute MI to treat frequent VPCs >6/min, multifocal or R on T. Lidocaine is the drug of first choice for the management of sustained VT where the patient is hemodynamically stable (Fig. 6-3) (VT >30 seconds or unstable signs

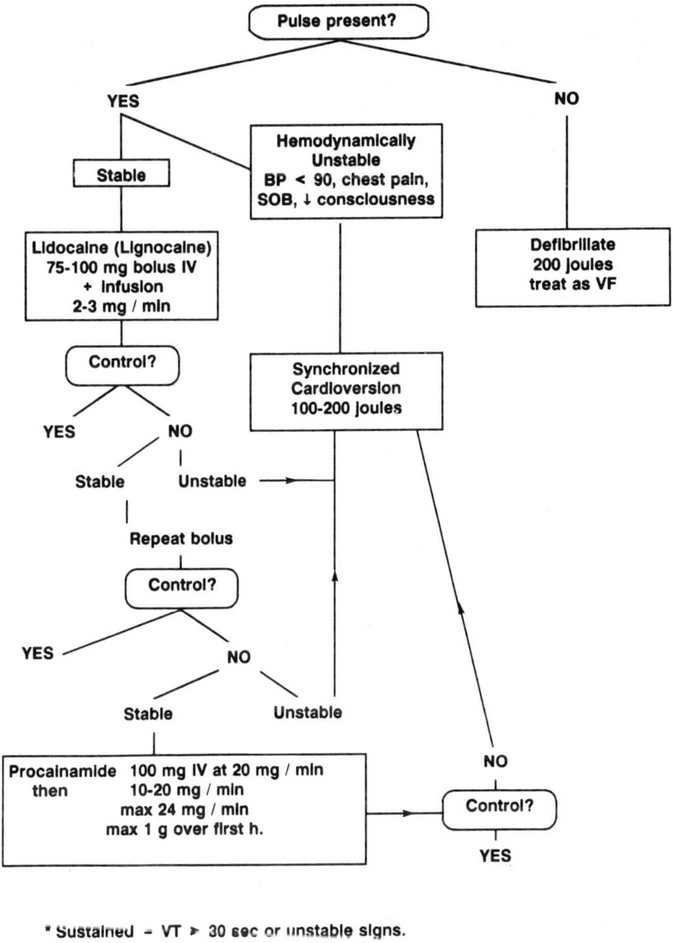

Figure 6–3. Management of sustained ventricular tachycardia.

= sustained). *Dosage:* IV rapid bolus 75–100 mg (1–1.5 mg/kg) with immediate infusion of 2–3 mg/min. A second bolus of 50–75 mg is administered within 5 min for VPCs, and earlier if VT persists. A further bolus may be required. In the presence of severe hepatic disease, CHF, or cardiogenic shock, the dose should be halved. A max infusion of 4 mg/min should be given only after careful reevaluation (see Tables 3-8 and 3-9).

Quinidine. Although quinidine has the feature of not precipitating CHF, the drug is not very effective in patients with malignancy arrhythmias and because of its high proarrhythmic effect, it has a small role in patients with low EF. The drug may precipitate torsades de pointes, decreases VF threshold, and may precipitate VF.

Procainamide. *Dosage:* Table 6-8. Indications include management of VT that fails to terminate with a second bolus of lidocaine (lignocaine).

Table 6–7
Drugs for Ventricular Arrhythmias, Adverse Effects, and Efficacy with Lethal Arrhythmias

DRUG	NEGATIVE INOTROPIC EFFECT	PRECIPITATES HEART FAILURE?	SERIOUS SIDE EFFECTS	EFFICACY WITH LETHAL ARRHYTHMIAS
Quinidine	+	No EF <25 yes +	Yes proarrhythmic ++++ precipitates torsades, VF, platelets ↓	Minimal
Procainamide IV oral	 +++ ++	Yes if EF <40	Yes agranulocytosis + lupus, torsades	Poor
Disopyramide	++++	Yes if EF <40	No; precipitates torsades +	Poor
Mexiletine	+	No EF <25, yes	No High minor effects Low proarrhythmic +	Minimal
Tocainide	+	EF <25 yes +	Yes agranulocytosis +++ pulmonary alveolitis	Poor
Encainide*	++	Yes if EF <30 +	No, but proarrhythmic ++++	Poor if EF <30
Felcainide*	+++	Yes if EF <35	No, but proarrhythmic ++++	Not recommended if EF <35
Propafenone	+++	Yes if EF <35	Yes; rare agranulocytosis + proarrhythmic ++	Not if EF <35
Amiodarone	+	No EF <25 yes +	Yes; low proarrhythmic +	Yes +++
Beta blocker	++	Yes if EF <35	No; not proarrhythmic**	Yes +++

EF = ejection fraction (%)
++++ = maximum effect
+ = minimal effect
* Not recommended for benign or potentially lethal arrhythmias
** Except sotalol mildly proarrhythmic

Chronic oral therapy is not advisable since the drug does not improve survival in this category of patients with ventricular arrhythmias. If the drug is prescribed, it should generally not be given for >6 months because of the incidence of drug-induced lupus and the occurrence of agranulocytosis, albeit rare. <u>*Adverse Effects:*</u> The IV preparation has moderate negative inotropic effects, and the oral preparation has a mild risk of precipitating CHF. Torsades de pointes is not uncommon. Lupus occurs in >33% of patients treated >6 months; agranulocytosis appears to occur more commonly with the sustained release preparation. <u>*Interactions:*</u> ACE inhibitors may enhance immune effects; cimetidine increases procainamide levels.

Table 6–8
Antiarrhythmic Drug Dosage

Quinidine:	200-mg test dose: If no hypersensitivity, syncope, or ↓ BP, 200–400 mg q 4h × 4 doses then q 6h then long-acting forms
Procainamide:	375–500 mg q 3h × 1 wk then, q 4h × 2–4 months. RF*
Disopyramide:	300 mg, then 150 mg q 6h. RF* SR 300 mg bid
Mexiletine:	200–400 mg then 2h later 200–250 mg q 8h RF* or MI q 12h or q 24h or elderly: 100–150 mg BID
Flecainide:**	50–200 mg bid max 400 mg daily RF* caution
Sotalol:†	160–240 mg daily × 1–7 days, then 160–240 mg once or twice daily. (investigational 320 to 720 mg daily for lethal arrhythmias, see Table 6–8 and text) RF*
Amiodarone:	200 mg tid or QID × 1–2 wk then 200 bid × 4–6 wk reduce weekly dose‡ by about 400 mg every 4 weeks until patient is taking 200 mg on 5–7 days per week (final maintenance according to Holters)

* Renal Failure: increase dosage interval
** See restrictions within text
† Other beta blocker dosages (see Table 1–3)
‡ Higher doses previously used in USA cause increased pulmonary toxicity
BID = twice daily
TID = three times daily
QID = four times daily
h = hours
q = every

Mexiletine (Mexitil) is a very weak antiarrhythmic agent and rarely shows salutary effects in the treatment of lethal arrhythmias. However, because of its weak negative inotropic effect, it can be combined in selected cases with sotalol, amiodarone, or quinidine if sinus node disease, hypotension, bradycardia, and A-V block are absent. The drug can precipitate CHF in patients with EF <24%.

Beta Blockers. β-adrenergic blocking agents are effective antiarrhythmic agents that have no proarrhythmic effects, with the exception of sotalol which, because of its unique Class III effects, is the most effective β-blocking antiarrhythmic agent.

Beta blockers are

- Effective in all grades of ventricular arrhythmias
- May not completely suppress VPCs, nevertheless, may prevent the occurrence of VF in the same individual
- Particularly useful for ventricular arrhythmias initiated by ischemia or catecholamine release
- Effective for supraventricular arrhythmias. (This aspect was discussed earlier in this chapter.)

Dosage: See Table 1-3 for oral, and Tables 2-7 and 3-4 for IV.

Atenolol, acebutolol, and nadolol at doses of 100, 600 and 120 mg,

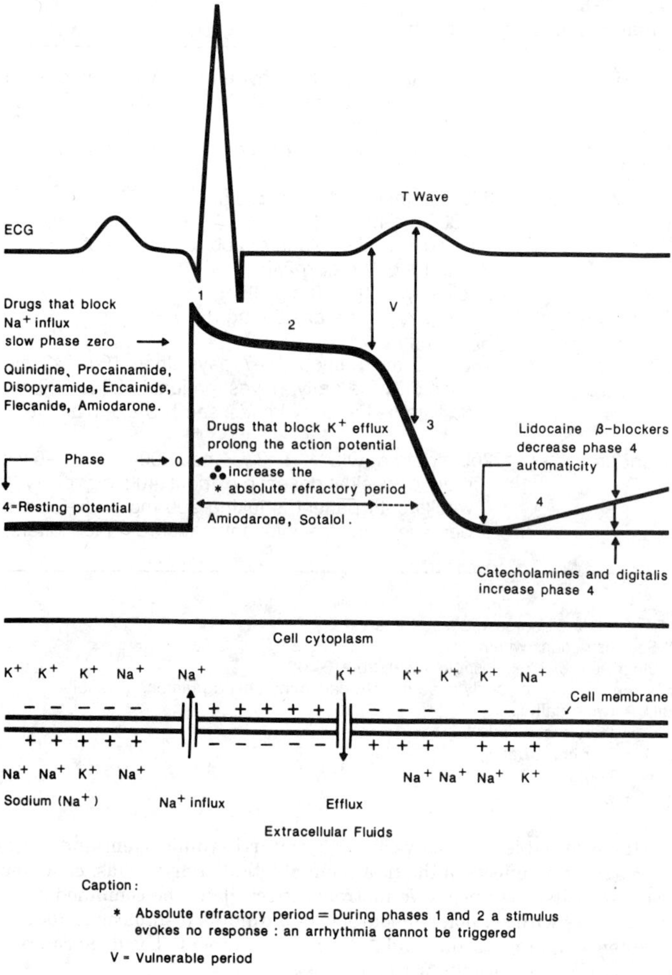

Figure 6–4. Antiarrhythmic drug action. From: Khan M Gabriel: Cardiovascular system, pharmacology. *In* Encyclopedia of Human Biology, Vol. 2. Edited by R. Dulbecco, San Diego, Academic Press, Inc., 1991, pp. 167–177.

respectively, have proven to be effective in suppressing ventricular arrhythmias. Both acebutolol 600 mg and atenolol 100 mg have been shown to be as effective as quinidine in controlling ventricular arrhythmias, and more effective than quinidine in suppressing exercise-induced ventricular arrhythmias. In one study, sotalol and propranolol caused ≤65% and 44% ↓ in VPCs, but sotalol caused ≤99% ↓ of ventricular couplets versus <50% ↓ obtained with propranolol

- In general, β blockers are avoided in patients with EF <30% because CHF may be precipitated. However, recent trials indicate benefit and relative safety of β blockers in the management of patients with EF

Table 6–9
Electrophysiologic Classification or Antiarrhythmic Drugs*

CLASS	EFFECT ON THE ACTION POTENTIAL (AP)†
I. Sodium channel blockers	
A. Sodium channel (+ +); blocks potassium efflux (+)	
Disopyramide	Slows phases zero (+ +)
Quinidine	Moderately prolongs the AP:
Procainamide	↑ repolarization time, ↑ QT
B. Sodium channel (+)	
Other effects	Minimal slowing phase zero (+)
Lidocaine (lignocaine)	Minimal narrowing of the AP
Mexiletine	↓ repolarization time
Moricizine (also IA IC actions)	
Tocainide	
C. Sodium channel (+ + + +)	
Encainide	Marked slowing phase zero:
Flecainide	Marked depression of upstroke
Lorcainide	Marked inhibitory effect on HIS-Purkinje conduction:
Propafenone	↑ QRS duration
	Shortens AP but only of Purkinje fibers: marked depression on conduction.‡
	Repolarization time unchanged.‡
II. Inhibition of the effects of sympathetic stimulation Beta-adrenergic blockers	No effect on AP or repolarization.§ ↓ phase 4 spontaneous depolarization: Decrease automaticity
III. Potassium channel efflux blockade	Slows phase zero (Class I effect)
Amiodarone + + + +, Also sodium block. Sotalol (+ +) (No sodium block and usual Class II effects) Bretylium partly Class III	Markedly prolongs the AP: Markedly prolongs repolarization time. ↑ QT; Amiodarone brings about a more uniform AP throughout the myocardium: Enhances EP homogeneity
IV. Calcium channel blockers	No effect
V. Alinidine	Investigational

* Modified from Vaughan Williams
† See Fig. 6–4
‡ May explain proarrhythmic effect
§ Except sotalol, Class III effect

+ = Minimal effect
+ + + + = Maximal effect
K = Potassium

as low as 22% who are at high risk for sudden death following episodes of monomorphic VT. Often a combination of acebutolol 200–400 mg or nadolol 40–80 mg with amiodarone proves effective and safer than amiodarone combined with a Class I agent

- Several clinical trials have shown sotalol to be a well-tolerated, effec-

tive antiarrhythmic agent in patients at high risk for sudden death. The drug may be effective in patients who did not benefit from multiple drug treatment. A dose of sotalol ranging from 160 to 720 mg with a mean dose of 240 mg is usually required for suppression that is more frequent in patients with VF, 58% versus 24% in patients with VT. When sotalol is used, it is necessary to maintain a normal serum K. Thiazide diuretics should not be used in combination. If a diuretic is necessary, it is advisable to give amiloride, a K-retaining diuretic
- Beta blockers and amiodarone are the only 2 antiarrhythmics that have been shown to cause prolongation of life in patients with potentially lethal or lethal arrhythmias

Amiodarone (Cordarone) blocks the efflux of K from myocytes and markedly prolongs the action potential, thus increasing repolarization time and the effective refractory period. Although the QT interval is prolonged, torsades de pointes is, in fact, a rare complication of amiodarone, mainly because the drug enhances homogeneity of the action potential throughout the myocardium. Fortunately, the drug has a very mild negative inotropic action that allows its use in patients with lethal arrhythmias, which often have underlying severe LV dysfunction with EF <30%. *Dosage:* IV for life-threatening arrhythmias: Infusion ≤5 mg/kg; usually 300 mg over 2 h with ECG monitoring; often given over 1/2 h if life is threatened; max dose 1.2 g in 24 h. Central venous cannulation is required for prolonged infusion. Additional 150-mg boluses can be given if required during the infusion. *Caution:* Hypotension may occur. Oral dosage: See Table 6-8. *Pharmacokinetics*

- About 50% of the oral dose is absorbed; bioavailability is 20–80% and plasma levels occur in 6–12 h. The lipophilic compound is extensively metabolized to desethyl amiodarone, which has pharmacologic activity. The drug is highly bound (95%) to protein, and widespread distribution occurs in most tissues, especially the liver, lungs, and adipose tissue. The concentration in the myocardium is about 20–40 times that in plasma. The volume of distribution is high; an adequate loading dose is necessary; half-life is about 30–110 days
- With dosages of 200 mg tid, a therapeutic effect is observed in 1–4 days, but increases ≤6 months; the action of the drug may persist for >50 days after cessation of therapy, although most side effects show a decrease after 4–7 days, depending on the oral loading dose. When given IV, a therapeutic effect is observed within a few minutes. A loading dose of 10–12 g in the first 2 weeks and maintenance of 400 mg qd 5 days weekly achieves steady-state plasma amiodarone and desethylamiodarone concentrations of 1.7 ± 1.3 and 1.1 ± 0.5 μg/ml, respectively, only after about 1 month of therapy. Patients usually experience therapeutic benefits to amiodarone at plasma concentrations <1.0 μg/ml, and toxicity is not often manifest with concentrations <2.0 μg/ml. The action of the drug appears to relate to tissue stores, and myocardial concentration is important

Indications

- Lethal ventricular arrhythmias: Sustained VT, recovery from VF, or cardiac arrest. Patients with a first occurrence of lethal arrhythmias in the absence of precipitating factors have about a 50% mortality. Survivors have a high mortality; some have a mortality of >90% in 1 year. The overall mortality in survivors of cardiac arrest is about 66% over 5 years. In these high-risk patients, amiodarone has a role. Alternatively, an antiarrhythmic device may be implanted. The BASIS indicated that in patients at high risk for sudden death (i.e., potentially lethal arrhythmias), amiodarone at low dose 200 mg qd caused a decrease in mortality in the first year in post-MI patients

- For conversion of acute AF to sinus rhythm, especially in patients with hypertrophic cardiomyopathy
- Paroxysmal AF that is highly symptomatic, with rapid ventricular rates refractory to other therapy and deemed bothersome and incapacitating
- WPW: Management of AF or atrial flutter with rapid ventricular rates due to anterograde conduction over the accessory pathway

Contraindications: Sinus bradycardia, sinus node disease, or A-V block (requires pacing to allow amiodarone therapy); hypokalemia; severe hepatic dysfunction; iodine sensitivity; pregnancy and breast feeding; porphyria. *Interactions*

- Class 1A antiarrhythmic agents prolong the QT interval and may induce torsades de pointes; also erythromycin increases the QT interval and must not be given concomitantly
- Oral anticoagulant activity is increased
- Verapamil and diltiazem may produce a sinus arrest or A-V block, and quinidine and digoxin levels increase
- Sotalol should not be used in combination, but any of the available β-blocking drugs can be combined with amiodarone
- Tricyclics and phenothiazines, including moricizine, may induce torsades de pointes
- Diuretics may produce hypokalemia and increase the risk of torsades

Adverse Effects

- Cardiac side effects: Severe bradyarrhythmias, asystole, and rarely torsades de pointes, especially in patients with a low serum K. The incidence of serious proarrhythmic effects in patients administered amiodarone is <1%
- Hypothyroidism or, less often, hyperthyroidism occurs in about 5% of patients. Asymptomatic corneal microdeposits develop in most patients after about 3 months of therapy
- Hepatitis with grossly elevated transaminase levels occurs very rarely but may progress to cirrhosis, which may be fatal; immediate discontinuation of amiodarone is necessary if hepatic transaminases rise to >3 times normal
- Photosensitivity, metallic taste, nausea, and vomiting; slate-grey skin, rarely seen, is related to high loading and maintenance doses
- Nervous system effects are common, especially sleep disturbance, twitching, and paresthesia, but they usually respond to decreases in dosage
- Pulmonary infiltrates and alveolitis should occur in <1% of patients with modern conservative dosing schedules

Necessary Monitoring: Because of the high potential for adverse effects, amiodarone should be administered in the hospital or out-patient setting under close supervision. Monitor at 2–4 weeks for 2–4 months, assessing the following

- Serum K and magnesium levels: If a diuretic is necessary, ensure that a K-sparing diuretic is used, or administer supplemental K
- ECG for bradyarrhythmias and QT prolongation
- Liver-function tests
- Free T_4, TSH, and T_3
- Digoxin serum assay and the dose of digoxin should be halved. If oral anticoagulants are used concomitantly, the dosage should be halved
- Amiodarone and desethylamiodarone plasma levels

- Request chest x rays at 3 and 6 months, then 6-monthly or annually thereafter, or earlier if dyspnea occurs
- Holter monitoring early in the course of therapy confirms arrhythmia suppression and is useful in screening for intermittent bradycardia

Torsades de Pointes

Torsades de pointes is a life-threatening arrhythmia often associated with a prolonged QT interval. The rate is usually 200-250/min. It is rarely precipitated by drugs that prolong the QT interval (quinidine, disopyramide, procainamide, sotalol, rarely amiodarone, tricyclics, astemizole, pentamidine), severe hypokalemia hypomagnesemia and the congenital QT prolongation syndrome. *Therapy*

- Immediately identify and withdraw the offending agent (antiarrhythmics and other drugs known to increase the QT interval)
- Rapidly correct K and magnesium deficiency
- Magnesium sulfate 1–2 g is usually highly successful, even in the absence of magnesium deficiency; 2 g (10 ml of a 20% solution) is given IV over 10 minutes and is followed by 4 g over 4–8 hours as an infusion of 30 mg/min. Also, a low K is corrected by KCl infusion. Magnesium is a cofactor of membrane Na, K, adenosine, triphosphatase, or Na pump known to keep the intracellular K-level constant. Magnesium sulfate given IV at higher doses occasionally causes marked hypotension. The substance also has a mild negative inotropic action. Patients with moderate to severe renal failure generally have high magnesium levels, and great caution is required in this situation
- Accelerating the HR is the simplest and quickest method to shortening the QT interval
- Temporary transvenous pacing is the safest and most effective method of management since the HR can be quickly and easily controlled for long periods. If available, atrial or atrial ventricular sequential pacing is preferable, but ventricular pacing is a simple procedure and the catheter obtains a more stable position with reliable capture. As an immediate measure, transthoracic pacing may be used while preparations are being made for electrode placement. If there is chronic bradycardia, the patient progresses to permanent atrial sequential pacing
- An infusion of isoproterenol 2–8 μg/min is sometimes used if pacing is not readily available. This agent is carefully infused to increase the HR to about 120/min. Isoproterenol is contraindicated in acute MI, angina, or severe hypertension. However, isoproterenol infusion needs to be carefully monitored to maintain a HR of 100–120. Myocardial ischemia may be precipitated, and the drug may precipitate VT or VF
- Amiodarone has been successfully used to manage torsades de pointes precipitated by sotalol or Class 1A agents. This approach requires further confirmation, however
- Patients with congenital QT or prolongation syndrome are best managed with β-adrenergic blockers because these agents reduce mortality. Phenytoin has a role if β blockers are contraindicated. Resistant cases are managed with permanent pacing plus β blockers or left stellate ganglionectomy. Isoproterenolol is contraindicated in the congenital QT prolongation syndrome.

Prevention of torsades depends on the removal of the cause and maintenance of normal K. Amiloride has Class III antiarrhythmic activity; the drug retains K and is the diuretic of choice in patients treated with agents that have the propensity to prolong QT interval.

It is important to recognize that polymorphic VT associated with a prolonged QT interval is termed torsades de pointes. When polymorphic VT occurs in the absence of prolonged QT, however, the condition must not be managed as torsades de pointes. It is important to differentiate the two conditions. Most patients with polymorphic VT and normal QT intervals have underlying CHD and are managed in the manner described previously.

Accelerating the HR shortens the QT interval. Thus, sympathetic stimulation with physical exertion or excitement often controls the acquired form of torsades de pointes. Sudden acceleration of HR, however, tends to provoke the occurrence of torsades de pointes in patients with congenital long QT syndrome. Although β blockers do not usually shorten the QT interval, they are the agents of choice in this syndrome and have been shown, in symptomatic patients, to reduce mortality. In patients with congenital long QT syndrome, with or without deafness, torsades de pointes represents the predominant form of VT. Agents that shorten the QT (e.g., Ca, K, lidocaine, digitalis) are not effective. Because syncope or sudden death occurs in these patients, consideration must be given for intervention with cervicothoracic sympathectomy or implantation of an AICD.

Bradyarrhythmias

Severe bradycardia-producing symptoms are usually treated with atropine 0.5–0.6 mg q 2 min to a max of 2–2.4 mg. However, when atropine is used to treat asystole prior to pacing, a dose of 1 mg is given immediately followed by a further 1 mg 2 min later. Mobitz type 2 block and complete heart block must be managed with ventricular pacing (Chap. 7).

Suggested Reading

Khan M Gabriel: Arrhythmias. *In* Cardiac and Pulmonary Management. Philadelphia, Lea & Febiger, 1993.

Nonpharmacologic Therapy for Cardiac Arrhythmias

7

Davendra Mehta and Sanjeev Saksena

TEMPORARY CARDIAC PACING

Indications Acute Myocardial Infarction

The use of temporary cardiac pacemakers in patients with acute MI is best understood by considering the vascular supply of the heart's conduction system. The sinoatrial node, which is located near the junction of the right atrium and the superior vena cava, is supplied by the sinoatrial nodal artery. This is a branch of the right coronary artery in 55% of individuals and of the circumflex artery in the remainder. The A-V node is supplied by the A-V nodal branch of the right coronary artery in approximately 90% of individuals, and by the left circumflex coronary artery in the remaining 10%. There is very little collateral blood supply for these structures. In contrast, the His bundle and proximal portions of both the left and right bundles have a dual blood supply from the A-V nodal artery and the septal branch of the LAD. This anastomosis can allow retrograde flow into the His bundle and the A-V node when the A-V nodal artery is blocked. The right bundle branch, however, is a compact structure and receives blood supply from the LAD. The left bundle branch is anatomically less discrete. The left anterior fascicle receives blood supply from the branches of the LAD and the left posterior fascicle from the A-V nodal and posterior descending arteries.

Conduction disturbances associated with right coronary artery occlusion depend on the site of occlusion. Occlusion proximal to the sinoatrial nodal artery can result in sinus node dysfunction, while occlusion more distally can result in A-V block at the level of A-V node. Therefore, A-V block might result from occlusion of the A-V nodal branch of the right coronary artery alone and is not necessarily associated with a sizable MI. Since the bundle branches are more diffuse, bundle branch block is usually associated with extensive anterior MI.

The decision to insert a temporary pacemaker in patients with acute MI depends on the location of the block, the extent of MI, and the presence of preexisting conduction system disease. Inferior infarction is usually associated with conduction disturbances proximal to the His bundle. Escape rhythms usually have a narrow QRS complex, tend to be fast and stable, and respond well to atropine. A-V block in these situations is usually transient. Indications for temporary pacing in these patients include a HR of <40 beats/min and symptoms of low cardiac output or bradycardia associated with angina or ventricular irritability. In asymptomatic patients with a stable escape rhythm despite complete A-V block, temporary pacemakers need not be inserted. However, the long-term prognosis of patients with inferior MI and high-degree A-V block is worse than in patients without A-V block.

New abnormalities of the conduction system distal to the A-V node are usually seen with anterior MI. Both high-degree A-V block and bundle branch blocks can be observed. In these cases, the escape rhythms are associated with a wide QRS complex, are slower and less stable, and usually do not respond to atropine. Frequently, they progress to complete A-V block. These patients also have extensive MI and often have signs of pump failure. As progression to complete A-V block contributes independently to morbidity and mortality, temporary cardiac pacing is performed more promptly than for inferior wall infarction. Pacing is recommended in patients who are at risk of complete A-V block and include

- Type II 2nd° A-V block
- New bifascicular block (RBBB with left anterior or left posterior block) or complete LBBB
- LBBB or RBBB with 1st° or 2nd° A-V block
- Alternating LBBB or RBBB
- Preexisting RBBB with new left fascicular block or 1st° A-V block

Drug-Induced Bradyarrhythmias Antiarrhythmic drugs, β-blocking agents, clonidine, Ca antagonists, digoxin, methyldopa, reserpine, and parasympathomimetic agents can lead to bradycardia as a result of sinus node dysfunction, sinus arrest, sinus exit block, and A-V nodal block at toxic levels. These arrhythmias may occur even at low or therapeutic levels as a result of idiosyncratic reaction or if the conduction system is previously diseased. Temporary cardiac pacing is indicated in these conditions for the duration of drug effects or until the drug effects are counteracted. If longterm therapy with these agents is needed, as in the case of some antiarrhythmic agents for ventricular arrhythmias, permanent cardiac pacing is indicated.

Temporary cardiac pacing is also indicated for immediate management of torsades de pointes or arrhythmias related to prolonged QT interval, which can be drug induced or drug exacerbated. Pacing has been demonstrated to reduce temporal dispersion of repolarization in this situation. Temporary overdrive pacing is used until reversible factors such as electrolyte imbalance or toxic drug levels have been corrected or permanent pacemaker insertion has been carried out. Overdrive pacing of the atrium or the ventricle has been shown to be effective and is the treatment of choice for management of these patients.

During Cardiac Catheterization Temporary cardiac pacing is used prophylactically in the cardiac catheterization laboratory when there is a risk of complete A-V block during the procedure. In patients with preexisting LBBB, right heart catheterization can result in transient complete A-V block. Thus, it is advisable to insert a temporary pacemaker prior to the procedure. Significant bradycardia and asystole can occur during injection of radiopaque dye into the right coronary artery. This risk is small in patients with a normal conduction system but may be higher in patients with preexisting sinoatrial or conduction system disease. Thus, prophylactic temporary pacing is recommended in the latter group. Prophylactic temporary cardiac pacemakers are inserted in all patients undergoing coronary angioplasty, because there is a significant risk of symptomatic bradycardia during balloon inflation in the right or circumflex coronary arteries.

Management of Tachycardias The use of temporary cardiac pacing in patients with tachyarrhythmias can be diagnostic or therapeutic. Simultaneous recording of the surface ECG and the atrial activity using

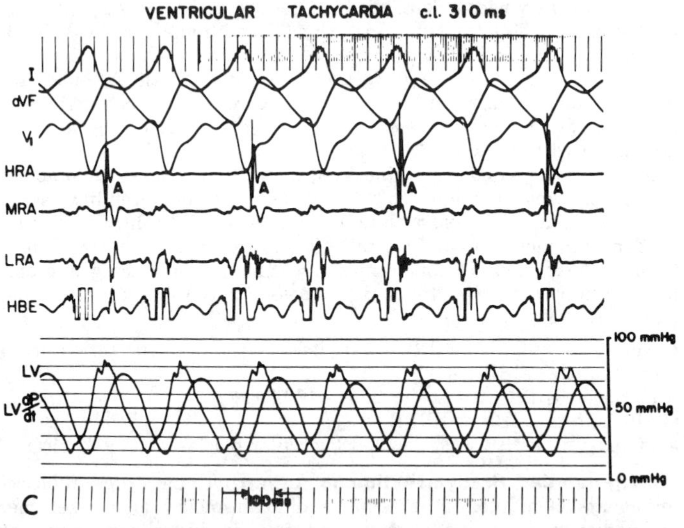

Figure 7–1. Three lead surface electrocardiogram, atrial and ventricular electrograms, and blood pressure recordings in a patient with broad complex tachycardia. There is complete dissociation between atrial (HRA = high right atrial; MRA = mid right atrial) and ventricular electrogram as seen on His-bundle recording (HBE). This confirms the diagnosis as ventricular tachycardia. Reproduced with permission from: Saksena S, Ciccone J, Craelius W, et al.: Studies on left ventricular function during sustained ventricular tachycardia. J Am Coll Cardiol, *4*:501–508, 1984.

a temporary pacing electrode is useful in studying A-V relationships. Such recordings are also useful in diagnosing broad complex tachycardia. V-A dissociation suggests the diagnosis of VT (Fig. 7–1). One-to-one V-A relationship suggests the diagnosis of supraventricular arrhythmia with aberration or pre-excitation but might also be seen in VT when associated with 1:1 retrograde conduction. Recording of atrial activity is also helpful in patients with other supraventricular arrhythmias; e.g., recording atrial rates of 250–300 beats/min, establishes diagnosis of atrial flutter, and in AF, fibrillating activity can be identified.

Electrical stimulation using temporary pacemakers might be helpful in terminating a wide range of tachycardias, including atrial flutter, sinoatrial, A-V nodal, and A-V reentrant tachycardias, and at times, sustained VTs (Fig. 7–2). Atrial or VF cannot be terminated by pacing. Pacing is used if the catheter is already in place or if drug therapy is ineffective and recurrent cardioversions are necessary due to frequent arrhythmia recurrence. Pacing at a rate slightly faster than the tachycardia (overdrive pacing) can terminate atrial flutter, A-V reentry, and VTs. Timed premature beats or pacing at rates slower than the tachycardia (underdrive pacing) can terminate reciprocating A-V reentrant and VTs.

In addition to terminating tachyarrhythmias, pacing can prevent tachyarrhythmias that are bradycardia dependent or those associated with prolonged QT interval (Fig. 7–3). In patients with frequent VPBs associated with sinus bradycardia, pacing at a rate 10–25% faster than

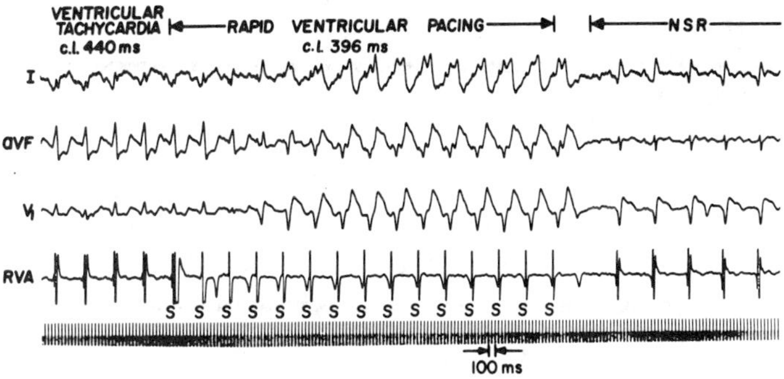

Figure 7–2. Termination of ventricular tachycardia (cycle length 440 ms) by overdrive ventricular pacing (cycle length 396 ms). First four complexes of the illustration represent ventricular tachycardia, followed by 15 beats of overdrive pacing at the right ventricular apex. Sinus rhythm ensues after termination of overdrive pacing. RVA = electrogram from the right ventricular apex. Reproduced with permission from: Saksena S, Chandran P, Shah Y, et al.: Comparative efficacy of transvenous cardioversion and pacing in patients with sustained ventricular tachycardia. Circulation, *772*:153–160, 1985.

the spontaneous rate can help reduce the frequency of VPBs. Atrial pacing can be used to convert a hemodynamically unstable atrial tachyarrhythmia such as atrial flutter to a hemodynamically more favorable arrhythmia such as AF, in which concealed conduction results in better control of the ventricular response.

Although in most instances temporary cardiac pacing is performed in the right ventricle, atrial pacing can prove to be a better choice in the following conditions

- Sinus node dysfunction without A-V block
- Overdrive pacing for atrial and junctional tachycardias
- Differential diagnosis of broad complex tachycardia
- Drug-induced sinus bradycardia
- Spontaneous or drug-induced prolonged QT interval and ventricular arrhythmias

Temporary dual chamber pacing is the choice for

- Patients with noncompliant ventricles that need temporary pacing
- Sizable acute MI (especially right ventricular infarction) and A-V block
- To assess the efficacy of a permanent dual chamber pacemaker, in a trial by measuring BP and cardiac output in ventricular and dual chamber pacing modes
- In patients who need temporary pacemakers for bradycardia or poor hemodynamic status in the immediate postoperative period

Methods of Temporary Cardiac Pacing

Temporary cardiac pacing can be established by transvenous, transthoracic, transesophageal, and epicardial approaches. The choice of a specific route depends on factors such as availability of the device, indica-

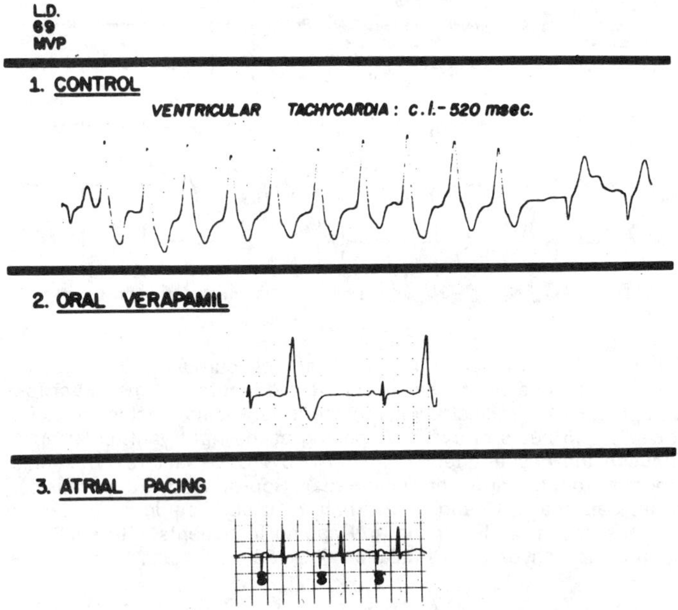

Figure 7–3. Suppression of frequent ventricular premature beats and nonsustained ventricular tachycardia by overdrive atrial pacing. 1 and 2) Runs of nonsustained ventricular tachycardia (cycle length 520 ms) that are partially suppressed by oral verapamil leading to ventricular bigemeny. 3) Atrial pacing at 72 beats per minute leads to total suppression of ventricular arrhythmia. Reproduced with permission from: Goldschlager N, Saksena S: Hemodynamic effects of cardiac pacing. *In* Electrical Therapy for Cardiac Arrhythmias: Pacing Anti-Tachycardia Devices, Catheter Ablation. Edited by: Saksena S, Goldschlager N. Philadelphia, W.B. Saunders, 1990, p 168.

tions for pacing, expertise of the physician, and the clinical situation. The transvenous approach is the most often used method.

Transvenous. External or internal jugular, subclavian, antecubital, and femoral venous approaches are most often used for introduction of pacing catheter electrodes. Under radiographic control, the electrode tip is positioned in the right atrial appendage or the right ventricular apex for stable atrial and ventricular pacing, respectively. In an emergency or in the absence of radiological facilities, a balloon-tipped flotation electrode catheter can be used to enter the right ventricle. A pacing threshold of <1 V is usually satisfactory. It increases over the following few days, probably due to tissue edema around the electrode tip. Although invasive when compared to transthoracic and transesophageal approaches, transvenous pacing is rapidly accomplished and is reliable when instituted. Atrial, ventricular, and dual chamber pacing can be achieved, and atrial and ventricular ECGs can be selectively recorded for diagnostic purposes. Once initiated, it causes little patient discomfort and is thus ideal for prolonged use. Complications include ventricular arrhythmias, especially in patients with acute MI, pericarditis, ventricular perforation, bleeding, pulmonary embolism, air embolism, pneumothorax when the subclavian vein is used for lead introduction, and local and systemic infections.

Transthoracic. This was the first modality to be used for temporary pacing. Gel patches are applied on the chest, one over the anterior precordium and the other over the lower part of the left scapula. These are connected to an external stimulator. It can be rapidly instituted but causes significant discomfort to conscious patients and is thus not ideal for prolonged use. Furthermore, it cannot be used for atrial pacing. This mode is only used in an emergency situation before a temporary transvenous pacemaker can be inserted.

PERMANENT CARDIAC PACING

Indications

Class 1 indications: Conditions in which a permanent pacemaker must be implanted, provided the condition is chronic or recurrent and not due to transient causes such as acute MI, electrolyte imbalance, or drug toxicity

- Acquired, symptomatic, chronic, or intermittent complete A-V block
- Congenital complete A-V block with significant bradycardia or symptoms due to bradycardia
- Symptomatic advanced (type II) 2nd° A-V block
- Bifascicular or trifascicular block with intermittent type II 2nd° A-V block, even without symptoms directly attributable to the A-V block
- Symptomatic (syncope, seizures, CHF, dizziness, or confusion) sinus bradycardia. It must be documented that the symptoms are directly related to bradycardia
- Drug-induced symptomatic sinus bradycardia, when there is no acceptable alternative to longterm use of drug therapy
- Sinus node dysfunction: This category includes tachycardia-bradycardia syndrome, sinoatrial block, and sinus arrest
- Potentially life-threatening ventricular arrhythmias secondary to bradycardia with or without symptoms
- Carotid sinus hypersensitivity with recurrent syncope associated with spontaneous events (like neck movements) provoking carotid sinus stimulation, or if carotid sinus pressure induces asystole of >3 seconds' duration in the absence of any medication that depresses the sinus or A-V node

Class 2 indications: Conditions in which pacemakers are frequently used, but there may be differences in opinion among experts with respect to their use for these conditions

- Asymptomatic acquired complete A-V block (permanent or intermittent) with ventricular rate of ≥40 beats/min
- Asymptomatic type II 2nd° A-V block
- Bifascicular or trifascicular block with syncope that is not proven to be due to intermittent complete A-V block, but other causes of syncope have been excluded
- Congenital complete A-V block with bradycardia but no symptoms
- Sinus node dysfunction with a HR of <40 beats/min, but there is no

clearly documented association between symptoms consistent with bradycardia and the actual occurrence of bradycardia

- Recurrent syncope without clear, provocative events and a hypersensitive cardioinhibitory carotid sinus response
- Overdrive pacing to prevent ventricular arrhythmias in patients with recurrent VT

Class 3 indications: Conditions for which there is general agreement that pacemaker therapy is not indicated

- 1st° or asymptomatic type I 2nd° A-V block
- Fascicular block with 1st° A-V block without symptoms suggestive of intermittent high-degree A-V block
- Sinus bradycardia or sinoatrial block without significant symptoms
- Asymptomatic sinus bradycardia, including those in which substantial sinus bradycardia (HR <40 beats/min) is a consequence of long-term drug treatment, which can be withdrawn or modified
- Hypersensitive cardioinhibitory response to carotid sinus stimulation in the absence of symptoms
- Recurrent syncope of undetermined cause, in the absence of a cardioinhibitory response

Specific Conditions

DISORDERS OF ATRIOVENTRICULAR CONDUCTION

First-degree A-V block. The PR interval comprises the sinoatrial, intra-atrial, A-V nodal, His Bundle, and His-Purkinje conduction intervals. The clinical significance of solitary prolongation of the PR interval depends on the site of conduction delay and the underlying cardiac condition. Isolated prolongation of PR interval, in most instances, is due to delayed conduction at the level of A-V node as a result of enhanced vagal tone or drug therapy (digitalis, β blockers, or Ca antagonists). It is generally a benign condition and is not an indication for permanent pacemaker therapy because it usually does not progress to symptomatic advanced A-V block. However, 1st° A-V block associated with either LBBB or RBBB, particularly of recent onset, usually reflects the pres-

---

Figure 7–4. Second-degree A-V block. Panel A: Three lead electrocardiogram illustrating Type I second-degree/Wenckebach A-V block. In an asymptomatic individual with this arrhythmia, permanent pacemaker is not indicated and a reversible cause should be eliminated. The level of block is usually above the His bundle. Panel B: Twelve lead electrocardiogram and a 3 lead (V_1 II, V5) rhythm strip of 2:1 Type II second-degree A-V block. Alternate P waves superimpose T waves and are best seen in leads II and V_1. Permanent pacing is indicated as A-V block in these patients and is usually below the level of His bundle. Panel C: Intracardiac recordings from the same patient with Type II second-degree A-V block seen in Panel B illustrating 2:1 infra-His block during atrial pacing. I and V_1 = electrocardiographic leads; RA = right atrial electrogram with atrial pacing; HIS-P and HIS-D = proximal and distal His bundle electrograms, respectively. His bundle recording show all atrial, His, and ventricular electrograms. First paced atrial beat is followed by an His complex and a ventricular electrogram while the second is followed only by an His bundle deflection and no ventricular electrogram illustrating an infra-His block.

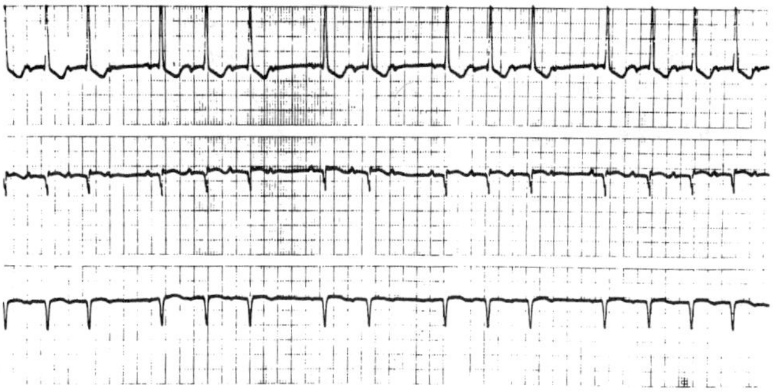

A. TYPE I 2ND DEGREE A-V BLOCK

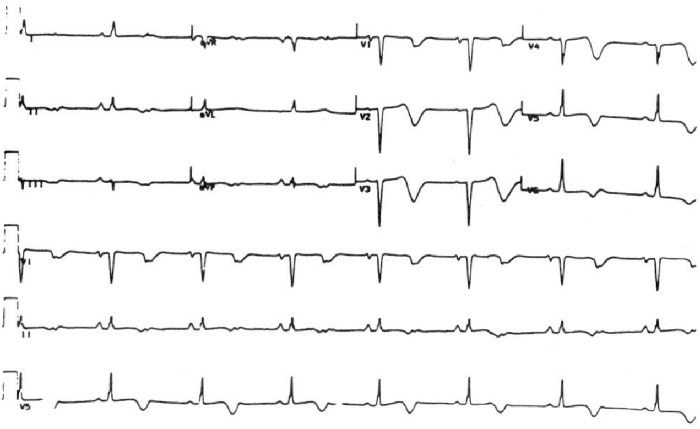

B. TYPE II 2ND DEGREE A-V BLOCK

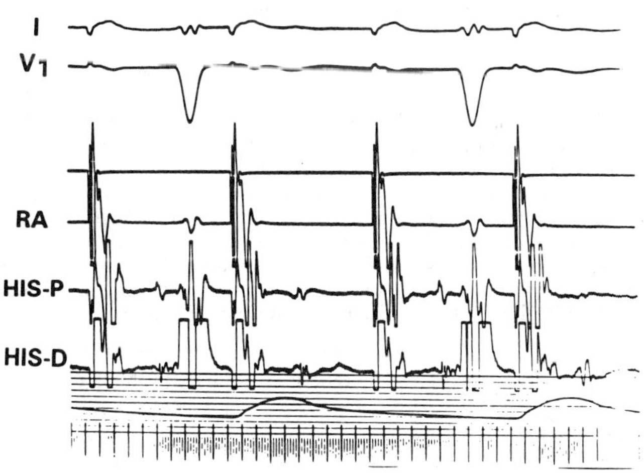

C. INFRA-HIS BLOCK DURING ATRIAL PACING

ence of infra-His conduction delay. This is an indication for implantation of a permanent pacemaker, especially when associated with symptoms or intermittent complete A-V block.

Second-degree A-V block. Type I 2nd° A-V block is most often observed in the setting of acute MI, after drug therapy (digitalis, β blockers, and Ca blockers), or when high vagal tone is present, as in trained athletes (Fig. 7–4A). It has also been reported in hypervagotonia related to specific maneuvers such as swallowing, deglutition, yawning, and micturition. Its prognostic significance depends on coexisting symptoms and heart disease. It is, most often, benign in nature. Isolated asymptomatic type I 2nd° A-V block does not warrant insertion of a permanent cardiac pacemaker. When associated with drug refractory hypervagotonia and resulting in serious symptoms such as syncope, permanent cardiac pacing is indicated. Type II 2nd° A-V block usually indicates the presence of conduction system disease beyond the A-V node (Figs. 7–4B and 7–4C). It is often due to isolated degenerative conduction system diseases but can be seen with regional or diffuse myocardial disease or acute MI. During acute MI, it may precede complete A-V block. Type II 2nd° A-V block unrelated to antiarrhythmic drug therapy is considered an indication for permanent cardiac pacing. The natural history of this bradyarrhythmia, even in initially asymptomatic individuals, is progression to severe bradycardia and related symptoms.

Complete (third-degree) atrioventricular block. Symptomatic advanced or complete A-V block is considered an indication for implantation of a permanent pacemaker, particularly when due to infranodal disease. 3rd° A-V nodal block can, at times, be asymptomatic, transient, or due to reversible factors. If stable or obviously reversible, permanent pacing can be deferred unless symptoms develop. There is a continuing debate about timing of pacemaker implantation in asymptomatic individuals with chronic stable complete A-V block. The nature of escape rhythm is often helpful in making a decision. Junctional escape rhythms, which are associated with a relatively narrow QRS complex, are often stable over time and responsive to physiological demands (Fig. 7–5). Escape rhythms originating in Purkinje or ventricular tissues are identified by wide QRS complexes, are less stable, and tend to have slow attenuated rate responsiveness to catecholamine stimulation. Hence, permanent pacing is recommended.

Fascicular blocks. There is considerable controversy concerning the rationale for permanent pacemaker therapy in patients with documented bifascicular and trifascicular block. Patients with advanced fascicular block and symptoms believed to be due to A-V block have a high mortality largely due to a significant incidence of sudden death. It has also been shown that although pacing relieves transient symptoms like presyncope and syncope, it may not reduce the frequency of sudden death. One predictor of progression of advanced fascicular block to complete A-V block is prolonged HV conduction interval. Patients with bifascicular block with a prolonged HV interval (>80 ms) develop A-V block more readily than patients who have a normal HV interval.

SINUS NODE DYSFUNCTION/SICK SINUS SYNDROME

The symptom complex of sinus bradycardia, sinus arrest, sinoatrial exit block, and/or paroxysmal atrial tachyarrhythmias is often referred to as "sick sinus syndrome." One or more types of sinus nodal bradyarrhythmias and atrial flutter, AF, or atrial tachycardia can be present

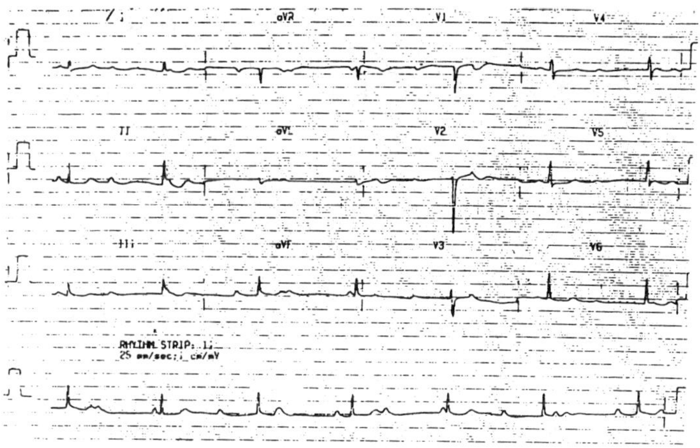

Figure 7–5. Twelve lead electrocardiogram from a young girl with congenital complete heart (A-V) block. The escape rhythm is high junctional and the QRS complexes are narrow. In this condition, permanent cardiac pacing is indicated only if the patient develops severe bradycardia or related symptoms.

in the same patient. Symptoms in these patients can be related to the tachycardia, the bradycardia, or both, but are most often due to the sudden changes in HR involved in conversion from one rhythm to another. These patients usually present with palpitations, weakness, dizziness, and syncope. About 1/3 of patients with sick sinus syndrome have conduction abnormalities involving the A-V node and the bundle branches.

Permanent pacemakers in patients with sick sinus syndrome are indicated in the presence of symptoms. Correlation of symptoms with a specific arrhythmia is essential, although this may be difficult in view of the intermittent nature of arrhythmias. Asymptomatic sinoatrial exit block, sinus bradycardia, and sinus pauses do not constitute an indication for permanent pacemaker therapy. There is disagreement about the absolute duration of the asystolic period that requires pacing. Sinus pauses of 3 seconds or sustained symptomatic sinus rates <40 beats/min in the awake patient are usually accepted as indications for permanent pacing. In such individuals prior to pacemaker implantation, it is essential to determine that symptoms are related to bradycardias before proceeding to pacemaker implantation. EP evaluation of sinus node function is performed in patients who are asymptomatic during detailed noninvasive monitoring, but it has low sensitivity. In North America, sick sinus syndrome accounts for 46% of all pacemaker implantations. Demand ventricular pacing has been performed widely for this condition. Demand atrial pacemakers are indicated for those patients with sick sinus syndrome who do not have any evidence of A-V conduction abnormality.

CAROTID SINUS HYPERSENSITIVITY

Mechanical stimulation of the carotid sinus region results in vagal stimulation with secondary sinus bradycardia and PR interval prolongation.

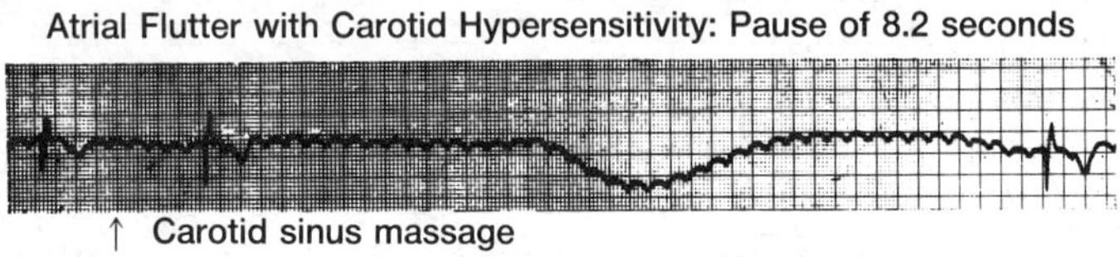

Figure 7–6. Electrocardiographic lead V_1 demonstrating carotid sinus hypersensitivity in a patient with atrial flutter. Right carotid sinus massage resulted in ventricular asystole with a pause of 8.2 seconds.

In some patients, these responses are exaggerated. Hyperactive carotid sinus responses result in excessive bradycardia (cardioinhibitory response) (Fig. 7–6) and/or hypotension (vasodepressor response). Ventricular asystole of 3 seconds or a ↓ in BP to 30–50 mm Hg without HR changes, especially when associated with symptoms, is considered abnormal. The incidence of the cardioinhibitory type of carotid sinus hypersensitivity is substantially higher than that of the vasodepressor type. Clinically, symptoms of dizziness, presyncope, and syncope are often precipitated by a tight neck collar, neck rotation, or neck extension. In patients with symptomatic cardioinhibitory carotid sinus hypersensitivity, permanent demand ventricular pacing usually eliminates symptoms but does not often benefit vasodepressor carotid sinus hypersensitivity.

Mineralocorticoid therapy, denervation of the carotid sinus, and ephedrine administration have also been shown to be effective in selected patients with vasodepressor carotid sinus hypersensitivity.

PERMANENT PACING IN ACUTE MYOCARDIAL INFARCTION

The management of bradyarrhythmias related to conduction disturbances in acute MI is determined by the site of the culprit MI, hemodynamic consequences of the arrhythmia, and arrhythmia duration after acute MI. The requirement for temporary pacing does not, by itself, indicate permanent pacing.

Inferior myocardial infarction. 1st° A-V block and Mobitz I 2nd° A-V block, if present, are usually transient, unassociated with hemodynamic disturbances, and do not require pacing therapy. A minority of patients will develop higher degree or symptomatic A-V block. Temporary pacing is indicated, particularly if the patient is hemodynamically unstable. If symptomatic 2nd° or 3rd° A-V block persists >2–3 weeks after MI, permanent pacemaking may be indicated.

Anterior myocardial infarction. Permanent pacing is generally indicated for: new onset bifascicular block; persistent Mobitz type II 2nd° or complete A-V block; transient Mobitz type II 2nd° or complete A-V block when associated bundle branch block (trifascicular block) is present. This is because of the substantial potential of these conduction disturbances for the development of complete A-V block. Patients with anterior wall MI who have A-V conduction and intraventricular conduction disturbances, except left anterior hemiblock, have a poor short- and long-term prognosis and an increased incidence of sudden death. The poor prognosis is primarily related to the extent of MI rather than to the A-V block itself. Mortality is high even with pacemaker therapy due to myocardial failure.

NONPHARMACOLOGIC THERAPY FOR TACHYCARDIAS

Ablation

Catheter ablation procedures involve delivery of radiofrequency current (same as used for electrocautery) at the target site in the A-V conduction system or accessory pathway. For the accessory pathways related to right A-V groove, catheters are placed in the right atrium; for posteroseptal accessory pathways, electrodes at the coronary sinus orifice deliver the ablative energy. For left-side freewall accessory pathways, electrode catheters are introduced retrogradely from the femoral artery into the left ventricle or transseptally from the right atrium and positioned across the left A-V groove at a previously localized site to deliver ablation energy. General anesthesia is not needed. With precise localization of the A-V pathway by EP study and in trained hands, ≥98% of accessory pathways can now be ablated using percutaneous catheter techniques with radiofrequency energy. Loss of pre-excitation with normalization of the PR interval and noninducibility of reentrant tachycardia are taken as markers of successful ablation. Incidence of complications with the use of radiofrequency ablation is low; complications include pericardial tamponade and occasional injury to the circumflex artery, as it lies in the A-V groove. Radiofrequency ablation is the preferred method of treatment for all A-V accessory pathways, irrespective of the location.

Supraventricular Arrhythmias. Underlying mechanisms for supraventricular arrhythmias have been previously discussed (Chap. 6). For the purpose of nonpharmacologic therapy, they can be classified into

- Atrial tachycardias (including automatic atrial tachycardia, atrial flutter, and fibrillation)
- PSVTs due to dual A-V nodal pathways
- PSVTs due to ≥1 accessory A-V bypass tracts

Current indications for catheter ablation include

- SVTs associated with severe symptoms or leading to life-threatening electrical or hemodynamic consequences such as syncope, ventricular failure, cardiomyopathy, and cardiac arrest (VF). VT and fibrillation are special risks for patients with WPW Syndrome and short antegrade refractory period of the pathway (<250 ms)
- Symptomatic patients without life-threatening problems who are refractory to multiple antiarrhythmic drugs
- Patients intolerant to antiarrhythmic drugs, despite their effective control of the arrhythmia
- Patient preference for nonpharmacologic therapy as an alternative to prolonged pharmacological treatment. This is particularly important in young patients, due to employment implications, and in female patients contemplating pregnancy

In AF, as well as most cases of atrial flutter and atrial tachycardias, control of symptoms can be achieved by ablation of the A-V junction (i.e., A-V node–His bundle) resulting in therapeutic complete A-V block or modification of A-V conduction. Insertion of a permanent pacemaker is necessary, especially when heart block is induced. Modification of A-V conduction is attempted but can culminate in complete A-V block. In some patients with atrial flutter and atrial tachycardia, it is possible to map the focus of atrial arrhythmia and selectively ablate it, thus leaving

A-V conduction intact and precluding the need for a permanent pacemaker.

It has recently become possible, based on better understanding of dual A-V nodal pathway anatomy, to modify the A-V node by catheter ablation or surgery and to eliminate 1 of the pathways without producing complete A-V block. Reentry is related to the presence of dual A-V nodal pathways. It is unclear if 1 of the pathways is an atrionodal tract or a partial extranodal circuit. If the area adjacent to the A-V node is carefully mapped, the extranodal/nodal circuit components are identified by activation of the adjoining atrial segment during tachycardia or ventricular pacing. Radiofrequency energy application in this area results in modification of 1 of the A-V node pathways' noninducibility of arrhythmia, and preserved A-V conduction via the alternate pathway. Success of this procedure is high, but there is always a risk of complete heart block. Selective ablation of the slow pathway is reported to have lower risk of heart block.

Ventricular Tachyarrhythmias. Therapeutic modalities for the management of ventricular tachyarrhythmias include antiarrhythmic drugs, implantable devices, catheter ablation, and surgery. The majority of ventricular arrhythmias are related to IHD, with or without myocardial scarring, and are reentrant in nature, as they can be initiated and terminated by programmed electrical stimulation of the heart.

Map-guided surgical ablation also offers a potential cure for VT and is presently the first line of nonpharmacologic treatment. Patients with drug-refractory VTs, in whom tachycardias can be induced and terminated by programmed electrical stimulation (reentrant tachycardia) and who have reasonably preserved LV function (LV EF >20–25%), are considered for surgical ablation. Sustained monomorphic VT that is hemodynamically stable with localized regional wall motion abnormality (scar or aneurysm) is ideal for map-guided surgical ablation. Nonsustained and polymorphic VTs and primary VF are not suitable for surgical ablation.

IMPLANTABLE CARDIOVERTER-DEFIBRILLATORS

These devices automatically detect ventricular tachyarrhythmias and deliver a shock via epicardial patch electrodes or endocardial lead electrodes, usually within 30 seconds or arrhythmia onset. For VT, the shock is synchronized, but the shock is asynchronous for VF. As the shock is directly delivered to the heart, energy required for internal cardioversion/defibrillation is 15–40 J, compared to 200–350 J required for external cardioversion. The new generation of implantable cardioverter-defibrillators, in addition, have antibradycardia pacing and algorithms for pace termination of VTs (Fig. 7-7).

Indications. Implantable cardioverter-defibrillators are indicated in any patient with hemodynamically unstable ventricular tachyarrhythmia that is unrelated to acute MI, electrolyte imbalance, or drug toxicity. Concerning the use of cardiac pacemakers, specific indications for cardioverter-defibrillator implantation can be divided into 3 categories. The current recommendations from the North American Society of Pacing and Electrophysiology are as follows:

Class I (should be implanted): One or more documented episodes of hemodynamically significant VT or fibrillation in a patient in whom EP

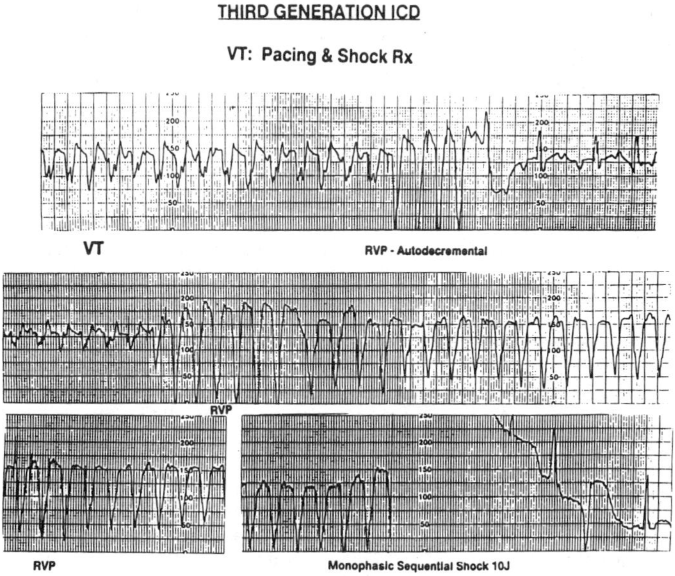

Figure 7–7. Holter recordings demonstrating termination of ventricular tachycardia by third-generation implantable cardioverter-defibrillator. Top tracing illustrates termination of ventricular tachycardia by a burst of overdrive ventricular pacing. Middle trace shows failure to terminate another similar episode of ventricular tachycardia by overdrive pacing with an increase in rate of tachycardia, which is finally terminated by a synchronized shock of 10 J delivered by the implanted device (bottom trace).

testing and ambulatory monitoring cannot be used to accurately predict efficacy of therapy. One or more documented episodes of hemodynamically significant VT or fibrillation in a patient for whom no drug is found to be effective or no drug is currently available and appropriately tolerated. Continued inducibility at EP study of hemodynamically significant VT or fibrillation despite best available drug therapy or despite surgery or catheter ablation if drug therapy has failed.

Class II (cardioverter-defibrillator can be used): One or more documented episodes of hemodynamically significant VT or fibrillation in a patient for whom drug efficacy testing is possible. Recurrent syncope of undetermined origin in a patient with hemodynamically significant VT or fibrillation induced at EP study, for whom no effective or tolerated drug is available or appropriate.

Class III (cardioverter-defibrillator should not be used): Recurrent syncope of undetermined cause in a patient without inducible tachycardias. Arrhythmias not due to hemodynamically significant VT or fibrillation. Incessant VT or fibrillation.

An implantable cardioverter-defibrillator system is composed of 2 sensing electrodes, 2 shocking (cardioversion/defibrillation) electrodes, and the device. Defibrillation leads can be epicardial patches or endocardial lead electrodes. Implantation of epicardial patch electrodes requires thoracotomy, and 2 or 3 patch electrodes are placed on the heart. Sensing/pacing leads can be epicardial or endocardial in location. Epicardial screw-in electrodes are used for sensing ventricular signals. Endocardial electrodes are usually inserted via the subclavian or cephalic veins into the right ventricle and atrium with a thoracic subcutaneous pouch. Before the leads are connected to the device, adequacy of lead function is tested. The minimal amount of energy required to reproducibly terminate induced VF is referred to as the "defibrillation threshold." A safety margin of ≥10 J between the defibrillation threshold and output of the device is desirable. The efficacy of the device in terminating ventricular arrhythmias is established before it is implanted in the abdominal pocket. Its efficacy is again confirmed by EP study prior to discharge. Perioperative mortality associated with cardioverter-defibrillator implantation using epicardial leads is 1–5%. This mortality rate is likely to ↓ with the use of transvenous defibrillation lead systems.

Following hospital discharge, patients are monitored every 2 months for appropriate device use and device status. Frequent use of shock therapy often indicates recurrent ventricular or uncontrolled supraventricular arrhythmias and the need for concomitant drug therapy. Appropriate device use for VT/VF is reported to occur in 50–75% of all implanted patients. This rate increases along with the length of follow-up. Initial shocks occurring >1 year after implant are common. Patients with implantable cardioverter-defibrillators can have a fairly normal lifestyle but are advised to refrain from driving due to the risk of syncopal VT/VF. Pulse generator longevity is currently 3–4 years. Replacement is usually necessary but can be based on device use; it is a debatable issue in patients who do not experience shocks for >5 years after implant. Another frequently encountered problem in the management of these patients is the occurrence of spurious discharges. These are shocks delivered by the device, usually in the absence of symptoms or during exercise. In most instances, these are related to supraventricular arrhythmias such as AF with a fast ventricular rate, sinus tachycardia, or recurrent nonsustained VT. They can usually be managed by device reprogramming and/or appropriate concomitant pharmacologic therapy. Less frequently, spurious shocks can result from lead fracture of the sensing electrodes, myopotential sensing, or the use of electrocautery. It is recommended to disconnect the implantable cardioverter-defibrillator device during surgery if clinically feasible.

Since their availability for clinical use in 1984, >15,000 cardioverter-defibrillators have been implanted throughout the world. Their use has been shown to be associated with low recurrent sudden death rates in survivors of cardiac arrest related to VT and VF. With the availability of antitachycardia pacing and better algorithms for antitachycardia pacing, the use of cardioverter-defibrillators is gradually expanding. High cost, however, remains an important limiting factor in their more extensive use. These devices can be anticipated to replace extensive drug testing procedures or high-risk surgical ablative procedures in patients with recurrent VT/VF.

Recent developments in device technology have made possible the availability of demand ventricular pacing, programmable tachycardia detection, and programmable tachycardia therapies in implantable cardioverter-defibrillator devices. A major advance has been the availability of nonthoracotomy defibrillation lead systems, which have obviated the need for thoracotomy in most patients. In a clinical report of 200 patients implanted with programmable pacemaker-cardioverter-defibrillators, device function permitted demand ventricular pacing for bradyarrhythmias, long Q-T interval or tachycardia suppression, as well as programmable (3–30 J) energy shocks for treatment of VT and VF.

VT or VF recognition is based on electrogram rate and required reconfirmation prior to shock delivery. The patients in this study were followed for ≤23 months. The incidence of sudden death during follow-up was 1%, with a total cardiac mortality of 6.5%. Perioperative mortality in this study, which used epicardial lead systems with a thoracotomy, was 5.5%. In another study, the longterm results of epicardial and endocardial lead systems were compared; 660 patients were implanted with a programmable pacemaker-cardioverter-defibrillator with either endocardial leads (226 patients) or epicardial leads. The perioperative mortality was 5.5% for epicardial leads and 0.4% for endocardial leads. This difference was statistically significant. Life table analysis showed improved total 1-year survival of 96.4% for endocardial leads versus 85.4% for epicardial leads ($p<0.001$).

Future devices are likely to have multiprogrammable parameters for pacing for tachycardias and bradycardias, shock therapy for tachycardias, and implantation using nonthoracotomy approaches.

Suggested Reading

Mehta D, Saksena S: Non-pharmacologic therapy for cardiac arrhythmias. *In* Khan, Gabriel M, Cardiac and Pulmonary Management. Philadelphia, Lea & Febiger, 1993.

Saksena S, Goldschlager N, eds. Electrical Therapy for Cardiac Arrhythmias. Philadelphia, W.B. Saunders, 1990.

Cardiac Arrest

8

M. Gabriel Khan

Sudden cardiac death is defined as sudden natural death caused by cardiac disease associated with the following

- An abrupt loss of consciousness within 1 h of onset of acute symptoms
- Known or unknown preexisting heart disease
- Unexpected time and mode of death

Hinkle and Thaler classify cardiac death as

- Class I: An arrhythmic death if circulatory failure follows the disappearance of the pulse. In these situations, the nature of the terminal illness is an acute cardiac event in >98% of victims, and VF or asystole has been observed to be the terminal event in approximately 83% and 17% of patients, respectively
- Class II: Circulatory failure death if the disappearance of the pulse is preceded by circulatory failure. This scenario is common in patients with terminal illnesses and usually is associated with a terminal bradyarrhythmia; asystole and VF have been observed in 67% and 33% of these patients, respectively

Cardiac arrest is defined as the abrupt cessation of cardiac pump function that will result in death that may be averted if prompt intervention is instituted. A number of cardiac disorders cause lethal tachyarrhythmias or failure of formation or transmission of the cardiac impulse that results in cardiac arrest, but the mechanisms that initiate these fatal arrhythmias are mostly unknown and diverse.

The basic cardiac causes of cardiac arrest include

- VF or pulseless VT: in at least 80%
- Asystole: 10%
- EMD: 5%
- Myocardial rupture, cardiac tamponade, acute disruption of a major blood vessel, and acute mechanical obstruction to blood flow

The AHA's long overdue "Improving Survival from Cardiac Arrest: The Chain of Survival Concept" involves early access, early CPR, early defibrillation, and early advanced care. Since prompt defibrillation is the single most effective lifesaving intervention for the majority of victims of cardiac arrest, the Advanced Cardiac Life Support Subcommittee and the Emergency Cardiac Care Committee of the AHA have approved the widespread distribution of AEDs, which are now required items in all ambulances or emergency vehicles engaged in the transit of cardiac patients. These lifesaving devices should be in housing complexes, stadiums, and at all large public gatherings.

CARDIOPULMONARY RESUSCITATION

Unless immediate defibrillation is possible (for example, in the CCU), early CPR is essential.

Basic Life Support/CPR Technique

- Rapidly establish that the patient is unconscious, unresponsive
- Activate the emergency medical service: Call 911 or alternative. This is the major change in the BLS guidelines advocated in 1992 (*JAMA* 268[16] [1992])
- Promptly verify that the patient is not breathing: Do head tilt-chin lift maneuver. Listen over the victim's mouth and nose: If breathless, give 2 initial breaths delivered over 1-1/2 to 2 seconds (Fig. 8–1)
- Determine that the carotid pulses are absent: Locate the larynx, slide 2 fingers into the groove between the trachea and the muscles at the side of the neck, press gently to avoid compressing the artery. If pulses

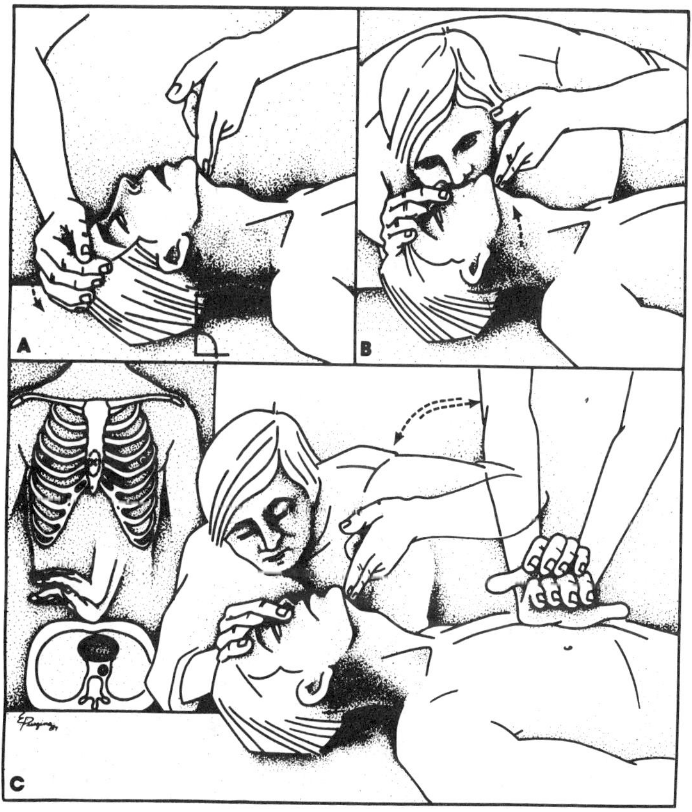

Figure 8–1. The ABCs of cardiopulmonary resuscitation. *A*. The airway is opened using the head tilt/chin lift technique. *B*. Breathing: the victim's nostrils are pinched closed and the rescuer breathes twice into the victim's mouth. *C*. Circulation: if no pulse is present, external chest compression is instituted at 80 to 100/minute. Two rescuers: 5 compressions to 1 ventilation. One rescuer: 15 compressions to 2 ventilations. Modified from: Khan M Gabriel: Cardiac Drug Therapy. 3rd Ed. London, W.B. Saunders, 1992.

are absent, commence chest compressions at a rate of 80-100/min (count "1 and 2 and 3 and . . . 15") then 2 ventilations (Fig. 8–1)
- In some European countries circulation-airway-breathing is the CPR technique

MANAGEMENT OF VENTRICULAR FIBRILLATION

Immediate defibrillation within 2–4 min of witnessed cardiac arrest and following either minimal or no CPR is the most important single therapy that may rescue patients in cardiac arrest without producing tragic iatrogenic brain damage from attempting full CPR and the unavoidable hesitations that occur in many settings of cardiac arrest

- Turn the monitor power on
- Apply conductive medium to defibrillator paddles and evaluate rhythm with the "quick look" paddles
- If VF is present, turn defibrillator power on: Be certain that the defibrillator is not in synchronous mode
- Select energy and charge the defibrillator
- Defibrillate using 200 J (see Fig. 8–2). During recharge of the defibrillator or administration of IV bolus drugs, CPR must be continued. Immediate defibrillation for the patient with VF is the key to success; intubation, establishment of IV lines, and administration of medications should commence only if the first series of DC shocks fails to restore a spontaneous circulation

Apply quick look paddles or press analyze:* VF confirmed switch to defibrillator (DF) Non-synchronized

Immediate		
1st shock	200 joules (J)	Check pulse, rhythm VF: CPR; recharge DF
2nd shock	300 J	VF persists: recharge DF
3rd shock	360 J Epinephrine 1 mg IV bolus	CPR IV line, intubate
4th shock	360 J Lidocaine 100 mg IV	VF: CPR, for 1 min (allow drug action)
5th shock	360 J Epinephrine**1, mg IV	VF VF persists, assess pH
6th shock	360 J Lidocaine 50 mg IV	VF: CPR allow 2 min
7th shock	360 J $NahCO_3$ 50 mEq IV bolus	VF: arrest $>$ 10 min pH $<$ 7.1
8th shock	360 Lidocaine 50–75 mg IV bolus	VF: CPR or bretylium 5 mg/kg allow 2–4 min
9th shock	360 J Lidocaine 50 mg IV + simultaneous infusion 2 mg/min	Conversion successful

* Semi-automated external defibrillator.
** high doses may be tried, 2,3,5 mg, 3 min apart (unproven)

Figure 8–2. Management of VF or pulseless VT.

If a defibrillator is immediately available and defibrillation is achieved within 4 min of cardiac arrest, longterm survival rates of 20–30% are possible. However, without prompt defibrillation, the survival rate ranges from 1 to 5% and is not acceptable.

Paramedic systems have been shown to achieve defibrillation in an average of 12 min, which is considered to be late defibrillation, resulting in about a 10% survival rate. Several countries and many communities in the United States have approved the use of AEDs by emergency medical technicians trained as first responders, after completion of a 40-hour training program. It is feasible to train ambulance personnel, firefighters, police officers, emergency volunteers, security guards, airline crews, designated attendants at stadiums, etc.

The operation of AEDs does not demand complex learning skills in rhythm analysis, and operation of the device can be mastered within hours. A single control activates the defibrillator to quickly analyze the cardiac rhythm, indicates that a shock is required, and on command, charges and delivers the shock.

In 4 communities in the United States, survival rates for patients in VF increased from an average of 4% to 18% with the use of emergency defibrillators by medical technicians.

DRUG THERAPY FOR CARDIAC ARREST

Epinephrine and other cardiac arrest drugs and their dosages are listed in Table 8–1.

Salutary effects of epinephrine are

- Increased myocardial contractility
- Elevated perfusion pressure
- Possible conversion of EMD to electromechanical coupling
- Improved chances for defibrillation
- Improved blood flow to the heart and brain when sinus rhythm is restored

Epinephrine is the drug of first choice, administered as an initial 1 mg IV bolus after the third shock fails to defibrillate. Intracardiac epinephrine is not recommended, except when IV or intratracheal routes are not possible. Failure to defibrillate should prompt the use of high-dose epinephrine (0.1 mg/kg) IV push q 3 min. High dose epinephrine appears necessary to maintain adequate diastolic BP in order to produce adequate coronary and cerebral perfusion, but two trials reported in the N Engl J Medicine 1992 indicate no improvement in survival. The drug produces peripheral arteriolar constriction and a ↑ in systemic vascular resistance, thus increasing aortic and coronary diastolic perfusion pressure. Also, coronary artery dilation occurs. Some studies indicate that phenylephrine or methoxamine may be superior to epinephrine for the management of cardiac arrest *Indications include:* Fine VF is made coarse and more susceptible to removal by electrical countershock; VF that fails to respond to countershock may respond following epinephrine; asystole and pulseless idioventricular rhythms; EMD.

Lidocaine (Lignocaine) is given, after a fourth shock fails to defibrillate, as a 100-mg IV bolus followed, after about 1 min of CPR, by a 360-J shock. If defibrillation is successful, give a 50-mg bolus of lidocaine and an infusion at 2 mg/min immediately (1–3 mg/min is the lower dose for the elderly or those with CHF; see Tables 3–8 and 3–9). An additional bolus is given 10 min later to maintain therapeutic lidocaine levels. Lidocaine is preferred to bretylium because trials have not shown brety-

Table 8–1
Cardiac Arrest Drugs

DRUG	DOSAGE	SUPPLIED	COMMENT
Epinephrine	IV bolus 1 mg repeated q 3-5 min.* Tracheobronchial 10 ml (1:10,000)	10 ml (1 mg in 1:10,000 dilution)	Do not give with $NaHCO_3$ in same IV
Sodium Bicarbonate	IV bolus 1 mEq (mmol)/kg, usually 50 mEq (mmol) initially; then ½ initial dose q 10 to 15 min	50 ml of 8.4% = 50.0 mEq (mmol) 1 Amp = 44 mEq	Not used routinely. Recommended for trial after 7th shock, pH <7.1, or 10 min. in asystole
Atropine	In asystole 1 mg q 2–5 min (max of 3 mg, 0.04 mg/kg) Bradycardia 0.5 mg q 5 min to 2 mg	10 ml = 1 mg 5 ml = 0.5 mg (UK, 1 ml amp = 0.6 mg or 1 mg)	
Lidocaine	75–100 mg IV bolus simultaneous infusion 2–3 mg/min	50 mg in 5 ml (1%) 100 mg in 10 ml (1%) 100 mg in 5 ml (2%)	
Bretylium Tosylate for VF	5 mg/kg IV bolus (undiluted). CPR, 1 min. If countershock fails, repeat 10 mg/kg (max 30 mg/kg)	500 mg in 10 ml amp (UK 50 mg/ml; 2 ml amp)	Hypotension Do not give epinephrine or norepinephrine simultaneously
Propranolol for VF Metoprolol	USA: 1 mg over 2–5 min (q 2–5 min to max 5 mg) UK: 1 mg over 2 min (q 2 min to max 5 mg) 5 mg IV over 5 min		Useful in recurrent VF if lidocaine fails
Calcium Chloride	5 ml 10% (5–7 mg/kg 250–500 mg) IV bolus, Repeat 10 ml IV in 5 min	10 ml 10% $CaCl_2$	*Not recommended* in cardiac arrest, except with hyperkalemia or post verapamil Do not give with $NaHCO_3$

q = every;* high doses may be tried (unproven) 2,3,5 mg, 3 min apart
Modified from: Khan M Gabriel: Cardiac Drug Therapy. 3rd Ed. London, W.B. Saunders, 1992.

lium to be superior and lidocaine does not produce severe hypotension, which is often seen with bretylium.

Sodium bicarbonate is no longer recommended for routine use during cardiac arrest of brief duration. However, after about 10 min of CPR and if a seventh shock fails to result in defibrillation, an IV bolus of sodium bicarbonate (50 mEq) is advisable. The drug should not be used simultaneously with CaCl or epinephrine. In the UK, sodium bicarbonate is usually given after failure of the fifth shock.

Calcium chloride is no longer recommended. The drug may be useful

- If asystole is caused by verapamil. Give 2.5–5 ml 10% CaCl or Ca gluconate IV bolus
- In the management of hyperkalemia causing arrest
- The substance is, however, of no value in EMD

Bretylium may be given if a third bolus of lidocaine fails. Give 5 mg/kg IV rapid bolus, then wait 2–4 min before attempting defibrillation. If conversion fails, give 10 mg/kg bolus, wait 5–10 min, and continue CPR before attempting further defibrillation because occasionally bretylium may take 5–10 min to be effective. Unfortunately, by that time, the heart is likely to be atonic. As discussed in Chapter 6, the role of bretylium has appropriately dwindled with the availability of amiodarone.

BRADYARRHYTHMIAS—ASYSTOLE OR EMD

Severe symptomatic bradycardia is usually treated with atropine, 0.5–0.6 mg repeated q 2 min to a max of 2.4 mg. When atropine is used to treat asystole prior to pacing, a dose of 1 mg is given immediately, followed by an additional 1 mg after 2 min. In severe bradycardia or A-V block without a QRS complex, atropine is worth a trial. No harm can ensue, because as if VF is precipitated by atropine; defibrillation may produce a stable rhythm to allow coronary perfusion prior to pacing. Be aware that VF may masquerade as asystole. Thus, rotate the monitoring electrodes and check the monitor to ensure that VF is not present. Give epinephrine with the hope that fibrillation may ensue, and then countershock.

Asystole in a heart that was beating forcefully minutes prior to the occurrence of asystole may complicate anterior infarction, and pacing may be lifesaving. However, asystole in the atonic heart (agonal) and EMD are usually due to irreversible myocardial damage and prognosis is very poor.

Management of EMD: Commence CPR, IV line, epinephrine (1 mg IV bolus), intubate, assess for cardiac rupture and tamponade.

Search for extracardiac causes of EMD

- Inadequate ventilation, including intubation of right main stem bronchus and tension pneumothorax
- Poor perfusion: Hypovolemia (JVP decreased), give fluid challenge. If the JVP is markedly elevated, suspect cardiac tamponade or massive pulmonary embolism
- Severe acidosis or hyperkalemia

CPR should be continued with the hope that 1 of these factors may be correctible. Mobitz Type 2 block and complete heart block must be managed with ventricular pacing (see Chap. 7). If there is asystole or severe bradycardia unresponsive to atropine, continue CPR, give epinephrine 1 mg IV or endotracheal and then 2, 4, 6, 8 mg at 1 min intervals. If there is no response, consider pacing. For severe hypotension with mild bradycardia, dopamine is advisable (see Table 4–6).

Selected Reading

Emergency Cardiac Care Committee and Subcommittees, American Heart Association: Guidelines for Cardiopulmonary Resuscitation and Emergency Care, II: Adult Basic Life Support. JAMA *268*:2184, 1992.

Khan, M Gabriel: Cardiac arrest. *In* Cardiac Drug Therapy. London, W. B. Saunders, 1992.

O'Nunain S, Ruskin J: Cardiac Arrest. Lancet *341*: 1641, 1993.

9

Hyperlipidemia

M. Gabriel Khan

DIAGNOSIS AND DECISION MAKING

Elevated Blood Cholesterol

- A total blood cholesterol level <200 mg/dl (5.2 mmol/l) is considered desirable. Individuals with cholesterol levels >350 mg/dl (9 mmol/l) are at high risk for the development of premature atheromatous occlusion of the coronary arteries and early manifestations of IHD; fortunately, this scenario is uncommon and the attention given to familial hypocholesterolemia in the 1960s to early 1980s is being focused on mild and moderate elevations of blood cholesterol
- The recommendations of the Adult Treatment Panel of the National Cholesterol Education Program for Classification of Patients are listed in Table 9–1. Most heart attacks occur in individuals with levels of 210–240 mg/dl (5.5–6.2 mmol/l); approximately 50% of adult Americans have cholesterol levels in this range. In individuals with borderline high cholesterol, a low level of HDL-C further increases the risk for CHD (Fig. 9–1)

Low-Density Lipoprotein Cholesterol

- LDL-C is the main culprit in CHD, but its measurement is more costly than that of total cholesterol. While total cholesterol can be measured in the nonfasting state, the measurement of LDL-C requires a 12- to 14-hour fasting specimen for accurate determination of the triglyceride level, which is required for the estimation of the LDL-C. An LDL-C <130 mg/dl (3.36 mmol/l) is desirable, >160 mg/dl (4.13 mmol/l) is considered high risk (Table 9–1)
- LDL-C is derived as follows:

$$\text{LDL (mg/dl)} = \text{total cholesterol} - \text{HDL} - (\text{triglyceride} \div 5)$$

$$\text{LDL (mmol/l)} = \text{total cholesterol} - \text{HDL} - (\text{triglyceride} \div 2.2)$$

- If the triglyceride value is above 400 mg/dl (4 mmol/l), LDL-C estimation using the above formula is not accurate

High-Density Lipoprotein Cholesterol

HDL-C determination is recommended in the initial screen because the level is vital in decision making concerning the management of hyperlipidemia. Data from the Framingham Study indicate that the mortality risk from CHD ↑ as HDL-C levels ↓. Every 1% ↑ in HDL-C ↓ CHD risk by about 2%, and each 1% ↓ in total cholesterol should produce a 2% ↓ in CHD risk. The HDL-C shows a strong inverse association with

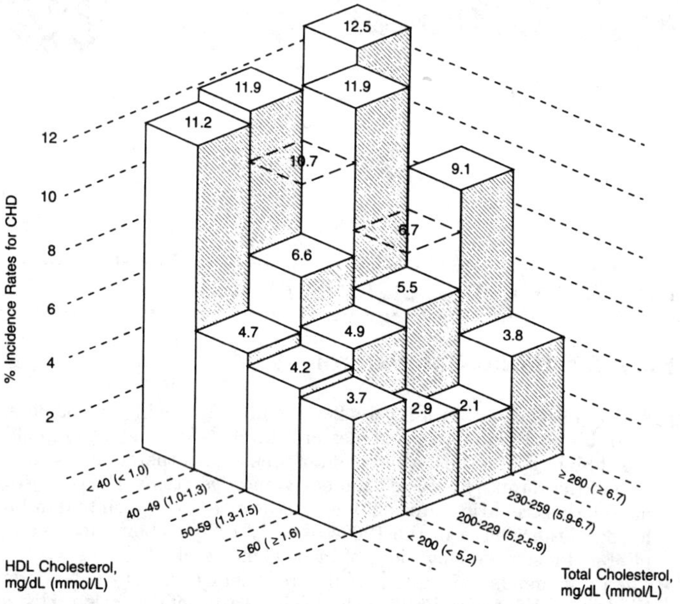

Figure 9–1. Incidence of coronary heart disease (CHD) in 4 years by high-density lipoprotein cholesterol (HDL-C) and total plasma cholesterol level for men and women free of cardiovascular disease. Modified from: Castelli WP, et al.: Incidence of coronary heart disease and lipoprotein cholesterol levels. The Framingham Study. JAMA, *256*:2837, 1986.

Table 9–1
Recommendations of the Adult Treatment Panel of the National Cholesterol Education Program for Classification of Patients

CLASSIFICATION BASED ON TOTAL CHOLESTEROL	CLASSIFICATION BASED ON LDL CHOLESTEROL
<200 mg/dl (<5.17 mmol/l) Desirable blood cholesterol	<130 mg/dl (<3.36 mmol/l) Desirable LDL cholesterol
200–239 mg/dl (5.17–6.18 mmol/l) Borderline-high blood cholesterol	130–159 mg/dl (3.36–4.11 mmol/l) Borderline–high-risk LDL cholesterol
≥240 mg/dl (≥6.21 mmol/l) High blood cholesterol	≥160 mg/dl (≥4.13 mmol/l) High-risk LDL cholesterol

LDL: low density lipoprotein
From the National Cholesterol Education Program, Adult Treatment Panel, January 1988.
From: Carleton RA, et al.: Report of the expert panel on population strategies for blood cholesterol reduction. Circulation, *83*:2161, 1991.

incidence of CHD at all levels of total cholesterol, including levels <200 mg/dl (5.2 mmol/l) (Fig. 9-1).

HDL-C and total cholesterol are initial screening tests and are not affected by food eaten within prior hours. A nonfasting specimen allows the sample to be taken immediately after the physician consultation and saves the time and cost of a return visit to a laboratory.

Elevated Blood Triglycerides

- Triglyceride-rich, VLDLs are secreted by the liver. The VLDL surface coat contains apolipoprotein (apo) B and other lipoproteins. VLDL triglycerides undergo hydrolysis by lipoprotein lipase
- Triglyceride levels >300–500 mg/dl (3–5 mmol/l) are considered borderline and levels >500 mg/dl (5 mmol/l) are considered high. Triglycerides are not routinely measured as a screening test. The independent contribution of triglyceride disappears once the risk of HDL has been taken into account
- ↑ triglycerides with LDL/HDL ratio >5 is associated with ↑ risk of CHD as indicated by the Helsinki and Münster (PROCAM) studies. In Germany and some European countries, screening includes cholesterol, HDL, triglycerides, and LDL/HDL

Causes of Hyperlipidemia

DIETARY FACTORS

Total cholesterol levels of 200–320 mg/dl (5.2–8.3 mmol/l) result from a complex interaction of polygenic and environmental factors. Although it is often assumed that excess dietary saturated fat intake is a major cause of elevated cholesterol levels, there is evidence that genetics is an important factor in most cases. A dietary history of increased saturated fat and/or total cholesterol intake must be ascertained.

UNDERLYING DISEASES

Diabetes, hypothyroidism, pancreatitis, nephrotic syndrome, obstructive jaundice, biliary cirrhosis, and dysproteinemia may be implicated in a minority of patients. Record the presence or absence of xanthelasma of the eyelids, xanthoma tendinosum, tuberosum, and planum. These lesions are mainly observed in patients with familial genetic severe hyperlipidemia. These individuals have a genetic abnormality characterized by cellular LDL receptor deficiency. Homozygote incidence is 1 in 1 million; they have few or no LDL receptors and a cholesterol range of 600-1200 mg/dl. Heterozygotes have about 50% of the total number of LDL receptors and a cholesterol range of 350-550 mg/dl. These patients are at very high risk for development of premature CHD. If the situation is suspected, screen 1st° relatives, parents, siblings, and children.

MEDICATIONS

Hormones, estrogens, progestins, contraceptive pills, anabolic steroids, and β blockers commonly alter lipid levels. In a menopausal woman, hormone deficiency will ↑ total cholesterol. Replacement therapy with premarin (0.625 mg), along with dietary measures, may suffice. Importantly, replacement hormone ↑ HDL-C levels.

Table 9–2
CHD Risk Factors Other Than LDL Cholesterol

- Male sex
- Family history of premature CHD (definite myocardial infarction or sudden death before age 55 in a parent or sibling)
- Cigarette smoking
- Hypertension
- Low HDL cholesterol concentration (below 35 mg/dl, 0.9 mmol/l confirmed by repeat measurement)
- Diabetes mellitus
- History of definite cerebrovascular or occlusive peripheral vascular disease
- Severe obesity (≥30% overweight)

CHD: coronary heart disease; LDL: low density lipoprotein; HDL: high density lipoprotein.
From: The National Cholesterol Education Program Report of the Expert Panel on Detection, Evaluation, and Treatment of High Blood Cholesterol in Adults. United States Department of Health and Human Services, Public Health Service, National Heart, Lung and Blood Institute. Publication No. (NIH) 88-2925 Bethesda, MD, 1988.

Diuretics may cause a mild ↑ in total cholesterol (1–4%) and a slight ↓ of HDL (approximately 1–10%).

Beta blockers, with the exception of those with ISA, ↑ triglyceride levels 10–30%. It is clear that LDL-C is not increased by β blockers.

Results of several studies evaluating the effect of β blockers on HDL-C have not been consistent. Propranolol caused a 6% ↓ in HDL-C in the BHAT study. Evidence to support the relatively neutral lipid effect of ISA β blockers was provided by the Treatment of Mild Hypertension Study (TOMHS); acebutolol (400 mg) administered qd to 77 patients caused no significant change in HDL after 1 year of therapy. Acebutolol, which has mild ISA, caused a 48% ↓ in post-infarction mortality in patients followed for 10 months. In patients with hyperlipidemia, acebutolol is the β blocker of choice.

DIETARY MANAGEMENT

- Dietary modification is expected to ↓ an elevated blood cholesterol by 7–15%, depending on the degree of adherence to a low saturated fat, low-cholesterol diet and should be tried for ≥6 months before drug therapy is considered except in patients with extreme hyperlipidemia, when both are needed. A weight reduction diet, however, ↓ triglycerides 25–50%.

Step 1 Diet (Expert Panel Recommendations)

- An average of ≤30% of total calories from total fat
- Saturated fatty acids should not be >10% of total calories
- 20% of total calories should be derived from the combination of polyunsaturated fatty acids and monounsaturated fatty acids. Polyunsaturated fatty acids should not be >10% of total calories
- <300 mg cholesterol qd

- Carbohydrates 50–60% of total calories
- Protein 10 to max 15% of calories
- Avoid: organ meats such as liver, kidney, sweetbreads, heart, or brain; heavily marbled steaks, salt pork, or duck; whole milk or whole milk products, cream, lard, and nonvegetable margarine; coconut oil or products containing coconut oil (such as nondairy creamers), palm oil, peanut oil, or peanut butter (see Table 9–3)
- Recommended foods: fruits, whole-grain products, beans, peas, vegetables, cereals; low-fat dairy products, including skim or low-fat milk, skim or low-fat butter (skim milk is a good source of Ca); fish such as salmon, mackerel, tuna, or cod, which contain an abundance of omega-3 fatty acids; moderate amounts of skinless chicken and lean red meat (up to 6 oz.) 2 or 3 times weekly. Shrimp contain a fair amount of cholesterol but no saturated fatty acids, provided that they are not fried in a batter. Vegetable oils such as safflower, sunflower, soybean, corn, and olive oil are recommended, but coconut, palm, rapeseed, and peanut oils are not. Walnuts contain a high amount of polyunsaturated fatty acid but are low in saturated fat. Oat bran has little specific cholesterol-lowering effect and is not superior to low-fiber dietary grain supplements

Step 2 Diet

- An average of ≤25% of total calories from total fat
- <7% of total calories from saturated fat
- Cholesterol 200–250 mg qd

The Step 2 diet is recommended for patients with cholesterol elevated to 275–310 mg/dl (7.1–8 mmol/l) after a 6-month to 1-year trial of the Step 1 diet.

DRUG THERAPY

Drugs are utilized only after an adequate trial of dietary therapy, a concerted effort by the patient and physician, and/or the assistance of a dietician or lipid clinic fail to adequately lower total cholesterol or LDL-C to the desired level (see Figure 9–2). When drugs are prescribed, dietary restrictions must be continued.

The United States Expert Panel on Detection, Evaluation and Treatment of High Blood Cholesterol in Adults recommends that drug therapy be considered in the following situations

- LDL-C ≥190 mg/dl (5 mmol/l) or a total cholesterol >280 mg/dl (7 mmol/l)
- LDL-C >160 mg/dl (4 mmol/l) or total cholesterol >240 mg/dl (6.2 mmol/l) and the presence of ≥2 risk factors (Table 9–2)
- LDL-C >130 mg/dl (>3.4 mmol/l) and manifestations of CHD: angina, MI, previous angioplasty or CABS

Since it is difficult for the human brain to recall decimals, the important numbers to remember for LDL-C, 4.13 and 4.9 mmol/l, have been altered to 4 and 5 mmol/l (Fig. 9–2). Drug therapy is strongly advised for LDL-C >130 mg/dl (3.4 mmol/l) in patients who have angina or who have had a heart attack, angioplasty, or CABS.

Table 9–3
Saturated Fat and Cholesterol Content of Foods

ITEM	CHOLESTEROL (mg)	TOTAL FAT (g)	SATURATED FAT (g)	NOT RECOMMENDED	**RECOMMENDED	USE SPARINGLY
MEATS						
beef liver	395	10	3		X	
kidney	725	11	4		X	
sweetbread	420	21	—		X	
lean beef	82	5	2			**
roast beef						
e.g., rib	85	33	14	X		¢
rump	85	21	9		X	
stewing	82	27	11	X		¢
" lean	82	9	4			**
ground	85	18	8	X		¢
steak						
sirloin	85	25	10	X		¢
" lean	85	5	2			*
veal	90	12	5			**
lamb, lean	90	7	4			¢
chop & fat	110	33	18		X	
ham						
fat roasted	80	28	7		X	
boiled						
sliced	80	18	5			¢
pork chop	80	30	12		X	
chicken						
breast & skin	72	6	1			**
drumstick (fried)	80	9	2			**
turkey	80	5	2			**

FISH					
sole	45	1	trace		**
trout	50	13	3		**
tuna	60	7	2		**
salmon					
fresh	42	7	1		**
canned	32	11	2		**
mackerel	85	10	2		**
halibut	54	6	trace		**
crabmeat	91	1	trace		¢
shrimp	130	1	trace		¢
lobster (450 g)	80	1	trace		¢
DAIRY PRODUCTS					
30 ml butter	460	25	16	X	
egg (50 g)	275	6	2		¢
substitute	0	0	0	**	
buttermilk†	10	2	1		
yogurt (250 ml)	16	3	2		**
whole milk					
250 ml	35	9	5		¢
2%	20	5	3		**
skim milk	trace	trace	trace		**
ice cream					
vanilla reg. (125 ml)	32	8	5		¢
rich (125 ml)	46	12	8	X	

(continued)

Table 9–3. *(continued)*
Saturated Fat and Cholesterol Content of Foods

ITEM	CHOLESTEROL (mg)	TOTAL FAT (g)	SATURATED FAT (g)	POLY-UNSATURATED	NOT RECOMMENDED	**RECOMMENDED	USE SPARINGLY
butter	30	11	7	trace			¢
lard	12	13	5	1	X		
cheese (1 oz)							
brick	27	8	6	trace			¢
blue	24			"		¢	
cheddar	30	10	6	"			¢
cottage†	2	.6	.5	"		**	
skim milk, processed 1 oz (30 g)	0	trace	trace	trace		**	
OILS							
corn oil	0	14	1	7		**	
rapeseed	0	14	1	3			
safflower	0	13	1	10		**	
sunflower	0	14	1	9		**	
soybean	0	14	2	7		**	
coconut	0	14	12	.2	X		
palm	0		7	.2	X		
olive	0	14	2	1		**	
peanut		14	2	4	X		
NUTS							
almonds	0	16	1	3		**	
brazil nuts	0	22	5	8	X		
cashews	0	13	3	2	X		
coconut	0	13	11	trace	X		
peanuts	0	17	3	4	X		
peanut butter	0	7.5	1.5	2	X		
pecans	0	21	2	5			¢
walnuts	0	19	2	11		**	

* Quantity is 3 oz (90 g) unless specified; 15 ml = one tablespoonful.
** Foods recommended contain less than 5 g saturated fat per 3 oz.
† Low-fat milk, 2%.
From: Khan M. Gabriel: Is cholesterol important again? *In* Heart Attacks, Hypertension and Heart Drugs. Toronto, McClelland-Bantam Inc., 1990. By permission of McClelland-Bantam Inc.

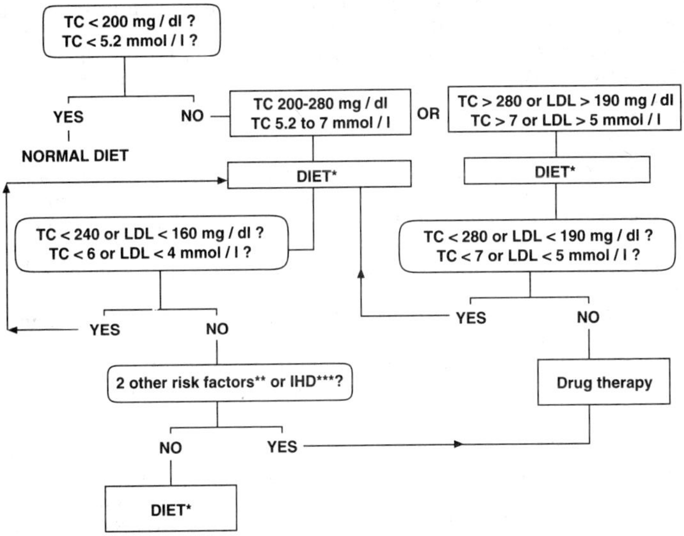

TC = Total Cholesterol
* = Step one therapeutic diet, see text
** = Table 9-2
*** = Presence of coronary angioplasty or bypass surgery
IHD = Ischemic heart disease

Figure 9–2. Guides for the management of high total or LDL cholesterol.

HMG-CoA Reductase Inhibitors

Available agents include lovastatin, simvastatin, and pravastatin. These agents are competitive inhibitors of HMG-CoA reductase, the enzyme catalyzing the early rate limiting step in the biosynthesis of cholesterol, conversion of HMG-CoA to mevalonate. A modest ↓ in intracellular cholesterol occurs, resulting in a ↑ in the number of hepatic LDL receptors that bring about clearance of circulating LDL-C. In the 48-week EXCEL Study of 8,245 patients with total cholesterol levels of 240–300 mg/dl (6.2–7.8 mmol/l) and LDL-C >160 mg/dl (4.1 mmol/l), the average changes from baseline for lovastatin (20, 40, and 80 mg qd) were –24%, –32%, and –40% for LDL-C and 6.6, 7.9, and 9.5% for HDL-C. The 20-mg twice-daily dose produced a more favorable trend compared to 40 mg each evening for both LDL and HDL-C.

Some regression and prevention of progression of atheroma have been observed with the use of HMG-CoA reductase inhibitors.

Lovastatin (Mecavor). *Supplied:* tablets; 10, 20, 40 mg. *Dosage:* 10–20 mg given as a single dose with the evening meal. ↑, if needed, to 20–30 mg bid, max 80 mg, after checking for efficacy and for increased hepatic transaminases and CK elevation.

Contraindications: women of childbearing age; pregnancy; breastfeeding; hepatic disease; concomitant use of cyclosporin, erythromycin, or other cytotoxic drugs; concomitant use of nicotinic acid or fibrates; porphyria; patients with myopathy or individuals engaging in strenuous physical exertion; patients < age 18.

Adverse Effects: Headaches in about 10%, stomach pain, flatulence, diarrhea, constipation, nausea, hepatic dysfunction with increased hepatic transaminases (2%), chest pain due to stomach disturbance or muscular aches. Myalgia, ↑ CK, myopathy (0.5%), and rhabdomyolysis have been observed in patients receiving concomitant niacin, gemfibrozil, other fibrates, cyclosporin, and other immunosuppressive drugs. Lens opacity observed in animals given high doses has not been a clinical problem, although minor lens opacification occurs. Rash is uncommon. Baseline transaminase, CK, and opthalmology assessment are advisable. If > a twofold ↑ in transaminases occurs, the drug should be discontinued.

Caution: Avoid in renal transplant patients on cyclosporin or immunosuppressives. Reduction in the dose of warfarin is usually required. Severe myositis may cause hyperkalemia in patients with renal insufficiency, particularly including longstanding diabetics who are also on ACE inhibitors.

Simvastatin (Zocor). *Supplied:* 5, 10, 20, 40 mg. *Dosage:* 5–10 mg with the evening meal, ↑ if needed in 8–12 weeks to 20 mg qd to a max of 40 mg once daily. Adverse effects and contraindications are similar to those for lovastatin. No effect on lens translucency has been observed.

Pravastatin (Pravachol; Lipostat, UK). *Supplied:* tablets; 10, 20 mg. *Dosage:* 10 mg with the evening meal, ↑ over 2–4 months to a max of 40 mg once daily or 20 mg bid. Contraindications and adverse effects are the same as those outlined for lovastatin, but hyperuricemia, urinary frequency, thrombocytopenia, leukopenia, and leukocytosis have been observed, albeit rarely. No lens disturbances have been recorded. Pravastatin is a hydrophilic compound and has primarily a hepatic site of action with little influence on cholesterol synthesis in other tissues. The fact that it does not cause cataracts in dogs at 100 mg/kg is probably related to its hydrophilic property.

HMG-CoA Reductase Inhibitors and Bile Acid Binding Resins

Several trials utilizing the combination of lovastatin, simvastatin, and pravastatin with cholestyramine or colestipol in patients uncontrolled by 1 agent alone have indicated a marked additive effect. The HMG-CoA reductase inhibitor must be given 1 h before or 4 h following the resin because bile acid resins interfere with absorption of these agents.

Bile Acid Binding Resins

The use of bile acid binding resins declined with the advent of HMG-CoA reductase inhibitors, but they have a role as combination therapy in patients with severe hyperlipidemia.

The Lipid Research Clinic trial showed no ↓ in cardiac or total mortality with the use of cholestyramine.

Action: Bile acid binding resins are not absorbed from the GI tract and act by binding bile salts in the gut; they are, therefore, bile acid sequestrants. This action causes cholesterol catabolism to bile acids and a ↓ in serum LDL-C. A decreased concentration of intrahepatic cholesterol stimulates the activity of LDL receptors that ↑ hepatic uptake of circulating LDL-C.

Cholestyramine (Questran). *Dosage:* 4 g (1 packet) bid with meals for 1–2 weeks, then 8 g bid or tid. It is advisable to prepare the daily dose at night; the bile acid binding resin is mixed with a noncarbonated beverage or orange drink and stored in the refrigerator for use the next day at meal times. Questran Light has an orange flavor and requires only about 75 ml liquid per packet.

Medications, especially digoxin, oral anticoagulants, diuretics, β blockers, thyroid hormone, and HMG-CoA reductase inhibitors, must be administered 1 h before or 4 h following the resin to prevent interference with absorption.

Adverse Effects: Constipation, abdominal cramps, and rarely mild malabsorption of fat-soluble vitamins.

Colestipol (Colestid). *Dosage:* 5 g bid in liquid; ↑, if necessary, at intervals of about 2 months to 25 g qd. The adverse effects are similar to those of cholestyramine.

Fibrates

These agents are activators of the enzyme plasma-lipoprotein-lipase. Fibrates cause a 1–15% ↓ in serum cholesterol, a 30–50% ↓ in triglycerides, and a 10–15% ↑ in HDL-C.

Gemfibrozil (Lopid). *Supplied:* capsules; 300 mg (600 mg Canada). *Dosage:* 300–600 mg 30 min before morning and evening meals.

Action: Gemfibrozil is a chemical homologue of clofibrate. The drug decreases hepatic production of VLDL triglyceride. Gemfibrozil causes a 30–40% ↓ in triglycerides, a 2–10% ↓ in serum cholesterol, and a 5–12% ↑ in HDL-C.

Indications include

- Severe hypertriglyceridemia, >1,000 mg/dl (10 mmol/l), that is unresponsive to dietary measures, exercise, and cessation of alcohol. In these patients, treatment is necessary to prevent pancreatitis
- Type III hyperlipoproteinemia that is associated with marked elevation of triglycerides
- Individuals with total cholesterol 250–300 mg/dl (6.5–7.9 mmol/l), and with 2 risk factors other than LDL, one of which is a low HDL-C <35 mg/dl (0.9 mmol/l)
- The use of gemfibrozil in patients with moderate hypercholesterolemia has gained support because of the results of the Helsinki Heart Study
- PROCAM has identified patients with LDL/HDL >5 and ↑ triglycerides as at high risk for CHD. This group may benefit from gemfibrozil therapy

Adverse Effects: bloating, cramps, diarrhea, muscle aching, eczema, ↑ in liver function tests, rarely a mild ↑ in blood sugar, and impotence. The lithogenic activity appears to be < that of clofibrate,

Caution: Reduce oral anticoagulant dose. Do not combine with HMG-CoA reductase inhibitors because of the risk of severe myositis and rhabdomyolysis. The drug is renally excreted. Reduce dose to 300 mg qd with renal failure.

Contraindications: Hepatic impairment, alcoholism, gallstones, pregnancy.

Fenofibrate. *Supplied:* capsule; 100 mg. *Dosage:* 100 mg qd or bid, max 400 mg qd. This prodrug is converted to fenofibric acid.

Adverse Effects; GI disturbances and dermatologic adverse effects occur in 7–14% of patients. Cholelithiasis. Abnormal liver function tests.

Rash, pruritus, urticaria or erythema, weight loss, impotence, alopecia, pancreatitis, hepatitis, and CK elevations.

Contraindications: Severe renal or hepatic impairment. Fibrates are excreted by the kidney and should be used with caution in patients with renal dysfunction. Gallbladder disease. Hypersensitivity to fenofibrate. Pregnancy, women of childbearing potential, and during lactation. Primary biliary cirrhosis.

Nicotinic Acid. *Supplied:* 50, 100, 500 mg. Assess transaminases and glucose levels. *Dosage:* 50 mg with the evening meal for 1 week, with 325-mg coated aspirin taken 30 min prior to prevent flushing. ↑ to 100 mg bid and, over months, slowly ↑ from 100 to 500 mg tid, always after meals.

Adverse Effects: Flushing, pruritus, nausea, abdominal pain, diarrhea, hepatic dysfunction, jaundice, exacerbation of diabetes, gout, palpitations, arrhythmias, hypotension, rarely pigmentation, and optic neuritis with blurred vision. Acute hepatitis is a dangerous complication of niacin, especially with sustained-release preparations.

Caution: Do not use in combination with HMG-CoA reductase inhibitors, because severe myositis may occur. Avoid the drug in patients with acute MI, CHF, gallbladder disease, jaundice, liver disease, peptic ulcer, and diabetes.

Suggested Reading

Khan M Gabriel: Hyperlipidemia. *In* Cardiac and Pulmonary Management. Philadelphia, Lea & Febiger, 1993.

Infective Endocarditis

10

M. Gabriel Khan

DIAGNOSIS

The diagnosis of infective endocarditis must be considered and excluded in all individuals with a heart murmur and fever of unknown origin. Infection of the heart valves may be caused by bacteria and, less commonly, fungi, Coxiella, or Chlamydia.

A few hours or days of fever, chills, and rigors are common with ABE. An insidious onset over weeks with fever, malaise, chills, and weight loss indicates SBE.

In a patient with a murmur and a fever of undetermined origin, 1 of the following precipitating or predisposing factors, if present, should produce a high index of suspicion of infective endocarditis

- Known valvular heart disease, especially rheumatic, bicuspid aortic valve or mitral valve prolapse, with significant regurgitation; Marfan's, floppy valve
- Prosthetic valve
- Recent dental or oropharyngeal surgical procedure
- Genitourinary instrumentation or surgery of the respiratory tract
- IV addiction
- Congenital heart disease: Patent ductus, VSD, Fallot's tetralogy, coarctation
- Prolonged use of IV catheters and hyperalimentation
- Burns
- Inflammatory and other bowel disease, suspect S. bovis. If this organism is isolated, exclude polyposis and carcinoma of the colon
- Hemodialysis

Infective endocarditis may occur, however, in the absence of previously known valvular disease or other precipitating factors, especially in elderly patients.

Physical Signs

- A heart murmur is usually present with SBE, absent in 1–5%
- A murmur may be absent in ≤15% of patients with ABE and not heard in about 33% of individuals with right-sided endocarditis, especially if care is not taken to listen for the murmur of tricuspid regurgitation
- A change in the quality or grade of the murmur is an unreliable indicator
- Intermittent medium- to high-grade fever is usually prominent, but in elderly or immunocompromised patients, fever may be mild or absent. Normal body temperature is lower in the elderly, 97°F (36°C) as opposed to 98°F (37°C) in individuals < age 70

- Finger clubbing takes about 6 weeks to appear, is seen only with SBE, and disappears a few weeks after successful treatment
- Osler's nodes, although uncommon, are pathognomonic, manifest as exquisitely painful, SQ papules, pea- to almond-sized on the palms and soles. Lesions disappear in 1–5 days and may be seen during adequate therapy
- Petechiae with pale centers may be observed on everting the upper eyelids. They may be seen in the oropharynx as retinal cotton wool exudates, canoe-shaped hemorrhages with white spots in their center (Roth's spots)
- Splinter hemorrhages may be due to trauma, but a ↑ in their numbers is relevant
- Splenomegaly is observed in about 50% of patients with SBE and in about 15% of those with ABE. The enlarged spleen may be painful and tender and can rupture. An ultrasound of the spleen is advisable in all cases of suspected infective endocarditis
- Pigmentation: pasty, café au lait complexion reverts to normal after treatment
- Janeway lesions are rare: 1–4 mm painless flat erythematous macules, nontender on the palms and soles, blanch on pressure

Investigations

- 4–6 blood cultures are taken over a 1- to 2-hour period and carry a 90% chance of recovering organisms
- Urinalysis often shows mild hematuria or increased RBCs and few RBC casts
- ↑ creatinine, urea, or BUN is nonspecific
- The ESR is virtually always elevated and can be 75–110 mm/h (Westergren) with SBE
- The rheumatoid factor is positive >50% of patients
- Anemia is seen in >30% of patients with SBE
- The WBC may be slightly ↑ or remain normal. There is almost always a shift to the left, however, with a ↑ in band forms
- Check Gram's stain of the blood, buffy coat for organisms

A sterile blood culture is observed in ≤25% of cases due to: prior antibiotic therapy; fastidious organisms (as with slow-growing streptococci); fungal infection (request fungal precipitins); Q fever (serology should be requested); chlamydia infection.

BACTERIA CAUSING ENDOCARDITIS INCLUDE:

- S. aureus is responsible for >85% of cases of acute endocarditis
- S. pneumoniae causing acute fulminant endocarditis is now rare. Gonococcus, pseudomonas, and S. marcescens may cause right-sided acute endocarditis
- Streptococci are implicated in 60–80% of subacute endocarditis
- Fecal streptococci, commonly termed "enterococci," cause ≤10% of infective endocarditis, but with a higher incidence in the geriatric population
- Nutritionally variant streptococci: S. anginosis, S. mitis, and similar organisms require special media for their growth

Table 10–1
Detection of Vegetations by Transesophageal vs. Transthoracic 2D Echocardiography

	OVERALL	>10 mm	6 to 10 mm	<5 mm
TEE	100%	100%	100%	100%
Transthoracic 2D Color Doppler	63%	70%	65%	25%

ECHOCARDIOGRAPHY IS OF MAJOR BENEFIT:

Transthoracic echocardiography detects approximately 63% of vegetations (see Table 10–1). S. aureus and some streptococci may produce small lesions of <5 mm, which are poorly detectable by transthoracic echocardiography.

TEE is superior to the transthoracic technique and can be crucial to the management of endocarditis (Table 10-1). Transthoracic 2-dimensional Doppler echocardiography gives poor detection of prosthetic heart valves, especially in the mitral position, and of calcific sclerotic native valves.

TEE has a role in the following

- Failure of transthoracic echocardiography to show vegetations in patients strongly suspected of having endocarditis
- All prosthetic heart valves
- Calcific sclerotic native valves
- Valvular destruction secondary to infective endocarditis, especially perivalvular abscesses

THERAPY

It is imperative that therapy be started immediately after 4–6 blood cultures are taken and relevant clinical information is forwarded to the microbiology laboratory.

Vegetations that are <1 cm are usually cured by 4–6 weeks of antibiotic therapy. Vegetations >1 cm that do not respond to 3 weeks of antibiotic therapy often necessitate surgery.

See Table 10–2, Chapters 17, 18, and 26 for a description of antimicrobial agents and therapy for various microorganisms.

Empiric therapy can be tailored based on the following.

Native Valve Endocarditis. In patients with native valve endocarditis, SBE presentation in patients < age 65 requires obvious coverage of S. viridans, which is the causative organism in ≤70% of cases, and fecal streptococci in ≤15%: penicillin (2 million U q 4 h IV) plus gentamicin (1.3–2 mg/kg q 8 h IV) until the organism has been defined and sensitivities and the MIC of the drug against the isolated organism are known.

Geriatric Endocarditis. As above, but in elderly patients, fecal streptococci are more common and occur in ≤25% of patients; it is advisable

Table 10–2
Prevention of Bacterial Endocarditis–Cardiac Conditions*

Endocarditis prophylaxis recommended
Prosthetic cardiac valves, including bioprosthetic and homograft valves
Previous bacterial endocarditis, even in the absence of heart disease
Surgically constructed systemic-pulmonary shunts or conduits
Most congenital cardiac malformations
Rheumatic and other acquired valvular dysfunction, even after valvular surgery
Hypertrophic cardiomyopathy
Mitral valve prolapse with valvular regurgitation
Endocarditis prophylaxis not recommended
Isolated secundum atrial septal defect
Surgical repair without residua beyond 6 months of secundum atrial septal defect, ventricular septal defect, or patent ductus arteriosus
Previous coronary artery bypass graft surgery
Mitral valve prolapse without valvular regurgitation†
Physiologic, functional, or innocent heart murmurs
Previous Kawasaki disease without valvular dysfunction
Previous rheumatic fever without valvular dysfunction
Cardiac pacemakers and implanted defibrillators

* This table lists selected conditions but is not meant to be all-inclusive.
† Individuals who have a mitral valve prolapse associated with thickening and/or redundancy of the valve leaflets may be at increased risk for bacterial endocarditis, particularly men who are 45 years of age or older.
From: Dajani AS, et al.: Prevention of bacterial endocarditis. Recommendations by the American Heart Association. JAMA, *264(22)*:2920, 1990. Copyright 1990, American Medical Association.

to use: Ampicillin/sulbactam (2 g q 4 h) plus gentamicin (1.3–2 mg/kg q 8 h). Penicillin is the second choice and an alternative to ampicillin/sulbactam, provided the SBE is present for <3 months. The dose interval of aminoglycosides must be increased in patients > age 65 or in individuals with renal impairment, and titrated to blood levels to avoid renal and ototoxicity. A predose level (trough) >2 μg/ml (2 mg/l) reflects decreased excretion rate and accumulation of the drug: extend the dosing interval. Keep predose level 1–2 μg/ml. Peak level 30 min post infusion 6–10 μg/ml, depending on sensitivities and type of organism.

Acute Endocarditis. Acute presentation requires coverage for S. aureus, which causes >85% of ABE and ≤50% occurring on valves not known to be abnormal, especially bicuspid aortic valves: cloxacillin (2 g IV q 4 h for 4–6 weeks) or nafcillin (2 g IV q 4 h for 4–6 weeks) or flucloxacillin (2 g IV q 4 h).

Prosthetic Valve Endocarditis. Infective endocarditis occurs in approximately 3% of patients within the first year of surgery and thereafter in about 1%/year. The incidence is highest in the first 2 months, and the most common organisms at that stage are S. epidermidis (in 25–30%) and S. aureus (in 20–25% of cases). S. epidermidis continues to be an important organism during the ensuing years but with a ↓ incidence. Within the first 2 months, gram-negative organisms, fungi, diptheroids, and enterococci are infecting organisms. S. epidermidis is nearly always methicillin resistant, and the use of vancomycin is necessary.

Dosage: Vancomycin 15 mg/kg IV q 12 h in combination with gentamicin 1–1.2 mg/kg IV q 8 h; the addition of rifampin 300 mg po q 8 h may cause a modest improvement in the cure rate but increases the incidence of toxicity.

Late prosthetic valve endocarditis should be treated in a similar method, as outlined, pending results of culture and sensitivities since the

Table 10–3
Prevention of Bacterial Endocarditis–Dental or Surgical Procedures*

Endocarditis prophylaxis recommended
- Dental procedures known to induce gingival or mucosal bleeding, including professional cleaning
- Tonsillectomy and/or adenoidectomy
- Surgical operations that involve intestinal or respiratory mucosa
- Bronchoscopy with a rigid bronchoscope
- Sclerotherapy for esophageal varices
- Esophageal dilatation
- Gallbladder surgery
- Cystoscopy
- Urethral dilatation
- Urethral catheterization if urinary tract infection is present†
- Urinary tract surgery if urinary tract infection is present†
- Prostatic surgery
- Incision and drainage of infected tissue†
- Vaginal hysterectomy
- Vaginal delivery in the presence of infection†

Endocarditis prophylaxis not recommended‡
- Dental procedures not likely to induce gingival bleeding, such as simple adjustment of orthodontic appliances or fillings above the gum line
- Injection of local intraoral anesthetic (except intraligamentary injections)
- Shedding of primary teeth
- Tympanostomy tube insertion
- Endotracheal intubation
- Bronchoscopy with a flexible bronchoscope, with or without biopsy
- Cardiac catheterization
- Endoscopy with or without gastrointestinal biopsy
- Cesarean section
- In the absence of infection for urethral catheterization, dilatation and curettage, uncomplicated vaginal delivery, therapeutic abortion, sterilization procedures, or insertion or removal of intrauterine devices

* This table lists selected procedures but is not meant to be all-inclusive.
† In addition to prophylactic regimen for genitourinary procedures, antibiotic therapy should be directed against the most likely bacterial pathogen.
‡ In patients who have prosthetic heart valves, a previous history of endocarditis, or surgically constructed systemic-pulmonary shunts or conduits, physicians may choose to administer prophylactic antibiotics even for low-risk procedures that involve the lower respiratory, genitourinary, or gastrointestinal tracts.
From: Dajani AS, et al.: Prevention of bacterial endocarditis. Recommendations by the American Heart Association. JAMA, *264(22)*:2920, 1990. Copyright 1990, American Medical Association.

offending organism is usually S. viridans, fecal streptococci, S. aureus, S. epidermidis.

Right-Sided Endocarditis is most common in IV drug addicts and may present with a pneumonic illness. Infecting organisms include: S. aureus (60%), S. epidermidis (10%), and Pseudomonas and Serratia (10%).

ORGANISM ISOLATED AND SENSITIVITIES DETERMINED

Once the microorganism has been isolated and antibiotic sensitivities are available, an appropriate antibiotic combination is selected. Organisms that commonly cause endocarditis and appropriate antibiotic combinations include the following

- S. viridans or S. bovis: If the MIC to penicillin is <0.1 mg/l, give: penicillin (IV 2 million U q 4 h for 2 weeks), then amoxicillin (po 500 mg q 6 h for 2 weeks) or ampicillin/sulbactam (2 g q 6 h for 2 weeks IV), then amoxicillin (po 500 mg q 6 h for 2 weeks)
- Partially sensitive S. viridans or S. bovis, MIC penicillin >0.1 mg/l: penicillin (3 million U q 4 h IV) plus gentamicin (1.3–2 mg/kg q 8 h IV for 2–4 weeks) or, from the third week, amoxicillin (500 mg po q 6 h for 2 weeks)
- S. fecalis, S. fecium, S. durans, or similar fecal streptococci are difficult to eradicate: If the length of illness is <3 months, give ampicillin/sulbactam (IV 2–3 g q 6 h for 4 weeks) plus gentamicin (1.3–2 mg/kg q 8 h) and monitor levels and adjustment for renal function. Gentamicin is given for 4 weeks. The combinations of ampicillin or penicillin

Table 10–4
Recommended Standard Prophylactic Regimen for Dental, Oral, or Upper Respiratory Tract Procedures in Patients Who Are At Risk*

DRUG	DOSING REGIMEN†
Standard regimen	
Amoxicillin	3.0 g orally 1 hour before procedure; then 1.5 g 6 hours after initial dose
Amoxicillin/penicillin-allergic patients	
Erythromycin	Erythromycin ethylsuccinate, 800 mg, or erythromycin stearate, 1.0 g orally 2 hours before procedure; then half the dose 6 hours after initial dose
or	
Clindamycin	300 mg orally 1 hour before procedure and 150 mg 6 hours after initial dose

* Includes those with prosthetic heart valves and other high-risk patients.
† Initial pediatric doses are as follows: amoxicillin, 50 mg/kg; erythromycin ethylsuccinate or erythromycin stearate, 20 mg/kg; and clindamycin, 10 mg/kg. Follow-up dose should be one half the initial dose. **Total pediatric dose should not exceed total adult dose.** The following weight ranges may also be used for the initial pediatric dose of amoxicillin: <15 kg, 750 mg; 15–30 kg, 1,500 mg; and >30 kg, 3,000 mg (full adult dose).
From: Dajani AS, et al.: Prevention of bacterial endocarditis. Recommendations by the American Heart Association. JAMA, *264(22)*:2920, 1990. Copyright 1990, American Medical Association.

and the β-lactamase inhibitor sulbactam have been shown to be the most active antimicrobials tested against gentamicin-resistant β-lactamase-producing S. fecalis

- S. aureus: Methicillin-sensitive strains constitute most cases of S. aureus endocarditis and are treated with nafcillin or cloxacillin (at doses given above) or flucloxacillin (IV 2 g q 4 h) plus gentamicin (1.3–2 mg/kg q 8 h IV), the dose to be monitored by levels. The dose is reduced in elderly patients and those with renal dysfunction, while the dosing interval is increased. Gentamicin is discontinued after 1 week, and nafcillin or flucloxacillin IV is continued for 3–4 weeks. The length of treatment is usually 4–6 weeks
- S. pneumoniae is highly sensitive to penicillin and is managed with penicillin G (2 million U q 4 h) for 2 or more weeks

For patients allergic to penicillin or methicillin-resistant S. aureus, give: vancomycin (15 mg/kg IV q 12 h given slowly over 6 h) for 4–6 weeks.

Table 10–5
Alternate Prophylactic Regimens for Dental, Oral, or Upper Respiratory Tract Procedures in Patients Who Are At Risk

DRUG	DOSING REGIMEN†
Patients unable to take oral medications	
Ampicillin	Intravenous or intramuscular administration of ampicillin, 2.0 g, 30 minutes before procedure; then intravenous or intramuscular administration of ampicillin, 1.0 g, *or* oral administration of amoxicillin, 1.5 g, 6 hours after initial dose
Ampicillin/amoxicillin/penicillin-allergic patients unable to take oral medications	
Clindamycin	Intravenous administration of clindamycin, 300 mg, 30 minutes before procedure and intravenous or oral administration of 150 mg 6 hours after initial dose
Patients considered high risk and not candidates for standard regimen	
Ampicillin, gentamicin, and amoxicillin	Intravenous or intramuscular administration of ampicillin, 2.0 g, plus gentamicin, 1.5 mg/kg (not to exceed 80 mg), 30 minutes before procedure; followed by amoxicillin, 1.5 g orally 6 hours after initial dose; alternatively, the parenteral regimen may be repeated 8 hours after initial dose
Ampicillin/amoxicillin/penicillin-allergic patients considered high risk	
Vancomycin	Intravenous administration of 1.0 g over 1 hour, starting 1 hour before procedure; no repeated dose necessary

* Initial pediatric doses are as follows: ampicillin, 50 mg/kg; clindamycin, 10 mg/kg; gentamicin, 2.0 mg/kg; and vancomycin, 20 mg/kg. Follow-up dose should be one half the initial dose. **Total pediatric dose should not exceed total adult dose.** No initial dose is recommended in this table for amoxicillin (25 mg/kg is the follow-up dose).

From: Dajani AS, et al.: Prevention of bacterial endocarditis. Recommendations by the American Heart Association. JAMA, *264(22)*:2921, 1990.

Monitor serum levels, peak 20–40 μg/ml 2 h post completion of infusion, trough levels 5–10 μg/ml. Reduce dose and ↑ the dosing interval in renal failure.

BACTERIAL ENDOCARDITIS PROPHYLAXIS

Recommendations from the AHA on the antibiotic prophylaxis of endocarditis are given in Tables 10–3 through 10–6. Recommendations from the Endocarditis Working Party of the British Society for Antimicrobial Chemotherapy are indicated in Table 10–7.

The recent changes include the following relevant points

- The AHA has adopted the British 1984 recommendation to replace penicillin with amoxicillin for dental procedures: amoxicillin 3 g po is given 1 h prior to dental procedures, including professional cleaning, then 1.5 g 6 h later
- Patients allergic to penicillin who can take oral medications are given the choice of erythromycin or clindamycin, 300 mg 1 h prior and 150 mg 6 h post procedure. This is a major improvement in prophylaxis, since erythromycin (at 800 mg as advised by the AHA or 1500 mg by the British group) causes severe nausea and/or abdominal discomfort. Also, the drug is not extremely effective for fecal streptococci

Table 10–6
Prevention of Bacterial Endocarditis–Regimens for Genitourinary/Gastrointestinal Procedures

DRUG	DOSING REGIMEN*
Standard regimen	
Ampicillin, gentamicin, and amoxicillin	Intravenous or intramuscular administration of ampicillin, 2.0 g, plus gentamicin, 1.5 mg/kg (not to exceed 80 mg), 30 minutes before procedure; followed by amoxicillin, 1.5 g orally 6 hours after initial dose; alternatively, the parenteral regiment may be repeated once 8 hours after initial dose
Ampicillin/amoxicillin/penicillin-allergic patient regimen	
Vancomycin and gentamicin	Intravenous administration of vancomycin, 1.0 g, over 1 hour plus intravenous or intramuscular administration of gentamicin, 1.5 mg/kg (not to exceed 80 mg), 1 hour before procedure; may be repeated once 8 hours after initial dose
Alternate low-risk patient regimen	
Amoxicillin	3.0 g orally 1 hour before procedure; then 1.5 g 6 hours after initial dose

* Initial pediatric doses are as follows: ampicillin, 50 mg/kg; amoxicillin, 50 mg/kg; gentamicin, 2.0 mg/kg; and vancomycin, 20 mg/kg. Follow-up dose should be one half the initial dose. **Total pediatric dose should not exceed total adult dose.**
From: Dajani AS, et al.: Prevention of bacterial endocarditis. Recommendations by the American Heart Association. JAMA, *264(22)*:2921, 1990. Copyright 1990, American Medical Association.

Table 10-7
Recommendations for Endocarditis Prophylaxis in the UK

(1) *Dental Extractions, Scaling, or Periodontal Surgery Under Local or No Anesthesia*

(a) For patients not allergic to penicillin and not prescribed penicillin more than once in the previous month:

Amoxycillin

Adults: 3 g single oral dose taken under supervision 1 hour before dental procedure
Children under 10: half adult dose
Children under 5: quarter adult dose

(b) For patients allergic to penicillin:

Erythromycin stearate

Adults: 1.5 g orally taken under supervision 1–2 hours before dental procedure plus 0.5 g 6 hours later
Children under 10: half adult dose
Children under 5: quarter adult dose

or

Clindamycin

Adults: 600 mg single oral dose taken under supervision 1 hour before dental procedure
Children under 10: 6 mg/kg body weight single oral dose taken under supervision 1 hour before dental procedure

Under general anesthesia

(c) For patients not allergic to penicillin and not given penicillin more than once in the previous month:

Amoxycillin intramuscularly

Adults: 1 g in 2.5 ml 1% lignocaine hydrochloride just before induction plus 0.5 by mouth 6 hours later
Children under 10: half adult dose

or

Amoxycillin orally

Adults 3 g oral dose 4 hours before anesthesia followed by a further 3 g by mouth as soon as possible after operation
Children under 10: half adult dose
Children under 5: quarter adult dose

or

Amoxycillin and probenecid orally

Adults: amoxycillin 3 g together with probenecid 1 g orally 4 hours before operation

Special risk patients who should be referred to hospital:

(i) Patients with prosthetic valves who are to have a general anesthetic
(ii) Patients who are to have a general anesthetic *and* who are allergic to penicillin or have had penicillin more than once in the previous month
(iii) Patients who have had a previous attack of endocarditis

Recommendations for these patients are:

(d) For patients not allergic to penicillin and who have not had penicillin more than once in the previous month:

Adults: 1 g amoxycillin intramuscularly in 2.5 ml 1% lignocaine hydrochloride *plus* 120 mg gentamicin intramuscularly just before induction: then 0.5 g amoxycillin orally 6 h later
Children under 10: amoxycillin, half adult dose; gentamicin 2 mg/kg body weight

(continued)

Table 10-7 *(continued)*

(e) For patients allergic to penicillin or who have had penicillin more than once in the previous month:
Adults: vancomycin 1 g by slow intravenous infusion over 60 min followed by gentamicin 120 mg intravenously just before induction or 15 min before the surgical procedure
Children under 10: vancomycin 20 mg/kg intravenously, gentamicin 2 mg/kg intravenously

(2) *Surgery or Instrumentation of Upper Respiratory Tract*
Recommended cover is as for 1*(a)* or 1*(e)*, but any postoperative antibiotic may have to be given intramuscularly or intravenously if swallowing is painful.

(3) *Genitourinary Surgery or Instrumentation*
For patients with sterile urine the suggested cover is directed against fecal streptococci and is as for 1*(d)* or 1*(e)* above. If the urine is infected prophylaxis should also cover the pathogens involved.

(4) *Obstetric and Gynecological Procedures*
Cover is suggested only for patients with prosthetic valves, and is as for 1*(d)* or 1*(e)* because of the risk from fecal streptococci

(5) *Gastrointestinal Procedures*
Cover is suggested only for patients with prosthetic valves and is as for 1 *(d)* or 1 *(e)*.

From: Simmons, NA et al.: Antibiotic prophylaxis of infective endocarditis. Recommendations from the Endocarditis Working Party of the British Society for Antimicrobial Chemotherapy. Lancet, *335*:89, 1990.

- Prophylaxis for mitral valve prolapse has caused confusion over the past 10 years. The AHA advises prophylaxis only for individuals with MR, i.e., presence of a mid to late or holosystolic murmur

Suggested Reading

Dajani AS, et al.: Prevention of bacterial endocarditis. Recommendations by the American Heart Association. JAMA *264*(22): 2920, 1990. Copyright 1990, American Medical Association.

Khan M Gabriel: Infective endocarditis. *In* Cardiac and Pulmonary Management. Philadelphia, Lea & Febiger, 1993.

Deep Venous Thrombosis

11

M. Gabriel Khan

DVT occurring in the lower limbs is often impossible to diagnose from the history and physical examination. Some patients present with pain and swelling of the calf or thigh; others are asymptomatic. The venous occlusion causes chronic passive congestion, and the muscle tissue becomes swollen with edema; a variable inflammatory response and perivascular hemorrhage may occur.

Differential diagnosis includes muscle tear, muscle cramps, ruptured Baker's cyst, external compression cellulitis without lymphangitis, and postphlebitic syndrome. The presence of risk factors lends strong support to the diagnosis: e.g., previous DVT, soft-tissue injury, the postoperative state, pregnancy, post partum, sudden immobilization for >3 days, fractured lower limb, obesity, oral contraceptives, estrogens, underlying malignancies, CHF, dehydration. Inciting factors are: venous stasis, endothelial injury, and hypercoagulability.

Because pulmonary embolism occurs commonly in patients with thrombosis of the femoral and iliac veins, this situation is considered serious and life threatening. Below-the-knee DVT that fails to extend above the knee rarely embolizes. It must be emphasized, however, that the incidence of postphlebitic syndrome is 30–40% with calf vein thrombosis.

INVESTIGATIONS

- Venography is the investigation of choice for DVT
- Impedance plethysmography (IPG) detects thrombosis above the knee. Because only approximately 30% of acute calf vein thrombi later extend above the knee, a first negative IPG would reveal the extension later if the test was repeated on day 2, days 5–7, and if needed, on days 10–14. If the IPG becomes positive, anticoagulation is commenced. Trials have shown this method to be effective, especially because extension above the knee is uncommon after day 7. In clinical practice, however, it is often difficult to arrange such tests for patients, except in specialized centers. Extension of thrombosis may occur and go unnoticed prior to the second or third IPG testing. IPG cannot distinguish old from fresh thrombi. Also, false positive results occur with CHF, compression by pelvic tumor, or a gravid uterus. Thus, loopholes exist that may allow medicolegal action. The IPG method of managing DVT is suited to some teaching hospitals
- Duplex scanning: Real-time B mode Doppler ultrasound imaging carried out by experienced staff is useful in detecting above-knee thrombosis, but an incomplete venous obstruction may not be detected

Table 11–1
Continuous Infusion Heparin

RATE (ml/hr)	UNITS (/hr)	UNITS (/24 hrs)
1. 21	840	20,160
2. 25	1000	24,000
3. 28	1120	26,880
4. 30	1200	28,800
5. 32	1280	30,720
6. 34	1360	32,640
7. 36	1440	34,560
8. 38	1520	36,480
9. 40	1600	38,400
10. 42	1680	40,320
11. 44	1760	42,240
12. 46	1840	44,160
13. 48	1920	46,080
14. 50	2000	48,000

20,000 units of heparin in 500 ml of 5% dextrose in water. If noncardiac, dilute in 0.9% saline. 1 ml equals 40 units.
* For each heparin order, specify both the rate of flow and the dose in units per hour.
Begin with No. 4, 1200 units/hr and adjust to maintain activated PTT at 1.5 to 2.5 times control value (usual therapeutic range 60 to 85 seconds; see text for the use of a nomogram).

THERAPY

After verifying a normal prothrombin time (PT) or INR, activated PTT, and platelets, commence the following.

Heparin

Dosage: IV bolus 100 U/kg, usually 5,000–7,500 U, then a continuous infusion of 15–25 U/kg/h (set up as suggested in Table 11–1). In practice, it is convenient to add 20,000 U of heparin to 1 liter of 0.9% saline or 5% dextrose water for cardiac patients. This diluted solution of heparin (20 U/ml) is safer for general use than a 40- to 50-U/ml solution, which can cause life-threatening hemorrhage if the infusion pump becomes defective and heparin is infused inadvertently. However, a 40 U/ml solution is commonly used. The physician should specify the rate of flow (e.g., 30 ml/h) and the dose (1,200 U/h) (Table 11–1). Commence the infusion at 1,200 U/h. Check the PTT 6 h after the bolus injection, and then ↑ or ↓ the infusion to maintain the activated PTT 1.5–2.5 times the mean control range that corresponds to a plasma heparin level of 0.2–0.4 U/ml (max 0.5 U/ml by protamine titration). The U.S. pharmaceutical units may be approximately 12% more potent than the international units used elsewhere. If either massive DVT or thromboembolism is suspected, the PTT should be determined 1 h after the bolus dose. If the PTT is near the control value, another bolus of heparin should be administered, because these patients may have a more rapid heparin clearance.

Curickshank, et al. have devised a standard heparin nomogram for the adjustment of IV heparin dosage. After a 5,000-U bolus, their advice is as follows

- Commence with IV heparin infusion 32 ml/h, 1,280 U/h (No. 5, Table 11–1)
- If the 6-hour PTT is 50–59, ↑ the rate 3 ml/h and repeat the PTT in 6 h
- If the PTT is 60–85, no change in rate, repeat the PTT next morning
- If the PTT is 86–95, ↓ the rate 2 ml/h, repeat PTT the next morning
- If the PTT is 96–120, hold the infusion for 30 min, ↓ the rate 2 ml/h, repeat the PTT in 6 h
- If the PTT is >120, hold the IV for 60 min, ↓ the rate 4 ml/h, and repeat the PTT in 6 h
- If during the first 48 h of therapy the PTT is subtherapeutic, <50 despite a heparin dose of 1,440 U/h or greater, administer a heparin bolus of 5,000 U and ↑ the rate 5 ml/h

At 24–48 h after the start of heparin therapy, a therapeutic PTT was achieved in 66 and 81%, versus 37 and 58% in a heparin control group. The nomogram has proven useful. A specific thromboplastin (Actin FS) was used to devise the nomogram, which could be adapted to other reagents; it is necessary to compare either the test reagents and the Actin FS reagent or the test reagent and the heparin assay.

When the PTT is in the desired range, monitor PTT once daily. The platelet count should be evaluated after the third day of heparin therapy.

Action: The anticoagulant activity of heparin requires a cofactor, antithrombin III. Heparin binds to lysine sites on antithrombin III and converts the cofactor from a slow inhibitor to a very rapid inhibitor of thrombin. The heparin-antithrombin III complex inactivates thrombin and factor X, as well as a number of coagulation enzymes. The principal anticoagulant effect of heparin-antithrombin III appears to be caused by inhibition of thrombin-induced activation of factor V and factor VIII. Almost 20 times more heparin is required to initiate fibrin-bound thrombin than to inactivate free thrombin. Thus, the prevention of the extension of venous thrombosis requires much higher concentrations of heparin than the prevention of thrombus formation.

Heparin inhibits some aspects of platelet function and increases the permeability of vessel walls. Heparin is poorly absorbed from the gut and must be given parenterally. Heparin bound to endothelial cells is internalized and depolymerized, and desulfation occurs in mononuclear phagocytes. The elimination route of heparin remains uncertain. The agent has an apparent half-life of approximately 30 and 60 min after a 25- and 75-U/kg IV bolus, respectively.

It is advisable to continue to treat patients with heparin IV if immobilization or precipitating factors persist. For below-the-knee DVT, 14 days of SQ calcium heparin appears to cause greater resolution of thrombosis compared to continuous heparin and deserves consideration. Calcium heparin, 250 U/kg SQ bid and adjusted to maintain PTT 1.5–2 times the control, has a role in below-the-knee DVT.

Adverse Effects: Thrombocytopenia caused by heparin occurs in ≤4% of patients. It is believed to be the result of immune sensitization to a heparin-platelet complex. This complication is associated with life-threatening arterial or venous thrombosis. Platelet counts should be assessed in patients administered heparin IV for a period >3 days. Osteoporosis may occur after 5 months of therapy. Alopecia is a rare adverse effect.

Interactions: High-dose IV nitroglycerin may ↑ the required dose of heparin possibly because of an alteration in the antithrombin III molecule.

Contraindications: Hemophilia and other hemorrhagic disorders; peptic ulceration, severe uncontrolled hypertension, severe hepatic disease, cerebral aneurysm, recent ophthalmic surgery, and pregnancy.

Oral Anticoagulants

Coumarins induce anticoagulation by inhibiting vitamin K epoxide reductase, which causes an accumulation of hepatic and circulating vitamin K epoxide and a depletion of vitamin KH_2, limiting the carboxylation and biologic function of vitamin-K-dependent coagulant proteins (prothrombin, factors VII, IX, and X) and anticoagulant proteins (protein C and protein S).

Warfarin, a 4-hydroxycoumarin compound, has some anticoagulant effect within 12–24 h, but peak activity is approximately 72 h, because it takes time to impair the biologic function of coagulant protein and to clear circulating clotting factors.

Because the half-life of factor VII is about 6-1/2 h and that of II, IX, and X is several days, peak warfarin effect is delayed (72–96 h). Importantly, protein C has a half-life as short as factor VII, and with depletion during the first 24–48 h of anticoagulant therapy, there is a theoretically heightened risk of thrombosis in the first 12 h of therapy. Therefore, for optimal salutary effects, heparin must be administered for 12 h before giving warfarin.

Because protein C has a short half-life, a 5-day overlap of IV heparin and warfarin is necessary to prevent a potentially thrombogenic effect, which can be caused by low levels of protein C during the period when the levels of factors II and X are normal (during the first 4 days of warfarin therapy).

Adverse Effects: Bleeding is common with a prothrombin ratio >2 or INR >3.5; if the INR is <3 with an ISI of 2.3, search for an underlying cause of bleeding. The risk of bleeding is increased in patients > age 65 and those who have occult GI lesions, renal failure, anemia from other causes, a history of cerebral vascular disease, ingestion of aspirin or NSAIDs. Rarely, skin necrosis occurs due to extensive thrombosis of capillaries and venules in SQ tissue. The pathogenesis of this unusual complication, which occurs between the third and seventh day of therapy, is undetermined but appears to be linked to the ↓ in biologic activity of protein C caused by coumarins.

Contraindications: Peptic ulcer or recent GI bleeding, pregnancy, severe and controlled hypertension, bacterial endocarditis.

Monitoring of oral anticoagulant effect: Measurement of the INR is recommended by the WHO and has become established in the UK and Europe, but has been adopted by only a minority of hospitals and laboratories in North America, where most physicians have used a PT ratio of 1.5–2.0 since the early 1970s and more recently 1.4–1.7, with further changes in the thromboplastins used. Physicians who have inadvertently continued to use the 1948 AHA guideline prothrombin ratio of 2.0–2.5 have noted an increased incidence of bleeding.

The laboratory-determined INR is the PT ratio that reflects the result that would have been obtained if the WHO reference thromboplastin had been used to perform the test in that laboratory.

$$\text{INR} = \frac{(\text{patient PT}}{\text{control PT})^{\text{ISI}}}$$

The INR is based, therefore, on 2 contributing factors: the PT ratio and the ISI. The ISI is a measure of the responsiveness of a given thromboplastin to ↓ in the vitamin-K-dependent coagulation factors. All reagent manufacturers should provide the laboratory with the ISI value.

Table 11–2
Suggested Therapeutic Range of INR and Corresponding Prothrombin Time Ratio for Anticoagulation

CLINICAL SITUATION	PROTHROMBIN TIME RATIO	INR	ISI
Deep venous thrombosis	1.4–1.7	2–3	2.0
	1.4–1.6	2–3	2.3
	1.3–1.5	2–3	2.6
Atrial fibrillation	1.4–1.6	2–3	As above
Prosthetic heart valves:			
mechanical	1.5–1.9	2.6–3.6	2.0*
tissue	1.4–1.5	2–2.3	

INR = International Normalized Ratio
ISI = International Sensitivity Index
* The laboratory should state the ISI of the thromboplastin used. (see Table 11–3, INR nomogram)

Rabbit-brain thromboplastins have an ISI of 2.0–2.6, and the INR should be determined with the consistent use of sensitive thromboplastins with similar ISI values. An INR of 2–3, the desired range of anticoagulation for the majority of clinical situations, utilizing a thromboplastin with an ISI of 2.3, gives a corresponding PT of 1.4–1.6. This is considered a moderate-intensity regimen that is adequate for the treatment of DVT. The suggested range of INR and the PT ratio for the management of some clinical situations are shown in Table 11–2; also see Table 11–3: PT ratio, INR conversion chart, INR nomogram.

Table 11–3
INR Nomogram

PT ratio										
3.0	3.74	4.66								
2.9	3.59	4.44								
2.8	3.44	4.23	5.19							
2.7	3.29	4.02	4.90							
2.6	3.15	3.81	4.61							
2.5	*3.00**	3.61	4.33	5.20						
2.4	*2.86*	3.41	4.06	4.83						
2.3	*2.72*	3.21	3.79	4.48	5.29					
2.2	*2.58*	3.02	3.53	4.13	4.84					
2.1	*2.44*	*2.82*	3.28	3.80	4.41	5.16				
2.0	*2.30*	*2.64*	3.03	3.48	4.00	4.59	5.28			
1.9	*2.16*	*2.26*	*2.79*	3.18	3.61	4.10	4.67	5.31		
1.8	*2.02*	*2.28*	*2.56*	*2.88*	*3.24*	3.64	4.10	4.61	5.19	5.83
1.7	1.89	*2.10*	*2.34*	*2.60*	*2.89*	3.21	3.57	3.97	4.42	4.91
1.6	1.76	1.93	*2.12*	*2.33*	*2.56*	*2.81*	3.09	3.39	3.73	4.10
1.5	1.63	1.76	1.91	*2.07*	*2.25*	*2.44*	*2.65*	*2.87*	3.11	3.38
1.4	1.50	1.60	1.71	1.83	1.96	*2.10*	*2.24*	*2.40*	*2.57*	*2.74*
1.3†	→1.37	→1.44	→1.52	→1.60	→1.69	→**1.78**	1.88	1.98	*2.08*	*2.20*
1.2	1.24	1.29	1.34	1.39	1.44	↑1.49	1.55	1.61	1.67	1.73
1.1	1.12	1.14	1.16	1.19	1.21	↑1.23	1.26	1.28	1.31	1.33
	1.2	1.4	1.6	1.8	2.0	↑**2.2**	2.4	2.6	2.8	3.0

Range of ISI values for most commercial thromboplastins (bracketed: 1.4–2.2)

* Italic numbers = Most Common INR Values
The nomogram is used to determine the INR from observed prothrombin ratio.
† Bold = Example (arrows): An observed ratio of 1.3 with thromboplastin of ISI 2.2 equals an INR of 1.78.
Adapted from: Leclerc J: Venous Thromboembolic Disorders. Philadelphia, Lea & Febiger, 1990.

Warfarin for Deep Venous Thrombosis. DVT that extends to the mid thigh but is noniliofemoral, occurring in patients where the precipitating factors are removed and early mobilization is attained, can be treated with early administration of oral anticoagulants. Warfarin is begun on the second night following the commencement of heparin, by which time the therapeutic level of heparin has been well maintained for >24 h and the diagnosis already established by venography at this stage. Because warfarin may take 24–96 h to achieve anticoagulation and the biologic activity of protein C is markedly limited within the first 24 h of warfarin therapy, resulting in an enhanced early thrombogenic state, Hull and Raskob advise that heparin and warfarin be overlapped for 5 days to prevent the potentially thrombogenic effect caused by the presence of nearly normal levels of factors II and X during the first 3 or 4 days of warfarin therapy. A similar duration of heparin therapy is obtained if an order is written to discontinue IV heparin when the PT or INR is in the therapeutic range for 2 full days.

Warfarin *Dosage:* 10 mg qd for 2 days, the third and daily dose is titrated to maintain the INR (2–3) or PT ratio (1.4–1.6, PT 1.4–1.6 times the control). The PT is often 16–19 seconds when the control PT is 12 seconds.

When the prothrombin time ratio or INR is in the desired range, overlap heparin for an additional 2 full days. Thus, heparin is given for a total of 5–6 days. With this method of heparin/warfarin therapy, the patient is usually ready to be discharged on the sixth day. A recent study has indicated that 9–10 days of heparin therapy is not superior to 5 days of heparin with overlapping warfarin in patients with submassive venous thrombosis. The short course of heparin reduces the length of hospital stay and is an important patient cost consideration but is not recommended for iliac vein thrombosis or major pulmonary embolism.

The warfarin dose should be given at bedtime; this allows the physician or nurse to alter the dose based on the result of the prothrombin time ratio or INR obtained during the day.

For iliofemoral thrombosis or major pulmonary embolus, warfarin is commenced on the fifth night of heparin therapy, which with 5 days overlap results in 10 days of heparin therapy. Warfarin is usually continued for 3 months, and the prothrombin time ratio is maintained in the range of 1.5–1.75 (INR = 2–3.2). Patients with isolated calf DVT are treated for 3 months, and the prothrombin time ratio is maintained at 1.4–1.5 (INR = 2–3). Patients presenting with a second DVT are treated for 1 year. Patients with recurrent DVT and underlying risk factors are administered warfarin indefinitely. Patients with a stable anticoagulant response should be maintained with an estimation of INR or PT every 4 weeks. Drugs that may ↑ or ↓ anticoagulant activity are listed in Table 11–4.

Thrombolytic Therapy

Acute massive pulmonary embolism and iliac or iliofemoral vein thrombosis, the latter of <14 days duration, should be managed with thrombolytic therapy to prevent a 60–70% incidence of postphlebitic syndrome and/or pulmonary embolism.

Streptokinase *Dosage:* Loading dose, 250,000 U IV over 30 min, maintenance infusion 100,000 U/h for 48–72 h in patients with iliofemoral vein thrombosis. In patients with pulmonary embolism, the infusion is continued 12–24 h. Following the infusion, the PTT should be main-

Table 11–4
Oral Anticoagulants–Drug Interactions

1. **Drugs that may enhance anticoagulant responses**
   - Alcohol
   - Alopurinol
   - Aminoglycosides
   - Amiodarone
   - Ampicillin
   - Anabolic steroids
   - Aspirin
   - Cephalosporins
   - Chloral hydrate
   - Chloramphenicol
   - Chlorpromazine
   - Chlorpropamide
   - Chlortetracycline
   - Cimetidine
   - Ciprofloxacin
   - Clofibrate (fibrates)
   - Co-trimoxazole
   - Danazol
   - Dextrothyroxine
   - Diazoxide
   - Dipyridamole
   - Disulfiram
   - Erythromycin
   - Ethacrynic acid
   - Fenclofenac
   - Fenoprofen
   - Flufenamic acid
   - Fluvoxamine
   - Liquid paraffin
   - Mefenamic acid
   - Methotrexate
   - Metronidazole
   - Monoamine oxidase inhibitors
   - Nalidixic acid
   - Naproxen
   - Neomycin
   - Penicillin (large doses IV)
   - Phenformin
   - Phenylbutazone
   - Phenytoin
   - Propylthiouracil
   - Propafenone
   - Quinidine
   - Sulfinpyrazone
   - Sulfonamides
   - Tetracyclines
   - Tolbutamide
   - Tricyclic antidepressants
   - Verapamil
2. **Drugs that may decrease anticoagulant response**
   - Antacids
   - Antihistamines
   - Barbiturates
   - Carbamazepine
   - Cholestyramine
   - Colestipol
   - Corticosteroids
   - Cyclophosphamide
   - Dichloralphenazone
   - Disopyramide
   - Glutethimide
   - Griseofulvin
   - Mercaptopurine
   - Oral contraceptives
   - Pheneturide
   - Phenobarbitone
   - Primidone
   - Rifampicin
   - Vitamins K_1 and K_2

Modified from: Khan M Gabriel: Cardiac Drug Therapy. 3rd Ed. London, W.B. Saunders, 1992.

tained at 1.5–2 times the control with the use of heparin (Table 11–1). Contraindications for SK or thrombolytic therapy are given in Chapter 3.

Urokinase. Although it is more expensive than SK, urokinase is nonantigenic and IV therapy is given for a much shorter duration. *Dosage:* IV bolus of 4,000 IU/kg over 10 min and continuous infusion of 4,000 IU/kg/h. Noninvasive studies should show a response in 24 h. Continue the infusion as long as there is continued improvement. Discontinue the infusion if no improvement is observed in 24 h or if there is no clot resolution over a 24-hour period. tPA also works well in this condition (see Chap. 3 for dosage).

Suggested Reading

Curickshank MK, Levine MN, Hirsh J, et al.: A standard heparin nomogram for the management of heparin therapy. Arch Intern Med *51*: 333, 1991.

Gallus A, Jackaman J, Tillett J, et al.: Safety and efficacy of warfarin started early after submassive venous thrombosis or pulmonary embolism. Lancet *2*:1293, 1986. Hirsh J: Review article. Oral anticoagulant drugs. N Engl J Med *324*:1865, 1991.

Hull RD, Raskob GE, Rosenbloom D, et al.: Heparin for 5 days as compared with 10 days in the initial treatment of proximal venous thrombosis. N Engl J Med *322*:1260, 1990.

Hirsh J: Drug therapy: Heparin. N Engl J Med *324*:1565, 1991.

International Committee for Standardization in Haematology, International Committee on Thrombosis and Haemotosis: ICSH/ICTH recommendations for reporting prothrombin time in oral anticoagulant control. Thromb Haemot *53*:155, 1985.

Leclerc J: Venous Thromboembolic Disorders. Philadelphia, Lea & Febiger, 1990.

Hull R, Raskob G, Pineo G, et al: A comparison of cubcutaneous low-molecular-weight heparin with warfarin sodium for prophylaxis against deep-vein thrombosis after hip or knee implantation. N Engl J Med *329*:1370, 1993.

Valvular Heart Disease and Rheumatic Fever

12

M. Gabriel Khan

AORTIC STENOSIS

Diagnosis

- The causes of aortic stenosis and the average survival of patients are given in Tables 12–1 and 12–2
- Diagnosis < age 30 is typical of congenital aortic stenosis. In patients > age 70, calcific aortic sclerosis due to degenerative calcification is common, and significant stenosis develops in <5% of these individuals. A bicuspid valve occurs in 2–3% of the population, with a male-to-female ratio of 4:1 and is predisposed to degenerative calcification. Between age 30 and 70, calcification of a bicuspid valve is the most common cause of aortic stenosis, and, much less frequently, cases of rheumatic valvular disease are encountered

Physical signs of significant aortic stenosis include

- A systolic crescendo-decrescendo murmur best heard at the lower left sternal border, the second right interspace, or occasionally at the apex, with radiation to the neck
- The longer the murmur and the later the peak of the crescendo-decrescendo, the greater the gradient
- The intensity of the murmur, in the absence of significant aortic regurgitation, is usually Grade 3 or greater, except if cardiac output is low, as with CHF; then, even a Grade 2 murmur may be in keeping with severe stenosis. Aortic regurgitation increases flow across the aortic valve and may produce a loud systolic murmur without stenosis
- An absent or very soft aortic component of the second sound (A2)
- An S4 gallop is usually present and is highly significant in patients < age 50
- A thrill is commonly present over the base of the heart or the carotid arteries; this indicates a murmur of Grade 4 or louder and may relate to the severity of aortic stenosis if aortic regurgitation is absent
- A thrusting, forceful apex beat of LVH; the apex beat is usually not displaced, except in patients with concomitant aortic regurgitation or with terminal LV dilation
- The carotid or brachial pulse in patients < age 65 shows a typical delayed upstroke. In the elderly, loss of elasticity in arteries often masks this important sign

The ECG in patients with moderate to severe stenosis often shows features of LVH. Chest x ray usually shows a normal heart size, with some rounding of the left lower cardiac border and apex; occasionally some posterior protrusion in the lateral view may suggest LVH. The heart size may be increased if cardiac failure supervenes or with concomitant

Table 12–1
Causes of Aortic Valvular Stenosis

Biscuspid calcific	60%*
Degenerative calcific	15%
Rheumatic	20%*
Other	5%

* Reverse in Asia, Africa, Middle East, Latin America

aortic regurgitation. A common hallmark of valvular aortic stenosis is post-stenotic dilation of the ascending aorta.

Echocardiographic features of moderate to severe aortic stenosis are indicated by the following

- Doppler peak systolic pressure gradient >60 mm Hg in the presence of a normal cardiac output
- Maximal instantaneous Doppler gradient >60 mm Hg (range = 64–165 mm Hg)
- Peak systolic flow velocity >4 m/s (range often observed = 4–7 m/s)
- Valve mean gradient >40 mm Hg (range in several clinical studies = 40–120 mm Hg)
- Valve area < about 0.75 cm^2 in an average-sized adult, 0.4 cm^2/m^2 of body surface area, severe or critical stenosis (Table 12–3)

Valve area >1.5 cm^2 indicates mild aortic stenosis, 0.75–1.4 cm^2 indicates moderate stenosis.

Severe aortic stenosis. The echocardiographic findings usually indicate a valve area <0.7 cm^2 in an average-sized adult and Doppler peak systolic pressure gradient >60 mm Hg, with a maximal instantaneous gradient in the range of 64–145 mm Hg. If the cardiac output is low or the valve gradient appears inadequate to account for symptomatology, the valve area index should be calculated (Table 12–3).

Patients with LV failure or LV dysfunction require emergency surgery. Others require prompt surgery. During the waiting period, dental work under antibiotic coverage should be completed. The patient should be instructed concerning the risk and strictness of longterm anticoagulant regimen.

Diuretics are indicated if CHF is present and digoxin is used if systolic dysfunction is documented. CHF is not a contraindication to surgery.

Coronary angiography is necessary in patients > age 35 or in those with chest pain.

Moderate aortic stenosis. Patients who have a valve area of 0.75–1.4 cm^2 are usually categorized as having moderate aortic stenosis.

Table 12–2
Average Survival in Patients with Moderate or Severe Aortic Stenosis

CLINICAL PARAMETERS	SURVIVAL YEARS
Left ventricular failure	1.5 to 2
Severe shortness of breath	2
Mild shortness of breath	3 to 4
Syncope	3
Angina	4 to 5

Table 12–3
Hemodynamic Parameters for Severe Aortic Stenosis

	AORTIC VALVE AREA* (cm^2)	AORTIC VALVE AREA INDEX (cm^2/m^2)	PEAK SYSTOLIC GRADIENT (mm Hg)	MEAN GRADIENT (mm Hg)
Severe stenosis	<0.75	<0.4	≥80	≥70
Probable severe	0.75–0.9	0.4–0.6	50–79	40–69
Uncertain	>0.9 to 1.2	>0.6	<50	<40

* = In an average-sized adult

However, the situation in patients with valve area of 0.75–1 cm^2 is regarded by some as a "fool's paradise" (see Table 12–3). Some determine severe stenosis by valve area of ≤0.9 cm^2 and/or valve area index ≤0.6 cm^2/m^2. Patients who have moderate aortic stenosis, if minimally symptomatic, should be regarded as being at high risk for development of complications during the following 1–2 years, especially if the EF is <50% or if there is hemodynamic evidence of LV decompensation. In a study of 66 patients who had moderate aortic stenosis, 31% with minimal symptoms experienced serious complications within 4 years. Also, patients who have EF <50% at catheterization appear to have ≤64% chance of complications due to aortic stenosis over a 4-year period. The absence of severe symptoms does not ensure a favorable outcome. The elderly, mildly symptomatic patient with degenerative calcific aortic stenosis of a moderate degree is at high risk. Thus, if underlying diseases such as respiratory failure, stroke, renal failure, anemia, or cancer are not present, surgery is recommended.

Truly asymptomatic patients with moderate or severe aortic stenosis are not offered surgery but should be followed closely for a change in effort tolerance and breathlessness or other cardiac complications.

The patient should be advised to carry on with activities that are normal and to report any changes immediately.

Patients with a moderate degree of aortic stenosis should be considered at high risk if they are mildly symptomatic, especially if the EF is ↓ or there is hemodynamic evidence of LV decompensation.

Surgical Therapy

Mechanical obstruction to the LV outflow due to significant aortic stenosis is a pressure overload situation that leads to progressive LVH, LV strain, and finally CHF or sudden death. Symptoms due to obstruction of outflow are usually the main indications for valve replacement in patients with moderate or severe aortic stenosis (see Table 12–4). In most of these patients, the valve area is <1.0 cm^2 and the peak systolic gradient is >60 mm Hg. Fortunately, the hypertrophied myocardium often retains mechanical efficiency, and once the valve is replaced, significant improvement in ventricular systolic performance occurs in most patients. Thus, CHF is not a contraindication to valve replacement. Patients with LV failure due to severe aortic stenosis and followed for >1 year because of intercurrent illness contraindicating surgery usually regain adequate LV function with later valve replacement. Since mortality is >50% in 1 year in patients with CHF, surgery should be done promptly.

Table 12–4
Indications for Aortic Prosthetic Valve Surgery

PARAMETERS	INTERVENTION
Severe Aortic Stenosis	
Aortic Valve area <0.75 cm^2	
Valve area Index <0.4 cm^2/m^2	
Symptomatic patients	
a. Heart failure or dyspnea	Emergency surgery
b. LV dysfunction or EF <50%	Urgent surgery
c. Angina	Urgent surgery
d. Syncope	Urgent surgery (Within a few weeks)
Asymptomatic patients	
Valve area as above	No surgery
Hemodynamic deterioration	
a. Left ventricular dysfunction	Fairly urgent (Within a few months)
b. Ejection fraction <50%	
c. Cardiomegaly or LVH on: ECG or echocardiography	
Moderate Aortic Stenosis	
Valve area 0.75 to 1.3 cm^2	
Symptomatic	
Heart Failure	Urgent surgery
Other symptoms or LV dysfunction or EF <50% (Follow up monthly)	Fairly urgent (Within a few months)
Truly asymptomatic (Follow up at least every 2 months)	Surgery (1–5 years) (if becomes symptomatic)

Indications for valve replacement include

- LV failure
- Shortness of breath
- Angina
- Presyncope or syncope not due to preload-reducing agents or other causes of syncope (see Chap. 15)

Patients with chest pain or those > age 35 require coronary angiography to assess the degree of atheromatous coronary stenosis and suitability for CABS. Young patients with LAD disease should be offered left internal mammary artery to LAD anastomosis or graft; in patients > age 65, vein graft is appropriately recommended by the ACC and the AHA Task Force.

Contraindications to surgery include

- Serious underlying disease, especially respiratory failure, cancer, severe renal failure, cerebrovascular accident with residual stroke, and contraindication to anticoagulant therapy
- Age > 80 is a relative contraindication, except in patients with robust health and excellent cerebral status. Severe intercurrent illness should weigh heavily against surgery, except in patients with CHF due only to severe aortic stenosis with a valve area <0.75 cm^2. Because angina may require a combination of valve replacement and bypass surgery if there is coronary artery obstruction, care must be taken to individualize the selection. The patient and family must understand the risks

Prosthetic valve choice. Problems exist with all types of valve prostheses; none is ideal. Scientific studies have indicated a superiority of mechanical valves over bioprosthetic valves, especially in patients < age 30 or at all ages in the mitral position, and mechanical valves are the obvious choice in patients with AF in whom anticoagulation is already necessary (Table 12–5). Importantly, Collins points out that of 1,117 isolated mitral valve replacements done at Brigham and Women's Hospital since 1971, 620 (54%) had AF and a need for anticoagulation. Bloomfield reiterates that 60% of mitral valves currently implanted in patients in the United States are mechanical; in 1988, the UK Registry reported that 68% of mitral valves implanted were mechanical. The surgeon's background and personal preferences, however, often dictate the choice of valve, taking into consideration the patient's age and the possible presence of contraindications to anticoagulant therapy. In underdeveloped countries, a mechanical valve is still considered first choice because it is preferable to monitor anticoagulation than to run the risk of 2 operations in 20 years (reoperation carries a >10% mortality and is costly). In the aortic position, it is expected that the durability of the mechanical valve is superior over a 10- to 20-year period because of a high reoperation rate with the use of bioprosthetic valves. The major disadvantage of mechanical valves is the small risk of bleeding due to anticoagulant therapy, and this must be weighed against possible reoperation over 7–15 years with a bioprosthetic valve.

It is well established that reoperation is required much more frequently with bioprosthetic valves, but the complications of thromboembolism, endocarditis, and valve obstruction are similar. A bioprosthetic valve may be considered a reasonable choice in patients > age 70 whose life expectancy may be shorter than that of the bioprosthesis. In patients in whom anticoagulants are contraindicated or compliance is expected to be poor, a prosthetic valve is appropriate. In women who intend to become pregnant, a bioprosthetic valve is advisable but a mechanical valve with the use of heparin SQ for the first 4 months and during the last few weeks of pregnancy is an alternative.

Accelerated calcification of glutaraldehyde-treated bioprosthetic valves in patients < age 30 is of concern. However, cryopreserved tissue valves are being tested and appear to maintain tissue flexibility with considerably less tendency to calcify.

Table 12–5
Choice of Valve Prosthesis

CLINICAL PARAMETERS	MECHANICAL VALVE	BIOPROSTHESIS
Age <30	First choice	Not recommended
Anticoagulant necessary as in atrial fibrillation	Natural choice	Not recommended
Anticoagulant contraindicated	Not recommended	First choice
Aortic valve replacement		
age 30 to 70	First choice	Second choice
over age 70*, sinus rhythm	Second choice	First choice
Mitral (all ages)	First choice	May be considered in patients over age 70 in sinus rhythm

* Higher risk of bleeding with anticoagulants, and average life span 10 years

Table 12–6
Prosthetic Valve Complications

CLINICAL PARAMETERS	MECHANICAL VALVE %	BIOPROSTHETIC (%)
Reoperation		
Veterans Administration* (10 year)	6.6	12
Scottish Study** (12 year)	8.5	37
Major bleeding (12 year)	19	7
Perivalvular leak	4.5	2
Major embolism	8.8	9
Endocarditis	3.7	4.6
Survival rate (12 year)	51.5	44.4

Modified from: * J Am Coll Cardiol, *176(2)*:41A, 1991. ** N Engl J Med, *324*:573, 1991.

Two studies compared the mechanical valve with the bioprosthesis. The Veterans Administration study reported 10-year follow-up in 575 patients randomized between mechanical valve and bioprosthesis: reoperation for primary valve failure was necessary in 35 patients fitted with bioprostheses, compared to 19 patients with mechanical valves; repeat surgery was performed for perivalvular regurgitation in only 6 bioprosthetic versus 13 mechanical valves. There was a significantly higher incidence of bleeding due to anticoagulant therapy in patients with mechanical valves.

A 12-year comparison in Scotland of the Bjork-Shiley spherical disc valve with bioprosthesis in 261 mitral, 211 aortic, and 61 in both positions indicated no difference in reoperation or survival at 5 years. However, at 12 years, reoperation was necessary in 68 (37%) patients with bioprosthetic valve and 17 (8.5%) with mechanical valve. Porcine valve failure was usually due to rupture of 1 or more cusps, causing severe regurgitation, with a much greater risk in the mitral position. Importantly, 16 patients died as a result of reoperation for porcine valve replacement. Also, valve failure may cause death before further surgical intervention. Using death and reoperation as endpoints for an actuarial assessment of survival with the original prosthesis intact, the survival rate in patients with Bjork-Shiley prostheses was 48%, versus a 30% survival rate in patients 12 years after porcine valve replacement. This effect was significant for mitral valves but inconclusive for the aortic position.

As a result of the study, the Scottish group advises that a bioprosthesis appears to be contraindicated in the mitral position; replacement in young patients should be with a mechanical valve, but an aortic bioprosthesis has a role in patients > age 70 who are in sinus rhythm.

The results of balloon aortic valvuloplasty have been disappointing and valve replacement is preferred even in the very elderly.

Complications of valve replacement. The major differences in complication rates in mechanical and bioprosthetic valves relate to the incidence of primary valve failure and major bleeding; primary valve failure is very high with bioprosthesis after 5 years, and major bleeding is a drawback of the mechanical valve (see Table 12–6).

AORTIC REGURGITATION

Over the past 25 years, there has been a major change in the pattern of underlying conditions associated with diseases causing aortic regurgi-

Table 12–7
Causes of Aortic Regurgitation

ACUTE	CHRONIC
Bacterial endocarditis	Rheumatic
Aotic dissection	Endocarditis
Prosthetic valve surgery	Congenitial: bicuspid valve, ventricular septal defect, sinus of valsalva aneurysm
Aortic balloon valvuloplasty	Aortic root dilatation: connective tissue disorder: Marfan's, ankylosing spondylitis, Reiter's syndrome, rheumatoid arthritis, lupus erythematosus
Trauma	Takayasu aortitis, cystic medionecrosis myxomatous degeneration, psoriatic arthritis, Behçet's syndrome, relapsing polychondritis, giant cell arteritis, osteogenesis imperfecta, ulcerative colitis
Rheumatic fever	Whipples disease
	Hypertension
	Arteriosclerosis
	Syphilis

tation. Whereas rheumatic fever and syphilis comprised 70% and 20% of cases, respectively, they now account for <30% and 1%. With the fall in prevalence of these diseases, bicuspid valve, endocarditis, and diseases causing aortic root dilation have emerged as the common causes (Table 12–7).

Diagnostic Hallmarks

With chronic aortic regurgitation, the left ventricle tolerates regurgitant volume overload and compensates adequately; an asymptomatic period of 10–30 years is not uncommon. Many patients with a moderate degree of aortic regurgitation deny shortness of breath on walking 3–5 miles and/or 3 flights of stairs. Complaints of shortness of breath on exertion, fatigue, palpitations, or dizziness are generally associated with moderate or severe regurgitation over a prolonged period or severe regurgitation of recent onset. Rarely, angina with diaphoresis occurs as the diastolic BP falls, frequently at night, causing a ↓ in coronary perfusion. Symptoms and signs of CHF at rest are late manifestations.

Hallmarks on physical examination include

- Typical collapsing pulse: Water-hammer or Corrigan's pulse or a bounding pulse. The underlying mechanism is a rapid ↑ in upstroke followed by an abrupt collapse due to a quick diastolic runoff from the arterial tree. Indeed, all conditions that cause a brisk runoff produce a collapsing or bounding pulse (Table 12–8). The collapsing quality is detected by the examiner placing his or her fingers or palm closed firmly over the radial pulse with the entire limb extended to the ceiling. Pulsus bisferiens, a double peak to the pulse, may be observed with the combination of aortic regurgitation and significant aortic stenosis
- The patient's head often bobs with each cardiac pulsation
- The BP reveals a wide pulse pressure due to a ↑ in systolic BP and a diastolic that is often <50 mm Hg. Occasionally, Korotkoff sounds persist to zero with diastolic arterial pressure still >60 mm Hg

Table 12–8
Causes of a Collapsing Bounding Pulse

CARDIAC CAUSES	NONCARDIAC CAUSES
Aortic regurgitation	Arterovenous fistula
Patent ductus arteriosus	Paget's disease
	Pregnancy
	Fevers
	Thyrotoxicosis
	Vasodilator drugs

- Arterial, neck pulsations are usually prominent
- Quincke's sign: Exerting mild pressure on the nail beds brings out intermittent flushing
- Finger pulsations: Collapsing pulsations in the finger pulps or tips
- Traube's sign: Pistol-shot sounds over the femorals
- Duroziez's sign: Compression of the femoral artery proximal to the stethoscope produces a systolic murmur and a diastolic murmur with distal compression

The apex beat is virtually always displaced downward and outward to the left, indicating LV enlargement in patients with moderate or severe aortic regurgitation. A diastolic thrill may be palpated in the second right interspace or third interspace at the left sternal border, where the murmur of aortic regurgitation is most prominent.

Hallmarks on auscultation include

- Typical high-pitched blowing, early decrescendo murmur begins immediately after the aortic second sound (A2). The early decrescendo murmur beginning immediately after A2 is unmistakable to the trained ear and is best heard with the diaphragm pressed firmly against the chest, with the patient leaning forward and the breath held in deep expiration. The listener should then listen to the murmur with the patient breathing normally and in the recumbent position in order to train the ear for detection of the softest diastolic murmur
- The degree of aortic regurgitation correlates best with the duration of the murmur and may be pan-diastolic with severe regurgitation
- Perforation of an aortic cusp may change the quality of the murmur to one that resembles the cooing of a dove
- A mid or late diastolic rumble at the apex, the Austin Flint murmur, may be heard as the regurgitant jet hits the anterior mitral leaflet, as it opens and closes during diastolc. The leaflet's shuddering can be heard with the stethoscope or observed with the help of Doppler echocardiography
- The A2 may be increased, decreased, or normal, and the accompanying aortic systolic murmur and thrill may represent flow rather than stenosis

The ECG commonly shows nonspecific ST-T wave changes, and with LVH, the pattern of LVH with volume overload is often present.

Chest x ray. In patients with moderate or severe aortic regurgitation, dilation of the left ventricle with elongation of the apex inferoposteriorly is almost invariably visible. Progressive further enlargement occurs over years in patients with severe aortic regurgitation. Dilation of the ascending aorta is common in Marfan's syndrome and other causes of aortic root dilation (Table 12–7). The typical appearance of linear eggshell calcification of the ascending aorta is a hallmark of syphilitic aortitis, which is now rare.

Echocardiographic findings include

- Detection of the type of aortic valve abnormality and underlying disease, e.g., aortic regurgitation due to bicuspid valve or vegetations caused by endocarditis
- LV chamber dimensions: estimates of LV volume and ventricular function measurements (LV end systolic dimensions, LV end diastolic dimensions, fractional shortening or EF)
- Dilation of the aortic root
- Aortic dissection
- Other valve disease
- Other associated states, e.g., perivalvular abscesses in infective endocarditis

Management of Chronic Aortic Regurgitation

Medical therapy plays an important role, since the timing of valve surgery presents an ongoing challenge for both physician and patient. A review of the natural history of the condition indicates that

- >75% of patients with moderate aortic regurgitation survive for ≥5 years
- >50% are alive 10 years after diagnosis
- >90% of patients with relatively mild aortic regurgitation survive >20 years
- As with aortic stenosis, the occurrence of CHF carries about a 2-year survival, while for angina survival is about 5 years

A VA study, completed in 1991, comparing the survival of 102 medically treated and 147 surgically treated patients with severe aortic regurgitation, and followed for 7.5 years, indicated that valve replacement may not prolong survival in these patients.

Valve replacement should be considered prior to irreversible myocardial deterioration. However, because timing is often difficult, close follow-up of the patient with minimal or absent symptoms is essential.

PHARMACOLOGIC AGENTS OF VALUE

Nifedipine. The unloading effect of nifedipine has been recently shown to be capable of reversing LV dilation and hypertrophy, and this agent may delay the need for valve surgery. In a study of 72 patients followed for 12 months, LV end diastolic volume index decreased from 136 ± 22–110 ± 19 ml/m^2, $p < 0.01$, and LV mass decreased from 142 to 115 g/m^2 (Fig. 12–1). A 25% ↓ of the mean LV wall stress and a ↑ in EF from 60 to 72% were observed.

Nifedipine is superior to hydralazine, which does not ↓ LV mass or significantly ↓ LV end diastolic or systolic dimensions. It appears that afterload ↓ with nifedipine in patients with moderate to severe aortic regurgitation and normal LV function can achieve a 5-year survival rate approaching 87%. The 5-year survival rate for aortic valve replacement is approximately 72%, and the surgical mortality is 5%.

Nifedipine is given preferably as the extended-release preparation: Procardia XL or Adalat XL, 30 mg once daily (see Chap. 1, Dosage). The extended-release formulation is preferable since the nifedipine capsule causes an early and transient peak effect; also, adverse effects are more frequent than those observed with the sustained-release preparation.

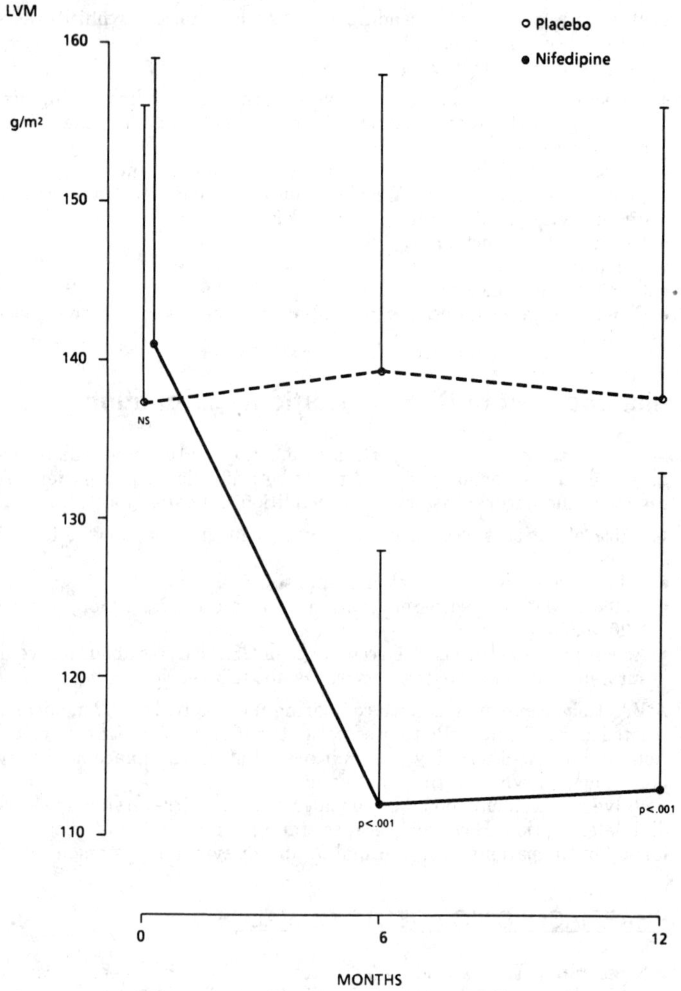

Figure 12–1. Changes in left ventricular mass (LVM) over time for the two study groups. LVM did not change in patients treated with placebo but decreased significantly in the nifedipine-treated patients. From: Scognamiglio R, et al.: Longterm nifedipine unloading therapy in asymptomatic patients with chronic severe aortic regurgitation. J Am Coll Cardiol, *16*:424, 1990.

Nifedipine has a mild negative inotropic effect that is somewhat offset by sympathetic stimulation. Verapamil and diltiazem are contraindicated because of their negative inotropic effects and their propensity to cause bradycardia, which can worsen nocturnal angina or CHF. Indeed, all vasodilators are not alike, and hydralazine has not proven useful. Prazosin and other $alpha_1$ blockers are contraindicated because postural hypotension and increased HR may occur; these agents do not ↓ LV mass or favorably alter LV systolic or diastolic dimensions.

ACE inhibitors have not been tested, but caution is necessary since these agents have a marked lowering effect on diastolic BP, which may worsen diastolic coronary perfusion in patients with aortic regurgitation, a situation that is prone to occur during sleep and can be deleterious in patients with significant, concomitant atheromatous coronary stenoses. These agents have been shown to be harmful in patients with angina and in patients with CHF in the presence of aortic regurgitation; ACE inhibitors should be avoided in patients who manifest angina or silent ischemia. Ca antagonists, unlike ACE inhibitors, do not usually cause a ↓ in BP in normotensive individuals (see Chap. 1).

Digoxin. This agent increases resting EF. Peak exercise EF increases with both digoxin and nifedipine but not with hydralazine. The combination of digoxin and nifedipine improves chronic hemodynamics in symptomatic and asymptomatic patients with severe regurgitation.

TIMING OF VALVE REPLACEMENT

- There is general agreement that symptomatic patients with severe chronic aortic regurgitation should have valve surgery in the absence of contraindications
- Valve surgery is not indicated in asymptomatic patients with severe chronic aortic regurgitation who have good effort tolerance and normal LV function

Between these 2 extremes is a large group of patients for whom firm data comparing the effect of prognosis of medical with surgical management are lacking, as are widely accepted criteria or a task force consensus that may guide the physician.

Patients with moderate or severe aortic regurgitation should be followed at least every 3 months. A careful history is necessary, including questioning of a spouse or relative who may be able to describe symptoms that are denied by the patient. A cardiovascular examination and ECG are done at each visit. Echocardiography is advisable every 6 months if LV end systolic dimension is >50 mm or if fractional shortening is <30%. A biannual exercise test is useful to assess functional capacity.

If symptoms manifest (dyspnea on mild or moderate exertion, orthopnea, or chest discomfort), cardiac catheterization is necessary for verification of echocardiographic dimensions with a view to surgery.

Patients with prolonged severe LV dysfunction and marked LV dilation are not expected to benefit from surgery. Although there are no fixed rules giving clear contraindications, surgery generally is not advisable in patients who have

- EF <30%
- Prolonged severe LV dysfunction (≥18 months)

In these patients, symptoms, signs, and hemodynamic parameters of LV dysfunction may persist or worsen after successful valve replacement. Patients with EF <45% and <1 year of LV dysfunction usually have a successful postoperative outcome, but those with EF <45% and prolonged LV dysfunction (>18 months) have a poor postoperative survival. Repeated radionuclide or echocardiographic assessment of EF and end systolic volume, especially at rest, is necessary for decision making. It must be emphasized that radionuclide EF is not accurate in patients with AF.

The role of the cardiologist is to consider interventional therapy prior to the occurrence of significant LV dysfunction. At this stage of careful follow-up, surgery is offered if LV function is impaired, if exercise capacity is reduced, or if LV dimensions are "highly abnormal" or show significant deterioration. Management of the asymptomatic patient with severe aortic regurgitation, depressed LV function, and abnormal dimensions, as indicated, should be individualized.

The following echocardiographic or catheter dimensions may be used to help serve in decision making regarding timing for valve surgery. No single estimation should be accepted for making decisions. Marked changes or rate of change at 3- or 6-month visits should guide the physician

- LV end systolic dimension of 50–55 mm Hg. A dimension >55 mm usually indicates LV dysfunction and, as outlined earlier, one does not wait for such ominous signals
- LV end diastolic dimension >70 mm
- LV end systolic volume index >60 ml/m^2; >90 ml/m^2 indicates severe LV dysfunction
- LV end diastolic volume index 140–150 ml/m^2; >180 ml/m^2 indicates severe LV dysfunction
- EF <50% or fractional shortening <30%; fractional shortening <25% indicates severe LV dysfunction, LV EF <45% represents moderately severe LV dysfunction, and <35% indicates very severe dysfunction

The asymptomatic patient with severe aortic regurgitation should meet ≥1 of the above criteria and should show a marked change from the evaluation done 4–6 months previously in order to be considered a candidate for surgery.

It must be reemphasized that no single measurement is ideal and that most of them must be obtained to enable the cardiologist to apply the best clinical judgment, taking into account other variables such as age, occupation, and intercurrent illness.

Preparations for surgery include attention to dental work under antibiotic cover. Coronary angiography is necessary in patients > age 35 or in those with angina.

The choice of prosthetic heart valve is discussed in this chapter under aortic stenosis. Elective valve surgery has a 3–6% operative mortality and emergency surgery >10%. The 5-year survival for valve implant is 60–85%.

MITRAL STENOSIS

Mitral stenosis is almost always due to previous rheumatic fever. It takes ≥2 years following the rheumatic episode for sufficient fibrosis and thickening of the valve to produce the typical murmur. Most patients remain asymptomatic for 15–20 years following an episode of rheumatic fever, which is subclinical in >50%.

Over the past 30 years, the problem of rheumatic valve disease has shown a marked decline in North America, the UK, and Europe. However, the disease is still endemic in much of Asia, Africa, the Middle East, Latin America, and the West Indies. Indeed, in these countries, significant mitral stenosis may emerge within a few years of the initial acute rheumatic fever and result in symptomatic disease in juveniles and young adults.

Diagnosis

- The patient with mild mitral stenosis, valve area 1.6–2.0 cm^2, may develop mild dyspnea on moderate to severe exertion but is usually able to do all normal chores; lifestyle is not altered. Symptoms progress slowly, if at all, over the next 5–10 years. However, infection, pregnancy, or tachycardias, including AF, may precipitate severe dyspnea

- Patients with moderately severe mitral stenosis, valve area 1–1.5 cm^2, usually have symptoms that affect or interfere with daily living. Dyspnea due to progressive pulmonary venous hypertension becomes bothersome. Breathlessness is precipitated by moderate activity such as walking 100 yards briskly, walking up an incline, or even running slowly for 20 yards. Some patients with mild mitral stenosis may reduce activities and tolerate symptoms for several years. Pulmonary infection or AF often precipitates pulmonary congestion, emergency room visits, or hospitalization. Cough, shortness of breath, wheeze, and hemoptysis may mimic bronchitis for several months because the subtle signs of mitral stenosis can be missed by the untrained auscultator. Palpitations are usually due to AF, and some patients may present with a very rapid tachycardia or systemic embolization
- Severe mitral stenosis, valve area <1 cm^2 and valve area index <1 cm^2/m^2, usually causes symptoms on mild exertion. The patient presents with ≥ 1 of the following symptoms: progressive dyspnea, palpitations, marked fatigue, and occasionally cough, hemoptysis, hoarseness, or chest pain. Progression may be rapid, with increasing edema, orthopnea, PND, and marked breathlessness. However, some patients tolerate dyspnea and are able to continue work that is not strenuous, at their own pace, for 3–12 months prior to interventional therapy. Fortunately, with mitral stenosis, patients with the most bothersome symptoms benefit the most from mitral valvotomy

PHYSICAL SIGNS

- On inspection, a malar flush is common in the presence of longstanding, moderately severe mitral stenosis
- A lower left parasternal lift of heave due to right ventricular hypertrophy may be present
- The apex beat is tapping in quality, usually not displaced
- A diastolic thrill localized to the apex beat may be palpated
- Auscultation reveals a loud slapping first heart sound and is so typical that it warns the examiner to search for other signs of mitral stenosis. Immobility of the cusps reduces this valuable sign
- The pulmonary second sound is intensified and this vibration associated with pulmonary valve closure is often palpable with significant pulmonary arterial hypertension
- An opening snap, a sharp high-pitched sound, is a hallmark of mitral stenosis. The opening snap is best heard with the diaphragm pressed firmly just internal to the apex beat and occurs from 0.04 to 0.14 seconds after the second heart sound. The opening snap may be heard over a wide area and, with severe mitral stenosis, usually occurs <0.08 seconds following the second heart sound, audible immediately rather than after a definite gap. The opening snap disappears if the valve becomes heavily calcified and nonpliable
- The loud slapping first heart sound and opening snap produce a particular cadence that alerts the examiner
- The opening snap is followed by a low-pitched, mid-diastolic rumbling murmur that is associated, if there is sinus rhythm, with presystolic accentuation, best heard with the bell lightly applied over the apex beat. The murmur often is localized to an area the size of a coin and can easily be missed; it is brought out by exercising the patient and

listening with the patient lying on the left side. Occasionally, critical mitral stenosis may cause a marked ↓ in transmitral flow, and the murmur may be hardly audible. There is evidence that in these cases, the disease and contracted chordae ↑ the impedance to ventricular filling so that the reduced mitral valve area is no longer the limiting factor
- The severity of mitral stenosis correlates best with the length of the murmur rather than the intensity

CHEST X-RAY HALLMARKS

- Straightening of the left heart border due to left atrial enlargement
- Larger than normal double density, seen through the right half of the cardiac silhouette, indicating left atrial enlargement
- Elevation of the left main stem bronchus caused by distension of the left atrium with widening of the angle between the 2 main bronchi
- Redistribution: restriction of lower lobe vessels and dilation of the upper lobe vessels
- If CHF is present, signs of interstitial edema are present: Kerley B lines due to lymphatic engorgement and fibrosis, perihilar haze, and eventually frank pulmonary edema are observed
- Fluoroscopy is no longer commonly done, but shows posterior displacement of the barium-filled esophagus
- The heart size on posteroanterior x ray is generally normal or near normal, and the lateral film should be assessed for right ventricular enlargement: "creeping up the sternum"

ELECTROCARDIOGRAPHIC HALLMARKS

- Signs of left atrial enlargement are common with moderate and severe mitral stenosis: broad bifid P waves in lead 2 and, more specifically, a ↑ in the P terminal force ($PTFV_1$) ≥40 millisec/mm, measured in V_1 (area subtended by the terminal negative portion of a biphasic P wave). Hazen, et al. have shown that when $PTFV_1$ is >40 millisec/mm, 95% of individuals had left atrial size >4 cm; when $PTFV_1$ is ≥60 millisec/ mm, 75% had left atrial size >6 cm
- Right axis deviation of 90–150° reflects severe mitral stenosis
- Right ventricular hypertrophy may be present with severe stenosis but does not correlate well with the degree of pulmonary hypertension
- AF is common with moderate longstanding rheumatic disease, with the left atrial size >4.5 cm, and is characteristically coarse in appearance

ECHOCARDIOGRAPHIC ASSESSMENT

- The mitral diastolic gradient can be defined
- Excellent quantification of mitral valve orifice area
- Left atrial enlargement is uniformly present, and the size can be accurately determined
- The degree of calcification of the mitral valve leaflets can be verified
- Decreased posterior leaflet movement is often observed
- The degree of right ventricular enlargement can be documented
- LV size is expected to be small
- Right ventricular systolic pressures reflect the degree of pulmonary hypertension
- The degree of concomitant MR can be assessed

A flat E to F slope or EF slope <10 mm/sec may indicate severe mitral stenosis, but this measurement is no longer used for quantitating the degree of obstruction. Marked alteration of the E to F slope may be observed in patients with aortic stenosis and regurgitation with no evidence of mitral stenosis and in patients with impaired LV filling caused by reduced LV compliance.

Medical Therapy

All patients should receive prophylaxis for the prevention of rheumatic fever for ≥25 years from the acute episode and up to age 45, whichever is the longest. Although pure mitral stenosis is rarely the site of endocarditis, trivial MR is often present, and endocarditis prophylaxis should be strongly enforced (see Chap. 10).

MILD MITRAL STENOSIS

- Patients are usually asymptomatic and should be followed annually. A chest x ray and echocardiogram are done initially, or if needed because of worsening symptomatology. Then, about every 5 years should suffice
- No treatment is indicated, except for advice on mild dietary salt restriction and avoidance of excessive weight gain and physically strenuous occupations

MODERATE MITRAL STENOSIS

- Moderate mitral stenosis, valve orifice area 1–1.5 cm^2, is usually mildly symptomatic. Salt restriction is advisable. K-sparing diuretics such as Moduretic (Moduret) ameliorate shortness of breath and prevent K and magnesium loss (see Chap. 5). If palpitations are bothersome or short runs of SVT are documented, a small dose of a β-blocking drug is useful: metoprolol 25–50 mg bid, atenolol 25 mg qd, or an equivalent dose of another β blocker should suffice. Digoxin is not indicated for patients with sinus rhythm or CHF with pulmonary congestion, except as prophylaxis against fast ventricular rates and pulmonary edema if AF develops
- Chest infections must be vigorously treated because hypoxemia increases pulmonary hypertension and may precipitate right CHF. Also, tachycardia may precipitate pulmonary edema
- If the patient is managing daily chores and enjoying a near-normal lifestyle, the interventional approach can await some progression of the disease or symptoms but is not delayed in very active patients who need to engage in strenuous work or sport. Marked limitation of lifestyle in such individuals may require early corrective measures. A patient with moderate mitral stenosis should be followed at least twice yearly, but annual echocardiography should suffice

SEVERE MITRAL STENOSIS

- Severe mitral stenosis, valve area corrected for body surface area (valve area index) <1 cm^2/m^2, usually requires interventional therapy within 3–6 months to abolish symptoms or ↓ complications and/or progressive ↑ in pulmonary vascular resistance
- AF with a fast ventricular response decreases LV filling and may

precipitate pulmonary congestion. Digoxin is indicated to control the ventricular response. Digoxin is discussed in detail in Chapter 5. If palpitations remain bothersome and the HR cannot be controlled with digoxin, as often occurs in very active individuals, the addition of a small dose of β-blocking drug is useful. The latter agents can also be used to ↓ sinus tachycardia that is easily provoked in some patients without AF. Many physicians regard the development of AF as an indication for intervention when stenosis is of moderate severity, because the prospects for permanent restoration of sinus rhythm ↓ rapidly with time from onset of arrhythmia
- The patient with AF must be anticoagulated, if no contraindication exists, because systemic embolization is common. Warfarin is given to maintain the prothrombin time, 1.25–1.5 times the control or INR 2–3 (see Chap. 11 for advice on anticoagulant control). These tests are done at least every 2 weeks until stabilized, then monthly should suffice. If contraindications to anticoagulant therapy exist, enteric coated aspirin (325 mg qd) is advisable

Interventional Management

Balloon valvuloplasty or surgery to relieve valvular obstruction is indicated for most symptomatic patients who have moderate to severe mitral stenosis, valve orifice <1 cm^2, as determined by Doppler echocardiography. The results of this technique correlate sufficiently well with catheterization data. Cardiac catheterization is not required in patients less than age 40, in whom IHD is not present or suspected, and who have typical, clinical features of mitral stenosis that are confirmed by Doppler echocardiography.

Mild mitral stenosis, valve area 1.6–2.0 cm^2, often remains minimally symptomatic ≥5–10 years. However, as explained earlier, in countries where rheumatic valve disease is endemic, tight mitral stenosis may emerge at a faster rate in the adolescent or young adult.

Moderately severe mitral stenosis, valve area 1–1.5 cm^2, usually does not require intervention, but decisions must be individualized. In these patients, intervention may be required in the following cases

- For symptomatic young patients engaged in strenuous activity
- If AF supervenes
- To allow a further pregnancy in a patient who manifested pulmonary edema in a previous pregnancy

Elective procedures are sometimes performed in women who anticipate pregnancy, but relief of obstruction may be required during the second and third trimester of pregnancy, because the valve orifice is no longer large enough to permit the necessary ↑ in cardiac output to occur without an unacceptable ↑ in left atrial and pulmonary venous pressures. Interventional therapy may take the form of: Surgical closed commissurotomy, surgical open commissurotomy, balloon valvuloplasty, or valve replacement.

Closed mitral commissurotomy was the technique of choice until the early 1970s for patients with severe mitral stenosis with noncalcified pliable valves. Open commissurotomy has largely replaced the closed technique, except in much of Asia, Africa, Latin America, and the West Indies, where closed valvotomy has remained the treatment of choice.

Undoubtedly, there will be a resurgence of closed commissurotomy in North America and Europe based on the recent survey entitled "Outcome Probabilities and Life History after Surgical Mitral Commissurotomy." In this study, Hickey, et al. compared the outcome in 236 open and 103 closed commissurotomies performed between 1967 and 1988. The survival rate at 1 month, 1 year, 5 years, and 10 years was 99.7%, 99%, 95%, and 87%, respectively, with outcomes being similar after closed and open commissurotomy. Thus, both techniques provide excellent relief, although eventual restenosis is usual over the ensuring 10 or more years post mitral valvotomy. Mitral valve replacement was required in 22% within 10 years of commissurotomy. In the entire study group, thromboembolism occurred in 33 (10% of 339 patients), and 9 (2.6%) patients had significant cerebral embolism.

Moderate to severe mitral stenosis accompanied by mild to moderate MR is not uncommon, and open repair with limited opening of the Tubbs dilator is considered an option for this category of patients.

MITRAL BALLOON VALVULOPLASTY

Percutaneous mitral balloon valvuloplasty appears to give hemodynamic results comparable with surgical closed commissurotomy, as shown by an 8-month follow-up study. The valve area is increased 100% from 1 cm^2 to 2 cm^2 in ≤77% of cases. A mortality of ≤2.7% has been reported by the Valvuloplasty Registry. The National Heart, Lung and Blood Institute 30-day follow-up report on 738 patients indicates an 83% overall clinical improvement and mortality of 3%; 4% of patients require valve surgery. An iatrogenic ASD has been reported to occur in 20–87% of patients, depending on criteria used for defining the ASD, which takes ≤6 months to close. However, the defect is usually small, the magnitude of the shunt being <2:1, and only few of these ASDs are clinically significant. Currently, complication rates are still high (see Table 12–9). The procedure should be done only by highly trained and experienced operators. In such hands, the procedure is first choice in appropriately selected patients for relief of severe mitral stenosis.

Mitral balloon valvuloplasty must have a mortality of <1% to be considered an acceptable alternative to surgical commissurotomy. The proper selection of patients and technical aspects are changing such that morbidity and mortality from the procedure are expected to fall.

The patient selection for mitral balloon valvuloplasty is crucial to obtaining a salutary effect with a minimum number of complications. The patients are usually selected based on 2D echocardiographic results. Ideally, the patients should have

- Very symptomatic severe mitral stenosis, mitral valve area <1 cm^3
- Noncalcified, mobile valve with no subvalvular fibrosis (echo score <8). Valve rigidity, valve calcification, thickening, and subvalvular

Table 12–9
Complications of Mitral Balloon Valvuloplasty

CLINICAL PARAMETERS	COMPLICATIONS, INCIDENCE (%)
Mortality	2.7
Emergency surgery	6.7
Cardiac tamponade	6.7
Embolism	2.7
Significant mitral regurgitation	13
Emergency valve replacement	4
Restenosis	16
Iatrogenic atrial septal defect	20 to 87

fibrosis are graded from 0 to 4, and the points are added together. The best candidates are patients who have an echo score <8. Contraindications include

- Bleeding disorder: Abnormal prothrombin time, prolonged PTT, increased bleeding time (the patient must discontinue aspirin compounds for ≥1 week prior to the procedure)
- Left atrial or appendage thrombus
- Recent embolization
- Severe mitral valve calcification of subvalvular fibrosis
- Moderate or severe MR
- Cardiothoracic deformity

TEE has a role in obtaining information needed for the selection of patients for balloon valvuloplasty such as calcification, thickening, mobility, and subvalvular fibrosis. Atrial or appendage thrombus is best visualized with TEE. The technique is also of value in assessing the magnitude of the ASD following the procedure.

MITRAL VALVE REPLACEMENT

A prosthetic valve implant may be required because of the presence of moderate to severe MR coexisting with mitral stenosis. Replacement may also be selected for management of heavily calcified and immobile valves, which are often conical in shape, when they are considered to be beyond repair at the time of surgery. In general, a mechanical valve is preferred in the mitral area. See earlier discussion of prosthetic valve choice and Table 12–5. In ≤50% of patients, AF is present; a mechanical valve is a natural choice because anticoagulants are necessary. In the young female who may wish to become pregnant, a bioprosthesis is sometimes recommended. However, a mechanical valve can be used in this situation with discontinuation of oral anticoagulants; heparin can be used SQ for the first 4 months of pregnancy and again for the last 3 weeks. Importantly, in the young patient, accelerated calcification of a bioprosthesis may occur. Calcification, as well as pannus formation, may require a second operation.

MITRAL REGURGITATION

While mitral stenosis is nearly always due to rheumatic disease, MR is a common valvular lesion caused by a number of conditions that alter the mitral valve apparatus: valve leaflets, annulus, chordae, and papillary muscles. Common causes of acute and chronic MR are given in Table 12–10.

Acute Mitral Regurgitation commonly occurs during acute MI, which causes papillary muscle dysfunction, and less commonly, chordal or papillary muscle rupture (see Chap. 4). Other causes of acute MR are listed in Table 12–10.

Chronic Mitral Regurgitation. Patients may tolerate a mild to moderate degree of MR for 10 or more years without the appearance of CHF. Chronic volume overload, however, causes slow progressive dilation and mild hypertrophy of the left ventricle. Characteristically, a loud holosystolic murmur is heard maximal at the apex with radiation to the axilla, accompanied by a third heart sound gallop if regurgitation is moderate

Table 12–10
Causes of Mitral Regurgitation

Cause	Mechanism
ACUTE:	
Myocardial infarction	Papillary muscle dysfunction
	Rupture chordae tendineae
	Rupture of papillary muscle
Mitral valve prolapse	Rupture chordae tendineae
	Rapid progression of prolapse
Endocarditis	Acute
	Rare subacute endocarditis
Chronic:	
Rheumatic	
Mitral valve prolapse	
Healed endocarditis	
Ischemic heart disease	
Functional dilatation	

to severe. In patients with posterior papillary muscle dysfunction causing MR, however, the murmur radiates anteriorly and is best heard at the left sternal border without radiation to the axilla.

Mild to moderate shortness of breath indicates pulmonary congestion or LV dysfunction and should be managed with afterload-reducing agents, particularly ACE inhibitors, to encourage forward flow at the expense of regurgitation. Small doses are advisable: captopril, 6.25 mg bid for several days, increasing slowly to avoid hypotension to a maintenance of 37.5 mg bid (max 75 mg in 2 or 3 divided doses or equivalent doses of enalapril).

If concomitant IHD with angina is present and LV dysfunction is not severe, nifedipine is preferred to ACE inhibitors, which may ↑ angina. Also, digoxin and the judicious use of diuretics in combination with nifedipine may be beneficial before considering early valve repair or valve replacement.

AF with a rapid ventricular response is managed with digoxin and anticoagulants to prevent embolization.

Progressive dyspnea is a late stage and CHF should be anticipated and prevented by timely surgical intervention.

Surgical Treatment

- The timing of valve surgery, whether for repair or replacement due to chronic MR, remains a trial in decision making, as with aortic regurgitation. Patients with mitral valve prolapse and acute complications are often suitable for valve repair
- There is an increasing tendency to attempt valve reconstruction. It is advisable to repair as many and as often as feasible, but success depends on the skill of the surgeon. For mitral stenosis and regurgitation, many valves are beyond repair and require replacement
- Surgery should be considered in patients who have moderately severe MR prior to the development of severe pulmonary arterial hypertension and prior to a ↓ in EF to <50%. The interpretation of EF has to be adjusted downward to take into account the low impedance to retrograde flow resulting from MR. A patient with severe MR and an EF <40% will have a prohibitively high surgical mortality and will fare better with afterload ↓ and digoxin. Because of the problems of

assessing EF in the presence of MR, other parameters of LV function have been used, including end systolic volume index >50 ml/m^2

- If surgery is done prior to the manifestations of the aforementioned parameters, survival, functional class, and LV systolic function should show significant improvement. If MR is moderately severe and LV dysfunction is present, it is hazardous to procrastinate. Early surgery is preferable
- In patients with predominant posterior leaflet prolapse, repair of the posterior leaflet followed by insertion of a nonflexible ring, as recommended by Carpentier, appears to be successful in preventing postoperative systolic anterior motion of the mitral valve
- In some patients with heavily calcified valves, the mitral valve annulus can be decalcified, and valve repair, decalcification, and annuloplasty should be considered based on Doppler echocardiographic data. TEE gives a more accurate visualization of the mitral valve, however, and is advisable in potential candidates; the latter is justifiable and cost-effective, especially in view of the difficult decision as to timing of surgery
- The tricuspid valve is also often severely incompetent; tricuspid annuloplasty is advisable in such cases
- Intraoperative TEE is of considerable value in assessing valve repair. The surgeon ensures excellent coapting edges and lines of closure; if the geometry is ideal, saline is pumped into the ventricle

MITRAL VALVE PROLAPSE

- Mitral valve prolapse is said to be a common condition affecting an estimated 5% of the U.S. population. The incidence of mitral valve prolapse has been exaggerated because of the inclusion of a large number of patients with a normal variant of mitral valve closure but with correct coaptation; leaflets may only billow slightly into the left atrium with normal coaptation. Also, the appearance may result from the normal saddle shape of the normal mitral ring
- The minor variant with a click, without a murmur and nondiagnostic echocardiographic features commonly labeled mitral valve prolapse, is subject to interpretation, and this "normal variant" disappears after age 40. Probably because of the inclusion of normal variants with billowing leaflets without true prolapse, the incidence of mitral valve prolapse is reported to be as high as 30% at age 10–20, 15% at age 30, 10% at age 50, 3% at age 70, and <1% at age 80. Under age 30, the female-to-male ratio is 3:1, but at age 70, both men and women are about equal. The incidence of significant mitral valve prolapse is about 6% in adult women and 3% in men
- Genuine mitral valve prolapse has a familial incidence of about 33%, as noted in 1st° relatives

Causes. These include

- In developed countries, the common underlying process is a degenerative nonrheumatic condition of unknown etiology described as a dyscollagenosis or myxomatous degeneration of the mitral valve. A ↑ in the spongiosa, myxomatous tissue, in the middle layer of the mitral valve leaflet, encroaches upon the fibrosa. The anterior and posterior leaflets become elongated, thickened, voluminous, and grossly redundant. The chordae become thin and elongated and have a propensity to rupture. Herniation of the posterior leaflet above the anterior leaflet may occur. A mural endocardial fibrous plaque is often observed beneath the posterior leaflet in patients who die suddenly from mitral valve prolapse. The mitral valve annulus is often dilated in patients with significant regurgitation, and in those patients who die suddenly, calcification and fibrosis of the annulus appears to be a common finding

- Myxomatous changes and mitral valve prolapse are associated with Marfan's, Ehlos-Danlos syndrome, and osteogenesis imperfecta
- Rheumatic heart disease, where this disease is still endemic. A dilated annulus allows elongation of chordae with, sometimes, prolapse of the anterior leaflet, but marked billowing or redundancy of leaflets are unusual
- Papillary muscle dysfunction due to IHD

Symptoms

Most patients are asymptomatic. Dyspnea is rather vague, often occurs at rest, and is commonly out of proportion with the degree of MR that is usually asymptomatic in >80% of patients. Extreme fatigue, dizziness, anxiety, panic disorders, palpitations, presyncope, syncope, and chest pain may occur without a satisfactory explanation. Psychogenic factors play a role in the varied symptomatology.

Some symptoms relate to the presence of autonomic dysfunction with increased levels of circulating catecholamine, and a hyperadrenergic state; in some patients, increased vagal activity is present. In this condition, there is a tendency for the sinus rate to ↑ steeply in the early part of exercise, and the high frequency of palpitations has been attributed to this pattern of response in these patients. It is not surprising, therefore, that Holter monitoring commonly shows sinus tachycardia, when palpitations are a complaint.

Signs

One or multiple mid or late systolic clicks of nonejection type may be constant or intermittent, changing with posture or maneuvers, but do not prove the existence of mitral valve prolapse. The timing of clicks may be misinterpreted as gallop sounds, but apart from their timing, clicks can be differentiated from a third heart sound by the high-pitched quality and by being most audible with a diaphragm. In some patients, the click is followed by a murmur; in others, only a murmur is present.

The murmur has typical features

- A typical late systolic murmur is unmistakable and confirms the diagnosis
- The murmur is usually crescendo-decrescendo, the auscultator gets the impression that the murmur is occurring synchronously with the second heart sound, and the murmur often extends through the aortic second sound
- A whoop, a short honking sound, or a sound of other musical quality may highlight the murmur, which changes in intensity depending on LV volume and BP
- The late systolic murmur or click is heard earlier and made louder by the following maneuvers that reduce LV volume: standing, tilting upright, valsalva, and tachycardia. Amyl nitrite decreases ventricular

volume and BP; therefore, the murmur is heard earlier but is made softer

- The murmur or clicks are heard later and are softer with maneuvers that ↑ LV volume or ↓ BP: squatting, bradycardia, β-blocking agents. Thus, the physician should listen to the patient lying, standing, and squatting because the murmur may be heard only on standing. With more severe MR, the duration of the murmur is longer and may become pansystolic
- When chordal rupture occurs, the murmur changes in quality and radiation
- The posterior mitral leaflet often has 3 scallops; rupture of the chorda to the middle scallop of the posterior leaflet is the most common chordal rupture. The resulting murmur radiates anteriorly, is maximal at the lower left sternal border, and radiates toward the upper right sternal edge. The crescendo-decrescendo quality may simulate an aortic systolic murmur. However, the late timing of the murmur of mitral valve prolapse is a distinguishing feature that differentiates the murmur from the early timing of aortic valvular murmurs
- Chordal rupture of the anterior leaflet causes the murmur to radiate to the posterior axilla
- The flail mitral valve produces a loud murmur, the intensity of which is characteristically accentuated over the spine and may be heard from the occiput to the sacral spine
- The MR jet can be identified by TEE; it moves in a counterclockwise direction with flail anterior leaflet, and clockwise with posterior leaflet involvement

Approximately 15% of patients with mitral valve prolapse have skeletal abnormalities: "straight back," pectus excavatum or carinatum, scoliosis, or some features of Marfan's syndrome.

Complications. These include

- Severe MR occurs in approximately 10% of patients with true mitral valve prolapse and is 5 times more common in men > age 45 than in women. Although mitral valve prolapse occurs most commonly in women, severe MR requiring surgery occurs in about 5% of men and <1.5% of women. Chordal rupture is a common occurrence in patients with severe MR
- Arrhythmias commonly occur and include VPCs, atrial ectopics, PSVT, and occasionally AF. Lethal arrhythmias have been reported (see Chap. 6)
- Sudden death, although rare, occurs in healthy young active individuals and is unexplained. Table 12–11 lists clinical and morphologic features in 15 patients who died suddenly secondary to mitral valve prolapse. These data and a review of previously reported studies on 63 patients indicate that patients with mitral valve prolapse who die suddenly have the following clinical and morphologic hallmarks
- Women aged 21–51, without significant MR (70%)
- Dilated mitral valve annulus (80%)
- Elongated anterior mitral valve leaflet (>80%)
- Abnormal elongated posterior mitral leaflet, often with herniation of the posterior leaflet above the anterior leaflet (approximately 80%)
- Fibrous endocardial plaque under the posterior mitral valve leaflet (≤75%)
- Significant, moderate to severe prolapse of the mitral valve (53%)
- Raptured chordae (33%)

- Significant, moderate or greater MR (10%)
- MR murmur (50%)
- A click is present (only 25–37%)
- Arrhythmia (>50%); VPCs (about 33%)
- The incidence of endocarditis in patients with true mitral valve prolapse is unknown but estimated to be about 1 in 6,000 in all patients with mitral valve prolapse and about 1 in 2000 of patients with MR (see Chap. 10)
- TIAs, stroke, retinal arteriolar occlusions, and amaurosis fugax are rare complications of mitral valve prolapse due to embolization of bland emboli. The exact incidence has not been accurately assessed

Therapy

- The physician must be careful in reassuring patients with mitral valve prolapse syndrome. Patients with billowing leaflets without genuine prolapse rarely get severe MR. Palpitations due to VPCs or occasionally runs of SVT usually require no drug therapy. Following reassurance, if episodes of VPCs or SVT are bothersome, and Holter monitoring demonstrates multiform VPCs, couplets or runs, nonsustained VT, or short bouts of SVT, a very small dose of a β-blocking drug is appropriate and the safest remedy. Metoprolol (25–50 mg bid) or atenolol (25–50 mg once daily) is advisable since both cause less fatigue than propranolol. Sotalol (80–160 mg once daily) is useful, but fatigue and the propensity to precipitate torsades de pointes, albeit rare, do not justify its use in this benign condition. Potentially lethal arrhythmias are rare with mitral valve prolapse and require higher doses of β blockers. Chest pain requires reassurance or the use of enteric coated aspirin (325 mg qd). If pain is bothersome or "angina like," a β-blocking drug should be administered with avoidance of nitrates, which reduce ventricular volume and thus ↑ the prolapse
- Small, bland emboli consisting of platelet and fibrin, which form in relation to the slightly abnormal valve apparatus, may cause TIAs or stroke. Management is with enteric coated aspirin (160–325 mg qd) or 1/4 of a regular 325-mg aspirin qd. If TIAs continue, it is advisable to add dipyridamole (75 mg tid). This drug is more effective when given on an empty stomach or 30 min before meals. However, it is expensive and of unproven value except when combined with aspirin. (The drug is ineffective when used without aspirin.)
- Severe MR due to mitral valve prolapse is managed with surgical reconstruction where possible, but in some cases, valve replacement is necessary. The same considerations apply as in other varieties of MR as discussed earlier in this chapter

RHEUMATIC FEVER

Rheumatic fever is now rare in North America and the Western world but is still prevalent in Asia, the Middle East, Africa, and Latin America, and is the most commonly acquired heart disease in childhood.

Clinical Features

The peak incidence is from age 5 to 15; rheumatic fever is uncommon < age 5 and virtually unknown < age 2. Symptoms are manifest 2–3

Table 12–11
Clinical and Morphologic Features in 15 Patients Dying Suddenly Secondary to Mitral Valve Prolapse

PT NO.	AGE (yr)	RACE	GENDER	MVP DIAGNOSED CLINICALLY	THE MARFAN SYNDROME	LOCATION OF DEATH	LAST ACTIVITY	AUSCULTATORY FINDINGS		
								SC	SM	SH
1	16	W	M	+	+	Basketball court	Sitting after playing	−	+	0
2	18	W	F	+	0	Home	Arguing	−	0	0
3	21	W	F	+	0	Work	Talking on phone	−	−	0
4	23	W	F	+	0	Work	Drinking water	+	+	0
5	26	W	F	+	0	Work	Talking	+	+	0
6	30	B	M	0	0	Work	Sitting alone	−	−	−
7	30	W	M	0	0	Golf course	Playing golf	−	−	0
8	40	W	F	0	+	Home	Playing with children	−	−	0
9	47	W	F	0	0	Home	Gardening	−	−	0
10	51	W	M	+	0	Restaurant	Sitting after fast dancing	+	+	0
11	53	W	F	+	0	Church	Sitting	−	−	0
12	53	W	F	0	0	Restaurant	Getting up to dance	−	−	−
13	55	W	F	+	0	Home	Standing	+	+	0
14	55	W	M	+	0	Home	Sleeping	−	+	0
15	69	W	F	0	0	Home	−	−	−	−

Table 12–11. *(continued)*

PT NO.	CHF	VFCS ON ECG	HW (g)	MV ANULUS (cm)	TV ANULUS (cm)	AML LENGTH (cm)	PML LENGTH (cm)	CHORDS MISSING	GRADE OF MVP (1–3+)	PLAQUE UNDER PML	MAC (0–4+)	VC PFO	REDUNDANT OF MEMBRANE
1	0	+	325	12.5	12	3	2.5	+	2	0	0	–	–
2	0	+*	220	9.6	11.5	2	1.5	0	1	+	0	0	0
3	0	–	360	14	–	3	1.5	+	2	0	1	–	–
4	0	–	280	10	9	2.5	2	0	3	+	0	+	+
5	0	0†	265	12	11	3	3	0	3	+	0	+	+
6	0	–	570	15.5	13	3	2.5	0	3	+	0	0	0
7	0	–	475	10	11	3	2	0	1	+	0	0	0
8	0	–	355	13	12	–	–	+	2	0	2	–	+
9	0	+	445	12.5	12.5	2.5	2	0	3	+	0	0	0
10	0	0	500	10.5	12	2	1.5	0	1	0	0	0	0
11	0	+	325	12.6	10.5	2.5	3	0	2	+	3	0	0
12	0	–	390	13.6	11	3.5	3	0	3	+	1	+	+
13	0	+	390	13	13	3	2.5	+	3	+	0	0	0
14	+	+	670	>12	14	3.5	2	0	3	+	0	+	0
15	0	–	400	15.4	14.5	2.5	3	+	3	+	0	0	0

* This patient had survived a cardiac arrest 2 years earlier; † this patient had a history of paroxysmal atrial trachycardia.

AML = anterior mitral leaflet; B = black; CHF = congestive heart failure; F = female; FO = fossa ovale; HW = heart weight; M = male; MVP = mitral valve prolapse; MAC = mitral annular calcification; PFO = patent foramen ovale; PML = posterior mitral leaflet; Pt = patient; SC = systolic click; SH = systemic hypertension; SM = systolic murmur; TV = tricuspid valve; VC = valvular competent; VPC = ventricular premature complex; W = white; + = present; 0 = absent; – = no information available.

From Dollar AL, et al.: Morphologic comparison of patients with mitral valve prolapse who died suddenly with patients who died from severe valvular dysfunction or other conditions. J Am Coll Cardiol, *17*:921, 1991.

weeks after Group A streptococcal pharyngitis, which causes a hyperimmune reaction in susceptible individuals.

Symptoms and signs include

- Fever for 2–3 weeks
- Anorexia
- Weight loss
- Arthritis in >80% of patients, especially in older patients. It takes the form of flitting or migratory polyarthritis. Pain, redness, and swelling usually occur in large joints, knees, elbows, wrists, and shoulders; notably, the last joint is rarely involved in other arthritides. A single joint is inflamed for about 1 day to 1 week; the pain resolves completely and then moves on to the second joint. There is typically no deformity of joints
- Sinus tachycardia
- SQ nodules in ≤12% of cases
- Erythema marginatum in ≤10% of individuals. This is an effervescent, nonpruritic rash with pink circumscribed circles with a pale center mainly involving the trunk
- Sydenham's chorea (St. Vitus dance), which may last for weeks to months, rarely for a few years
- Pancarditis, which is more common in the young, who have minimal or no arthritis. When rheumatic fever "licks" the joints, the disease often spares the heart
- New murmurs, friction rub, cardiomegaly, and CHF, which indicate pancarditis
- An apical pansystolic murmur Grade I-II, which is common with valvular involvement and is usually accompanied by the Carey-Coombs murmur. A short, low-pitched rumbling, mid diastolic apical murmur. Its presence serves to distinguish the systolic murmur of carditis from common innocent systolic murmurs that are typically early or mid systolic vibratory murmurs or a scratchy short ejection systolic murmur located between the pulmonary area and the lower left sternal edge
- 1st° A-V block or, rarely, bundle branch block

Therapy

- Prophylaxis of rheumatic fever requires aggressive treatment of the initial attack of pharyngitis with oral penicillin G, 500 mg immediately then 250 mg qid for 10 days, or I.M. benzathine penicillin G, 1.2 million U in patients >60 lbs. and 600,000 U for patients <60 lbs. Erythromycin (250 mg qid) or clindamycin (150 mg q 8 h) is administered to patients allergic to penicillin
- Arthritis is controlled with enteric coated aspirin (100 mg/kg qd) in 4 divided doses to achieve a blood level of 20–25 mg/dl. Corticosteroids should be avoided because they produce no better results than aspirin
- Pancarditis requires modified bedrest for several weeks until signs of carditis are improved or unchanging. The sedimentation rate should revert to normal, and the C-reactive protein should become negative. Enteric coated aspirin should be given if fever and carditis are present, as well as for arthritis. Corticosteroids are not usually indicated and are used only if carditis is progressive with manifestation of cardiomegaly and CHF. When required, prednisone (60–80 mg/day; 1.0–1.5 mg/kg/day) is administered in 4 doses for a period of 4–6 weeks. The dose is then reduced slowly with maintenance of aspirin. The possibility of steroid rebound may be reduced by employing aspirin as overlap-

ping therapy with steroids for 2–3 weeks, during which time the steroids are weaned off. Pericarditis should be managed with aspirin

- Secondary rheumatic fever prevention is important to prevent recurrence since valvular damage is more intense with each recurrence of rheumatic fever. Management is with benzathine penicillin G (1.2 million U I.M. q 4 weeks), commonly used in North America and Europe; in endemic areas, 3 weekly injections are advisable. Penicillin is continued for at least 20 years after the initial attack of rheumatic fever or to age 45, whichever occurs first. Patients allergic to penicillin are treated with sulfonamides: 1 g of oral sulfadiazine daily for patients >60 lbs. and 0.5 g once daily for patients <60 lbs., with liberal fluid intake

Suggested Reading

Bernard Y, Etievent J, Mourand JL: Long-term results of percutaneous aortic valvuloplasty compared with aortic valve replacement in patients more than 75 years old. J Am Coll Cardiol *20*: 795, 1992.

Khan M Gabriel: Valvular heart disease and rheumatic fever. *In* Cardiac and Pulmonary Management. Philadelphia, Lea & Febiger, 1993.

Pericarditis/Cardiac Tamponade

13

M. Gabriel Khan

PERICARDITIS

The common causes of pericarditis are listed in Table 13–1. The division into obvious causes based on the presence of an easily recognizable underlying disease, and causes that are not obvious, but easily excluded by history and physical and finally nonspecific pericarditis probably caused by viral infections, provides for easy recall.

Chest pain

- Is typically retrosternal or left precordial
- Occasionally radiates to the trapezius ridge (a radiation that does not occur with angina)
- May radiate to the neck or left arm and may simulate angina or MI
- At times is localized to the epigastrium or left upper quadrant
- Is sharp, pleuritic, but may be described as an oppressive, dull, vague ache
- Is increased by deep inspiration, coughing, swallowing, recumbency
- Is relieved by sitting and leaning forward

Genuine shortness of breath or forced, shallow breathing due to pain, as well as palpitations, are common features. Underlying infection may cause fever and myalgia.

A pericardial friction rub is characteristically

- Heard between the lower left sternal edge and apex
- Localized to any area or over most of the precordium
- Heard with the diaphragm pressed firmly against the chest wall, with the patient leaning forward with the breath held
- Absent if effusion develops

The 4 stages of ECG abnormalities are given in Table 13–2

- Sinus tachycardia is common and may be the only ECG finding if ST elevation has resolved and the T waves remain normal
- ST segment elevation, when present, is concave upward with no T wave inversion. With MI, the ST segment is convex, often with Q waves present, and the T waves begin to invert before the ST segment normalizes

Echocardiography is necessary to detect and quantitate associated pericardial effusion and to assess tamponade.

Idiopathic and Viral Pericarditis

Most cases of idiopathic pericarditis are caused by viral infections (Table 13–1). The patient should be hospitalized and observed for tamponade.

Table 13–1
Causes of pericarditis

- Obvious causes (Underlying diseases)
  - Post MI
    - early
    - late (Dressler's)
  - Renal failure
  - Neoplastic
  - Tuberculosis
  - Septicemia (purulent)
  - Endocarditis
  - Collagen disease
    - rheumatic fever, rheumatoid arthritis, lupus, scleroderma
  - Trauma
    - ↓ Iatrogenic
      - surgery
      - catheter
      - pacemaker
- Not obvious (but easily excluded by history and physical examination)
  - Drugs
    - anticoagulants
    - cromolyn
    - daunorubicin
    - dantrolene
    - hydralazine
    - isoniazid
    - methysergide
    - minoxidil
    - procainamide
    - phenytoin
  - Radiation
  - Myxedema
- Viral infections
  - Coxsackie B_5 B_6
  - Echovirus
  - HIV, Epstein-Barr
  - Influenza, mumps, varicella, rubella (Mycoplasma)
- Idiopathic
  - Probable viral

The occurrence of tamponade is manifested by: Hemodynamic compromise; elevation of the JVP; pulsus paradoxus; and usually hypotension, which may mask pulsus paradoxus.

Echocardiography helps confirm the pericarditis or tamponade. Pericardiocentesis is not done routinely, even with moderate-sized effusions, if tamponade is not present. If pain is bothersome, the patient should rest in bed and chair for a few days, followed by slow ambulation over 1–2 weeks.

Table 13–2
Electrocardiographic Clues to Pericarditis

STAGE I (hours to days)	Widespread ST segment elevation 2–5 mm concave upward LI, II, III, V_2–V_5; reciprocal depression AVR V_1
STAGE II (few days later)	ST and PR segments isoelectric, upright or flattened T
STAGE III	After normalization of ST segment, diffuse T wave inversion occurs
STAGE IV (days to weeks)	T waves normalize, rarely remain inverted

Management of Pain. Pain is relieved by aspirin or other NSAIDs: Ibuprofen, 400 mg q 6 or 8 h, Indomethacin, 25–50 mg q 8 h, or Naproxen, 250 mg tid for 4–10 days. Modified bedrest and increasing dosage of NSAIDs with adequate gastric cytoprotection usually brings relief of pain without major adverse effects.

It is not advisable to commence corticosteroids solely for the relief of pain, because these agents may ↑ viral replication. Corticosteroids are indicated when there is total failure of high-dose NSAIDs used over several weeks and with relapsing pericarditis not controlled by NSAIDs.

Dexamethasone. Dosage: IV 4 mg may relieve pain in a few hours.

Prednisone. Dosage: 60 mg qd for a few days, ↓ by 10 mg q 3–5 days until a dose of 15 mg is reached. If symptoms are controlled, it is advisable to give 15 mg on alternate days for 5 days, and then 10 mg alternate days for 5 days, 5 mg alternate days for 5 days, and discontinue. The course of prednisone should be tapered as quickly as feasible. NSAIDs are added at adequate dosage when the corticosteroid dose has reached 15 mg qd, and gastric cryoprotective agents are used if there is a history of previous peptic ulceration or if gastric symptoms are present.

Approximately 25% of patients experience recurrence; if effusion develops, the risk of tamponade is high. In the absence of CHF or tamponade, patients with severe recurrent chest pain unrelieved by adequate doses of NSAIDs may require corticosteroids for control of pain, fever, and shortness of breath. Alternate-day therapy carries less risk of adverse effects.

Pericarditis Due to Specific Causes

Post-infarction pericarditis. Acute pericarditis occurs in approximately 10% of patients within 12 h to 10 days after infarction. The pain may be confused with post-infarction angina, extension of infarction, or pulmonary embolism. Most cases occur on the third or fourth day post infarction. Chest pain is best treated with aspirin. NSAIDs such as indomethacin, ibuprofen, and naproxen should be avoided because they appear to interfere with the healing of infarcted tissue and have been shown to cause infarct expansion and to accelerate remodeling.

Dressler's Syndrome occurs in <0.1% of patients, usually weeks or months after MI, and may be an immune reaction. Pleuritic chest pain, fever, friction rub, leukocytosis, and increased sedimentation rate simulate nonspecific pericarditis. Enteric coated aspirin, 650 mg bid or tid for 1–2 weeks, should suffice. If pain remains bothersome or is recurrent, NSAIDs should be tried. Occasionally, corticosteroids are necessary and should be given as prescribed under Idiopathic and Viral Pericarditis.

Purulent pericarditis usually occurs during septicemia caused by pneumococcus, meningococcus, hemophilus, gonococcus, and other organisms. Pericardiocentesis is indicated in patients suspected of purulent pericarditis in order to isolate microorganisms and determine sensitivities and the appropriate choice of antibiotics. Cardiothoracic surgical assistance often is required for open pericardial drainage or creation of a pericardiopleural window.

Tuberculous pericarditis. In Asia, Africa, the Middle East, Latin America, and some nonindustrialized countries, tuberculosis is the most common cause of pericarditis. In North America and Europe, tuberculosis is responsible for about 4%, 7%, and 6% of acute pericarditis, tamponade, and constrictive pericarditis, respectively. Diagnosis requires isolation of myocobacterium tuberculosis in pericardial fluid or a histologic examination of pericardial tissue or proven active tuberculosis in other organs. Tuberculous pericarditis is more common in blacks, is commonly seen in patients with AIDS, and has a peak incidence in patients 30–60 years of age.

Symptoms and signs include

- Cough
- Weight loss
- Dyspnea, occasionally orthopnea
- Fever, chills, and night sweats sometimes for several months before signs of pericarditis occur
- Cardiomegaly
- Possibly a pericardial friction rub plus signs of tamponade
- Hepatomegaly (>90% of patients)
- Ascites (fairly common)
- Cardiac arrhythmias, especially AF or flutter

Echocardiographic and CT examination may reveal pericardial effusion and pericardial thickening.

The patient should be hospitalized, observed for tamponade, and given therapy with isoniazid (300 mg), pyridoxine (50 mg), rifampin (600 mg), and ethambutol (15 mg/kg) qd for at least 9 months, allowing a minimum of 6 months of drug treatment following culture conversion. The combination of isoniazid (300 mg) and rifampin (600 mg) qd for 9 months has been shown to produce a satisfactory response in 95% of patients with extrapulmonary tuberculosis (see Chapter 18).

Corticosteroid therapy is indicated for recurrent or persistent pericardial effusion in patients receiving adequate courses of antituberculous therapy. This therapy may cause the avoidance of pericardial resection, which appears to be required in 7–40% of patients adequately treated with antituberculous drugs. Although some series show a high incidence of pericardial constriction, pericardiectomy is not routinely recommended. In a study by Strang, et al., only 17 of 240 patients treated with prednisolone in addition to antituberculous drugs for 11 weeks required pericardiectomy, and prednisolone therapy reduced overall mortality from 14% to 3%. <u>Dosage:</u> Prednisone or prednisolone, 40–60 mg qd in 2 divided doses.

Uremic pericarditis. Pericardiocentesis is required only if there is suspicion of purulent infection or tamponade. The condition usually subsides with more frequent dialysis. Recurrent effusions uncontrolled by dialysis may respond to instillation of triamcinolone into the pericardial sac.

The instillation of sclerosing agents is of benefit in some patients with neoplastic pericarditis.

CARDIAC TAMPONADE

Tamponade may occur acutely secondary to

- Chest trauma. An individual who has sustained recent chest trauma and appears in shock with increased venous pressure should be suspected of having cardiac tamponade
- Acute MI with freewall rupture
- Dissecting aneurysm

Acute or subacute presentations occasionally occur with

- Neoplastic involvement

- Nonspecific pericarditis
- Uremia or purulent infections

Sudden progressive severe shortness of breath, chest tightness, or dysphagia may herald the shock-like state. The JVP is usually elevated; hypotension and tachycardia are usually present.

Diagnostic Hallmarks

Significant pulsus paradoxus is usually detectable, except when severe hypotension or elevation of the diastolic pressure of either ventricle is present; for example, with uremic pericarditis and hypertension. Thus, the physician should not be lulled into a sense of false security by the absence of paradoxus. Pulsus paradoxus is an exaggeration of the normal inspiratory decline of systemic arterial pressure. To determine the presence of significant pulsus paradoxus, the patient's respirations are observed while slowly deflating the BP cuff. Initially, the Korotkoff sound is heard only on expiration, but as the cuff pressure is lowered, Korotkoff sounds are heard during inspiration; the difference in systolic BP recorded at the commencement of the Korotkoff sounds in inspiration and expiration is an estimate of pulsus parodoxus. Normally, this difference is <10 mm Hg. Pulsus paradoxus >12 mm Hg is significant. Muffled heart sounds represent another hallmark.

Pulsus paradoxus may be observed in several conditions, including

- Severe COPD
- Status asthmaticus
- Pneumothorax
- Massive pulmonary embolism

However, in COPD and asthma, the JVP falls normally on inspiration. With right ventricular infarction, the venous pressure is high but increases on inspiration (Kussmaul's sign), and pulsus paradoxus is absent. Massive pulmonary embolism may produce a shock-like state with markedly elevated JVP and represents a diagnostic challenge, but the clinical setting usually assists in differentiating the 2 conditions.

Cardiac tamponade and cardiogenic shock secondary to acute MI may be difficult to differentiate, and both may occur during the course of massive infarction, but tamponade is uncommon. Heart sounds may be faint in both conditions.

Severe CHF causing marked elevation of JVP can be confused with cardiac tamponade. It is important to differentiate the 2 conditions, since the use of diuretics is contraindicated in the presence of tamponade. Because the most common cause of right HF is left HF, pulmonary congestion is usually detectable with the presence of crackles, third heart sound, radiologic evidence of pulmonary congestion, and LV failure. Pulsus paradoxus is not a feature of severe CHF, and the presence of a prominent V wave in the venous pulse indicates tricuspid regurgitation and CHF.

Cardiac regional tamponade causing hemodynamic deterioration may occur within the first 2 weeks of cardiac surgery or in conditions causing adhesions and loculation. In these situations, pulsus paradoxus may be absent and the echocardiogram may fail to show effusion all around the heart. In patients with suspected cardiac tamponade, urgent echocardiography is mandatory.

Echocardiographic features include

- An early finding of right atrial collapse, which occurs in most cases except regional tamponade, in which right or left atrial collapse may be observed
- Right ventricular collapse

Therapy

- Maintenance of an adequate preload so as to generate stroke volume. Thus, diuretics and preload-reducing agents such as nitrates and ACE inhibitors must be avoided. Volume expansion with saline and even transfusion with packed red cells may provide hemodynamic stability until pericardiocentesis is accomplished. It is important to maintain volume expansion so that right atrial pressure may be maintained above intrapericardial pressure in order to prevent right atrial or ventricular collapse
- Pericardiocentesis carried out by an experienced cardiologist under echocardiographic control or by a cardiac thoracic surgeon. An indwelling pericardial catheter with multiple side holes may be used for drainage and for installation of antibiotics, triamcinolone, or chemotherapeutic agents. Failure of pericardiocentesis is usually due to a posteriorly located effusion. Reaccumulation of fluid and recurrent tamponade are indications for subxiphoid pericardial window drainage carried out by a cardiothoracic surgeon

CONSTRICTIVE PERICARDITIS

The proper management of constrictive pericarditis begins with correct diagnosis. Common causes include

- Neoplastic disease, especially carcinoma of lung, or breast asbestosis and lymphoma
- Mediastinal irradiation
- Nonviral pericardial infections
- Viral pericarditis
- Tuberculosis
- Post-cardiac surgery
- Chest trauma
- Connective tissue diseases
- Chronic renal failure and dialysis

Diagnostic Hallmarks

- If the JVP is both markedly and chronically elevated and the history and physical examination fail to suggest an apparent cardiac cause in the presence of a small quiet heart, then a restrictive syndrome must be considered, the most common cause being constrictive pericarditis. Neck vein examination should reveal Kussmaul's sign, which may be difficult to elicit when the venous pressure is severely elevated. The venous pulse usually has a prominent y-descent, coincident with the early rapid diastolic filling of the ventricle. A prominent x-descent, coincident with filling of the atrium, is often observed in patients with sinus rhythm. The exaggerated x- and y-descents give the venous pressure a characteristic M- or W-shaped pattern (Table 13–3)
- Auscultation should reveal the presence of an early high-frequency third heart sound (S3) caused by abrupt cessation of early diastolic filling. This sound, referred to as a pericardial knock, occurs earlier than the conventional third heart sound of CHF and has a sharp, high-pitched quality that is easily heard with the diaphragm and may

Table 13–3
Constrictive Pericarditis vs. Restrictive Cardiomyopathy

	CONSTRICTIVE PERICARDITIS	RESTRICTIVE CARDIOMYOPATHY
Clinical Features		
Heart size	Usually normal	Usually large
Heart impulse	Quiet	LV and/or right ventricular dilatation
JVP	M pattern*	M pattern
Kussmaul's sign	Present	Present
Systolic (v) waves	Absent	Present (tricuspid regurgitation)
Systolic murmurs	Rare	Common
S3 gallop**	Present	Present (except in amyloid)
Chest X-Ray	Clear lung fields	Similar
	Normal heart size	Similar or moderately enlarged
	Pericardial calcification (50%)	Rare Myocardial calcification not uncommon
ECG	P mitrale	Uncommon
	Atrial fibrillation 33%	Common
	Conduction defects uncommon	Common
	Flat or inverted T waves common	Widespread T wave inversion common
	May show low voltage	Low voltage common
	Q waves very rare	QS precordial leads, pseudoinfarction pattern common
Echocardiogram	Thickened pericardium	
	Calcified pericardium	No pericardial calcification, myocardial calcification
	Normal septal motion	
Systemic Disease (associated)	Tuberculosis	Amyloid; sarcoid; tuberculosis (See text)
CT or MRI scan	Thickened pericardium	Normal pericardium

* Due to exaggerated x- and y-descents
** Pericardial knock

mimic an opening snap or early filling sound heard in endomyocardial fibrosis

- AF occurs in approximately 33% of cases of constrictive pericarditis
- The presence of marked ascites, occurring days to weeks before the presence of significant edema, points strongly to constrictive pericarditis and serves to distinguish the condition from CHF, in which prominent edema occurs, followed weeks later by mild ascites. In a few

patients with longstanding constriction and congestion, protein-losing gastroenteropathy may ensue

- Patients who present with noncalcific constrictive pericarditis pose a diagnostic problem. Table 13-3 gives diagnostic points for constrictive pericarditis versus restrictive cardiomyopathy

Investigations

A few or all of the following investigations may be required to ascertain the diagnosis

- Chest x ray may show pericardial calcification, especially of the apex and posteriorly, which is best seen on lateral views. The heart size is usually normal
- ECG is virtually always abnormal but nonspecific and shows diffuse flat or inverted T wave in >75% of patients; the depth of inversion of the T waves is usually proportional to the degree of pericardial adher-

Table 13–4
Catheterization Data

PARAMETERS	CONSTRICTIVE PERICARDITIS	RESTRICTIVE CARDIOMYOPATHY
Diastolic pressure	Equalization of early & late diastolic pressures	LV > right* Rarely LV-right and resembles constrictive pericarditis
LVEDP-RVEDP ≥6 mm Hg (predictive value 87%)**	Usual finding (few exceptions)	Usually >6, but significant overlap
LA pressure	Equal right	Higher than right; may equalize with severe tricuspid regurgitation
RV pressure square root sign	Always present: early dip and plateau during diastole	Present, but may disappear with therapy
Pulmonary hypertension	Mild	Moderate or severe
RV systolic pressure ≥52 mm Hg** (predictive value 71%)	Usual finding	Wide range (30 to 85 mm Hg)
RVEDP/RV systolic ≥0.38** (predictive value 83%)	Usual finding	Variable, significant overlap

LV = left ventricular
RV = right ventricular
EDP = end diastolic pressure
LA = left atrial
* = both measured simultaneously
** = modified from Vaitkus PT, Kussmaul WG: Constrictive pericarditis versus restrictive cardiomyopathy: A reappraisal and update of diagnostic criteria. Am Heart J, *122*:1431, 1991.

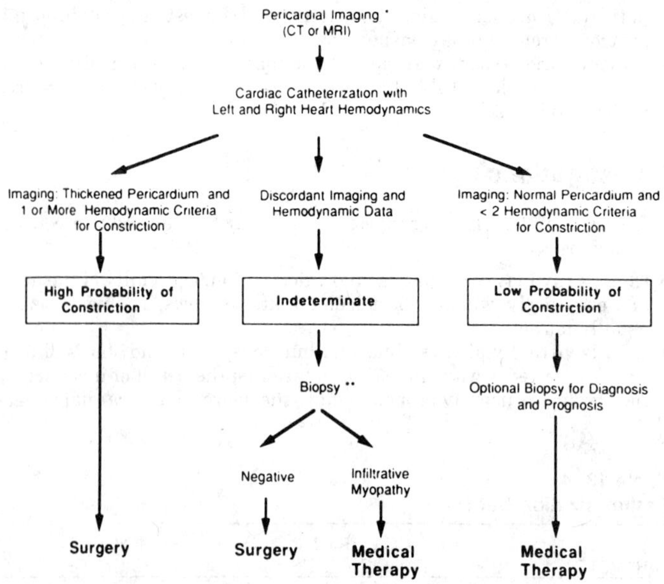

Figure 13–1. Algorithm for evaluating patients with a clinical profile consistent with construction or restriction. *If chest x-ray films reveal a calcified pericardium, more sophisticated imaging modalities (i.e., CT or MRI) are unnecessary. **If endomyocardial biopsy is unavailable, surgery should be pursued in this setting. From: Vaitkius PT, et al.: Constrictive pericarditis versus restrictive cardiomyopathy: A reappraisal and update of diagnostic criteria. Am Heart J, *122*:1431, 1991.

ence to the myocardium, which may make stripping difficult. Low voltage is present in approximately 50% of cases, along with P-mitral. AF is present in approximately 33% of patients

- Echocardiography is of limited value in identifying thickened pericardium, unless calcification is present. Doppler echocardiography shows typical Doppler features in both mitral and hepatic vein flow in approximately 85% of patients with constriction amenable to surgery
- Ultrafast cine-CT and/or MRI fairly accurately assess pericardial thickness, pericardial impingement on the right ventricle, and the degree of dilation of the vena cavae and hepatic veins
- Cardiac catheterization findings are listed in Table 13–4. Elevation and equalization of all diastolic pressures and the dip and plateau or square root sign are typical findings, but these may be observed in some patients with RCM. As outlined above, CT and MRI are useful in differentiating these 2 categories of patients (see Fig. 13–1 and Table 13–3)
- It is important to avoid diuretics prior to catheter studies, because Na and water loss may cause equalization of left and right ventricular filling pressures in patients with RCM

Therapy

Surgical pericardiectomy is needed when medical therapy, with the judicious use of diuretics and digoxin for control of the ventricular response in patients with AF, fails to reduce markedly elevated JVP and when symptoms are persistent and bothersome. Early surgical mortality is approximately 5%. In patients with severe calcific disease, recovery may be delayed for weeks or months. If constriction and restriction are both present, pericardiectomy may not cause symptomatic improvement.

Suggested Reading

Vaitkus PT, Kussmaul WG: Constrictive pericarditis versus restrictive cardiomyopathy: A reappraisal and update of diagnostic criteria. Am Heart J *122*:1431, 1991.

Cardiomyopathy, Specific Heart Muscle Disease

14

M. Gabriel Khan and John F. Goodwin

Cardiomyopathy is defined as heart muscle disease of unknown cause. Cardiomyopathies are classified as: hypertrophic, dilated, and restrictive.

Heart muscle disease from known causes, particularly infiltrative or systemic disease, formerly termed secondary cardiomyopathy, is currently referred to as specific heart muscle disease and is discussed at the end of this chapter.

HYPERTROPHIC CARDIOMYOPATHY

HCM refers to a condition in which massive ventricular hypertrophy occurs in the absence of any definite cause. The term hypertrophic cardiomyopathy is preferred because not all affected patients have idiopathic hypertrophic subaortic stenosis or features of hypertrophic obstructive cardiomyopathy. Approximately 33% of patients have no significant LV outflow tract gradient at rest or on provocation.

The myofibrillar disarray commonly seen in HCM is believed to be caused by an aberration of catecholamine function in the heart of the embryo. Familial cases show an autosomal dominant trait linked to chromosome 14q1.

Pathophysiology

- Most patients show asymmetric hypertrophy of the septum and a hypertrophied nondilated left and/or right ventricle. But the septum may be diffusely hypertrophied or only in its upper, mid, or apical portion. Hypertrophy extends to the freewall of the left ventricle
- Decreased compliance and incomplete relaxation of the left ventricle cause impedance to diastolic filling
- Rapid, powerful contraction of the hypertrophied left ventricle expels most of its contents in the first half of systole. This hyperdynamic systolic function is apparent in most patients with HCM
- The anterior leaflet of the mitral valve is displaced toward the hypertrophied septum. MR is virtually always present in the obstructive phase of the disease. Therefore the sequence of events is: eject, obstruct, leak. A variable LV outflow pressure gradient at rest occurs in approximately 35% of patients. A further 25% develop a similar gradient precipitated by conditions that ↑ myocardial contractility or ↓ ventricular volume. Thus, diuretics and other causes of hypovolemia and preload-reducing agents that ↓ the volume of the small ventricular cavity may increase gradients.
- Fibrosis and occlusive disease in small coronary arteries and arterioles may occur. The major coronary arteries are wide and patent unless

occlusive atherosclerotic coronary disease occurs as a chance association

Clinical Hallmarks

- Dyspnea caused by raised LV end diastolic pressure
- Angina resulting from reduced diastolic coronary perfusion
- Presyncope or syncope during exercise, normal activities, or at rest, not simply related to failure to ↑ cardiac output on exercise
- May present with palpitations or symptoms and signs of CHF

Table 14–1 gives the predominant symptoms and signs and their approximate incidence. General physique is usually normal and well developed. The palpable left atrial beat preceding the LV thrust is a most important sign, since it can occur in the absence of gradient or murmur.

The murmur has typical features

- Crescendo-decrescendo starts well after the first heart sound and ends well before the second. It is best heard between the apex and left sternal border
- Radiates poorly to the neck
- Intensity increases with maneuvers or drugs that ↓ preload (valsalva, standing, amyl nitrate) and decreases in intensity with a ↑ in afterload (squatting, hand grip, phenylephrine)
- Easy to distinguish from aortic valvular stenosis, in which the murmur starts soon after the first heart sound and radiates well to the neck

Table 14–1
Clinical Hallmarks of Hypertrophic Cardiomyopathy

SYMPTOMS AND SIGNS	APPROXIMATE INCIDENCE (%)	FACTORS
Dyspnea	80	Diastolic dysfunction
Angina	60	Decreased coronary reserve, small vessel disease, or associated CHD
Presyncope	50	Even at rest
Syncope	20	Post-exertional and normal activities
Sudden death/annual		
Adult	2.5	Mainly arrhythmic
Children	6	
Annual mortality	4	
Brisk carotid upstroke	90	
Atrial fibrillation	15	
Left atrial beat	50	
Left ventricular thrust	60	
4th heart sound	50	
3rd heart sound	30	
Systolic murmur, late onset crescendo-decrescendo	90	Begins well after S1 Little or no radiation to neck or axilla, outflow gradient
Mitral systolic murmur	50	Mitral regurgitation, radiates to axilla

An MR murmur is often heard in the last half of the systole with radiation to the axilla. It is usually associated with an outflow tract gradient. A mitral diastolic rumble may be detected.

It must be emphasized that the physical examination may be relatively unremarkable in HCM; attention is necessary to elucidate 3 subtle signs: rapid carotid upstroke, abnormal cardiac impulse, and gallop sounds.

HCM causes a brisk carotid upstroke because of the dynamic LV emptying, giving an ill-sustained quality, whereas aortic valvular stenosis produces a slow-rising pulse, with a delayed carotid upstroke.

Supraventricular arrhythmias occur in 20–50% of patients, and ventricular arrhythmias occur in almost all patients.

Unfortunately, the pathophysiologic mechanism of sudden death remains unresolved. Patients presumed to be at risk for sudden death include those who

- Are <20 years of age at time of diagnosis
- Are <20 years of age and have a family history of HCM and sudden death
- Have potentially lethal ventricular arrhythmias, sustained VT, nonsustained VT, and frequent multiform ventricular ectopics
- Have a history of syncope
- Have severe exertional dyspnea or orthopnea in association with ventricular arrhythmias

Studies indicate that death cannot be predicted adequately by the following conventional criteria.

The presence of sustained, or nonsustained, VT, or of multiform ventricular ectopy reflects a high risk, but in childhood, the absence of potentially lethal ventricular arrhythmias on 48-hour Holter monitoring must not be interpreted as a lowered risk. Mildly symptomatic or asymptomatic patients who die suddenly have marked LVH. Some evidence indicates that mildly symptomatic patients who have HCM with mild LVH have a low incidence of sudden cardiac death. The commencement of AF with loss of atrial function may precipitate pulmonary edema or hypotension

- AF occurs in approximately 15% of patients with HCM. The loss of atrial systole with a fast ventricular response may precipitate pulmonary edema and, occasionally, severe hypotension. The outcome for patients with HCM and AF is not as bleak as envisaged in the 1970s and 1980s, however. The outlook is not significantly worse for patients with AF and failure to convert than it is for patients with sinus rhythm. Functional class does deteriorate with the onset of AF, but it improves with conversion and control of ventricular response or when chronic AF with controlled ventricular response is achieved
- The chest x ray may be normal but often shows some left atrial enlargement; the left ventricle ranges from normal to severe enlargement. Aortic valve calcification is absent in HCM, but annular calcification of the mitral valve occurs
- ECG findings: Virtually always abnormal (95%) in patients with significant symptomatic HCM and about 80% abnormal in asymptomatic patients. AF in 15%; an additional 33% have paroxysmal episodes. Other supraventricular and ventricular arrhythmias, nonsustained VT is common, but sustained VT occurs in approximately 3%. Deep, narrow Q waves in about 30% in leads II III AVF, V5–V6 or in I, AVL V5–V6, rarely V1–V3 which may mimic infarction. Intraventricular conduction delay in >80%. High QRS voltage LVH. Diffuse T wave changes in some patients or T waves of LVH. Giant inverted T waves, very high precordial QRS voltage with apical HCM. ST segment

Table 14–2
Echocardiographic Hallmarks of Hypertrophic Cardiomyopathy

1. Disproportionate septal thickness, septum to posterior wall ratio >1.5
2. Left ventricular myocardial segment >1.5 cm in thickness
3. Poor septal contraction, hypercontractile free posterior wall
4. Systolic anterior motion of the mitral valve when outflow tract gradient >30 mm Hg
5. Mid systolic aortic valve closure
6. Small left ventricular cavity, typically with virtual elimination in systole
7. Mitral regurgitation frequently present
8. Left ventricular outflow tract gradient at rest in about 35% of patients

depression in some. PR interval occasionally short; pre-excitation may be seen

- Two-dimensional echocardiographic observation of a LV myocardial segment of ≥1.5 cm thickness in a normal-sized adult is considered diagnostic, if there is no other evident cause (Table 14–2 gives echocardiographic hallmarks). Asymmetric hypertrophy is supporting evidence. Myocardial mass increases with age and size. Continuous-wave Doppler echocardiography defines the degree of LV outflow-tract gradient
- A 48-hour Holter monitor is necessary because a 24-hour study detects <50% runs of nonsustained VT. Repeated studies may be required. Where facilities exist, a signal-averaged ECG is advisable, especially in younger patients. In this subgroup, an abnormal signal-averaged ECG appears to be a marker for sudden death. Further studies are necessary to confirm the role of the signal-averaged ECG in patients with HCM

Therapy

Management of the patient with HCM includes counseling and entails screening of all 1st° relatives of newly diagnosed cases. An ECG, chest x ray, and echocardiogram should usually suffice to identify affected individuals, but cases can still be missed.

Holter monitoring and/or examination of relatives is important

- Patients must be instructed to avoid strenuous competitive exercise because it can cause sudden death. A ↓ in ventricular volume or ↑ in ventricular contractility increases the outflow gradient. Thus, dehydration and the use of preload-reducing agents, such as diuretics, nitrates, or ACE inhibitors, should be avoided
- Beta agonists ↑ contractility and are contraindicated
- Digoxin increases contractility and its use should be avoided, except in the management of chronic AF, a fast ventricular response uncontrolled by amiodarone, β blockers, or verapamil. Also useful in patients with end-stage disease with CHF (see Table 14–3)
- Drugs that ↓ myocardial contractility or produce myocardial relaxation, particularly β blockers and Ca antagonists, play a major role in the control of symptoms
- Patients without significant obstruction with moderate MR and end-stage disease with CHF and ventricular dilatation may benefit from the judicious use of ACE inhibitors (Table 14–3)

Clinical trials have documented the role of β blockers in the manage-

Table 14–3
Pharmacologic and Surgical Interventions for the Obstructive and End-Stage Phase of Hypertrophic Cardiomyopathy

INTERVENTION	OBSTRUCTIVE PHASE	END STAGE
Negative inotropes		
Beta blockers	Yes (especially with latent obstruction)	Small dose considered
Verapamil	Yes	Contraindicated
Disopyramide	Yes	Contraindicated
Digoxin	Contraindicated	Needed & useful
Diuretics	Contraindicated	Needed & useful
Afterload-reducing agent:		
ACE inhibitors	Contraindicated	Of some benefit in patients with ventricular dilatation and heart failure
Surgery	Myectomy	Transplant

ment of HCM. Beta blockers and verapamil are equally effective for the management of symptoms, but β blockers generally are safer and therefore are considered first-line therapy. Beneficial effects of β-adrenergic blocking drugs include the following

- ↓ in myocardial contractility causes a ↓ in "venturi" effect and therefore less gradient
- Relief of dyspnea in about 40% of patients
- Significant relief of angina in 33–66% of patients
- The HR should be maintained between 55 and 60 beats/min; this results in an improvement in coronary filling because of prolongation of the diastolic interval
- Improvement in diastolic dysfunction
- Partial control of supraventricular and ventricular arrhythmias

Contraindications for individual β blockers: see Chapters 1 and 2.

Propranolol. _Dosage:_ 10 mg tid, ↑ slowly to 120 mg tid. A slow buildup of the dosage to 320 mg may be required or an equivalent dose of atenolol or metoprolol.

Calcium antagonists. Verapamil enhances LV diastolic filling by improving ventricular relaxation, actions similar to those produced by β-adrenergic blockade. Considerable experience with verapamil is now available, but the initial high expectations have not materialized and the drug has caused deaths. Verapamil decreases dyspnea and increases exercise capacity in some patients but does not appear to improve survival; it is contraindicated in patients with end-stage disease associated with ventricular dilatation and CHF. _Dosage:_ 40 mg tid or 80 mg bid, ↑ slowly over weeks to 120 bid under close observation. Preferably, administration of the drug is begun in the hospital setting. _Adverse Effects:_ High-grade A-V block, asystole, sinus arrest, acute pulmonary edema, hypotension. _Contraindications:_ Orthopnea or PND (deaths have occurred in these patients as a result of verapamil use); CHF and/or end-stage disease (Table 14–3); sick sinus syndrome; A-V block and conduction defects. _Interactions:_ See Table 1–8.

Amiodarone has gained widespread acceptance as a major advance in the management of patients with AF and, in others, to reduce the incidence of ventricular arrhythmias and sudden death where the risk is assessed to be high. See Chapter 6 for indications, dosage, and adverse effects.

Sotalol is a useful alternative to amiodarone. *Dosage:* 80 mg bid increasing to 240 mg/day if needed.

Anticoagulants are indicated in all patients with AF, to prevent embolism at the time of DC conversion, and when waiting for amiodarone to produce conversion. Patients who remain in AF while on amiodarone should receive anticoagulants, but with careful monitoring of INR or prothrombin time since amiodarone enhances the activity of coumarins and life-threatening bleeding can be precipitated.

Surgery/septal resection, mitral valve surgery. Indications include the following

- Patients who have had adequate trials of β blockers, verapamil, or amiodarone plus β blocker and remain severely symptomatic with angina and dyspnea
- Outflow gradient >50 mm Hg at rest
- Moderate or severe MR
- Very thick ventricular septum
- High LV end diastolic pressure

Sequential AV pacing reduces symptoms and improves hemodynamics. Surgery, which is only palliative, causes an 8% early and about 12% late mortality but depends on the expertise of the surgical team. When surgery is indicated, a septal myotomy/myectomy is performed. Surgery does not reduce mortality, but a significant number of patients obtain relief from anginal symptoms. The Düsseldorf experience shows an encouraging ↓ in sudden death and syncope following successful myotomy/myectomy. Mitral valve replacement is indicated only for severe MR. Transplantation may be considered for intractable symptoms.

DILATED CARDIOMYOPATHY

A diagnosis of DCM should be considered in a patient with CHF, documented global hypokinesis and dilation of the left and/or right ventricles, and reduced systolic function in the absence of evidence of CHD, congenital, specific valvular, hypertensive, or specific heart muscle disease, and chronic excessive alcohol consumption. DCM is not due to alcohol but can be exaggerated by it.

Clinical Hallmarks

- Progressive dyspnea on exertion appears over weeks or months, culminating in orthopnea, PND, and edema, which are common features. Physical signs of right and LV failure are prominent in late cases. The extremities tend to be cool and pale due to vasoconstriction
- The apex beat is displaced downward and outward to the left due to LV dilatation
- Left lower parasternal lift or pulsation indicates RV dilatation
- The JVP may be elevated and may show a systolic wave of tricuspid regurgitation
- A soft Grade I–II/VI systolic mitral murmur and a soft tricuspid systolic murmur are commonly present because of mitral and tricuspid

regurgitation as a result of dilation of the ventricles and valve rings as well as papillary muscle dysfunction
- S4 and S3 are constantly present, as well as sinus tachycardia; thus, a summation gallop is a frequent finding
- The loud S3 is present in virtually all cases and is often heard when CHF is absent. This hallmark serves to differentiate DCM from a Class 4 ventricle due to CHD where a soft S3 is heard during episodes of CHF, but is frequently absent or quite soft when the individual is assessed not to be in CHF, and in the absence of LV aneurysm
- BP is frequently low; hypotension carries a poor prognosis

Aortic systolic or diastolic murmurs are usually absent and serve to exclude specific valvular heart disease as a cause of the severe CHF but aortic regurgitation occasionally occurs in DCM. These are signs of advanced disease. Echocardiographic diagnosis can be made before overt CHF has developed.

- ECG features include: sinus tachycardia and flat or inverted T waves. Modest LVH may be masked by low voltage. AF occurs in about 25%; LBBB is observed in a significant minority. Poor R wave progression (V2–V4) or Q waves of pseudo infarction may suggest an incorrect diagnosis of IHD (Table 13–3)
- Chest x ray: The heart is enlarged and 4-chamber enlargement is commonly present. There is usually evidence of a raised left atrial pressure in the pulmonary vascular pattern. Pleural effusions may be present
- Echocardiographic features include: severe dilation of both ventricles; global hypokinesis and commonly paradoxical movement of the septum; increased end systolic and end diastolic dimensions; EF usually <35%; EF 10–30% in the presence of CHF; atrial enlargement and ventricular thrombi; a small pericardial effusion
- Endomyocardial biopsy: Used as a research tool to exclude suspected known heart muscle disease and to detect evidence of myocarditis or viral particles
- Holter monitoring carried out for 48 h helps to define patients with potentially lethal ventricular arrhythmias

Therapy

- The most important aspect of DCM management is the prevention and control of CHF, arrhythmias, and embolization. The standard management for CHF should be instituted: bed-to-chair rest for several days; oxygen and a sedative at night to allow restful sleep, which adds to the patient's comfort and reduces the workload of the failing myocardium; salt restriction. Avoidance of alcohol is necessary in all patients with CHF and especially in the patient with a Class 3 or 4 ventricle, because alcohol decreases the EF. Patients should be assessed for the presence of macro-ovalocytes, decreased platelet counts, and increased levels of gamma glutamyltransferase, which may indicate alcohol damage
- Digoxin provides some benefit in CHF patients in sinus rhythm and is indicated for AF with uncontrolled ventricular response (see Chap. 5). The dose should be adequate, but care is needed to avoid digitalis toxicity. In patients with refractory CHF, IV dobutamine may cause temporary "improvement."
- Diuretics play a vital role in the relief of symptoms. The 3 groups of drugs—diuretics, digoxin, and ACE inhibitors—are complementary
- ACE inhibitors have made a major contribution to survival of patients

with CHF; however, diastolic dysfunction in patients with DCM tends to worsen with ACE inhibitor therapy. The dosage and pharmacologic profile of ACE inhibitors are given in Table 1–5. **Captopril** (Capoten). Dosage: 3–6.25 mg test dose; if hypotension is not precipitated, give 6.25 mg bid for 1–2 days and ↑ to 12.5 mg bid. Then over days to weeks, ↑ to 25 mg bid to a max of 50 mg bid. A dose >75 mg provides little added benefit for these patients and there is a risk of lowered diastolic pressure with consequent poor coronary perfusion that may trigger an arrhythmic death

Beta-adrenergic blockers. Judicious use of β blockers appears, however paradoxically, to benefit some patients with DCM, especially individuals with resting sinus tachycardia and/or diastolic dysfunction. Removal of sympathetic drive on myocytes and restoration toward normal of the downgrading of β-adrenergic receptors in CHF appear to provide benefits.

Reduction in HR decreases myocardial O_2 demand and also improves coronary blood flow. Prevention of arrhythmias, with even modest ↓ in sudden deaths, is a potential benefit of careful β-adrenergic blockade. Clinical trials have shown mixed results, however, and large-scale trials are underway.

Fortunately, all β blockers are not alike, and 2 recent reports of studies using agents that have vasodilating properties (bucindolol and labetalol, an $alpha_1$ β blocker) indicate beneficial effects that must be assessed in large-scale trials.

Administration of bucindolol (25–200 mg qd) caused a ↑ in EF from 2.5% to 35% and improved functional class in 17% of 20 patients over 2 years.

- Warfarin is advisable in most patients to prevent embolization from atrial and ventricular thrombi; it is essential if there is AF. Pulmonary embolism and systemic embolization occur fairly frequently and worsen the dismal prognosis. In addition, immobilization during periods of CHF predisposes deep vein thrombosis and pulmonary emboli (see anticoagulation control, Chap. 11)

RESTRICTIVE CARDIOMYOPATHY

This major abnormality is a restriction of ventricular filling, thus a ↑ in filling pressures. RCM is a member of the group of diastolic CHF in which diastolic function is impaired earlier and more severely than systolic function. The usual abnormality is impaired relaxation and compliance. Restrictive pathophysiology may occur at the pericardial, myocardial, or endomyocardial level.

The most common cause of RCM is endomyocardial fibrosis, especially in tropical regions. Myocardial involvement by amyloid, not associated with multiple organ involvement, is the most common cause of RCM in the Western world. Cardiac disease resulting from amyloid-associated multiple organ involvement, sarcoid, hemochromatosis, eosinophilic syndromes, scleroderma, Adriamycin toxicity, and infectious agents, including tuberculosis, causing restrictive physiology is considered specific heart muscle disease. HCM may produce diastolic abnormalities similar to those in RCM.

Clinical Hallmarks

- Intermittent fever, shortness of breath, cough, palpitations, edema, and tiredness
- Hypereosinophilia with abnormal eosinophil degranulation is seen in temperate climates (hypereosinophilic heart disease)
- Hypereosinophilia is less severe in tropical endomyocardial fibrosis
- Symptoms and signs of CHF and of moderate to severe mitral and tricuspid regurgitation due to involvement of the papillary muscles serve to differentiate RCM from constrictive pericarditis, as does the greater degree of cardiac enlargement on chest x ray in the former condition (Table 13–3)
- During the early stages, endomyocardial fibrosis may mimic the hemodynamic and clinical features of constrictive pericarditis. Table 13–4 gives hemodynamic differences, but significant overlap occurs
- The chest x ray in patients with endomyocardial fibrosis may show calcification of the right or left ventricular apical myocardium
- Echocardiogram shows obliteration of the apices of the ventricles by echogenic masses. Also, myocardial calcification may be detected, and in later stages, mitral and tricuspid regurgitation may require echocardiographic assessment
- The idiopathic endocardial fibrosis and associated thrombus may progressively obliterate the left or right ventricular cavities. Severe enlargement of the right atrium may occur

Therapy

- Steroids may be helpful in the early acute inflammatory phase associated with hypereosinophilia, but medical therapy is unrewarding
- Anticoagulants are necessary because thromboembolism is common
- Restriction to filling does not respond to digoxin, diuretics, or vasodilators, and all 3 medications are relatively contraindicated. Arrhythmias may respond to small doses of β blockers, and potentially lethal arrhythmias may require amiodarone therapy
- Resection of masses of obliterating endocardial tissue with valve repair has produced apparent relief in some patients with endomyocardial fibrosis for a few years
- Cardiac transplantation may require consideration in intractable cases

SPECIFIC HEART MUSCLE DISEASE

- Specific heart muscle disease usually produces a dilated form of cardiomyopathy with impaired systolic function
- Restrictive physiology is seen with amyloid, sarcoid, neoplasm, radiation, scleroderma, hemochromatosis, and eosinophilic endomyocardial disease, in which eosinophilia is usually present. Rarely, myocardial tuberculosis is present with restrictive features. Amyloid heart disease and endomyocardial fibrosis are usually considered examples of RCM, but when cardiac involvement is associated with multiple organ disease, they qualify as specific heart muscle disease
- The findings of systemic disease of other organs, especially the liver, lymph nodes, and skin, which can be easily submitted to biopsy, assist

in defining the underlying cause. Endomyocardial biopsy is often required but may not be helpful in patchy disease such as sarcoid

- Treatment should be directed at the underlying disease. Occasionally, cardiac pacing is required for the management of complete heart block due to involvement of conduction tissue by sarcoid, scleroderma, or hemochromatosis
- Other heart muscle diseases include involvement due to infectious disease: Chagas due to Trypanosoma cruzi is transmitted by a triatoma bug. The disease is prevalent in South America but does occur in the southern United States
- The incidence of HIV is increasing, and myocarditis with pericardial effusion and cardiac tamponade is now surfacing in victims of AIDS. Myocardial involvement might be due to the HIV virus; although this is unproven, involvement by Kaposi, opportunistic infections, and effects of medications must also be excluded
- Rare involvement of cardiac muscle is seen with alcohol abuse, polymyositis, progressive muscular dystrophy, Friedreich's ataxia, and Fabry's disease
- Deficiency disorders, such as Beri-beri or selenium deficiency
- Drugs, especially cocaine and toxins, may affect the myocardium; known toxins include cobalt (beer), chloroquine and emetine, phenothiazines, methysergide, and cancer chemotherapeutic agents (Adriamycin, daunorubicin, doxorubicin, cyclophosphamide); also, methyldopa, and phenindione rarely cause a hypersensitivity myocarditis. Overdose with toxic doses of acetaminophen or cocaine may cause myocardial necrosis and arrhythmias, including torsades de pointes
- Treatment of these disorders involves removal and treatment of the infective agent or toxin where possible

Suggested Reading

Goodwin JF and Olsen E. (Eds) Cardiomyopathies—Realisations and Expectations. Heidelberg, Springer-Verlag, 1993.

Khan M. Gabriel, Goodwin JF, Cardiomyopathy. *In.* Cardiac and Pulmonary Management. Philadelphia, Lea & Febiger, 1993.

Syncope

15

M. Gabriel Khan

Syncope (transient loss of consciousness as a result of inadequate cerebral blood flow) is a common problem representing ≤1% of medical admissions to general hospitals and ≤3% of emergency room diagnoses. Its causes are often elusive; the following points deserve attention

- An obvious cardiac cause can be defined by the history, physical examination, ECG, and Holter monitoring in approximately 10% of cases (see Fig. 15–1 and Table 15–1)
- Vasodepressor (vasovagal) syncope, the common form being the simple faint, accounts for >35% of cases of syncope. It is therefore most important to exclude this benign problem
- Unexplained syncope constitutes a large group of cases >(35%), but in patients who have structural heart disease and unexplained syncope, EP testing helps identify a significant number of cardiac causes and ↑ the total cardiac cause of syncope to approximately 22%
- In patients with unexplained syncope, if structural heart disease is not present, EP testing is rarely diagnostic; the head-up tilt test is useful (Fig. 15–1)
- Syncope may be the clue to possibly life-threatening underlying cardiac diseases
- Cardiac syncope carries a 24% incidence of sudden death in 1 year; the incidence is <2% in the remaining 78% of individuals. One-year mortality of patients with cardiac syncope is 15–30%, versus <2% for individuals with unexplained syncope and without structural heart disease
- Figure 15–1 gives an algorithmic approach to the diagnosis of syncope
- Dizziness is often a feature of presyncope and has several causes that are difficult to determine. Figure 15–2 indicates steps to consider
- Postural hypotension is an important cause of syncope. It commonly occurs because of a ↓ in preload and often occurs in patients on cardiac medications that cause venous pooling. Less often, syncope has a neurogenic cause, being a troublesome feature of autonomic neuropathy (Table 15–2)

It must be reemphasized that head-up tilt testing has a role in defining the cause of unexplained syncope in patients without structural heart disease. The result may be expedited by the simultaneous administration of IV Edrophonium; in patients < age 50, isoproterenol is used in some centers, but a study by Kapoor et al. questions the low specificity of this test.

These intensive investigations result in the prevention of some of the deaths associated with syncope, although syncope remains unexplained in a minority of patients.

The management of syncope entails the elucidation of the cause so that appropriate advice, medications, or corrective measures may be employed to prevent bodily injury or threat to life. Since most cardiac causes pose a threat to life, it is important to use a methodical approach to solving the cause of syncope in a given individual. This medical solu-

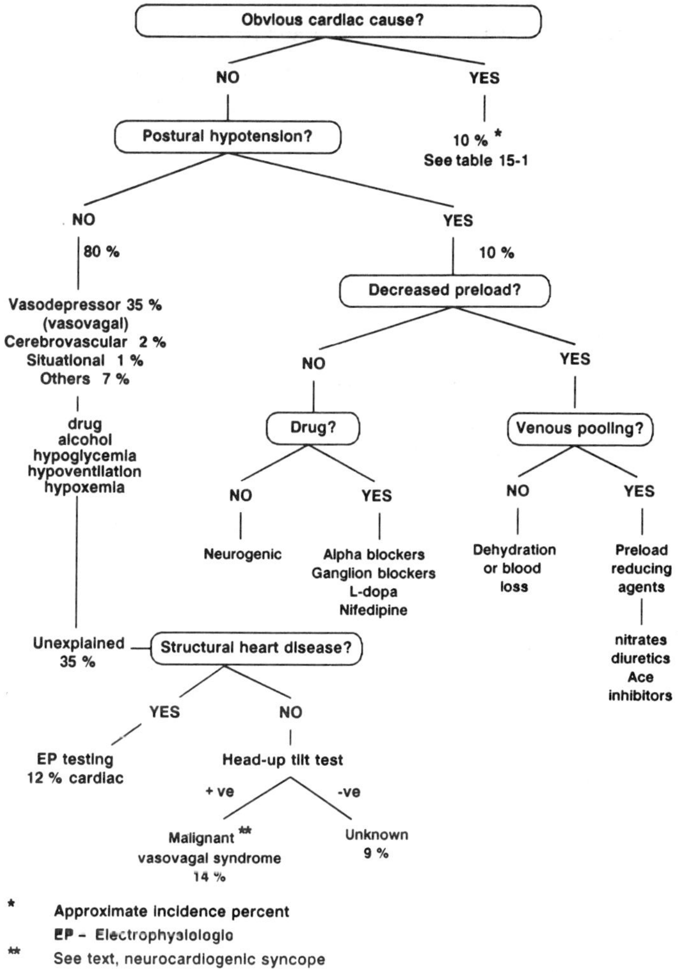

Figure 15–1. Algorithm for the assessment of syncope.

tion calls for sound knowledge of basic internal medicine and cardiology and should commence with a detailed history and physical examination.

Who should be admitted to a hospital

- Patients with suspected cardiac cause
- Patients with significant bodily injury
- The elderly patient in whom a readily identifiable cause is lacking
- Recurrent syncope of undetermined etiology
- Recurrence of syncope while awaiting investigation

A detailed relevant history and physical examination are mandatory

- Check the BP on the patient recumbent for >3 min and then on standing, to elicit postural hypotension
- Determine the BP in the arms and legs

Table 15–1
Obvious Cardiac Causes of Syncope and Approximate Incidence

CAUSES	APPROXIMATE INCIDENCE
Tachyarrhythmias	45%
Sustained and Nonsustained VT	
Torsades de pointes	
Atrial fibrillation	
Supraventricular tachycardia	
Long QT syndrome	
WPW syndrome	
Pacemaker mediated	
Bradyarrhythmias	35%
Sinus Node dysfunction	
(Sick sinus syndrome)	
AV block: second and third degree	
Drug induced	
Carotid sinus syncope	3%
Obstruction to stroke volume	10%
Aortic stenosis	
Hypertrophic cardiomyopathy	
Tight mitral stenosis	
Atrial myxoma or thrombus	
Cardiac tamponade	
Prosthetic valve dysfunction	
Pulmonary embolism	
Pulmonary hypertension	
Pulmonary stenosis	
Others	7%
Mitral valve prolapse	
Myocardial infarction	
Severe ischemic heart disease	
Coronary artery spasm	
Pacemaker syndrome	
Aortic dissection	
Fallot's tetralogy	

- Listen for bruits over the subclavian and carotid arteries
- Look for finger clubbing and cyanosis as signs of congenital cyanotic heart disease
- Perform a full cardiovascular examination. Check for LVH, presence of thrills, the murmur of aortic stenosis, HCM, mitral stenosis, mitral valve prolapse, and the presence of prosthetic heart valve (see Table 15–1 and Chap. 12)
- Assess for tachyarrhythmias and bradyarrhythmias

The history should exclude the most common cause of faint, i.e., vasodepressor syncope. All known causes of syncope should be methodically excluded (see Fig. 15–1)

After exclusion of postural hypotension, vasodepressor syncope, and cerebrovascular and situational causes, request the following

- CBC, electrolytes, blood urea, serum creatinine, and serum Ca. These routine tests are not usually helpful
- Chest x ray
- ECG

- Echocardiogram
- 24- or 48-hour Holter monitoring is advisable but has a low yield

Vasodepressor (Vasovagal) Syncope. The simple faint is the most common cause of syncope and is easily recognized. Vasodepressor syncope virtually never occurs in a patient in the recumbent position. Precipitating circumstances are almost always present and typically occur in young individuals and occasionally in older patients in the setting of exhaustion, hunger, prolonged standing or sitting in a hot crowded room, and sudden severe pain or trauma, venipuncture, fright, and sudden emotional stress.

The simple faint usually gives a warning of seconds to minutes: a feeling of weakness, nausea, vague upper abdominal discomfort, diaphoresis, yawn, sighing, hyperventilation, unsteadiness, blurring of vision, an awareness prior to fainting. Importantly, vertigo is not a symptom associated with a simple faint. Thus, a good history identifies the faint and may save expensive and time-consuming investigations.

The constant findings in vasodepressor syncope are

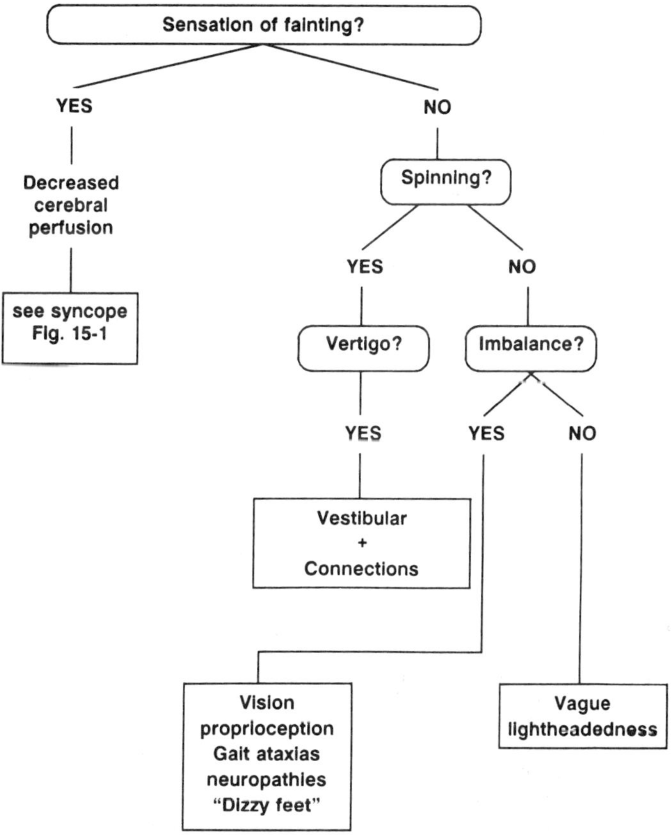

Figure 15–2. Algorithm for evaluating patients with dizziness.

Table 15–2
Noncardiac Causes of Syncope

CAUSE	APPROXIMATE INCIDENCE
1. Vasodepressor (vasovagal)	35%
2. Postural hypotension	10%
A. Decrease preload	
a) Venous pooling, caused by extensive varicose veins, post-exercise vasodilation venous angioma in the leg. Drugs: nitrates, diuretics, ACE inhibitors	
b) Decreased blood volume: blood loss; dehydration: vomiting, diarrhea, excessive sweating, Addison's disease	
B. Drug induced	
a) alpha blockers	
b) Ganglion blockers	
c) Bromocriptine	
d) L-dopa	
e) Nifedipine	
C. Neurogenic decrease autonomic activity	
a) Bedrest	
b) Neuropathies/diabetes	
c) Shy Drager syndrome	
d) Idiopathic	
D. Mastocytosis	
3. Cerebrovascular disease	2%
Transient ischemic attack	
Subclavian steal	
Basilar artery migraine	
Cervical arthritis, allanto-occipital dislocation compression vertebral artery	
4. Situational	1%
Cough, sneeze, micturition, defecation	
5. Others	7%
Drugs/alcohol	
Hypoglycemia	
Hypoxemia	
Hypoventilation	
Hysterical	
6. Unexplained	35%
Malignant vasovagal syndrome (Neurally mediated syncope) 30–60% of otherwise unexplained	

- A sudden marked fall in total peripheral resistance, resulting in a drastic fall in BP
- Decreased cerebral perfusion, causing loss of consciousness
- Loss of consciousness usually occurs within 10 seconds of onset of diminished perfusion
- Return of consciousness in seconds to minutes if the individual remains flat with the legs elevated
- Injuries are most uncommon with vasodepressor syncope

The exclusion of epilepsy is relatively easy, but occasionally syncope may be confused with akinetic seizures. Bradycardia in association with seizures has been described. The aura, if any, in epilepsy is transient but tells a story. Injuries, including lip and tongue biting, and incontinence with a prolonged postictal state are not seen with vasodepressor syncope.

Because cardiac sympathetic overstimulation, vigorous LV contraction, and stimulation of intramyocardial mechanoreceptors (C fibers) appear to be important underlying mechanisms in the genesis of unexplained syncope without structural heart disease, β blockers have been given as rational therapy and have proven successful in some patients with this disabling form of syncope, known as malignant vasovagal syndrome, neurocardiogenic syncope, or neurally mediated syncope (Fig. 15–1). Atenolol (25 mg) or metoprolol (100 mg) daily may produce a salutary response. Esmolol IV may be used to predict the outcome of oral β-blocker therapy.

Postural Hypotension. Several cardiac medications may cause orthostatic hypotension, particularly in the elderly. Assess the following

- Check the BP with the patient recumbent for ≥3 min and then on standing; a ↓ in systolic pressure of ≥20 mm Hg represents orthostatic hypotension
- Check for evidence of ↓ in preload, which may manifest itself by venous pooling that may occur on sudden standing after vigorous exercise or because of extensive varicose veins. Preload-reducing agents, particularly nitrates, ACE inhibitors or alpha_1 blockers may be implicated. Blood loss and dehydration are obvious causes, but an occult cause of the latter is Addison's disease
- If conditions causing a ↓ in preload are not present, inquire about the use of medications that cause arterial dilation (particularly alpha_1-adrenergic blockers such as prasozin and labetalol), ganglion-blocking drugs, L-dopa, bromocristine, and rarely nifedipine
- If drug use is excluded, postural hypotension may be caused by autonomic imbalance or neurologic diseases. Complete bed rest and a lack of leg exercise, plus a ↓ in autonomic activity, commonly result in postural hypotension. Neuropathy, especially due to diabetes, Shy Drager, and other neurologic problems must be excluded

Standing from a recumbent or sitting position causes immediate pooling of blood in the lower limbs and a consequent fall in BP that normally triggers a baroreceptor response, sympathetically mediated vasoconstriction, and a ↑ in HR. As indicated above, conditions that impair baroreceptor function and ↓ sympathetically mediated alpha_1 vasoconstriction may precipitate postural hypotension.

Orthostatic hypotension as a consequence of autonomic neuropathies and autonomic failure is difficult to treat successfully. It may respond to increased Na intake or fludrocortisone (Florinef), 0.1–0.2 mg qd. The management of orthostatic hypotension caused by autonomic failure can be successfully managed in properly selected patients with midodrine (Amatine), a selective peripherally acting postsynaptic alpha_1 adrenergic agonist. Salutary effects are caused by a ↑ in arterial and venous tone; venous pooling is prevented. Initial dosage: 2.5 mg tid with monitoring of supine BP, then increased in 2.5-mg increments at weekly intervals to a max of 10 mg tid. Caution is needed because the action of midodrine is identical to that of other alpha adrenergic receptor stimulants such as methoxamine or phenylephrine; a ↑ in total systemic resistance may cause supine hypertension that can precipitate CHF, myocardial ischemia, infarction, or stroke in susceptible individuals. Supine hypertension is more common during the initiation of midodrine therapy; during the titration period, adverse effects include supine hypertension, which may cause headaches and pounding in the ears. Reflex bradycardia may occur, and caution is needed when the drug is combined with agents that cause bradycardia (digoxin, β blockers, diltiazem, and verapamil). Urinary retention is an important adverse effect in elderly males. The drug is contraindicated in patients with significant CHD, CHF, renal failure, urinary retention, thyrotoxicosis, and pheochromocytoma. Midodrine is renally excreted, and care is necessary to ↓ the dose and ↑ the dosing interval in patients with renal dysfunction.

In patients who are not responsive to midodrine or fludrocortisone and have sustained injuries, atrial pacing with a HR of 100/min may afford some amelioration if combined with increased salt intake, fludrocortisone, elevation of the head of the bed during sleep, and full-length leotards to enhance venous return.

A release of histamine, prostaglandin D, and other vasodilators from mast cell proliferation (mastocytosis) causes vasodilation, and is a rare cause of postural hypotension.

Instruct the patient to change posture slowly and to engage in calf muscle flexion prior to standing. Elevating the head of the bed and gradually changing posture may provide a salutary response.

Aortic Arch Syndrome. Pulseless disease (Takayasu's disease) is an arteritis-producing occlusion of the aortic arch vessels, and syncope may result. The BP is lower in the arms than the legs.

Tachyarrhythmias. The major determinant in cardiac syncope is a ↓ in cardiac output due to reduced HR or ineffectual cardiac contractions secondary to arrhythmia. A diagnosis of cardiac syncope connotes a guarded prognosis with a mortality of ≤24% in 1 year, although this varies greatly according to the mechanism of the arrhythmia. Early diagnosis with appropriate therapy is lifesaving. Obvious causes of cardiac syncope are listed in Table 15–1.

Sustained rapid VT (i.e., VT duration >30 seconds) or symptomatic nonsustained VT commonly causes syncope. When VT is not apparent on the ECG rhythm strip or Holter monitoring, the underlying mechanism may be revealed by EP testing.

AF or other SVT with fast ventricular rates may cause syncope, especially in the elderly, or when rapid rates supervene in patients with WPW Syndrome.

Aortic Stenosis, Hypertrophic Cardiomyopathy. Syncope in aortic stenosis is typically exertional and suggests significant disease with life expectancy of 1–3 years. With HCM, syncope may be precipitated by exercise but can occur with normal activities or at rest (see Chaps. 12 and 14).

Sinus Node Dysfunction, Sick Sinus Syndrome. Severe bradycardia (30–40/min), sinus arrest, and brady- or tachyarrhythmias may cause lightheadedness, dizziness, confusion, memory loss, or presyncope. ≥1 of these associated symptoms usually produce a 1- to 10-second warning prior to syncope; however, syncope can occur without warning in this category of patients, and injuries may occur.

The setting is usually IHD with old infarction. The ECG may be normal or show evidence of old infarction, bradycardia, or sinus arrest. A 48-hour Holter gives about a 70% chance of detecting a significant arrhythmia, with symptoms noted in the patient's diary, as opposed to <48% with a single 24-hour Holter monitoring. Fairly often, repeat 48-hour Holter monitoring is necessary once or twice over a couple of weeks to identify a bradyarrhythmia that is symptomatic. Treatment of sinus node dysfunction is given in Chapter 7. Sinus node dysfunction and severe bradycardia causing presyncope or syncope may be due to drug therapy that inadvertently depresses sinus node function. Verapamil, diltiazem, digitalis, β blockers, Class 1 antiarrhythmic agents, amiodarone, and especially their combinations may cause severe bradycardia, A-V block, and asystole in susceptible individuals. Discontinuation of the causative agent or agents is unfortunately rarely practical, and pacing is usually indicated.

A-V Block, Stokes-Adams Attacks. Patients with Mobitz Type II or 3rd° A-V block may suddenly have an occurrence of transient asystole or VF with complete cessation of cerebral blood flow. Since VF is instantaneous, the cerebral circulation is suddenly deprived of perfusion, resulting in loss of consciousness usually without warning. Episodes can happen on sitting, lying, or walking. The unconscious patient appears very pale and, on arousal, becomes flushed as blood rushes to the head. When a patient is assessed hours or days later, ECG may show manifestations of Mobitz Type II or complete A-V block, RBBB or LBBB, or bilateral disease. Cardiac pacing should be instituted (see Chap. 7).

Prolonged QT Syndrome. Recurrent syncope in children and young adults with a positive family history may be due to prolonged QT syndrome. Episodes of life-threatening arrhythmias appear to be precipitated by increased sympathetic stimulation. Thus, β blockers have a role in management, despite a tendency for bradycardia in many of these patients. Propranolol in doses of 80–160 mg qd or a similar noncardioselective β blocker without agonist activity is preferred.

When recurrent syncope is uncontrolled by β blockers, combined pacing and β-blocker therapy may be required. In uncontrolled cases, excision of the left stellate ganglion may be a last resort.

Electrophysiologic Study

A provocative EP study is useful in revealing a cardiac cause in approximately 12% of patients with unexplained syncope. Approximately 21% of these patients with negative studies are subsequently diagnosed as having intermittent high-degree A-V block or sinus node disease. Caution is therefore necessary because an EP study is not a sensitive test to expose symptomatic bradycardia.

EP studies have been shown to initiate sustained monomorphic VT in approximately 18% of patients and nonsustained VT in approximately 23%. Nonsustained VT, especially if only for a few seconds duration, carries a minimal risk in patients with syncope and requires no arrhyth mia therapy. Patients with syncope and sustained monomorphic VT do not appear to benefit from antiarrhythmic therapy, and the incidence of syncope is not reduced except when amiodarone is used as therapy.

EP studies appear to be justifiable in patients who have a high probability of induction of sustained monomorphic VT

- Post-MI patients with unexplained syncope
- LV EF <30%
- LV aneurysm
- Complex ventricular ectopy on Holter

Head-up Tilt Testing

Head-up tilt testing has a role in delineating the pathophysiology, diagnosis, and management of patients with no detectable heart disease and unexplained syncope.

"Malignant" vasovagal syndrome or neurocardiogenic syncope, also termed neurally mediated syncope, occurs abruptly with no prodrome.

Fitzpatrick and Sutton call this tilt-inducible syncope "malignant" vasovagal syndrome because of the history of trauma in association with abrupt syncope, which occurs without a prodrome. Less than 50% of patients have been noted to have injured themselves prior to seeking medical attention. These patients have features that distinguish them from individuals who succumb to the simple faint; particularly prominent is the lack of warning and the occurrence of injuries.

Forty to seventy percent of patients with unexplained syncope experience syncope on being tilted 60° for 45 min. There is no standard protocol for the test, but current recommendations indicate the need for

- At least 60° tilt
- Duration of 45 min
- Use of foot plate support rather than saddle
- Isoproterenol infusion improves sensitivity with decreased tilt time of 10 min at 80° tilt. The use of isoproterenol has the disadvantage of dosing difficulty and reduced specificity. Isoproterenol is not recommended, however, in patients > age 50 because of adverse cardiac effects. Schienman et al. prefer the use of edrophonium IV (10 mg). Where edrophonium results in a negative head-up tilt test, isoproterenol does not reveal a positive test. In a study by Kapoor et al., isoproterenol infusion resulted in a nonsignificant difference in the rate of positive tests in 20 young patients with unexplained syncope and controls matched by age, sex, and absence of underlying heart disease.

Head-up tilt using 60° for 45 min does not appear to be useful in youthful subjects with typical vasovagal syncope, but in this group, the clinical diagnosis is usually apparent.

In unexplained syncope, both head-up tilt testing and EP evaluation are complementary and can identify the underlying cause in approximately 74% of patients presenting with unexplained syncope.

Beta-Adrenergic Blocker Therapy

Patients without structural heart disease and neurocardiogenic syncope respond to β-adrenergic blocking drugs. These agents have been shown to prevent neurocardiogenic syncope in 50–75% of patients. Atenolol (25 to max 50 mg), metoprolol sustained release (100 mg), or nadolol (20 mg) is effective. Propranolol is beneficial, but adverse effects are often bothersome. Sra et al. have shown esmolol to be effective in predicting the outcome of head-up tilt response to oral metoprolol. All patients who had a negative head-up tilt test response with esmolol IV had a negative test during oral metoprolol therapy.

Like β-adrenergic blockers, disopyramide has a negative inotropic effect, a tendency to ↑ peripheral vascular resistance, and produces a salutary response in about 15% of patients in whom syncope is caused by a hypotensive bradycardic response. Disopyramide (100–150 mg) sustained release bid may be tried in patients without structural heart disease and in patients who have failed to respond to β blockers.

Suggested Reading

Akhtar M, Jazayeri M, Sra J: Cardiovascular causes of syncope. Identifying and controlling trigger mechanisms. Postgraduate Medicine *90*: 87, 1991.

Fitzpatrick A, Sutton R: Tilting towards a diagnosis in recurrent unexplained syncope. Lancet *1*:658, 1989.

Fitzpatrick AP, Theodorakis G, Vardas P, et al.: Methodology of head-up tilt testing in patients with unexplained syncope. J Am Coll Cardiol *17*:125, 1991.

Kapoor WN, Brant N: Evaluation of syncope by upright tilt testing with isoproterenol. A nonspecific test. Ann Intern Med *116*:358, 1992.

Khan M Gabriel: Syncope. *In* Cardiac and Pulmonary Management. Philadelphia, Lea & Febiger, 1993.

Sra JS, Murthy VS, Jazayeri MR, et al.: Use of intravenous esmolol to predict efficacy of oral beta-adrenergic blocker therapy in patients with neurocardiogenic syncope. J Am Coll Cardiol *19*:402, 1992.

Bronchodilators/Asthma/ Chronic Obstructive Pulmonary Disease

16

Susan K. Pingleton, Diana S. Dark, Gerald R. Kerby, and Lewis J. Wesselius

BRONCHODILATORS

- Bronchodilators are available in several different dosage forms: Aerosol, oral, and IV
- Currently, there are 3 types of systems used to generate aerosols for clinical use: jet nebulizers, ultrasonic nebulizers, and MDIs
- The most widely used nebulizer is the MDI. This pressurized canister dispenses a single bolus of an aerosol, either a suspension or a solution. In a suspension system, fine crystals of medications are embedded in a propellant and released when the device is actuated. In solution systems, the formulation consists of a homogeneous mixture of medications and cosolvents in propellants
- In addition to pressurized canisters, several types of powder MDIs also exist. The 2 most common are the Spinhaler and Rotahaler. The Spinhaler mechanism consists of a capsule that is inserted into a propeller-driven turbine. After the capsule is punctured, inhaling through the canister causes the propeller to rotate and the capsule to vibrate, thus releasing the contents in a turbulent airstream. Usually, 1 single inspiration at high speed will dispense all of the drug. The Rotahaler uses a slight variation of this technique. Inspiration causes the chamber to spin, and a cutting block opens the capsule and releases the powdered drug in a spiral airstream. Both the Spinhaler and Rotahaler dispense relatively large quantities of drug and can be used by patients who have difficulty mastering the techniques required to use a pressurized device
- It is important for as much medication to enter and remain within the airways as possible. Inspiratory flow rate is the most critical variable and should be kept low (approximately 1 l/sec), inhaling over approximately 5 seconds, and inspiration should be followed by a 5- to 10-second period of breath holding. This low inspiratory flow rate reduces unwanted impaction in the oropharynx; breath holding facilitates deposition by gravity. Proper aerosol technique is most important (Table 16–1)

The bronchodilators discussed in this chapter will be grouped according to the following classifications

- β-adrenergic agonists
- Anticholinergic agents
- Methylxanthines

A comparison of various bronchodilators is presented in Table 16–2.

Table 16–1
Patient Instruction for Optimal MDI Use

- Remove cap from inhaler
- Shake inhaler for a few seconds
- Hold inhaler upright and tilt head back slightly
- Place inhaler between lips* or approximately 2 cm in front of open mouth. Alternatively, a spacer device can be used
- Take a deep breath and exhale completely
- Begin inhaling slowly and immediately press down on top of inhaler to deliver aerosol medicine
- Complete inhalation and hold breath for 5 to 10 seconds
- Wait at least 2 to 3 minutes then repeat above for subsequent puffs

* Recommended for anticholinergic drug, ipratropium bromide, to avoid contact with eyes, or use a spacing device

Beta$_2$-Adrenergic Agonists

β agonists provide the foundation for acute reversal therapy of obstructive airway disease. The rapidity with which they work make them the first choice of physicians and patients. The beneficial effects of epinephrine in the treatment of asthma were described early in the 20th century.

Table 16–2
Comparison of Bronchodilators

	BETA ADRENERGIC AGONISTS	ANTICHOLINERGICS*	METHYLXANTHINES#
ETIOLOGY OF ASTHMA			
Allergic	+ + + +	+ +/−	+ +/−
Emotional	+ +	+ + I I	+/−
Exercise-induced	+ + + +	+/−	+ +/−
Intrinsic	+ + +	+ +/−	+ +/−
Irritant-induced	+ + + +	+ + +	+ +/
CHRONIC OBSTRUCTIVE PULMONARY DISEASE			
Emphysema	+/−	+ + +	+ +/−
Bronchitis	+ + +	+ + +	+ +/−
ACTION			
Onset	Fast (5 min)	Slow (1–2 hrs)	Variable
Duration	Variable	Variable	Long
ADVERSE EFFECTS			
Arrhythmia-potential	+ + +	+/−	+ + + +
Hypokalemia	+ +	−	+/−
Nausea	+ +	−	+ + + +
Tachycardia	+ + + +	+/−	+ +
Tremor	+ + +	−	+ + +

* Ipratropium bromide will be compared as it is the safest and most frequently prescribed.
# Oral preparations will be compared

Subsequently, numerous other agents similar in structure but more β_2 selective have been developed and tried by several routes with variable degrees of success. The greatest benefit of the β_2-selective agonists may not be in the bronchodilatory capabilities but rather in the diminution of the adverse cardiac side effects. With the advent of β_2-selective agonists, the use of nonselective β agonists such as isoproterenol, metaproterenol, and isoetharine has become inadvisable.

PHARMACOLOGY AND MECHANISMS OF ACTION

- β agonists are structural analogs of norepinephrine
- Modification of the ring constituents generally results in prolongation of action, while modification of the terminal amine confers β selectivity
- Aerosolized β_2 agonists have a relatively short time to onset of action, generally within 15 min. Oral formulations have an onset of action in the range of 30 min–1 h, which depends on GI absorption. The duration of action depends on the formulation of the ring constituent and varies with each compound
- β_2-agonist stimulation of bronchial smooth muscle results in relaxation and, consequently, bronchodilation. This effect is believed to be mediated by ↑ intracellular cyclic AMP levels. Increased cyclic AMP leads to a ↓ in cytosolic Ca and smooth muscle relaxation. Virtually all β receptors in the bronchial smooth muscles are of the β_2 subtype
- Both β_1 and β_2 agonists ↑ mucus secretion from submucosal glands. β_2-agonist stimulation increases ion transport in epithelial cells which, in turn, leads to ↑ water secretion. β-receptor stimulation may thereby improve mucociliary clearance
- The secretion of histamine and other mast cell mediators appears to be modulated by β_2-adrenergic stimulation, as is pulmonary vasoconstriction
- Lastly, β-adrenergic receptors are found throughout the alveolar walls. Approximately 2/3 are of the β_2 subtype. While stimulation of these alveolar β receptors results partly in stimulation of surfactant secretion by Type II pneumocytes, the function of β receptors in other cell populations is not yet clearly defined

Adverse Effects are much more prevalent when nonspecific β agonists are used

- Common β_1 side effects include tachycardia, palpitations, and muscle tremors
- Hypokalemia may also result from β-agonist use. This appears to be mediated by β_2-receptor stimulation of a membrane-bound Na/K ATPase. This hypokalemic response has been implicated in the development of cardiac arrhythmias and is speculated to have a role in sudden death in patients with asthma. It would be prudent, therefore, to closely monitor serum K in those patients given frequent high-dose β_2 agonists concomitantly with K-losing diuretics. This would be especially true of patients at risk for cardiac arrhythmias, such as those with CHF or IHD

Dosages of β_2-selective agonists are given in Table 16–3. The recommendations in Table 16–3 are intended for use in mild to moderate obstructive airway disease. More frequent dosing intervals of the shorter-acting β_2-selective agonists (salbutamol, terbutaline) are indicated in more severe obstructive disease, specifically status asthmaticus. In this case, the dosing intervals may be decreased to q 30–60 min, although this

Table 16–3
Beta$_2$ Agonist Preparations

BETA$_2$ AGONIST	FORMULATION	DOSAGE
Albuterol (USA)	Tablet; 2 mg	Up to 4 mg qid
Salbutamol (Canada, UK)	Tablet; 24 mg	Up to 4 mg qid
Ventolin (USA, Can, UK)	Syrup; 2 mg/5 ml	Up to 4 mg qid
	Repetabs; 4 mg (ext. release)	Up to 16 mg bid
Proventil (USA)		
Aerolin (UK)	MDI; 90 mcg/puff	2 puffs q 4–6 hrs
Salbulin (UK)	Solution; 0.25%	2.5 mg/3 ml q 4–6 hrs
	Solution; 0.5%	2.5 mg/3 ml q 4–6 hrs
	Rotocaps; 200 μg	200 mcg q 4–6 hrs
Bitolterol	MDI 350 μg/puff	2–3 puffs q 4–6 hrs
Tornalate (USA)		
Fenoterol	MDI; 180–360 μg/puff	1–2 puffs q 6–8 hrs
Berotec (Canada, UK)		
Pirbuterol	MDI; 200–400 μg/puff	1–2 puffs q 6 hrs
Maxair (USA)		
Exirel (UK)		
Reproterol	MDI; 500 μg/puff	1 puff q 6 hrs
Bronchodil (UK)		
Rimiterol	MDI; 400–600 μg/puff	1 puff q 6 hrs
Plumadil (UK)		
Terbutaline	Tablet; 2.5 mg	2.5–5 mg q 6–8 hrs not >15 mg/day
Brethaire (USA)	Tablet; 5 mg	
Brethine (USA)	Solution; 1 mg/ml	Nebulizer 1–2 mg q 4–6 hrs
Bricanyl (USA, Can, UK)		Subcutaneous—0.25 mg repeated in 15–30 min
		Not >0.5 mg q 4 hrs IV—Not recommended
	MDI; 200 μg/puff	2 puffs q 4–6 hrs

should be done only in hospitalized, monitored patients. Some clinical situations require reductions in dosage and dosing interval, most notably in patients with heart disease or those receiving monoamine oxidase inhibitors and/or tricyclic antidepressants.

CLINICAL APPLICATIONS

- β_2-agonist therapy is most effective in the treatment of asthma and in the prevention of exercise-induced (and other forms of) bronchospasm. β_2 agonists are the cornerstone of emergent therapy for the management of acute asthma and exacerbations of COPD. The role of regular β_2-agonist use in chronic stable asthma is less certain. As-needed administration of β_2 agonists in conjunction with inhaled corticosteroids is preferable therapy in patients with stable disease
- There is data suggesting beneficial effects in chronic airflow obstruction with less reversibility. These beneficial effects include improvements in objective measurements of airway function, improvements in exercise capacity, and improvements in overall subjective quality-of-life measurements. However, while β_2 agonists are clearly superior

to anticholinergics in asthma, anticholinergics have equivalent, if not greater, effects in most patients with chronic bronchitis and emphysema. This is particularly true for patients with "fixed" obstructive airway disease

Anticholinergics

Two forms of anticholinergic bronchodilators are most commonly used: Atropine (as SO_4 and methonitrate salts) and ipratropium bromide (Atrovent, Iprafen).

PHARMACOLOGY AND MECHANISM OF ACTION

- Anticholinergic bronchodilators act through antagonism of the muscarinic receptor
- Stimulation of these receptors is believed to be responsible for "resting" bronchomotor tone
- Muscarinic receptors are found predominantly in the larger, central airways, and the anticholinergics are believed to exert their greatest bronchodilatory effects on these airways
- Anticholinergics appear to mediate the bronchoconstrictive effects of certain stimuli, including cholinergics (carbachol and metacholine), cold air, and psychogenic stimuli
- Anticholinergic bronchodilators have little or no effect on those bronchoconstrictive effects believed to be the result of inflammatory mediators, e.g., histamine. This makes them theoretically less effective for antigen-induced bronchoconstriction, as is frequently seen in asthma
- Compared to β agonists, the anticholinergics have a delayed onset of action, with maximal response occurring in 1–2 h. However, the duration of action is longer, with the effects being maintained for ≤6 h

Adverse Effects of anticholinergic alkaloids are easily predicted and result from their antagonism of the muscarinic receptor

- Inhalation of atropine may result in mouth dryness, dry skin, mydriasis, tachycardia, urinary retention, flushing, GI disturbances, and visual blurring. These symptoms are dosage dependent. Higher doses (>5 mg) result in CNS excitement, fever, headache, weakness, slurred speech, bowel and bladder dysfunction, delirium, and eventually coma
- There have also been reports of decreased mucociliary clearance secondary to the use of atropine. The mechanism of this effect is multifactorial

Adverse effects do not seem to be a problem with ipratropium bromide, whose use is much less frequently associated with side effects, even in large doses. It has been estimated that dosages 100 times > currently used for bronchodilatory effects would be necessary to produce significant side effects

- The most common complaints associated with ipratropium bromide use are a bitter taste, mouth dryness, and throat or tracheal irritation. These are usually well tolerated, and the incidence is significantly decreased when a spacer device is used
- One adverse effect that is clinically significant is mydriasis after inadvertent aerosol delivery to the eyes. This can result in acute angle closure glaucoma, in addition to unnecessary diagnostic evaluation by individuals not aware of this side effect

The difference in the side effect profiles of the 2 anticholinergics is the result of structural differences. Atropine is a tertiary ammonium compound with a neutral charge, while ipratropium bromide is a quaternary ammonium compound with a positive charge. The charge difference makes ipratropium bromide relatively lipid insoluble, resulting in markedly decreased systemic absorption of ipratropium bromide as compared to atropine. With the advent of ipratropium bromide in most markets, the use of atropine salts has waned.

Ipratropium bromide (Atrovent, Iprafen). Dosage: 2–4 puffs via metered dose inhaler q 6 h. Each actuation of the MDI contains 40 μg of ipratropium. Higher doses have been shown to be beneficial in patients with COPD with essentially no ↑ in adverse effects. An inhalant solution (250 μg/ml) is available in Europe and Canada for use as a wet aerosol with a recommended dose of 100–500 μg q 4 h. This agent is often given in combination (salbutamol 0.5 ml in 2 ml ipratropium q 4–6 h).

CLINICAL APPLICATIONS

- In diseases such as chronic bronchitis and emphysema, the use of ipratropium bromide may result in therapeutic effects comparable to or even > those of the β-adrenergic agonists
- In addition, the combined effect of ipratropium bromide and β_2 agonists appears to be better than either drug alone. This synergistic effect appears to be active in asthma as well. Ipratropium bromide also appears to act synergistically with methylxanthines. The 3 agents together have also been shown, in some instances, to be more effective than any single agent or combination of agents
- In patients with fixed obstructive pulmonary disease unresponsive to β-agonist therapy (specifically emphysema), ipratropium use may not show an improvement in FEV_1 but it results in a ↑ in vital capacity, with subsequent decreased work of breathing and hence symptomatic improvement
- Tachyphylaxis does not appear to develop with ipratropium therapy in contrast to β-agonist therapy
- Older patients with obstructive airway disease appear to have a better clinical response to ipratropium than to β agonists
- The effects of ipratropium bromide have a longer duration of action when compared to the presently available β_2 agonists, although longer-acting β_2 agonists are currently undergoing trial (see Table 16–2)
- While the effects of ipratropium bromide in asthma are less clear, there currently exists a considerable amount of data to support its use in asthmatic patients. Specifically, in those patients whose symptoms are not controlled by β_2-agonist or theophylline therapy, a trial of ipratropium bromide is indicated as an adjunct to these therapies

Theophylline

Theophylline is a methylxanthine and has been in use in obstructive airway disease since the early 20th century. Its use has decreased since its time of greatest popularity in the 1970s and 1980s.

PHARMACOLOGY AND MECHANISMS OF ACTION

The precise mechanism of action of bronchodilation by methylxanthines is not well defined, but the primary effect appears to be relaxation of smooth muscle in the bronchial walls

- Initial research was concentrated on the inhibition of phosphodiesterase. However, other phosphodiesterase inhibitors currently in use in clinical medicine (e.g., dipyridamole) do not result in bronchodilatory effects similar to those of theophylline
- Other proposed mechanisms of bronchodilatory action have included antagonism of adenosine receptors, prostaglandin antagonism, altered metabolism of smooth muscle, and stimulation of catecholamine release
- In addition to its bronchodilatory effects, theophylline may ↑ diaphragmatic contractility and reduce diaphragmatic fatigue
- There is evidence of improved biventricular cardiac performance as well
- Theophylline may stimulate hypoxic ventilatory drive, enhance mucociliary clearance, inhibit mast cell mediator release, and ↓ PA vasoconstriction
- There are data to suggest an anti-inflammatory mechanism of theophylline in the therapy of asthma. It appears to be effective in blunting the late asthmatic response to bronchial challenge. This action of theophylline requires further definition

Most theophylline preparations are primarily hepatically metabolized, with the exception of dihydroxypropyl theophylline, which is excreted unchanged in the urine. Unlike other bronchodilators, theophylline use is best guided by serum concentrations

- Multiple studies have shown that the bronchodilatory effects are relatively insignificant in most patients at a serum level of <10 μg/ml (10 mg/l or 55 μmol/l)
- At levels >20 μg/ml (20 mg/l or 110 μmol/l), toxic effects often emerge
- Thus, it is recommended that serum concentrations of 10–20 μg/ml (10–20 mg/l or 55–110 μmol/l) define the therapeutic endpoints
- Benefit may be observed in some patients at lower serum theophylline concentrations, in the range of 6–10 μg/ml (6–10 mg/l or 35–55 μmol/l). This is seen predominantly in patients who receive theophylline in addition to β-agonist therapy. The benefits deal primarily with subjective measures of improvement, such as patient's perception of disease activity, quality of life, and decreased hospital admissions

Adverse Effects are generally dose related and are much more prevalent at plasma concentrations >20 μg/ml (20 mg/l or 110 μmol/l)

- The most common side effects include abdominal discomfort, nausea, vomiting, diarrhea, headache, tremor, and restlessness
- A mild diuretic effect and ↑ gastric acid secretion may also occur
- Insomnia and other disturbances of sleep pattern have been reported
- While these symptoms are bothersome to patients and may result in noncompliance, they are rarely life threatening
- However, theophylline, even at therapeutic concentrations, has been associated with cardiac dysrhythmia, including atrial and VPCs, AF, and perhaps most commonly, multifocal atrial tachycardia. At higher concentrations, seizures and more malignant cardiac arrhythmias may occur, which can be lethal, albeit rare

Side effects can be evident in some patients at any serum concentration but are distinctly more common with levels >30 μg/ml (30 mg/l or 165 μmol/l). Adequate monitoring and maintenance of theophylline levels in the therapeutic range lessens these adverse drug manifestations.

Dosage: A partial list of available oral formulations is shown in Table

Table 16–4
Common Oral Theophylline Preparations

PRODUCT NAME	FORMULATION
ANHYDROUS THEOPHYLLINE COMPOUNDS	
Bronchodyl	Capsule; 100 and 200 mg
Aerolate	Liquid; 150 mg/15 ml
Aerolate III	Capsule; 65 mg
Aerolate Jr	Capsule; 130 mg
Aerolate SR	Capsule; 260 mg
Constant-T	Tablet; 200 and 300 mg
Elixophyllin	Capsule; 100 and 200 mg Elixir; 80 mg/15 ml
Elixophyllin SR	Capsule; 125 and 250 mg
Quibron-T	Tablet; 300 mg
Quibron-T/SR	Tablet; 300 mg
Resbid	Tablet; 250 and 500 mg
Slo-bid	Capsule; 50, 75, 100, 125, 200, and 300 mg
Slo-Phyllin	Capsule; 60, 125, 250 mg Tablet; 100 and 200 mg Syrup; 80 mg/15 ml
T-PHYL	Tablet; 200 mg
Theo-24	Capsule; 100, 200, 300 mg
Theochron	Tablets; 100, 200, 300 mg
Theoclear L.A.	Capsule; 130, 260 mg
Theoclear 80	Syrup; 80 mg/15 ml
Theo-Dur	Tablets; 100, 200, 300, 450 mg
Theo-Dur Sprinkle	Capsule; 50, 75, 125, 250 mg
Theolair	Tablet; 125 and 250 mg Liquid; 80 mg/15 ml
Theolair-SR	Tablets; 200, 250, 300, 500 mg
Theostat	Syrup; 80 mg/15 ml
Uniphyl	Tablet; 400 mg
DIHYDROXYPROPYL THEOPHYLLINE COMPOUNDS	
Dilor	Tablet; 200 and 400 mg Syrup; 100 mg/15 ml Injectable; 250 mg/ml
Lutyllin	Tablet; 200 and 400 mg Syrup; 100 mg/15 ml Injectable; 250 mg/ml
ETHYLENEDIAMINE THEOPHYLLINE COMPOUNDS	
Aminophyllin	Tablet; 100 and 200 mg
Somophyllin	Liquid; 105 mg/5 ml

16–4. While dosage must be individualized for the patient and the underlying illness, rough estimates of oral dosing are as follows

- Oral loading dose: 5 mg/kg ideal body weight
- Oral maintenance dose: 10 mg/kg ideal body weight/day, divided into 3 doses, depending upon formulation

Oral dosage must be adjusted to maintain serum level of 10–20 μg/ml (10–20 mg/l or 55–110 μmol/l).

IV dosing estimates and clinical scenarios requiring dosage adjustment are given in Table 16–5. Theophylline drug interactions are listed in Table 16–6.

Table 16–5
Dosing Guidelines for Intravenous Theophylline

INTRAVENOUS DOSAGE

5–6 mg/kg ideal body weight given over 20–30 minutes if no theophylline preparation used in the last 24 hours

2–3 mg/kg ideal body weight given over 20–30 minutes if a theophylline preparation used in the last 24 hours

Maintain an infusion rate of **0.4–0.6 mg/kg** ideal body weight per hour with the following adjustments in dosing due to other clinical circumstances:

INCREASE DOSAGE 0.6–0.8 mg/kg/hr	**DECREASE DOSAGE 0.3–0.4 mg/kg/hr**
Children	Elderly
Cigarette Smoker	Hepatic Insufficiency
Hyperthyroidism	Hypothyroidism
Marijuana Use	Congestive Heart Failure
High Protein Diet	Febrile Illness
Medications (Table 20–6)	Medications (Table 20–6)

Serum theophylline concentration should be determined approximately 6 hours after initial infusion and dosage adjusted accordingly. A general rule is adjustment of dose by 25% to achieve an increment or decrement of 5 μg/ml (5 mg/l or 27.5 μmol/l) in serum theophylline concentration.

CLINICAL APPLICATIONS

- Although it has little effect on the airways of normal individuals, theophylline ameliorates bronchoconstriction in individuals with asthma
- The bronchodilatory effects add to those of β agonists and anticholinergics, but theophylline is a less effective bronchodilator than either agent alone

There is a subset of patients with asthma who experience symptoms during the nocturnal hours and have disrupted sleep secondary to these symptoms. In these patients, there has been some improvement in symptoms and sleep with bedtime dosing of a 24-hour theophylline preparation.

The beneficial effects of theophylline in patients with chronic bronchitis and emphysema are less clear. There does appear to be subjective symptomatic improvement in patients with chronic bronchitis, but objective improvement in airflow is lacking

- Theophylline should be considered for use in patients with asthma and chronic bronchitis who have failed optimal inhalation therapy prior to the initiation of systemic steroids. However, the decision to begin theophylline therapy versus steroid therapy should include a knowledge of possible drug interactions and underlying disease states that alter theophylline pharmacokinetics. In some cases, the toxicity of shortterm systemic steroids will be < the toxicity of theophylline and may therefore be the preferred alternative

ASTHMA

Asthma is a disease of the airways characterized by ↑ responsiveness of the trachea and bronchi to a wide range of stimuli. Intermittent symp-

Table 16–6
Theophylline Interactions

DRUG	EFFECT	RESPONSE
Allopurinol	Decrease theophylline clearance	Decrease dose of theophylline
Barbiturates	Increase theophylline clearance	Increase dose of theophylline
Carbamazepine	Increase theophylline clearance	Increase dose of theophylline
Corticosteroids	Variable metabolic effects	Monitor theophylline levels
Coumarins	Interferes with assay method for serum level resulting in falsely low values	No adjustment in dose necessary
Diltiazem	Slight decrease in theophylline clearance	Possible decrease in theophylline dose
Erythromycin	Decrease theophylline clearance	Decrease dose of theophylline
Estrogens	Decrease theophylline clearance	Decrease dose of theophylline
H_2 Blockers		
Cimetidine	Decrease theophylline clearance	Decrease dose of theophylline
Ranitidine	No effect	No adjustment
Famotidine	No effect	No adjustment
Influenza Vaccine	Decrease theophylline clearance	Decrease dose of theophylline
Interferon	Decrease theophylline clearance	Decrease dose of theophylline
Isoniazid	Decrease theophylline clearance	Decrease dose of theophylline
Isoproterenol	Increase theophylline clearance	Increase dose of theophylline
Lithium	Increase lithium clearance	Increase dose of lithium
Mexiletine	Decrease theophylline clearance	Decrease dose of theophylline
Nicorette	No effect	No response
Oral contraceptives	Decrease theophylline clearance	Decrease dose of theophylline
Pancuronium	Decrease pancuronium responsiveness	Increase dose of pancuronium
Phenytoin	Increase theophylline clearance	Increase dose of theophylline
Quinolones	Decrease theophylline clearance	Decrease dose of theophylline
Tobacco smoking	Increase theophylline clearance	Increase dose of theophylline
Troleandomycin	Decrease theophylline clearance	Decrease dose of theophylline
Verapamil	Decrease theophylline clearance	Decrease dose of theophylline
Vidarabine	Decrease theophylline clearance	Decrease dose of theophylline

toms of cough, chest tightness, and wheezing usually alter in severity, either spontaneously or due to treatment. The widespread airway narrowing results from a combination of smooth muscle contraction, inflammation, edema, and mucous secretion. *Airway inflammation is present in virtually all patients with asthma* and, with widespread mucous plugging of airways, is a constant finding in patients who have died of status asthmaticus.

The complex forces that combine to cause asthma result in certain macroscopic and microscopic features that are common to those who have died from this disease

- Overinflated lungs that do not deflate upon opening the thoracic cavity
- Widespread airway plugging with thick mucus
- Airway wall thickening
- Upper lobe bronchiectasis (sometimes)
- Little evidence of emphysema
- *Infiltration of airway walls by inflammatory cells, particularly eosinophilic infiltration*
- Epithelial desquamation
- Smooth muscle hypertrophy
- Basement membrane thickening; subepithelial deposition of collagen

Other features of asthma include mucus gland hyperplasia and ↑ goblet cell numbers. Patients with asthma who are asymptomatic appear to have varying degrees of the abnormalities noted above.

Asthma Triggers

Allergens. Allergic asthma depends upon IgE response modulated by B and T cell lymphocytes and the interaction of mast-cell-bound IgE with antigen. Small amounts of antigen reach distal airways, where mast cells interdigitate with epithelial cells. There is usually an immediate response, resulting in bronchoconstriction, followed in some patients by a late-phase response 6–10 h later. Once contracted, the mast cells and other cells release mediators that cause constriction, edema, and vascular congestion

- Major airborne allergens include house dust, mites, and pollens
- Asthmatics who respond to allergens usually have a fair number of antigens that can trigger their disease
- The role of different foods (cow's milk, monosodium glutamate, preservatives, food coloring agents, etc.) are not clearly defined, although some individuals may react strongly
- Symptoms can be continual or seasonal, depending on the antigen

Pharmacologic Agents that trigger asthma include drugs such as aspirin, tartrazine dye, β blockers, and sulfating agents

- Nasal polyps, rhinorrhea, and asthma comprise a syndrome that has been associated with aspirin use in some patients
- Sulfating agents such as potassium bisulfite and sodium bisulfite, sulphur dioxide, and others are widely used in the fresh-food industry and may cause symptoms in some

Environmental and Air Pollution. Climatic conditions can ↑ the concentration of allergens and cause exacerbation of asthma. Occupational asthma refers to patients who develop symptoms while in the work place in response to some specific trigger. These symptoms will often improve when the patient is out of the offending environment, but chronic problems can also occur. Specific agents include

- Wood and vegetable dusts, such as western red cedar
- Metal salts, such as platinum, chrome, and nickel
- Pharmaceutical agents, including antibiotics, piperazine, and cimetidine
- Industrial chemicals and plastics, such as toluene, isocyanate, phthalic acid, ethylenediamine, and others
- Biologic enzymes, including detergents
- Animal and insect dusts, serums, and secretions

The underlying mechanisms for airway obstruction in occupational asthma include the formation of specific IgE, the direct release of factors causing bronchoconstriction by the offending agent, and direct airway stimulation.

Infections. Respiratory infections by viruses and bacteria are the most common causes of asthma exacerbation. Respiratory syncytial and parainfluenza virus are major offenders in children, while rhinovirus and influenza virus are most common in adults. The reason that viruses induce asthma is unclear, but bronchial hyperresponsiveness may last $\leq$8 weeks. Bacteria are less common than viruses as triggers of asthmatic exacerbation but can superinfect a prior viral process.

Exercise and Stress. Physical exertion can worsen asthma, and the first episode often occurs with exercise in children. This acute process may be due to thermal changes in the intrathoracic airways as heat and water are transferred from tracheal mucosa to the inspired air. High ventilation may lower airway temperature further, especially in colder, dryer air, and worsen symptoms. Hence, ambient temperatures and the level of exertion may correlate with the degree of obstruction. Activities such as cross-country skiing or ice skating usually produce more symptoms than swimming. Objective evidence suggests that psychological features play a role in asthmatic symptoms. These interactions are complex but may be related to vagal efferent activity mediating airway caliber. The extent of the influence of psychological factors on asthma is unclear.

Diagnosis

Symptoms and signs include

- Symptoms include: Dyspnea; chest tightness; wheezing, cough; exercise intolerance; rhinitis, sinusitis; nasal polyposis; atopic dermatitis. The hallmark of asthma is the variable nature of respiratory symptoms that are caused by the changing degree of airway obstruction. The marked variability in degree of airway obstruction is the main factor distinguishing asthma from other forms of chronic obstructive lung disease. Typically, symptoms in asthma are episodic. In some cases, the patient's clinical history may be so characteristic of asthma that a presumptive diagnosis of asthma can be comfortably made on the history alone. It is important to remember, however, that "not all that wheezes is asthma" and, in most cases, it will be necessary to have objective data to support a clinical diagnosis. Other features of medical history include: Positive family history for allergies/asthma (50%); aspirin sensitivity (5–10%); frequent association with sinusitis
- Pertinent findings of the physical examination include: Nasal polyps and scattered or diffuse wheezes with prolonged expiration in the chest
- Differential diagnosis of asthma includes: Emphysema, bronchitis, CHF, pulmonary emboli, foreign body in airway, aspiration, carcinoid syndrome, bronchiectasis, laryngeal edema, hyperventilation syndrome, factitious wheezing, and cystic fibrosis

Table 16–7
Changes in the Arterial Blood Gases

SEVERITY OF ATTACK	MILD	MODERATE	SEVERE	VERY SEVERE
pH	↑	↑	normal	↓
PaO_2	normal	↓	↓	↓
$PaCO_2$	↓	↓	normal	↑

Clinical data indicating severe asthma include

- Previous ICU admission, frequent emergency room visits, or hospital stay >4 days for treatment of documented severe asthma
- Recent oral corticosteroid use for exacerbation
- Brittle asthma
- Extreme dyspnea with inability to speak more than a few words
- Pulsus paradoxus >18 mm Hg
- Use of accessory muscles and paradoxical thoracoabdominal motion
- Diaphoresis
- Inability to lie supine
- HR >120 beats/minute
- Respiratory rate >30
- Absence of audible wheezing in a patient with severe exacerbation of asthma
- PaO_2 <60 mm Hg
- $PaCO_2$ ≥40 mm Hg
- PEFR or FEV_1 <30% of predicted for adults
- Failure of PEFR to improve ≥10% after initial treatment

Pulmonary function testing may be normal in patients with asthma if they are in remission at the time of testing. When patients are symptomatic, however, abnormalities in pulmonary function should be present

- FEV_1: ↓
- FEV_1/FVC: ↓
- Typically, a ≥20% ↑ in FEV_1 is noted after administration of an inhaled bronchodilator
- Total lung capacity: Normal or ↑
- Residual volume: ↑
- Normal or ↑ diffusion capacity (transfer factor)

ABGs may be normal if the patient is in remission at the time of testing. If the patient is symptomatic, however, ABGs will demonstrate abnormalities, the pattern of abnormalities indicating the disease severity. The ABGs may be useful, therefore, in determining the aggressiveness of treatment and the need for close monitoring of patients in the hospital or in the intensive care unit (Table 16–7).

Chest x ray is generally of little value in making a diagnosis of asthma. In asthmatics presenting with an acute attack, the chest x ray generally appears normal or demonstrates hyperinflation. The main value of the chest x ray is to rule out densities and/or atelectasis secondary to mucus plugging and other diagnostic possibilities, such as pneumothorax or pneumonia.

Therapy of Asthma

The available agents can be classified as bronchodilators, functioning primarily to directly reduce bronchoconstriction (see Table 16–3), or

Table 16–8
Inhaled Corticosteroids*: Aerosol Metered Dose Inhaler

PRODUCT	SUPPLIED	DOSAGE†
Beclomethasone		
Beclovent	50 μg/puff	2 puffs 2–4 times daily
Venceril	100–200 μg/Rotacap	
Becloforte	250 μg/puff	1–2 puffs 2 times daily
Becotide (UK)	50 μg/puff	2 puffs 2–4 times daily
	200 μg/puff	1–2 puffs 2–4 times daily
	100–200 μg Rotacaps	2–4 times daily
Budesonide		
Pulmicort Turbuhaler‡	100–400 μg/puff	1–2 puffs 2–3 times daily
Flunisolide	250 μg/puff	1–2 puffs 2 times daily
Bronalide		
Bronkolid		
Aerobid		
Triamcinolone acetate§	100 or 200 μg/puff	2–4 puffs 2 times daily

* Not recommended for acute attacks
† Dose inhaled 10–20 minutes after $beta_2$ agonist inhalation. Dose > 1500 μg/daily; risk adrenal suppression and osteoporosis
‡ Pulmicort chlorofluorocarbon-based inhaler replaced by Pulmicort Turbuhaler (non-chlorofluorocarbon) in some countries
§ High dosage of fluorinated agents may rarely cause myopathy

as anti-inflammatory agents (corticosteroids or cromolyn), *decreasing airway inflammation, which is the primary stimulus for bronchoconstriction and bronchial hyperresponsiveness.* Inhaled corticosteroids are listed in Table 16–8. Some patients with chronic, stable asthma have symptoms even with multi-drug treatment (inhaled steroids, β_2 agonists, theophylline, cromolyn, or ipratropium). In these patients, oral corticosteroids have a role (Table 16–9).

Table 16–9
Treatment of Chronic, Stable Asthma

PATIENT TYPE	AGENTS RECOMMENDED
1. Only occasional dyspnea, such as with exercise	$Beta_2$ agonist inhaled as needed
2. Chronic cough without airway obstruction	Inhaled steroid regularly
3. Frequent or prolonged episodes of dyspnea	Inhaled steroid regularly and $beta_2$ agonist as needed
4. Asthma not controlled by inhaled steroids and $beta_2$ agonists	Consider cromolyn and adding ipratropium

STATUS ASTHMATICUS

Refers to an asthmatic episode that does not respond to usual initial therapy and is severe enough to threaten life. This form of asthma is a medical emergency and requires intensive treatment and monitoring. The history is usually one of poorly controlled asthma that progresses over days or weeks, although in some cases there will be a more abrupt onset (see p. 276 and Table 16–7 for clinical data and ABGs indicating severe asthma). Initial treatment in the emergency room for patients with acute, severe asthma should include inhaled β_2 agonists and IV corticosteroids; for status asthmaticus ipratropium is added with aminophylline given consideration.

Beta$_2$ agonists. β_2-selective agents should be given frequently by inhalation, e.g., q 20 min over the first hour

- Inhaled β_2 agonists: Albuterol (Salbutamol) 2.5–5 mg (0.5–1 ml of 0.5% solution)
- Subcutaneous β agonists: Epinephrine (1:1000) 0.3–0.5 ml, avoid in older asthmatics (>40) and anyone with a history of heart disease; Terbutaline 0.24–0.50 mg

Corticosteroids. In patients with severe asthma, early use of IV corticosteroids is warranted. The optimal dose of corticosteroids is not known, but doses of 80–125 mg of methylprednisolone repeated q 6–8 h have been recommended. Patients who have responded to IV steroids can be safely switched to comparable doses of oral steroids. Because oral doses of steroids are frequently significantly lower than IV doses, however, it is wise to carefully monitor the clinical response of the patient during the switch from IV to oral steroids. Following discharge from the hospital, oral steroids should be tapered carefully with frequent determination of PEFR to monitor for any deterioration in pulmonary function. Inhaled steroids are not useful in the treatment of acute, severe asthma, but should be used to aid in the weaning process of oral steroids. Inhaled steroids have a role in patients with asthma requiring β_2 agonists >3 times daily for control.

Corticosteroids ↑ the effectiveness of β_2 agonists and have been shown to induce the formation of new β_2 receptors in the human lung.

Anticholinergics. Several studies have demonstrated some benefit from adding nebulized ipratropium bromide to treatment with inhaled β_2 agonists in acute, severe asthma. Given the safety and lack of significant side effects associated with the use of ipratropium, it is a reasonable adjunct to treatment in patients who have demonstrated a limited clinical response to β_2 agonists and corticosteroids. *Dosage:* Ipratropium (via nebulizer) 500 μg/2 ml unit; administer 2 ml q 4 h; in severe asthma, give q 2 h for 4 doses then 4–6 h under supervision. When the patient has been stabilized, a metered-dose inhaler (20 μg puff, 1–4 puffs 3–6 times daily) may be required.

Methylxanthines. There is little objective evidence that addition of methylxanthine therapy adds any significant benefit to patients treated with β_2, agonists and IV or oral corticosteroids. IV aminophylline therapy is controversial. Some studies have demonstrated that although there was no therapeutic benefit, a significant ↑ in treatment toxicity (including nausea and palpitations) was associated with the addition of methylxanthine therapy. There appears to still be a role for methylxanthines in chronic treatment of asthma, but it appears that these agents do not have a clear role in the treatment of acute, severe asthma. In patients who are being treated chronically with methylxanthines and present with acute, severe asthma, it is reasonable to obtain a serum theophylline level and, if subtherapeutic, administer aminophylline or theophylline to bring serum levels to a safe therapeutic range (10–15 μg/ml, United States; 10–20 mg/l, UK; 55–110 μmol/l, Canada).

Supplemental oxygen. This should generally be provided by nasal cannula to these patients. Oxygenation should be monitored by pulse oximetry; O_2 flow rates can then be titrated to maintain O_2 saturation >90%. In some cases, a higher inspired concentration of O_2 provided by a high-flow face mask may be required. In severely obstructed patients, it is important to obtain frequent ABGs, in addition to following oximetry, to determine whether there are progressive increases in arterial CO_2 that would indicate impending ventilatory failure.

Mechanical ventilation. Endotracheal intubation and mechanical ventilation of patients in status asthmaticus are last-resort treatments indicated in patients with impending ventilatory failure. Indications for intubation include

- Inability to maintain airway control, resulting in progressive ↑ in arterial CO_2 tension to elevated levels (particularly >50 mm Hg)
- Altered mental status
- Clinical evidence of respiratory muscle fatigue (paradoxical movement of diaphragm)
- Refractory hypoxemia, acidemia, or seizures

Mechanical ventilation of asthma patients may be complicated by very high airway pressures, which may lead to barotrauma. Mortality associated with mechanical ventilation for status asthmaticus has been reported to be relatively high (5–23%). Controlled hypoventilation, which uses lower tidal volumes and a lower respiratory rate and tolerates some hypercarbia while maintaining oxygenation, may result in a lower mortality. In general, the tidal volume and respiratory rate should be adjusted to maintain peak airway pressures at <50 cm H_2O (see Chap. 20).

OUTPATIENT MANAGEMENT OF THE SEVERE ASTHMATIC

Optimal outpatient management of patients with severe asthma should include routine assessment of PEFR, as the presence or absence of symptoms may not accurately reflect lung function. The patient should possess, and learn to use, a peak flow meter. Appropriate adjustments in inhaled medications or in oral corticosteroids should be made if the PEFR falls significantly. Patients should be instructed to obtain emergency medical assistance if the PEFR falls dramatically (<150 l/min). Monitoring PEFR on a regular basis will help limit any delay in initiating treatment for bronchospasm. This approach may help reduce mortality that may result from delayed initiation of treatment for bronchospasm in some asthmatics.

Features that characterize patients at ↑ risk for asthma-associated death include

- Age >55 years
- Prior history of ICU admission, intubation, or respiratory acidosis
- Hospitalization for asthma in last year
- Recent withdrawal from systemic steroids
- Psychological or psychosocial problems
- Lack of access to health care
- Inadequate medical management

CHRONIC OBSTRUCTIVE PULMONARY DISEASE

COPD is a generic term used to describe the condition of patients with expiratory airflow obstruction. The diseases usually included under the heading COPD are chronic bronchitis and emphysema, which both have varying degrees of expiratory airflow obstruction.

Chronic Bronchitis

The definition of chronic bronchitis is based on a clinical symptom complex: Cough with sputum production for 3 months of the year over 2 consecutive years in the absence of other causes with or without expiratory airflow obstruction. The pathophysiology is described as chronic excessive secretion of mucus with hypertrophy of the subepithelial tracheobronchial mucous glands. The goblet cells are another source of excessive mucous secretion. Studies have demonstrated that the mucous glands are ↑ in size. The Reid Index, or ratio of gland to bronchial wall thickness, is the most common means of measuring mucous gland enlargement

- The ↑ bronchial smooth muscle present in chronic bronchitis has been determined to result from smooth muscle hyperplasia. A correlation has been demonstrated between ↓ FEV_1 and ↑ amounts of smooth muscle in the major airways. ↑ amounts of smooth muscle are related neither to bronchodilator response nor to methacholine responsiveness in surgically resected lung
- Bronchoscopy and bronchoalveolar lavage performed on patients with chronic bronchitis demonstrated ↑ inflammation of the tracheobronchial tree compared to that of asymptomatic smokers or normal individuals. Bronchial samples of the lavage demonstrated ↑ nutrophils. Airway nutrophilia was associated with sputum production, airway obstruction, and cigarette smoking
- Bronchial walls are thickened with encroachment on the airway lumen. Patients with severe obstruction had double the bronchial wall width internal to the cartilage/lumenal diameter of that in patients without obstruction. Most series have reported that the ↑ in bronchial wall thickness resulting from mucous gland hypertrophy is minimal

Emphysema

Emphysema is defined as the abnormal, permanent enlargement of the airspace distal to the terminal (nonrespiratory) bronchioles with concomitant destruction of their walls without obvious fibrosis. Emphysema can be classified as follows

- Centriacinar emphysema: This form of emphysema involves the respiratory bronchioles with scarring and focal dilation of the bronchiole and adjacent alveoli, and exists as centrilobular and focal emphysema. Centrilobular emphysema is most frequently associated with prolonged cigarette smoking. It usually involves the posterior upper lobes and is the most common clinically expressed form of emphysema. Focal emphysema is associated with exposure to biologically inactive dust and is uniformly distributed throughout the lung
- Panacinar emphysema: This form of emphysema involves dilation of all the respiratory airspaces and of the secondary lung lobule with either diffuse or focal involvement. The diffuse form may be associated

with deficiency of protease inhibitors (α_1-antitrypsin deficiency), and the lung bases are involved more often than the upper lobes

Risk Factors for COPD

- Cigarette smoking: Smoking is by far the most important single factor associated with the development of COPD. Only a portion of chronic smokers, however, show an accelerated decline in FEV_1. Chronic cough and sputum occur independently of the development of airflow obstruction
- Air pollution: Exposure to particulate matter is related to symptoms of chronic bronchitis and ↓ in pulmonary function. Exposure to irritants can lead to cellular changes and acute respiratory infection or may enhance allergic response
- Occupational exposure: Exposures to both organic and inorganic dust may lead to symptoms of chronic bronchitis. Any effect that such exposure may have on the development of airflow obstruction has been difficult to demonstrate in cross-sectional studies; however, most longitudinal studies show the accelerated decline in indices typical of an airflow associated with chronic dust exposure. The effect is more pronounced in smokers
- Atopy: The role of immunologic response and airway hyperresponsiveness in the development of COPD is important. The immunologic precursors to COPD are in part genetically determined. Bronchial reactivity may be a precursor to obstructive airway disease. A relationship exists between COPD prevalence and serum IgE levels
- Heredity: Hereditary factors, such as deficiency of protease inhibitors (α_1-antitrypsin deficiency), have been related to the development of emphysema. Prevalence of this deficiency has been shown by blood donor studies to be 350 per 1,000,000. Nonsmoking patients may remain asymptomatic with little abnormality of lung function through their 6th–7th decades of life; however, smokers with protease inhibitor deficiencies may experience severely limited respiratory function by age 40

Diagnosis

- Dyspnea or acute chest illness with cough, sputum production, chest tightness, and wheezing may be of sufficient magnitude to bring the patient to seek medical attention. This condition usually occurs in the 6th–7th decade of life. Chronic bronchitis and emphysema often coexist and are reviewed together in the remaining sections
- The dyspnea is usually of insidious onset
- Smoking of >20 cigarettes/day for ≥25 years is often present. Hemoptysis may occur and, if so, is usually associated with the development of purulent sputum in a lower respiratory tract infection. Recurrent symptoms of cough, ↑ and/or purulent sputum, wheeze, and dyspnea are common
- Active accessory muscles (scalenes and sternomastoids) are a consistent finding with significant airflow obstruction because of the inability of the diaphragm to produce the force required for inspiration
- Pursed lip expiration is a common feature in patients with severe airflow obstruction
- Examination of patients with emphysema often demonstrates a barrel chest, caused by air trapping, and thus a prominent sternal angle, horizontal ribs, and a ↑ anteroposterior diameter. Also seen is a low

diaphragm with limited motion or decreased excursion. Normal diaphragmatic excursion is approximately 5–6 cm

- Indrawing of the intercostal space is a sign of hyperinflation of the chest
- Paradoxical abdominal and diaphragmatic movement during respiration indicates diaphragmatic fatigue or weakness. Patients with exacerbations of COPD who manifest this sign are more likely to require ventilator assistance
- Hoover's sign (paradoxical inward movement of the lateral costal margin) may be observed and is caused by horizontal rather than vertical (downward) diaphragmatic contraction that results from the flat position of the diaphragm. Hoover's sign is not a sign of diaphragmatic fatigue
- Tracheal tug (the downward movement of the thyroid cartilage and trachea with each inspiration) may be observed
- Wheezes (rhonchi), which are musical sounds produced by the rapid passage of air through a bronchus that is narrowed to the point of closure, may be heard. The walls of the bronchus oscillate between closed and barely open positions and generate audible sound. Wheezes are typically expiratory but may occur in both inspiration and expiration. Although wheezes vary in pitch, inferences as to the size of the airways involved cannot be made from the pitch
- Cardiac dullness is decreased
- Reduction in breath sounds is marked
- Central cyanosis and signs of cor pulmonale—jugular venous distension, hepatojugular reflux, hepatomegaly, and pedal edema—are apparent
- Signs of hypercapnia (asterixis, chemosis, and fundal vessel dilation), usually without papilledema, are important indicators of elevated $PaCO_2$
- A forced expiratory time of >6 seconds indicates airflow limitation. This maneuver is performed by placing the stethoscope over the trachea and requesting the patient to expire from full inspiration to full expiration. Normally the patient should be able to expire completely in <6 seconds
- Finger clubbing is not a feature of COPD and, if present, should alert the physician to other possible causes, such as bronchiectasis and carcinoma

The chest x ray may reveal the marked and persistent overdistension of the lungs that is strongly suggestive of emphysema; however, the sensitivity of chest radiography for the detection of emphysema is poor. The diaphragms are often low and flattened in emphysema. An enlarged retrosternal airspace (>3.5 cm) and a deep anteroposterior diameter of the chest may be present

- Hyperinflated, hypertransradiant lungs, as well as a large and small bullae, are seen
- Excessively rapid tapering of the vascular shadows, with narrow-angle branching and general oligemia resulting from loss of pulmonary vessels, is apparent
- A narrow, seemingly elongated heart is not uncommon
- The chest x ray of the patient with chronic bronchitis may be normal or may demonstrate accentuation of the normal bronchovascular markings
- Heart size is not a sensitive indicator of cor pulmonale
- The chest x ray may be suggestive of emphysema if air trapping, hyperinflation, vascular deficiency, and bullae are present, but these findings are often not present until late in the course of the disease

Pulmonary function testing reveals

- FEV_1 is ↓. An FEV_1 <70% of that predicted for age-, sex-, and height-matched controls is abnormal and indicates airflow obstruction
- The ratio of FEV_1 to FVC of <70% with incomplete reversibility indicates an airflow obstruction. Moderate airflow obstruction is evidenced as an FEV_1/FVC ratio of <65%, whereas severe airflow obstruction is evidenced as an FEV_1/FVC ratio of <60% with a markedly ↓ FEV_1 (<0.75 l)
- The FVC may be normal or may ↓ in proportion to any ↑ in the residual volume
- The diffusing capacity for carbon monoxide (DL_{CO}) is usually ↓ in emphysema and often remains near normal in chronic bronchitis
- ABGs may be normal or may show varying degrees of hypoxemia or hypercapnia, depending on the type of disease and the point in its natural course. Patients with predominant chronic bronchitis typically develop hypoxemia and hypercapnia earlier in the progression of airflow obstruction than do patients with predominant emphysema, who may have normal or near-normal ABGs despite severe airflow obstruction (FEV_1 <0.75 l). In such patients, development of hypercapnia is often a preterminal sign

Therapy

Therapy should be directed at

- Improvement of reversible airflow obstruction
- Treatment of complications in COPD
- O_2 therapy
- Pulmonary rehabilitation
- Prevention
- Home care

Improvement of reversible airflow obstruction involves treatment of bronchospasm, mucosal inflammation, and infection and control of abnormal and excessive mucoid or mucopurulent secretions that occur with varying degrees of clinical significance at different times in the same patient. A careful clinical assessment of the patient and examination of the sputum often provide hints as to which of these components of airway obstruction is contributing most to the current exacerbation.

Salutary effects of pharmacological therapy are obtained in most patients with the use of bronchodilators. Occasionally pulsed corticosteroids are used in combination with antibiotics during exacerbations when bacterial infection is deemed present. The main classes of compounds used in the treatment of COPD are

- β_2-adrenergic agonist (see Table 16–3)
- Anticholinergic agents (see Table 16–1)
- Methylxanthines (see Tables 16–4, 16–5, and 16–6)
- Corticosteroids (see Tables 16–8 and 16–10)

Antibiotic use includes the following

- The use of antibiotics in an exacerbation of COPD has been demonstrated in various studies to be both beneficial and of little benefit. The initial infection in most patients with an acute exacerbation of COPD is most commonly viral. Because of impaired mucociliary clearance, bacterial superinfection occurs in a substantial proportion of patients. Accurately differentiating those patients whose course will be improved by antibiotics from those who will receive no benefit is difficult or impossible. The administration of a broad-spectrum anti-

Table 16–10
Corticosteroids and Bronchodilators

NAME	PREPARATION	ROUTE OF ADMINISTRATION
Methylprednosolone (Solu-Medrol)	80 to 125 mg q 6 hrs	Intravenous
Prednisolone (Medrol)	Variable (initial 20–40 mg qd)	Oral
Dexamethasone (Decadron)	4–10 mg qd to qid	Intravenous, oral
Prednisone	Variable (40–60 mg qd to bid)	Oral
ANTICHOLINERGIC AGENTS:		
Atropine	1–3 mg q 6 hrs	Nebulized aerosol
Ipratropium bromide (Atrovent)	2–4 puffs qid	Metered dose inhaler
BETA$_2$ AGONISTS:		
(See Table 16–3)		
METHYLXANTHINES:		
(See Tables 16–4, 16–5, 16–6)		

microbial agent to a patient who is producing purulent, copious sputum during an exacerbation is a reasonable addition to therapy. Currently recommended antibiotics include trimethoprim/sulfa, amoxicillin/clavulanate, or tetracycline (see p. 306).
- Sputum culture is not helpful or necessary in most exacerbations. If the patient fails to improve with first-line therapy, culture should be obtained because the emergence of drug-resistant organisms, especially Pseudomonas, may occur after repeated courses of antibiotics. Choice of antibiotics when drug-resistant organisms are present should be guided by sensitivity testing

As potent anti-inflammatory drugs, corticosteroids may be useful in the treatment of active bronchial inflammation. Judicious use is mandatory because of the well-known deleterious side effects of longterm, high-dose corticosteroids

- Hospitalized patients with acute exacerbations causing respiratory failure should receive high-dose IV methylprednisolone, 250–500 mg/24 hr. *Supplied:* vials, 40 or 125 mg; convenient to give 80–125 mg q 6 h. After 48 h, the dose may be halved daily until a dose of 40–60 mg is reached. The patient is then changed to oral prednisone, and the dosage is tapered
- Outpatients with exacerbations associated with acute, purulent bronchitis often benefit from a short, pulsed dose of oral prednisone. A dose of 40–60 mg/day for 5 days without tapering is frequently successful in accelerating improvement in airflow obstruction. If obstruction flares when corticosteroids are stopped, a tapering schedule may be needed
- Patients with severe airflow obstruction (FEV$_1$ <1 l) deserve 1 controlled trial of corticosteroids to determine whether they are 1 of the approximately 20% who show substantial improvement in airway obstruction. Prednisone administered 40–60 mg/day for 2–4 weeks is an adequate trial (Table 16–10). The trial must be controlled by baseline and post-therapy measurements of FEV$_1$. A response is deter-

mined by improvement in airflow obstruction. Most patients show subjective improvement because of the euphoric effect of the drug. Maintenance of a therapeutic response requires chronic corticosteroid therapy

- Inhaled corticosteroids are commonly ineffective in patients with COPD, even in those who improve with systemic therapy. The lack of effect is probably caused by poor peripheral aerosol distribution
- Patients requiring chronic corticosteroid therapy to maintain improved airway function should be tapered to the lowest possible single daily dose or tried on alternate-day administration (1 dose q 48 h) to minimize side effects. Measures to prevent weight gain, hyperglycemia, and osteoporosis are important

Treatment of Complications

Acute exacerbations. The patient has ↑ dyspnea, chest tightness, and wheezing usually accompanied by ↑ cough and sputum production. The most common cause is acute lower respiratory infection, usually viral. Exposure to respiratory irritants may also cause an exacerbation. Treatment depends on the severity of the baseline disease and of the exacerbation. Severity is best judged by peak flow measurement, spirometry, and/or ABGs in addition to symptoms. An increasing order of intensity of therapy involves

- ↑ frequency of inhaled bronchodilators
- Antibiotic administration
- Use of pulsed corticosteroids
- O_2 if PaO_2 <55 mm Hg
- Mechanical ventilation for ventilatory failure with consideration of the patient's and the family's wishes

Pulmonary thromboembolism. An estimated 20–40% of patients with exacerbation of COPD experience acute pulmonary thromboembolism. (See Chap. 22.)

Pneumothorax. Spontaneous pneumothorax rarely causes the exacerbation of COPD and is most often secondary to the rupture of a bulla or bleb. Identification of a pneumothorax can be lifesaving. The chest examination often reveals decreased breath sounds on the side of the pneumothorax. The affected side of the chest is often more hyperresonant than the contralateral side, but this finding is difficult to ascertain clinically. If tension is involved, the trachea may be shifted to the opposite side of the pneumothorax and hemodynamic deterioration may arise emergently.

Respiratory drive depression. Neuromuscular abnormalities; sedative/hypnotic medication; narcotic analgesics; metabolic alkalosis, which may be caused by diuretics that induce hypochloremia and elevated bicarbonate levels; hypocalcemia; hypomagnesemia; hypophosphatemia.

Oxygen therapy. The predominant pathophysiologic mechanism leading to hypoxemia and hypercapnia in COPD is ventilation/perfusion mismatching leading to ↑ numbers of gas-exchanging units with low V/Q ratios. In addition, when the work of breathing exceeds respiratory muscle capacity for work, generalized hypoventilation occurs, either acutely or chronically, thus further worsening both hypoxemia and hypercapnia. Hypoxemia may be acutely lethal. Chronic hypoxemia leads

Table 16–11
F_IO_2/FLOW RATE EQUIVALENTS

NASAL CANNULA FLOW RATE (L/MIN)	APPROXIMATE F_IO_2 (%)
1	23
2	27
3	30
4	33
5	36
6	40

to pulmonary hypertension, polycythemia, cognitive impairment, and premature death.

Types of O_2 therapy include

- Nasal cannula: The most comfortable, generally most suitable means for O_2 therapy in COPD (Table 16–11). Less likely to be removed by patients
- O_2 masks: Venturi masks achieve the most accurate control of F_IO_2. Rebreather and nonrebreather masks can achieve F_IO_2 between 40 and 80%. All masks are somewhat uncomfortable and more likely to be removed
- Endotracheal intubation with mechanical ventilation: Can achieve F_IO_2 of 100%. Necessary when adequate oxygenation cannot be achieved without hypercapnia with respiratory acidosis severe enough to cause somnolence or coma
- O_2-conservation devices: Pulsed flow devices and reservoir devices both conserve O_2 by avoiding the wasted O_2 that does not reach the alveolar level or is delivered during expiration

O_2 therapy is indicated during acute exacerbations when the PaO_2 is <60 mm Hg or the $SaFO_2$ is <90%. The dose of O_2 required is generally low unless pneumonia or pulmonary embolism is present

- In the absence of hypercapnia, the dose of O_2 is not critical. A PaO_2 >65 mm Hg or SaO_2 >90% is adequate
- Hypercapnic patients may depend on their hypoxic drive to stimulate respiration. O_2 therapy may result in worsening hypercapnia and respiratory acidosis. Many such patients can be successfully treated with carefully controlled F_IO_2 achieving a PaO_2 of 55–65 mm Hg without producing clinically significant respiratory acidosis. A Venturi mask or pediatric O_2 flowmeter may be used to achieve a more precise F_IO_2
- If a PaO_2 of 55 mg Hg cannot be achieved without clinically significant respiratory acidosis, mechanical ventilation may be required. Clinically significant respiratory acidosis is best judged by cerebral effects (somnolence, coma, inability to cooperate with therapy) rather than by any arbitrary level of $PaCO_2$ or pH
- Hypoxemia can be rapidly lethal or deleterious. Respiratory acidosis can be tolerated for several hours. O_2 should never be discontinued in a patient with respiratory failure who has a rising Pa_CO_2
- The duration of O_2 therapy for acute exacerbation is unpredictable. Some patients require several weeks of O_2 therapy to restore their previous level of PaO_2. If the PaO_2 is <55 mm Hg at the time of discharge, home administration of O_2 should be arranged with a repeat ABG measurement taken in 2–4 weeks to determine when or whether O_2 therapy can be discontinued

Stable patients with COPD who remain hypoxemic despite optimal med-

ical therapy benefit from longterm O_2 therapy. Documented benefits are improved survival, decreased pulmonary artery pressure and polycythemia, improved cognitive function, improved exercise tolerance, decreased dyspnea, and fewer hospitalizations. O_2 is usually delivered via nasal cannula. O_2-conservation devices may ↓ the cost of O_2 and extend the duration of use for a portable O_2 system.
Guidelines for longterm O_2 therapy include

- $PaO_2 \leq 55$ mm Hg or $SaO_2 < 88\%$ at rest breathing air
- $PaO_2 < 60$ mm Hg or $SaO_2 < 90\%$ at rest breathing air in, patients with cor pulmonale, pulmonary hypertension, or polycythemia
- $PaO_2 \leq 55$ mm Hg or $SaO_2 < 88\%$ during exercise or sleep
- Dose: O_2 flow sufficient to raise PaO_2 to 65 mm Hg or $SaO_2 \geq 90\%$
- Duration: At least 15 h/day unless only needed during exercise or sleep

Prevention

Educational and psychosocial measures that lead to a choice not to smoke are the most cost-effective in approaching the problem of COPD. The accelerated rate of decline in FEV_1 that occurs in susceptible smokers appears to return to a normal rate once smoking has stopped, even when early airflow obstruction is present. Surveys of ex-smokers suggest that a physician's advice is the single most important factor leading to smoking cessation. Other adjunctive measures, such as self-help, group counseling, hypnosis, and nicotine substitution, may benefit selected patients. Although far less important than smoking, inhaled irritants and dusts accelerate the normal aging decline in FEV_1, especially in patients who smoke. Measures to control atmospheric and occupational pollution and protection of workers need to be taken.

Patients with COPD should receive an annual vaccination against influenza. Unvaccinated patients may benefit from amantadine during an influenza epidemic. Vaccination with a multivalent pneumococcal vaccine is recommended. Revaccination is now advised after 6 years (see Chapter 17).

In the rare patient with COPD caused by α_1-antitrypsin deficiency (at 1%), replacement therapy should be considered. When therapy should be started is uncertain, but most clinicians advise beginning when the patient shows early signs of emphysema. Whether the progression of far-advanced disease is affected by replacement is uncertain.

Selected Reading

Pingleton SK, Nelson ME, Dark DS. Bronchodilators. *In* Khan M Gabriel, Cardiac and Pulmonary Management. Philadelphia, Lea & Febiger, 1993.

British Thoracic Society and others. Guidelines for the management of asthma: a summary. BMJ *306*:776, 1993.

Ferguson GT, Cherniack RM: Management of Chronic Obstructive Pulmonary Disease. N Engl J Med *328*:1017, 1993.

Bacterial Pneumonia

17

Joseph P. Lynch, III and Galen B. Toews

COMMUNITY-ACQUIRED PNEUMONIA

Microbiologic Cause

- S. pneumoniae (pneumococcus) is the single most important pathogen responsible for CAP in all age groups, accounting for 30–70% of cases. M. pneumoniae has been implicated as the causative agent in 20–30% of CAP in young adults (< age 35), but accounts for only 1–9% of CAP in older adults
- Legionella and Chlamydia spp each account for 2–6% of CAP, but the incidence of these pathogens has been variable among geographic regions
- In recent studies, H. influenzae has been the second or third most common pathogen, accounting for 5–18% of CAP in adults
- GNB (predominantly Enterobacteriaceae) have been implicated in 3–8% of cases in recent series; even higher prevalence rates have been noted in elderly patients, residents of chronic care facilities, or patients with significant underlying diseases
- S. aureus accounts for 3–8% of CAP in adults, usually in patients with staphylococcal carriage risk factors (nursing home residence, advanced age, IV drug abuse, chronic dialysis) or in association with epidemics of influenza
- Moraxella (Branhamella) catarrhalis, which has only recently been recognized as an important pathogen in exacerbations of bronchitis, accounts for 1–2% of CAP
- Viruses, particularly influenza, parainfluenza, and adenovirus have been implicated in as many as 5–15% of CAP; most cases occur during the winter months
- No specific pathogen can be identified in 30–60% of CAP

Clinical and Radiographic Features

- Clinical and radiographic features of CAP may suggest certain pathogens but are not specific. An abrupt onset associated with high fever, a shaking chill, pleuritic chest pain, and lobar consolidation on physical examination and chest x ray is highly characteristic of bacteremic infections caused by S. pneumoniae. Identical features, however, may be observed with other bacteria, such as H. influenzae, E. coli, Klebsiella, or Legionella spp. Admittedly, this type of presentation is rare with Mycoplasma or Chlamydia
- Many of the "classic" features of acute bacillary pneumonia may be absent, particularly in elderly or debilitated patients. Nearly 25% of patients > 65 years old with pneumonia are afebrile; leukocytosis is present in only 50–70%. Clinical features of pneumonia in this context

may be subtle; lethargy, fatigue, nausea, anorexia, or deterioration in overall condition may be the predominant features. Unfortunately, delay in recognition and treatment of pneumonia may be disastrous. Mortality associated with CAP in the elderly population is 10–25%

- Chest radiographic changes in CAP are variable. Patchy bronchopneumonic infiltrates are most common
- Dense lobar consolidation with air bronchograms occurs in <33% of patients
- Pleural effusions complicate CAP in 10–25% of patients, and are not etiologically specific
- Cavitation, rare with S. pneumoniae, Mycoplasma, or Chlamydia, suggests such pathogens as S. aureus, Klebsiella (or other GNB), anaerobes, or nonbacterial causes, such as mycobacteria, fungi, or neoplasm
- An air fluid level is most characteristic of an anaerobic or mixed aerobic/anaerobic lung abscess
- Basilar interstitial or reticulonodular infiltrates suggest Mycoplasma spp; however, frank lobar pneumonia indistinguishable from bacillary pneumonias may also be seen in as many as 1/3 of the cases of Mycoplasma spp. Small (2–3 cm) patchy bronchopneumonic infiltrates have been stated to be characteristic of M. catarrhalis, but also may be observed with a wide range of pathogens
- Radiographic features may favor certain pathogens, but significant overlap exists. Thus, smears and cultures of sputum, blood, or pleural fluid (when present) are important to substantiate a specific microbiologic diagnosis

Etiologic (Cultural) Diagnosis

Despite a relatively low sensitivity and specificity, sputum smears and cultures should be obtained in all cases of suspected or proven pneumonia. The sputum gram stain is most useful for distinguishing predominantly gram-negative from gram-positive organisms, but is not specific for a unique organism

- Sputa demonstrating numerous leukocytes, rare or absent contaminating epithelial cells, uniform morphologic and staining characteristics of microorganisms, and many intracellular organisms within leukocytes may guide therapy. For example, lancet-shaped diplococci in pairs suggest S. pneumoniae, clumps of gram-positive cocci suggest S. aureus, gram-negative coccobacillary forms in a smoker may suggest H. influenzae, and gram-negative rods are characteristic of Klebsiella spp or other Enterobacteriaceae
- In most instances, however, mixed gram-negative and gram-positive organisms are observed. Even when a dominant pathogen is noted, the reliability of sputum smears is inexact
- Caution should be taken when basing initial therapy solely on a sputum gram stain
- In bacteremic cases of pneumonia, the pathogen can be isolated in only 40–60% of sputum cultures. Higher rates of isolation can be expected if a "good quality" sputum is obtained, but in clinical practice a pathogen can be isolated from sputum cultures in only 25–50% of cases of pneumonia (including nonbacteremic cases)
- Identification of the microorganisms on sputum cultures may take 2 or 3 days; even longer delays can be expected for antimicrobial susceptibility profiles
- The value of sputum cultures is further confounded because potential pathogens, such as S. pneumoniae and H. influenzae, may be part of normal oral flora. Thus, the isolation of a potential pathogen from

sputum does not prove that the isolated pathogen is responsible for pneumonia. This inconclusiveness may be particularly true in pneumonia caused by atypical pathogens, Legionella spp, or anaerobes; in such instances, only normal oral flora may be isolated on routine sputum cultures

In summary, Gram's stain and cultural results may be useful as guides to the diagnosis in some cases, but are frequently nondiagnostic and may even be misleading.

TYPICAL PNEUMONIAS

Streptococcus Pneumoniae

- S. pneumoniae remains the most common cause of CAP (accounting for 30–60% of cases) and, with Legionella spp, has been associated with the most fatalities resulting from CAP. S. pneumoniae has been implicated in only 15–30% of CAP in most recent series, but these data underestimate its true frequency, because no causative pathogen was identified in 50–70% of cases. Pneumococcal pneumonia has a predilection for the elderly patient and for patients with pre-existing disease, such as ethanol abuse and COPD. It can also affect previously healthy individuals in all age groups
- S. pneumoniae and M. pneumoniae are the 2 most common causes of CAP in adults < age 35
- S. pneumoniae is the leading cause of pneumonia in all age groups (including the elderly). Thus, therapy for CAP (irrespective of age and presence or absence of underlying disease) should always include coverage for S. pneumoniae
- Classic features include a temperature of >103°F, drenching sweats, chills, purulent sputum, pleuritic chest pain, and lobar consolidation. These features occur in 50–70% of persons with bacteremic pneumonia caused by S. pneumoniae, but do not distinguish pneumococcal pneumonia from other bacillary pneumonias
- Many of these manifestations are absent in non-bacteremic forms, in the elderly population, or in patients with serious associated diseases
- A single shaking chill, often stated to be a hallmark for pneumococcal pneumonia, occurs in <10% of patients; recurrent chills are more common
- Blood-tinged sputum occurs in as many as 15% of patients
- Constitutional symptoms, myalgias, nausea, vomiting, and prostration may be prominent. Headache is a common early feature; stiff neck may reflect meningeal spread. Diarrhea, seen in 20–30% of cases of legionellosis, occurs in <10% of cases of pneumococcal pneumonia
- Bacteremia occurs in 15–30% of patients; higher rates have been noted among patients with dense lobar consolidation and rigors

The course of pneumococcal pneumonia is highly variable, but may be fulminant. Mortality in bacteremic cases of pneumococcal pneumonia is 15–30%, and has not changed significantly over the past 3 decades. Multilobar involvement, respiratory failure requiring mechanical ventilatory support, extrapulmonary spread (endocarditis, meningitis), leukopenia, age > 60 years, and certain serotypes (e.g., type 3 strains) have been associated with even higher mortality rates

- The demonstration of lancet-shaped, gram-positive diplococci on sputum gram stain supports the diagnosis, particularly when intracellular forms are present within leukocytes. Sputum cultures are positive in only 40–60% of bacteremic cases. Peripheral blood leukocytosis or left shift on differential count occurs in >80% of patients; leukopenia has been noted in ≤33% of alcoholic or debilitated patients, and has been associated with a worse prognosis

- Chest x rays demonstrate lobar consolidation with air bronchograms in 30–60% of patients; patchy bronchopneumonic infiltrates occur as commonly. Pleural effusions have been noted in ≤20% of patients; empyema occurs in <5%

THERAPY

- Penicillin G, 4.8–10 million U IV until clinical improvement and defervescence have been achieved
- Penicillin VK, 500 mg qid po, then can be substituted for a full 10- to 14-day course—*Alternative Therapy:* Erythromycin, 500 mg q 6 h, or doxycycline, 100 mg bid, IV or po; Virtually all β-lactams, clindamycin, and TMP/SMX are active against S. pneumoniae

Despite the lack of firm data supporting efficacy, vaccination with the 23-valent vaccination should be administered to patients at risk for S. pneumoniae. Revaccination is now advised after 6 years.

Hemophilus Influenzae

- H. influenzae is a pleomorphic gram-negative rod that accounts for 5–15% of pneumonias, both community acquired and hospital acquired. Both typeable (encapsulated, primarily type B) and nontypeable (nonencapsulated) strains are capable of causing disease
- H. influenzae is a common commensal and may be part of normal oral flora; 20–40% of healthy individuals harbor H. influenzae in the oropharynx, and colonization rates of 50–70% have been demonstrated among smokers with COPD
- H. influenzae characteristically affects smokers, or elderly debilitated patients, but may also affect previously normal hosts
- Clinical features of H. influenzae pneumonia are indistinguishable from those of other bacillary pathogens. Lobar or segmental bronchopneumonic infiltrates are characteristic. Mortality rates of 10–20% have been reported with bacteremic pneumonia caused by H. influenzae; higher rates have been noted in immunosuppressed or debilitated individuals
- Pleomorphic gram-negative rods are characteristic on Gram's stain. Because H. influenzae is often part of normal oral flora, however, distinguishing infection from colonization may be difficult. The diagnosis of lower respiratory tract infection caused by H. influenzae may be further confounded by the fastidious growth requirements of the organism, and other bacteria may overgrow the culture plates. Thus, even in bacteremic cases of H. influenzae pneumonia, sputum cultures have been positive for the organism in only 40–60% of patients

THERAPY

- Ampicillin/sulbactam, cefuroxime, ceftriaxone
- Oral agents (amoxicillin/clavulanate, cefuroxime axetil, TMP/SMX) may be acceptable for mild infections in young, otherwise healthy individuals or following initial parenteral therapy

Alternative Agents:
- TMP/SMX, fluoroquinolones, newer macrolides (azithromycin, clarithromycin)
- Ampicillin, only for β-lactamase-negative strains; activity of erythromycin is marginal

Moraxella (Branhamella) Catarrhalis

- M. catarrhalis (formerly termed Neisseria catarrhalis or Branhamella catarrhalis) has long been recognized as part of the normal bacterial flora of the upper respiratory tract and as an important pathogen in otitis media and sinusitis (particularly in children); it accounts for 1–3% of CAP, especially in patients with COPD
- M. catarrhalis is of low virulence, and respiratory tract infections caused by M. catarrhalis are typically mild, manifesting as exacerbations of chronic bronchitis or purulent tracheobronchitis. Pneumonia occurs in only 5–20% of cases of M. catarrhalis infections and is usually mild
- Morphologically, M. catarrhalis resembles other Neisseria species; kidney bean-shaped gram-negative diplococci are characteristic on Gram's stain

THERAPY

- Cefuroxime (po or IV), ampicillin/sulbactam, amoxicillin/clavulanate

Alternative Therapy:
- TMP/SMX, erythromycin, tetracycline, quinolones

ATYPICAL PNEUMONIAS

- Pneumonia caused by M. pneumoniae, Chlamydia pneumoniae (TWAR), and viruses may be grouped under the term "atypical pneumonias." These pathogens are considered atypical because they lack many of the cardinal features of acute bacterial pneumonia, such as leukocytosis, pleuritic chest pain, rigors, and consolidation findings. Cough is often nonproductive, and extrapulmonary features, such as sore throat, arthritis, myalgias, GI symptoms, headache, and viral prodromal symptoms, may dominate the clinical picture. M. pneumoniae has a predilection for previously healthy, young individuals; Chlamydia-TWAR and viruses affect all age groups. Mycoplasma and Chlamydia spp are usually mild and self-limited; fatalities are rare
- Bibasilar interstitial infiltrates or small, patchy, subsegmental infiltrates are characteristic findings on chest x ray of pneumonia caused by M. pneumoniae or Chlamydia-TWAR; however, classic lobar pneumonia indistinguishable from bacillary pneumonias may occur in ≤20% of patients. Although characteristic clinical and radiographic features exist, none reliably discriminates between atypical and typical bacillary pathogens

Mycoplasma Pneumoniae

- M. pneumoniae, a cell-wall-deficient microbe within the class Mollicutes, is a pathogen of low virulence that accounts for 2–14% of CAP. M. pneumoniae has a striking predilection for younger patients and often spares older individuals, thereby suggesting that pre-existing antibody or prior exposure may confer lasting protection
- M. pneumoniae has been implicated in 20–30% of pneumonias in adolescents and adults < age 35. By contrast, Mycoplasma accounts for only 2–9% of pneumonias among adults of ages 40–60, and for only 1–3% of pneumonias among adults > age 60. Mycoplasma has rarely been implicated as a nosocomial pathogen
- Epidemics of Mycoplasma have been described in university dormitories, military institutions, schools, and families; prolonged close contact is usually necessary for transmission of infection. Pneumonia caused by M. pneumoniae occurs in only 3–10% of exposed individuals
- Despite the frequency of M. pneumoniae in certain populations, its importance as a serious pulmonary pathogen is overrated, because pneumonia caused by M. pneumoniae is usually mild and rarely life threatening. Bronchitis and upper airway symptoms are the predominant features of infections from M. pneumoniae. Radiographically evident pneumonia can be demonstrated in only 5–15% of infected individuals and rarely warrants hospitalization
- The onset of mycoplasmal pneumonia may be insidious, however, and the course may be protracted. Typical features include fever, malaise, headache, and an intractable, hacking cough, which may be productive or nonproductive. Features commonly observed in acute bacillary pneumonia, such as pleuritic chest pain, rigors, and lobar consolidation, are uncommon. Rhinorrhea, sore throat, earache, and hoarseness occur in 25–50% of mycoplasmal infections. On physical examination, erythema of the oropharynx and tender cervical lymphadenopathy can be appreciated in 30–50% of patients. Rhonchi and a few scattered crackles may be detected on auscultation; frank consolidation findings are rare. Bullous myringitis, a frequently emphasized feature of mycoplasmal pneumonia, occurs in 3–7% of patients. Nausea, vomiting, diarrhea, myalgias, and arthralgias occur in 20–45% of patients, but do not distinguish mycoplasmal pneumonia from pneumonias caused by bacteria, Legionella, or Chlamydia spp. Skin rashes occur in 10–15% of patients with mycoplasmal pneumonia; diffuse maculopapular rash, petechiae, urticaria, erythema nodosum, and erythema multiforme have been described
- Rare (1–3% of patients) complications of mycoplasmal infections include encephalitis, neurologic symptoms, myocarditis, pericarditis, and hemolytic anemia
- Chest x-ray findings are variable. Diffuse or patchy interstitial infiltrates or patchy bronchopneumonia are most characteristic. Frank lobar consolidation with air bronchograms is evident in <15% of patients. Cavitation does not occur. Small pleural effusions have been noted in 5–15% of patients. Peripheral blood leukocyte counts are usually normal, but neutrophilia or a left shift in the differential count occurs in 60–80% of patients. Cold agglutinin IgM antibodies have been demonstrated in 40–70% of patients. Cold agglutinins, however, may be positive in 10–15% of viral or bacterial pneumonias and, thus, are of limited diagnostic value
- Serum CF antibody directed against Mycoplasma spp is the preferred test because of its high specificity and sensitivity. A fourfold titer ↑ from acute to convalescent sera or single titers of >1:128 are considered diagnostic of recent or active infection. Indirect fluorescent anti-

body and ELISA methods have been applied to detect IgM antibodies against M. pneumoniae; neither technique has been shown to be superior to CF titers

THERAPY

- Erythromycin, 250–500 mg qid po or IV
- Doxycycline, 100 mg bid po or IV; tetracycline, 250 mg qid. *Alternative Agents:* fluoroquinolones (e.g., ciprofloxacin, ofloxacin); azalides (e.g., azithromycin); clarithromycin (Biaxin) (because Mycoplasma spp lack a cell wall, β-lactams and other cell wall-active antibiotics have no significant activity against Mycoplasma.)

Chlamydia Pneumoniae (TWAR)

- Clinical features of Chlamydia-TWAR pneumonia are similar to those of M. pneumoniae: Fever and cough occur in 50–80% of patients; severe sore throat, often with hoarseness, has been noted in >33% of patients and may be the presenting feature
- Chest x rays typically demonstrate small (2–3 cm), patchy bronchopneumonic infiltrates; dense lobar consolidation is rare. Pleural effusions are rare in young adults but may be observed in ≤20% of older adults (many of whom may have coexisting organisms). Peripheral blood leukocyte and differential counts are usually normal
- The illness is usually mild (albeit often protracted). Tetracyclines or erythromycin may shorten the duration of illness
- Diagnosis of Chlamydia-TWAR pneumonia may be made by culture, DFA staining of sputum, or by serologic methods. The micro-IF assay measures both IgM and IgG titers and is the most accurate serologic test. IgM antibody titers >16 or IgG titers >512 suggest recent or active infection; lower titers of IgG antibody suggest previous infection. The micro-IF test has been positive in >90% of culturally confirmed cases and is >95% specific. Antibodies do not appear until ≥10 days after the onset of illness, however, and titers may peak at 6–12 weeks. CF studies are less sensitive; ≤30% of patients with culturally confirmed infections have nondetectable CF antibodies. A fourfold ↑ in CF titer, or single antibody titers >64, are considered evidence of recent infection

THERAPY

- Doxycycline or tetracycline po for 14–21 days. *Alternative Therapy:* erythromycin, 500 mg qid (less effective than tetracyclines); fluoroquinolones, azalides (highly active in vitro, but limited data in vivo). β-lactams and aminoglycosides have no significant activity

Legionella Spp

- Legionella spp are endemic in the community and account for 2–10% of CAP. The prevalence of nosocomial legionellosis appears to be lower, but has been implicated in ≤10% of pneumonias in some centers
- Nosocomial acquisition has been linked to contamination by L. pneumoniae of the hospital water distribution system. Environmental control measures aimed at eradicating Legionella spp from hospital water supplies have been highly efficacious in limiting nosocomial legio-

nellosis. Advanced age, renal failure, cigarette smoking, ethanol abuse, organ transplantation, and serious underlying disease have been associated with a higher prevalence of legionellosis and a predilection for more severe disease (including respiratory failure and fatalities)

- Legionella spp have been associated with severe respiratory failure in 20–40% of patients and with fatality rates of 10–30%
- Clinically, pneumonia caused by Legionella spp may be indistinguishable from other bacterial pneumonias. Diffuse alveolar infiltrates, patchy bronchopneumonic infiltrates, or lobar consolidation may occur. Pleural effusions occur in <10% of patients; cavitation has been described, but is rare

Several features that occur more commonly with pneumonia caused by Legionella spp than with pneumonia caused by other pathogens may provide clues to the diagnosis. These include

- Progression of pneumonia while taking antimicrobials (particularly penicillins or cephalosporins)
- Hyponatremia in 20–50% of patients
- Neurologic symptoms (confusion, lethargy, headache) in 20–30% of patients
- GI symptoms (principally nausea, vomiting, diarrhea) in 20–40% of patients
- Elevations in serum transaminases in 20–40% of patients

Although characteristic, these features do not distinguish legionellosis from other types of pneumonia

- Legionella spp are gram-negative rods but are difficult to visualize on conventional Gram's stains. In addition, Legionella spp have fastidious growth requirements; thus, specialized media are required for culture. The diagnosis requires demonstration of the Legionella organisms by DFA or cultures of expectorated sputum, tracheal secretions, or BAL. The organisms can be identified also in tissue by using Dieterle silver stains or DFA. Newer diagnostic techniques, such as ELISA or radioimmunoassay for urinary antigen or gen-probe detection of L. pneumophila in respiratory secretions, have been developed, but the role of these adjunctive techniques has not been established. Measurements of serum antibodies against Legionella spp by the indirect fluorescent technique are invaluable to determine the prevalence of legionellosis in prospective epidemiologic surveys, but are of no value in individual patients, because results may not be available for ≥2–4 weeks. A single titer of 1:256 or a fourfold or greater ↑ in specific antibody titer is considered diagnostic of acute infection

THERAPY

- Erythromycin, 1 g q 6 h IV; 500 mg qid po may be substituted once clinical improvement and defervescence have occurred; 21 days of therapy are optimal
- Rifampin, synergistic in vitro; consider combining with erythromycin in seriously ill or immunocompromised host: *Alternative Therapy:* doxycycline, 100 mg bid IV followed by oral administration once patient's condition has improved; ciprofloxacin, ofloxacin, azalides, TMP/SMX (highly active in vitro; limited data in man). β-lactams and aminoglycosides are not active against Legionellae spp

EMPIRIC (INITIAL) THERAPY

In most cases of pneumonia, therapy is empiric, based on the probability of certain pathogens being involved. Initial treatment for CAP (undertaken while waiting for cultural confirmation) should be sufficiently broad to cover most likely pathogens while avoiding polypharmacy or excessively expensive or toxic antimicrobials. Choice of empiric therapy must be modified based on such clinical features as age, the presence or absence of underlying disease, radiographic appearance, prior use of antimicrobials, and severity of the pneumonic process. (See Fig. 17-1)

Young, Previously Healthy Adults

Pneumonia in previously healthy young adults (<age 35) can be successfully treated with a variety of agents, including penicillin G, ampicillin, ampicillin/sulbactam, erythromycin, doxycycline, or cefuroxime. M. pneumoniae has been implicated in 20–30% of CAP in this population; S. pneumoniae has been implicated in 30–60%. Chlamydia, Legionella spp, and H. influenzae each account for 2–6% of cases, viruses for 5–15%, and Enterobacteriaceae or S. aureus for <2% of CAP in previously healthy young adults. In view of the limited spectrum of microbes involved in this patient population, relatively narrow spectrum (and less

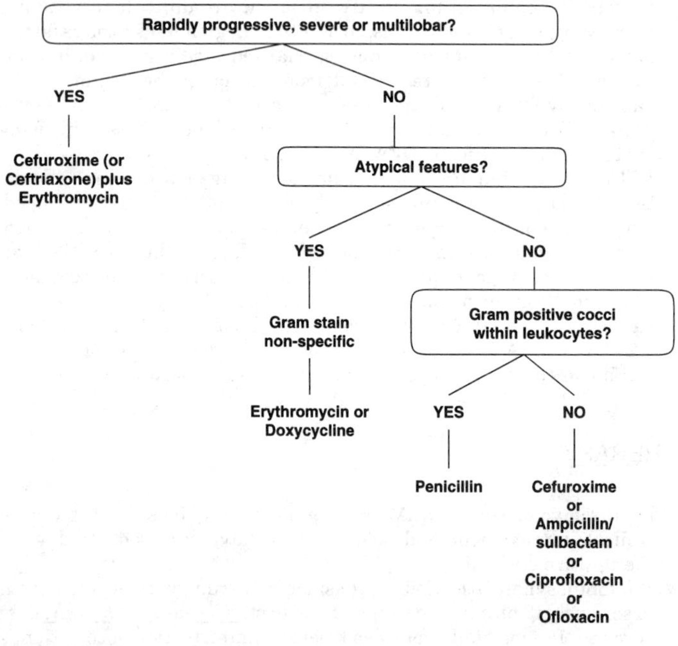

Figure 17–1. Antibiotic therapy for community-acquired pneumonia. (M. Gabriel Khan/Joseph P. Lynch, III. 1993)

expensive) agents can be considered. The choice of agent depends in part on the clinical and radiographic presentation

- If a lobar process is evident and a sputum Gram's stain demonstrates predominantly gram-positive cocci within leukocytes, treatment with penicillin G or ampicillin may be adequate. These agents fail to cover atypical pneumonias (e.g., those caused by Mycoplasma, Legionella, and Chlamydia spp), but have excellent activity against S. pneumoniae and other streptococci (see Fig. 17–1)
- When a sputum Gram's stain or clinical course is nonspecific, treatment with erythromycin or doxycycline to provide coverage against atypical pathogens may be appropriate. These agents are also active against S. pneumoniae but provide marginal coverage against H. influenzae
- When atypical pneumonia is unlikely based on clinical grounds, and Gram's stain is nondiagnostic, the use of broader-spectrum agents, such as ampicillin/sulbactam or cefuroxime, is reasonable. These antimicrobials are highly active against S. pneumoniae, H. influenzae, S. aureus, and certain Enterobacteriaceae

Elderly Patients or Those with Underlying Disease

- In the elderly patient or debilitated patient of any age, enteric GNB and H. influenzae may account for ≥20% of pneumonias. Taken together, GNB, H. influenzae, and S. aureus cause at least as many cases of CAP in this patient population as does S. pneumoniae
- In these "at-risk" patient populations, treatment strategies must encompass these pathogens
- Broader-spectrum agents are needed to encompass S. pneumoniae, H. influenzae, M. catarrhalis, and Enterobacteriaceae (principally E. coli, Klebsiella, and Proteus spp)
- Penicillin G and ampicillin do not provide adequate coverage against GNB or H. influenzae and are not recommended
- Ampicillin/sulbactam (Unasyn) provides ↑ activity against H. influenzae, E. coli, and Klebsiella spp, but has limited activity against other GNB
- Cefuroxime (a second-generation cephalosporin) and ceftriaxone (a third-generation cephalosporin) are advisable empiric treatment of pneumonia for these "at-risk" patients
- Exceptionally broad spectrum agents, such as antipseudomonal penicillins or imipenem, are efficacious but too expensive to justify as first-line therapy
- Ciprofloxacin has broad-spectrum activity against GNB and H. influenzae and has been used with success in community-acquired and nursing home-acquired pneumonias. The activity of ciprofloxacin against S. pneumoniae and anaerobes is marginal, however; thus, this agent should be restricted to patients in whom the presence of these pathogens is unlikely. Specific therapy against M. pneumoniae (e.g., erythromycin or doxycycline) is usually not warranted for elderly patients, because <2% of cases of CAP in this age group are caused by Mycoplasma spp
- For rapidly progressive, multilobar, or severe pneumonias, however, combination therapy with a broad-spectrum β-lactam, such as cefuroxime or ceftriaxone, to cover H. influenzae, S. aureus, and Enterobacteriaceae, together with erythromycin to cover Legionella and Mycoplasma, is appropriate (see Fig. 17–1)

NOSOCOMIAL PNEUMONIA

Microbiology and Pathogenesis

Pneumonia develops in 0.5–2% of hospitalized patients and has been associated with a mortality rate of 30–60%

- In striking contrast to CAP, S. pneumoniae and M. pneumoniae account for only 3–8% of pneumonias in hospitalized patients. Enteric GNB are responsible for 70–85% of nosocomial pneumonias. Enterobacteriaceae (predominantly Klebsiella and Enterobacter spp) have been implicated in 30–50% of nosocomial pneumonias; 15–20% are caused by Pseudomonas aeruginosa. H. influenzae is responsible for 3–8% of nosocomial pneumonias. A host of other aerobic enteric GNB, such as Providencia, Citrobacter, Morganella, and Acinetobacter spp, may each account for an additional 2–5% of cases. Aerobic gram-positive organisms, such as Staphylococcus spp (S. aureus and S. epidermidis) and streptococci account for 10–25% of nosocomial pneumonias. A disproportionate number of gram-positive infections, however, occur in patients with intravascular devices, such as Hickman catheters, A-V shunts, and hemodialysis shunts, and in neurosurgical patients or patients receiving hyperalimentation via indwelling central lines
- The dominant mechanism by which nosocomial pneumonia occurs is via aspiration of endogenous oropharyngeal bacilli into the tracheobronchial tree. Oropharyngeal and tracheal colonization with enteric GNB is markedly ↑ in hospitalized patients and in patients with serious underlying diseases, and is an important precursor of infection

Diagnosis

The diagnosis of nosocomial pneumonia may be difficult, particularly in ICU patients or postoperative surgical patients, because infiltrates on the chest x ray may be seen with other concurrent disorders, such as CHF, atelectasis, pulmonary embolism, or ARDS. Pneumonia complicates ARDS in 50–75% of patients; persistence or progression of respiratory failure in ARDS may reflect concomitant pulmonary suppuration, which may not be evident clinically

- The hallmarks of bacterial infection may be lacking in critically ill or debilitated patients unable to mount an adequate host response. Pleuritic chest pain, high fever, and chills are usually lacking; chest x rays often demonstrate only minimal, patchy infiltrates that mimic fluid overload or CHF. Frank consolidation with air bronchograms or cavitation, the cardinal findings of suppurative infection, is present in a distinct minority of patients. Thus, a high index of suspicion is required to make a diagnosis of lower respiratory tract infection in a timely fashion
- The development of unexplained leukocytosis (or left shift), worsening dyspnea, purulent tracheobronchial secretions, or new infiltrates on chest x ray warrants an aggressive approach
- A Gram's stain of expectorated sputum or tracheal secretions should be done to assess a predominant organism, but one should avoid overreliance on sputum/tracheal aspirates, smears, and cultures in dictating therapeutic strategy. Potential pathogens may be demonstrated on culture of tracheal aspirates in 60–100% of pneumonias, but cultures are also positive in most patients without clinical evidence of infection. Thus, specificity is low (<20%)

- Blood cultures should be done, even though only 5–10% of nosocomial pneumonia cases are bacteremic. Unfortunately, in many cases, a precise microbiologic diagnosis is never established, despite appropriate cultures
- Invasive diagnostic techniques, such as FB with a sheathed catheter (PB) and BAL and quantitative cultures have been employed to define more accurately the microbacteriologic aspect of nosocomial pneumonia. A "negative" study does not reliably exclude pneumonia. The routine application of FB with PB or BAL in suspected nosocomial pneumonia and the modification of therapy according to these results have not reduced either morbidity or mortality

Therapy

Because the diagnostic techniques used to ascertain the microbiologic cause of pneumonia remain inexact, treatment of nosocomial pneumonia often remains empiric. In view of the potentially lethal nature of nosocomial pneumonia, it is advisable to initiate therapy with broad-spectrum parenteral antibiotics pending identification of the responsible organism(s). Selection of antibiotics in this context should take into account findings on sputum Gram's stain, host and environmental factors that may point to specific pathogens, the known frequency of specific isolates in the hospital or ICU setting, and antimicrobial susceptibility patterns within institutions (and individual ICUs). Antimicrobial therapy can be switched to a narrower-spectrum agent once a definitive microbiologic diagnosis has been established.

Patients who have recently received parenteral antimicrobial agents are at risk of acquiring highly resistant organisms, such as Pseudomonas aeruginosa, Acinetobacter, Serratia spp, and methicillin-resistant staphylococci. Antibiotic resistance patterns may vary widely within hospitals or even within ICUs within hospitals, depending on previous trends of antibiotic use.

Monotherapy may be as effective as combination therapy in some circumstances, but the efficacy of monotherapy for nosocomial gram-negative pneumonia (particularly when P. aeruginosa has been implicated) has not been convincingly established. This area remains controversial.

EMPIRIC THERAPY (PRIOR TO IDENTIFICATION OF A SPECIFIC ORGANISM)

In view of the relatively high prevalence of Pseudomonas aeruginosa as a cause of nosocomial pneumonia in mechanically ventilated patients, *initial empiric* therapy in this context should include coverage against P. aeruginosa

- Combination therapy with an antipseudomonal broad-spectrum β-lactam, such as ceftazidime, piperacillin, ticarcillin/clavulanate, or imipenem/cilastatin, and an aminoglycoside (typically gentamicin because of its lower cost) is preferred as initial therapy. If contraindications to aminoglycosides exist, monotherapy with ceftazidime or imipenem may be adequate
- Ciprofloxacin can be substituted for the β-lactam if the patient is allergic to penicillin
- Agents with broad-spectrum gram-negative activity but without antipseudomonal activity, such as ceftriaxone, cefotaxime, and ceftizoxime, may be adequate in noncritically ill, nonventilated patients in whom the risk of infections caused by Pseudomonas spp is lower. First- or second-generation cephalosporins, ampicillin, or ampicillin/sulbac-

tam are not adequate for the *initial empiric* treatment of nosocomial pneumonia. Aminoglycosides *alone* are not adequate for the treatment of gram-negative bacterial pneumonia

MODIFICATION OF ANTIMICROBIAL THERAPY

The initial (empiric) antimicrobial therapy should be reassessed once cultural results are available (usually by 48–72 h) and the clinical course has been clarified. The appropriate agent(s) depends on the suspected (or confirmed) organism(s) and the microbiologic susceptibility results for each individual patient (see Table 17–1). For infections caused by P. aeruginosa, combination therapy with an extended-spec-

Table 17–1
Therapy for Specific Pathogens Causing Nosocomial Pneumonia

SPECIFIC PATHOGENS	PREFERRED THERAPY
Acinetobacter caloaceticus	TMP/SMX, antipseudomonal penicillins, imipenem/cilastin, ceftazidime, aminoglycosides, and the fluoroquinolones are usually highly active (choice of agent depends on results of susceptibility testing)
	Combine with an aminoglycoside to confer synergistic killing
Enterobacter species	Imipenem (combine with aminoglycoside)
	Antipseudomonal penicillin (combine with aminoglycoside)
Escherichia coli	Ampicillin/sulbactam, cefuroxime, or cefotetan (these agents are highly effective and less expensive than third-generation cephalosporins, imipenem, or aztreonam)
	Ampicillin (only for beta-lactamase-negative strain). <u>Alternative Agents:</u> TMP/SMX, ciprofloxacin, aztreonam, imipenem
Klebsiella pneumoniae	Second- or third-generation cephalosporins (monotherapy is adequate) <u>Alternative Agents:</u> Imipenem, ciprofloxacin, aztreonam, TMP/SMX
Serratia marcescens	Third-generation cephalosporin (combine with aminoglycoside). <u>Alternative Agents:</u> Imipenem, aztreonam, ciprofloxacin, TMP/SMX
Pseudomonas aeruginosa	Piperacillin or ceftazidime (combine with aminoglycoside)
	Imipenem (reserve for resistant strains; combine with aminoglycoside). <u>Alternative Agents:</u> Ciprofloxacin, aztreonam
Pseudomonas cepacia	TMP/SMX, ciprofloxacin, aztreonam (depending on susceptibility)
	Aminoglycosides may confer synergistic killing in some strains. <u>Alternative Agents:</u> Ceftazidime, chloramphenicol (Virtually all isolates are resistant to imipenem)
Xanthomonas Maltophilia	TMP/SMX (ciprofloxacin also acceptable) <u>Alternative Agents:</u> Antipseudomonal penicillins, ceftazidime (only a minority are susceptible). Addition of aminoglycosides does not confer synergy, although some antibiotic combinations (e.g., ciprofloxacin plus ceftazidime) may.

Table 17–1 *(continued)*

SPECIFIC PATHOGENS	PREFERRED THERAPY
Streptococci (other than enterococcus)	Penicillin G or ampicillin Combined with aminoglycoside for life-threatening infections. *Alternative Agents:* Third-generation cephalosporins, imipenem (highly active but expensive) Erythromycin, clindamycin, vancomycin for patients allergic to penicillin
Group D Streptococci (enterocci)	Ampicillin (or vancomycin) combined with an aminoglycoside (Cephalosporins are uniformly resistant)
Staphylococcus aureus	Oxacillin or cloxacillin (only for methicillin-susceptible strains) Vancomycin (uniformly active for both methicillin-susceptible and methicillin-resistant strains). *Alternative Agents:* clindamycin, imipenem, cefazolin
Methicillin-resistant Staphylococcus aureus	Vancomycin, *Alternative Agents:* TMP/SMX, clindamycin, imipenem
Coagulase-negative staphylococci (Staphylococcus epidermidis)	Vancomycin Nafcillin (only for susceptible strains)

trum penicillin (e.g., piperacillin or ticarcillin), ceftazidime, or imipenem/cilastin plus an aminoglycoside is warranted. Other third-generation cephalosporins, such as cefotaxime, ceftizoxime, and ceftriaxone, extended-spectrum penicillins, or imipenem/ cilastin provide excellent activity against most other enteric GNB. First- or second-generation cephalosporins may be substituted for more expensive agents if a specific organism has been isolated and shown to be susceptible. If highly susceptible pathogens, such as E. coli, Klebsiella, and Proetus spp, are isolated and the patient is improving, the aminoglycoside may be discontinued. For highly virulent strains, such as Pseudomonas aeruginosa, Serratia, Acinetobacter, and Enterobacter spp, the synergistic microbiocidal activity achieved with combination therapy is important to maintain for the duration of therapy.

Preferred combination therapy for specific pathogens is given in Table 17–1. Irrespective of the agent(s) utilized, duration of therapy for nosocomial pneumonia must be adequate to avoid recrudescent infection. Treatment is usually necessary for a *minimum* of 10 days; a more prolonged course (extending for ≥21 days) may be appropriate for more virulent pathogens, such as Pseudomonas aeruginosa, or for complicated, severe, or protracted cases.

ANAEROBIC PLEUROPULMONARY INFECTIONS

Epidemiology

Aspiration of many oropharyngeal bacilli may lead to a spectrum of pleuropulmonary manifestations, including acute pneumonitis, necrotizing pneumonia with cavitation, lung abscess, and empyema. The predominant oropharyngeal anaerobes include Bacteroides melaninogenicus, Fusobacterium nuclcatum, peptococcus, peptostreptococcus, and microaerophilic streptococci. B. fragilis and species within the B. fragilis group (e.g., B. ovatus, B. vulgatus, and B. thetaiotaomicron) account for 10–15% of isolates. Anaerobes have been implicated as either sole or concomitant pathogens in 60–97% of aspiration pneumonias or primary lung abscesses and in 6–15% of pneumonias in the community.

Clinical Features

Aspiration pneumonia should be considered in patients with primary neurologic or esophageal disease; common associated conditions include ↓ level of consciousness, alcohol or drug abuse, general anesthesia, previous strokes, seizures, periodontal disease, and the presence of NG, endotracheal, and tracheostomy tubes. Aspiration pneumonia preferentially involves the dependent segments of the lung (posterior segments of the upper lobes and superior segments of the lower lobes) as a result of gravitational forces; however, basilar infiltrates may also occur. Community-acquired aspiration pneumonia often exhibits an indolent course, evolving over 1–3 weeks. Cough, sputum production, and low-grade fever are characteristic. The hallmarks of acute bacillary pneumonias, such as chills, rigors, pleuritic chest pain, and consolidation findings, are usually lacking. In fact, constitutional signs, such as weight loss, anemia, and generalized weakness, may be the presenting features. The course of aspiration pneumonitis may be more fulminant, however, particularly when S. aureus or enteric GNB are present concomitantly. Chest x rays typically demonstrate patchy infiltrates without clear evidence for consolidation; persistence of the pneumonic infiltrate may lead to necrosis and cavitation. An air-fluid level indicates a lung abscess.

Microbiology

Clarification of the microbiologic cause of aspiration pneumonia (or lung abscess) is usually difficult. Expectorated sputum cultures often grow only normal oral flora because concomitant upper respiratory tract flora usually overgrow any anaerobes that may be present. Foul-smelling, putrid sputum is a clue to the presence of anaerobes but is only present in 1/3 of patients. Gram's stain of expectorated sputum or empyema fluid may demonstrate a mixture of both gram-negative (e.g., Bacteroides spp, Fusobacterium nucleatum) and gram-positive (e.g., streptococci, peptococci) organisms; however, these findings are nonspecific and of limited value. Only percutaneous needle aspiration, transtracheal aspirates, or thoracentesis can be considered reliable sources for anaerobic cultures. Because of the invasive nature of percutaneous needle aspiration or transtracheal aspiration, however, these procedures are not recommended for microbiologic diagnosis of aspiration pneumonia or lung abscess. Pioneering studies in the early 1970s by Gorbach, Finegold, and Bartlett (using transtracheal aspirates) elegantly delineated the organism(s) responsible for aspiration pneumonia or primary lung abscess in the community. Of primary lung abscesses, 50% were caused by pure anaerobes; 47% by a mixture of anaerobes and aerobes, and 3% predominantly by aerobes.

Therapy

Antibiotic therapy is almost always sufficient for management of anaerobic pneumonitis or lung abscess; drainage of abscess cavities usually can be accomplished by expectoration of sputum and local percussion and drainage. Progression of the infection to the pleural space may result in empyema; in such cases, aggressive drainage (employing a surgical empyema tube) in addition to antibiotics is required.

The decision as to initial therapy must be individualized. In view of its lower cost, penicillin G 8–12 million U daily is a reasonable first choice for patients with mild disease. Clindamycin is preferred for seriously ill patients with lung abscess or for patients who have failed initial therapy with penicillin. Metronidazole (Flagyl) has exquisite activity against anaerobes (including B. fragilis) in vitro, but has been associated with a high failure rate when used as monotherapy for pulmonary anaerobic infections and is not recommended.

Alternative agents: Cefotetan, antipseudomonal penicillins or imipenem (may be particularly useful when infection with enteric GNB coexists).

ANTIMICROBIAL AGENTS

Beta-Lactams

This class of agents includes penicillins, cephalosporins, carbapenems, and monobactams; the 4-membered β-lactam ring (usually fused to a second ring) is integral to the structure. Modifications or substitutions of the β-lactam ring may alter antimicrobial activity or resistance to β-lactamases.

PENICILLINS

Since the introduction of penicillin for clinical use in 1941, the penicillin group of antibiotics has remained key to the treatment of pulmonary infections. Penicillins have excellent bactericidal activity and relatively low toxicity. The basic structure of the penicillin group of antimicrobials consists of a β-lactam ring fused to a 5-membered thiazolidine ring; modification of the side chains attached to the β-lactam ring may alter the antimicrobial spectrum, β-lactamase, stability, and pharmacokinetics. Many of the newer penicillins are modifications of ampicillin. Substitution of a carboxy group for an amino group on ampicillin produced the carboxypenicillins, carbenicillin, and ticarcillin. Substitution of a ureido group for the carboxy group produced the ureidopenicillins (piperacillin, mezlocillin, azlocillin)

- *Mechanism of action:* Penicillins interfere with bacterial cell wall (peptidoglycan) synthesis and activate endogenous autolytic enzymes, inducing cell lysis. Killing of GNB requires that penicillins penetrate outer portions of the bacterial cell wall and combine with key PBPs on the inner membrane of the bacteria
- *Antimicrobial resistance:* The most common mechanism of resistance to penicillins is via β-lactamases. β-lactamases are produced by both gram-negative and gram-positive bacilli and hydrolyze the β-lactam ring, thereby inactivating penicillin
- *Toxicity:* Adverse effects include maculopapular rash, eosinophilia, drug fever (particularly with ampicillin and methicillin), bleeding disorders with high doses of carbenicillin and ticarcillin, and seizures when in high doses (particularly in presence of renal failure)

Benzyl-penicillin (penicillin G)

- *Antimicrobial spectrum:* Outstanding activity against S. pneumoniae (pneumococci), S. pyogenes (group A), all other β-hemolytic streptococci, most S. viridans, and group D streptococci (enterococcus spp). More than 80% of staphylococci are resistant. Anaerobes (with exception of β-lactamase [+] strains of B. fragilis) are exquisitely sensitive. Active against gram-negative cocci, such as Neisseria meningitidis and N. gonorrhoeae. No significant activity against H. influenzae or enteric GNB. No activity against Mycoplasma, Chlamydia, Legionella spp; most M. catarrhalis are now resistant
- *Dosage:* 4.8–10 million U of aqueous crystalline penicillin G IV qd in 4–6 divided doses; oral penicillin (the K salt of phenoxymethyl penicillin [Penicillin VK]) can be substituted in a dose of 500 mg qid once clinical response and defervescence have occurred
- *Indications:* Drug of choice for pneumonia caused by S. pneumoniae and most other streptococci: One of the choices for empiric therapy for suspected lung abscess (clindamycin may be superior). Therapeutic for infections caused by enterococci (S. faecalis and S. faecium); however, these streptococci are inhibited but not killed by penicillins alone. Thus, must be combined with either rifampin or an aminoglycoside

Because of its limited spectrum, penicillin G is not suitable as empiric therapy for CAP except when S. pneumoniae is strongly suspected from a compatible clinical picture and confirmatory Gram's stain (see Fig. 17-1). Penicillin G has no therapeutic role for nosocomial pneumonia.

ANTISTAPHYLOCOCCAL PENICILLINS

The semisynthetic penicillins were developed for treatment of β-lactamase-producing staphylococci resistant to penicillin G; the addition of an acyl side chain prevented disruption of the β-lactam ring by β-lactamases. The 3 semisynthetic penicillins available for parenteral use are methicillin (Staphcillin, Celbenin), nafcillin (Nafcil, Unipen), and oxacillin (Prostaphlin)

- *Antimicrobial spectrum:* Active against most staphylococci, including β-lactamase-producing strains. Not active against methicillin-resistant staphylococci. Less active than penicillin G against streptococci and other penicillin-susceptible organisms. No significant activity against anaerobes. No activity against GNB, Chlamydia, Mycoplasma, or Legionella spp
- *Toxicity:* Similar to that of penicillin, but also includes interstitial nephritis. Intensely irritating to veins (phlebitis)
- *Dosage:* 1–2 g IV q 4–6 h; oral antistaphylococcal penicillins (cloxacillin or dicloxacillin) can be substituted in some patients when clinical response has occurred (dose, 250–500 mg qid)
- *Indications:* In view of their limited spectrum of activity, the antistaphylococcal penicillins should be reserved for patients with pneumonia caused by susceptible strains of staphylococci. Other agents are preferred for other pathogens. Nafcillin, oxacillin, and methicillin are equivalent in efficacy, but side effects (particularly interstitial nephritis) are most frequent with methicillin. Thus, nafcillin and oxacillin are preferred agents

AMINOPENICILLINS

The aminopenicillins (ampicillin, amoxicillin) were the first of the penicillins to have activity against GNB. Ampicillin (the first of the aminopenicillins) was developed by adding an amino group to the benzylpenicillin molecule; other agents (amoxicillin, bacampicillin) were later developed. These agents have significant activity against H. influenzae and selected enteric GNB. Ampicillin and amoxicillin have no activity against Klebsiella pneumoniae and indole-positive Proteus spp, and can no longer be considered reliable against H. influenzae or E. coli. Antimicrobial resistance to these agents has ↑ dramatically over the past decade, even among isolates that previously were highly susceptible, such as H. influenzae, M. catarrhalis, and E. coli. These factors have relegated ampicillin and amoxicillin to secondary roles in the treatment of pneumonia

- *Antimicrobial spectrum:* Excellent activity against gram-positive cocci (including S. pneumoniae, other streptococci, enterococci) and anaerobes (comparable to penicillin G). Active against Neisseria spp, β-lactamase-negative strains of H. spp (not against β-lactamase-producing H. influenzae, which comprise 10–20% of isolates), 60–70% of E. coli, and Proteus mirabilis. Fails to cover β-lactamase-producing strains of M. catarrhalis. No significant activity against Klebsiella, Enterobacter, Serratia, indole-positive Proteus, or Pseudomonas spp. No activity against Chlamydia, M. pneumoniae, or Legionella spp
- *Toxicity:* Similar to that of penicillin G except higher incidence of diarrhea and GI symptoms (10–15%) and skin rash (3–5%)
- *Dosage:* Ampicillin 1–2 g IV q 6 h; in some patients, oral ampicillin 500 mg qid (or amoxicillin 500 mg tid) can be substituted once a clinical response to IV therapy has been demonstrated
- *Indications:* Pneumonia caused by a susceptible strain of H. influenzae, E. coli, or Proteus mirabilis. Infections caused by enterococci (combine with an aminoglycoside). Because of the limited spectrum of ampicillin and amoxicillin, other agents are preferred for empiric therapy of CAP or nosocomial pneumonia

BETA-LACTAMASE INHIBITORS

Clavulanate and sulbactam inhibit β-lactamases produced by certain gram-positive and gram-negative bacteria (e.g., H. influenzae, Klebsiella pneumoniae, staphylococci), but lack intrinsic antibacterial activity. The addition of these β-lactamase inhibitors to the parent compound (ticarcillin, ampicillin, amoxicillin) extends the spectrum of activity of these agents to include β-lactamase-producing strains resistant to the parent compound alone. Clavulanate and sulbactam do not improve the activity of the parent compound for β-lactamase-negative strains or bacteria that are resistant by mechanisms other than β-lactamase production. In addition, neither clavulanate nor sulbactam affects β-lactamases of the type 1 Richmond-Sykes classification produced by Pseudomonas aeruginosa, Enterobacter, Morganella, and Serratia spp. These agents are not adequate for infections caused by MRSA.

Ampicillin/Sulbactam (Unasyn). The addition of sulbactam to ampicillin extended the spectrum of ampicillin to include β-lactamase-producing strains of S. aureus, M. catarrhalis, H. influenzae, B. fragilis, Klebsiella, E. coli, Proteus, and Acinetobacter spp. Ampicillin/sulbactam (Unasyn) is less active against Enterobacteriaceae than are third-generation cephalosporins

- *Antimicrobial spectrum:* Excellent activity against gram-positive bacteria (including S. aureus, streptococci, and enterococci) and anaerobes (inhibiting >95% of strains, including B. fragilis). Active against M. catarrhalis, Neisseria spp, H. influenzae, E. coli, Klebsiella spp, and Proteus mirabilis. Not active against Pseudomonas aeruginosa, Serratia, Enterobacter spp, or difficult-to-treat gram-negative infections

- *Dosage:* Supplied as 3-g or 1.5-g vials for IV use in fixed 2:1 ratio of ampicillin to sulbactam; dose, 1.5–3 g q 6 h (pharmacokinetics similar to those of ampicillin)
- *Indications:* Most useful for polymicrobial infections including anaerobes. Reasonable as empiric therapy for CAP in nonimmunocompromised hosts. Less useful for nosocomial pneumonia because of its lack of activity against Pseudomonas aeruginosa and limited spectrum of activity against gram-negative bacteria. Excellent for pelvic and abdominal infections

Amoxicillin/Clavulanate (Augmentin). This combination was the first of the penicillin/β-lactamase inhibitors available for clinical use (marketed in the United States in 1984). It is available only in oral form

- *Antimicrobial spectrum:* Spectrum of ampicillin/amoxicillin plus β-lactamase-producing strains of H. influenzae, E. coli, Proteus, Klebsiella, M. catarrhalis, and S. aureus. No activity against Pseudomonas aeruginosa, Serratia, Enterobacter, Citrobacter, and MRSA
- *Toxicity:* Similar to that of ampicillin or amoxicillin
- *Dosage:* 250–500 mg tid
- *Indications:* Useful as oral empiric therapy for mild CAP (in patients at low risk for more resistant gram-negative bacteria) or following initial therapy with a parenteral agent

ANTIPSEUDOMONAL PENICILLINS

Carbenicillin (Geopen, Pyopen), a carboxypenicillin produced by substituting a carboxyl group for the amino group on ampicillin, extended the gram-negative spectrum of ampicillin and was the first of the penicillins with significant activity against Pseudomonas aeruginosa. Substitutions on carbenicillin resulted in ticarcillin (Ticar), which had even broader gram-negative activity. Attachment of ureido groups to the acyl side chain of ampicillin led to the "ureidopenicillins," which include piperacillin (Pipracil), mezlocillin (Mezlin), and azlocillin (Azlin). Antipseudomonal penicillins are effective in the treatment of CAP, nosocomial pneumonias, and serious nosocomial sepsis, and as empiric treatment of sepsis in immunocompromised, granulocytopenic hosts

- *Antimicrobial spectrum:* Antipseudomonal penicillins are broad-spectrum agents active against most GNB, including β-lactamase-negative H. influenzae, most Enterobacteriaceae, indole-positive Proteus, Providencia, Morganella, and Pseudomonas aeruginosa. The activity of antipseudomonal penicillins against E. coli is less predictable (only 80–90% of isolates susceptible) than that of third-generation cephalosporins. As many as 20–40% of Enterobacter spp are resistant. The carboxypenicillins (ticarcillin, carbenicillin) are not reliable against Klebsiella, Serratia spp, or enterococci; the ureidopenicillins, particularly piperacillin, have generally good activity against these pathogens. Piperacillin and mezlocillin have excellent activity against Klebsiella spp (>80% of isolates susceptible), whereas only 10–30% of Klebsiella spp are susceptible to carbenicillin, azlocillin, and ticarcillin. Compared to the other penicillins, piperacillin has slightly greater activity (lower MIC) in vitro, and is the most active agent against Pseudomonas aeruginosa. Whether these in vitro differences result in improved efficacy in vivo has not been established. Timentin represents a fixed combination of 3 g of ticarcillin and 100 mg of clavulanate K (a β-lactamase inhibitor). The clavulanate binds to β-lactamases secreted by staphylococci, B. fragilis, M. catarrhalis, H. influenzae, Klebsiella spp, Proteus spp, and certain enteric GNB and thus extends the spectrum of activity of ticarcillin to include these β-lactamase-producing organisms. Clavulanate, however, does not affect type 1 β-lactamases, such as those released by certain strains of Pseudomonas, Serratia, Citrobacter, and Enterobacter spp. Thus, clavulanate does not improve (and may actually reduce) the activity of ticarcillin against these strains. In addition, clavulanate does not improve the activity of ticarcillin against strains of bacteria resistant by mechanisms other than β-lactamase production (e.g., changes in the permeability of the cell wall). The activity of ticarcillin/clavulanate is no > that of ticarcillin alone against susceptible, β-lactamase-negative strains. Thus, for susceptible organisms, ticarcillin alone is preferable and is less expensive than ticarcillin/clavulanate (Timentin). Ticarcillin/clavulanate exhibits good activity against staphylococci in vitro (including MRSA), but treatment failures in vivo suggest that it is not adequate for proven infections caused by MRSA (irrespective of in vitro susceptibility data). Ticarcillin/clavulanate (Timentin) has only modest activity against enterococci. Activity of the antipseudomonal penicillins against streptococci and most gram-positive bacteria is good, but less effective than that afforded by penicillin G or ampicillin. None of these agents (except for ticarcillin/clavulanate [Timentin]) is effective against β-lactamase-producing strains of staphylococci. MRSA are invariably resistant. Anaerobic activity is generally excellent, but is less than the anaerobic activity of metronidazole or clindamycin; β-lactamase-producing strains of B. fragilis may be susceptible only to ticarcillin/clavulanate (Timentin). The major "holes" in coverage are E. coli, Enterobacter spp (resistance rates in nosocomial settings of 15–30%), and staphylococci (β-lactamase producing and MRSA)

- *Toxicity:* Adverse effects include skin rash, hypokalemia, and Na load (particularly with disodium salts carbenicillin and ticarcillin; 4.7 mEq of Na/g for carbenicillin and ticarcillin; only 1.8 mEq/g for mezlocillin and piperacillin). Prolonged bleeding time and abnormalities in coagulation tests, especially in uremic patients, are noted with carbenicillin, which is no longer used
- *Dosage:* 3–4 g IV q 4–6 h (3.1 g q 4–6 h for ticarcillin/clavulanate)
- *Indications:* Piperacillin or ticarcillin/clavulanate (Timentin) may be used as first-line agents for empiric therapy of nosocomial pneumonia, serious nosocomial sepsis, or when Pseudomonas aeruginosa is a consideration (e.g., cystic fibrosis, mechanical ventilation, previous antimicrobials, granulocytopenia, immunocompromised hosts). Ticarcillin/clavulanate has superior gram-positive activity but slightly less gram-negative activity compared to piperacillin; overall, these agents are therapeutically equivalent for serious nosocomial infections. Both agents are superior to mezlocillin or azlocillin in this context. Combination therapy with an aminoglycoside may provide synergy and is recommended. Antipseudomonal penicillins are not recommended for CAP. P. aeruginosa is rarely a consideration in this context, and less expensive agents (e.g., cefuroxime, ceftriaxone, ampicillin/sulbactam) provide adequate coverage against community-acquired respiratory pathogens, including most Enterobacteriaceae

CEPHALOSPORINS

- *Antimicrobial spectrum:* Broad-spectrum activity against both gram-negative and gram-positive bacteria. Gram-positive activity (particu-

larly against staphylococci) is best with cefazolin and modest with succeeding generations; ceftazidime has poor activity. Adequate against most streptococci (including S. pneumoniae), but generally less active than penicillins; ceftazidime is least active. Anaerobic activity is modest (only cefoxitin, cefotetan, and moxalactam) and < that of penicillins. First-generation cephalosporins have marginal activity against H. influenzae; the second-generation cephalosporins (cefoxitin and cefotetan) have modest activity. Cefamandole is active only against ampicillin-susceptible strains. Cefuroxime and all third-generation agents are highly active. Activity against enteric GNB improves with each succeeding generation (particularly against Enterobacteriaceae). First-generation cephalosporins are active against most strains of E. coli, Proteus mirabilis, and Klebsiella pneumoniae, but do not typically cover Enterobacter, Citrobacter, Serratia, Providencia, Proteus vulgaris, and Morganella spp. These species are variably sensitive to cefuroxime, cefotetan, and cefoxitin; most are inhibited by third-generation agents. Only ceftazidime and cefoperazone have significant activity against Pseudomonas aeruginosa. Acinetobacter calcoaceticus is usually resistant to all cephalosporins, although some strains are susceptible to ceftazidime. None of the cephalosporins is active against enterococci, MRSA, chlamydia, mycoplasma, or Legionella spp
- *Toxicity:* Adverse effects include hypersensitivity reactions, fever, rash (1–5%), and nonspecific GI symptoms (5–10%). The presence of methylthiotetrazole group in position 3 with cefamandole, cefotetan, cefoperazone, and moxalactam is associated with hypoprothrombinemia. Only moxalactam has been associated with significant risk of clinical bleeding

FIRST-GENERATION CEPHALOSPORINS

- *Mechanism of action:* Cephalosporins bind to PBPs and interfere with bacterial cell wall (peptidoglycan) synthesis
- *Antimicrobial spectrum:* The first-generation cephalosporins for parenteral use include cephalothin (Keflin), cephapirin (Cefadyl), cephradine (Velosef), and cefazolin (Ancef, Kefzol). Only cefazolin is currently used. Cefazolin has limited activity against H. influenzae, and its activity against Enterobacteriaceae (including Klebsiella pneumoniae and E. coli) is inconsistent. The spectrum of oral cephalexin (Keflex) is similarly narrow. First-generation cephalosporins are not recommended for empiric treatment of either community- or hospital-acquired pneumonia. Cefazolin should be restricted to uncomplicated pneumonias caused by an organism that is highly susceptible to this agent
- *Dosage:* 1 g q 8 h

SECOND-GENERATION CEPHALOSPORINS

These agents include cefuroxime (Zinacef, Cefurox), cefamandole (Mandol), cefonicid (Monocid), cefoxitin (Mefoxin), and cefotetan (Cefotan) for parenteral use; cefaclor (Ceclor) and cefuroxime axetil (Ceftin) are available for oral administration. Cefamandole is no longer used, and cefoxitin has largely been replaced by cefotetan, except for antimicrobial surgical prophylaxis

- *Antimicrobial spectrum:* Second-generation cephalosporins have broader activity against gram-negative bacteria (including most E.

coli, Klebsiella, Proteus spp, and H. influenzae) compared to first-generation agents. Activity against staphylococci is modest, but is excellent against S. pneumoniae and most streptococci (other than enterococci)

Cefuroxime (Zinacef, Cefurox). Cefuroxime, a broad-spectrum agent with excellent activity against common respiratory pathogens, has supplanted cefamandole as the cephalosporin of choice for empiric treatment of CAP. Several features favor the use of cefuroxime over cefamandole: greater β-lactamase stability; lack of the methylthiotetrazole side chain, which has been associated with prolongation of prothrombin time and risk of bleeding; superior CNS penetration; and slightly longer half-life (q 8 h vs q 6 h dosing)

- *Antimicrobial spectrum:* Active against S. pneumoniae, S. aureus, H. influenzae, Klebsiella pneumoniae, and oral anaerobes
- *Dosage:* 0.75–1.5 g IV q 8 h; can switch to oral formulation, cefuroxime axetil (Ceftin), after an initial response to parenteral cefuroxime
- *Indications:* Cefuroxime is excellent for empiric therapy of CAP in adults, including elderly patients and patients with underlying disease. Cefuroxime has excellent CNS penetration. It is not recommended for nosocomial pneumonia (unless a susceptible pathogen is identified) because alternative agents (third-generation cephalosporins, antipseudomonal penicillins, imipenem) have broader activity against gram-negative bacteria

Cefuroxime axetil (Ceftin) for oral use is more active than cefaclor against M. catarrhalis and H. influenzae and is an ideal agent for completing a course of therapy after an initial brief course of IV cefuroxime (dose of cefuroxime axetil is 500 mg bid).

Cefonicid (Monocid). Cefonicid may be comparable to cefuroxime but has been used sparingly for the treatment of lower respiratory tract infections. Few studies have evaluated cefonicid in this context. The antimicrobial activity of cefonicid is no > that of cefuroxime. Ceftriaxone (a third-generation cephalosporin that has greater gram-negative activity) can also be dosed once daily. Thus, there is little advantage of cefonicid over cefuroxime or ceftriaxone, agents that have been widely used for empiric therapy of CAP. Neither cefuroxime nor cefonicid has any role in nosocomial pneumonias

- *Antimicrobial spectrum:* Similar to that of cefuroxime, but slightly less active than cefuroxime against staphylococci, H. influenzae, and Enterobacteriaceae
- *Dosage:* 1–2 g IV/I.M. q 24 h

Cefotetan (Cefotan). Cefotetan, a cephamycin, has superior anaerobic activity as compared to that of other cephalosporins, but less activity against H. influenzae. It is particularly suited for aspiration pneumonias or polymicrobial infections involving anaerobes and enteric GNB

- *Antimicrobial spectrum:* Superior anaerobic activity (including β-lactamase-producing B. fragilis); less activity against H. influenzae as compared to that of cefuroxime
- *Toxicity:* Has methylthiotetrazole side chain; theoretic risk for bleeding (low)
- *Dosage:* 1–2 g q 12 h
- *Indications:* Empiric therapy of community-acquired or nursing home-acquired pneumonias in alcoholic patients, patients with esophageal disease, or patients in whom aspiration is suspected (particularly when polymicrobial anaerobic/gram-negative bacillary infections are a consideration)

THIRD-GENERATION CEPHALOSPORINS

Within this group, cefotaxime (Claforan), ceftizoxime (Cefizox), and ceftriaxone (Rocephin) have similar antimicrobial spectra and may be therapeutically equivalent. The activity of cefotaxime may be slightly greater against S. aureus as compared to that of the other agents; none is active against Pseudomonas aeruginosa. Ceftazidime (Fortaz, Tazidime, Tazicef) and cefoperazone (Cefobid) are the only cephalosporins with significant activity against P. aeruginosa; however, these agents have inferior activity against anaerobes, S. aureus, and gram-positive bacteria compared to that of cefotaxime, ceftizoxime, and ceftriaxone. Moxalactam is no longer used because of bleeding complications associated with its use

- *Antimicrobial spectrum:* Third-generation cephalosporins extend the gram-negative spectrum of second-generation agents to include Serratia, Morganella morganii, Providencia spp, and Citrobacter spp in addition to E. coli, Klebsiella spp, and Proteus mirabilis. Despite widespread use over the past decade, the activity of third-generation cephalosporins against E. coli, Klebsiella spp (K. pneumoniae, K. oxytoca), Proteus spp, Serratia, Hemophilus spp, Neisseria, and Providencia has remained excellent (>95% susceptible). All the third-generation agents are extremely active against H. influenzae and other Hemophilus spp, such as H. parainfluenzae, including β-lactamase-producing isolates. Some strains (10–20%) of Citrobacter freundi are resistant. Enterobacter spp (E. cloacae, E. aerogenes) are a major weakness; 20–40% of strains produce β-lactamases that hydrolyze cephalosporins. The prevalence of resistant strains of Enterobacter spp has ↑ dramatically within the past decade, particularly in centers in which use of third-generation cephalosporins is high. Among the cephalosporins, only ceftazidime and cefoperazone have significant activity against Pseudomonas aeruginosa. Activity against Pseudomonas cepacia is variable; some strains are inhibited by ceftazidime, but most are resistant to other agents. Xanthomonas maltophilia is generally resistant. Activity against Acinetobacter spp is variable; usually ceftizoxime, ceftriaxone, and cefoperazone exhibit poor activity; some strains are susceptible to cefotaxime or ceftazidime. Third-generation cephalosporins are highly active against M. catarrhalis. Gram-positive activity is variable; cefotaxime (and its diacetyl metabolite) is the most active; ceftazidime is the least active. Cefotaxime, ceftizoxime, and ceftriaxone are highly active against streptococci, including S. pneumoniae, S. pyogens, hemolytic streptococci, S. mutans, S. milleri, S. sanguis, S. mitis, S. bovis, and the viridans group of streptococci. These agents are also moderately active against methicillin-sensitive S. aureus; ceftazidime exhibits fair to poor activity. MRSA and enterococci (S. faecalis, S. faecium) are invariably resistant to cephalosporins (irrespective of in vitro susceptibility testing). Anaerobic activity of third-generation cephalosporins is fair. The activity is modest against mouth anaerobes (peptococci, peptostreptococci, Bacteroides melaninogenicus), but is fair to poor against the B. fragilis group. Moxalactam and ceftizoxime are the most active agents in this class; ceftazidime is the least active

Cefotaxime (Claforan). Cefotaxime is an excellent agent for empiric therapy of nosocomial pneumonias because of its broad-spectrum activity, low toxicity, and relatively low cost compared to that of other third-generation cephalosporins. Its lack of activity against Pseudomonas aeruginosa makes it less than ideal for treatment of ICU-acquired pneumonias unless this pathogen has been excluded

- *Antimicrobial spectrum:* Broad-spectrum antimicrobial activity comparable to that of ceftriaxone and ceftizoxime; cefotaxime's activity against S. aureus may be superior to that of these agents
- *Distinguishing features:* The desacetyl metabolite of cefotaxime (desacetylcefotaxime) has excellent antimicrobial activity similar to that of the parent compound, but has a longer half-life and confers improved activity against staphylococci (including S. epidermidis). It is synergistic with cefotaxime against susceptible strains of Enterobacteriaceae. Cefotaxime, ceftriaxone, and ceftizoxime penetrate well into the CSF and can be used to treat meningitis
- *Dosage:* 1–2 g IV q 8 h
- *Indications:* Cefotaxime is an excellent empiric agent for nosocomial pneumonia arising outside the ICU when Pseudomonas aeruginosa is not a major consideration, and is acceptable treatment for documented pneumonia caused by E. coli, Klebsiella, Proteus, Serratia, H. influenzae, and other susceptible organisms. Because of its inadequate activity against P. aeruginosa, cefotaxime (or ceftriaxone or ceftizoxime) is not recommended for empiric treatment of pneumonia in mechanically ventilated patients suffering from complications and residing in ICUs

Ceftriaxone (Rocephin). Because of its broad-spectrum antimicrobial activity and prolonged half-life, which permits once-daily dosing, ceftriaxone is one of the most widely used antibiotics, both in the community and nosocomial setting

- *Antimicrobial spectrum:* Similar to that of cefotaxime and ceftizoxime
- *Toxicity:* Ceftriaxone is primarily eliminated by the biliary system. Compared to other cephalosporins, ceftriaxone causes slightly ↑ GI symptoms and diarrhea. High concentrations in bile may lead to biliary sludge (biliary pseudolithiasis) and symptoms resembling cholelithiasis
- *Dosage:* 1–2 g q 24 h (q 12 h dosing is not recommended because any cost advantage achieved with once-daily dosing is negated by more frequent administration; cefotaxime or ceftizoxime is less expensive when administered in a comparable dose q 8 h)
- *Distinguishing features:* The prolonged half-life of ceftriaxone allows once-daily dosing; 90% protein binding as compared to 15–35% for ceftizoxime and cefotaxime. Ceftriaxone has excellent penetration into the CSF, as do cefotaxime and ceftizoxime
- *Indications:* The antimicrobial spectrum of ceftriaxone is exceptionally broad, and thus this agent may be useful in the empiric therapy of community- or hospital-acquired pneumonias. Because of its prolonged half-life, which permits once-daily dosing, ceftriaxone may be used as initial therapy for CAP in nursing homes or in patients with underlying diseases because coverage is excellent against S. pneumoniae, most Enterobacteriaceae, and H. influenzae. I.M.-administered ceftriaxone (1 g q 24 h) may permit outpatient administration in the clinic or emergency department, with follow-up doses at 24 h. Subsequent therapy can be converted to an oral agent once clinical improvement has occurred. This strategy may limit the need for hospitalization among patients deemed to require parenteral antibiotic therapy. Ceftriaxone may be useful in the nosocomial setting as well, but its lack of significant activity against Pseudomonas aeruginosa makes this agent less appropriate for treatment of ICU-acquired pneumonia

Cefoperazone (Cefobid). Cefoperazone has broad-spectrum antimicrobial activity and is the only cephalosporin other than ceftazidime to have excellent activity against Pseudomonas aeruginosa. Cefoperazone has been successfully used as empiric therapy for nosocomial pneumonia. Significant gaps in the spectrum exist, however. Cefoperazone is less consistently active against common GNB, such as E. coli and Klebsiella, as compared to cefotaxime, ceftriaxone, and ceftizoxime, and its activity against Pseudomonas aeruginosa is < that of ceftazidime. Thus, we rarely use cefoperazone, prefering these other agents (the specific choice depends on suspected or confirmed organisms)

- *Antimicrobial spectrum:* Excellent activity against P. aeruginosa (> that of either ceftriaxone or ceftizoxime but < that of ceftazidime); less consistent activity against some Enterobacteriaceae, including E. coli and Klebsiella spp, and less β-lactamase stability compared to that of other third-generation cephalosporins. Modest activity against anaerobes and gram-positive bacilli (< that of cefotaxime)
- *Toxicity:* Contains methylthiotetrazole chain, and thus has potential for bleeding resulting from prothrombin deficiency
- *Dosage:* 1–2 g q 8–12 h
- *Distinguishing features:* Excreted primarily via biliary route (75%); 90% protein bound

Ceftazidime (Fortaz, Tazidime, Tazicef). Ceftazidime is the most active cephalosporin against Pseudomonas aeruginosa and has excellent activity against most GNB. Its activity against gram-positive bacilli and anaerobes is less than that of other cephalosporins. This agent is most appropriate when P. aeruginosa is a consideration

- *Antimicrobial spectrum:* Excellent activity against P. aeruginosa; comparable to other third-generation cephalosporins against Enterobacteriaceae and aerobic GNBs; least active of the cephalosporins against staphylococci, gram-positive cocci, and anaerobes
- *Dosage:* 1–2 g IV q 8 h
- *Indications:* Cornerstone of therapy for pneumonia when Pseudomonas aeruginosa is suspected or documented (e.g., in mechanically ventilated patients, patients in ICU, patients with cystic fibrosis or neutropenia)

When P. aeruginosa is not a prime consideration, less expensive third-generation cephalosporins (e.g., cefotaxime, ceftizoxime, or ceftriaxone) that have better gram-positive and anaerobic activity are preferable to ceftazidime.

Cefixime (Suprax). Cefixime is the only third-generation cephalosporin that can be administered orally. Cefixime is more active than second-generation agents against enteric GNB, but has poor activity against staphylococci and anaerobes and fails to cover Pseudomonas spp. The role of this agent in the treatment of community-acquired and nosocomial pneumonias has not yet been established.

Carbapenems

The carbapenems represent a new class of β-lactams that differ from the penicillins by the substitution of a carbon atom for sulphur at position 1 and an unsaturated bond between carbon atoms 2 and 3 in the 5-membered ring. Carbapenems also have unique side chains that confer remarkable resistance to a variety of β-lactamases and provide antipseudomonal activity.

Imipenem/Cilastatin (Primaxin). The only carbapenem currently in clinical use is imipenem. Because imipenem is not stable to renal dedrogenases and its degradation products may be nephrotoxic, it is administered with a fixed combination of the dehydropeptidase inhibitor, cilastin

- *Antimicrobial spectrum:* Imipenem has the broadest spectrum of activity among all β-lactams. It is active against most GNB, including multiply resistant Pseudomonas aeruginosa, Serratia spp, and Acinetobacter spp, but Pseudomonas cepacia and Xanthomonas maltophilia are nearly invariably resistant. Imipenem is highly active against gram-positive cocci (including both methicillin-sensitive and MRSA strains); however, the MIC90 for MRSA isolates may be 8–400 times the MIC90 for susceptible strains, and vancomycin is preferred for MRSA. The activity of imipenem against S. faecium and methicillin-resistant S. epidermidis is inconsistent; anaerobic activity (including B. fragilis species) is outstanding
- *Toxicity:* Imipenem may induce seizures. Although the risk of seizures is low (<0.5%) among patients with normal renal function and no underlying neurologic disease, considerably higher seizure rates (10–20%) have been noted among patients with renal failure who are receiving conventional dosages or who have underlying CNS disease. In this context, imipenem is not recommended. Superinfection or colonization with Xanthomonas maltophilia or Pseudomonas cepacia may complicate therapy
- *Dosage:* 0.5–1.0 IV q 8 h. In view of the exquisite sensitivity of most organisms to imipenem. Initiate therapy at 500 mg q 8 h, and reserve higher doses (to a max of 1,000 mg q 6 h) for serious infections caused by Pseudomonas aeruginosa or pathogens with a relatively high MIC
- *Distinguishing features:* The extraordinarily broad antimicrobial spectrum of imipenem may relate to its ability to penetrate well through the outer cell envelope of GNB, its high affinity for PBP targets, and its resistance to a wide variety of β-lactamases. Imipenem is not hydrolyzed by penicillinases or cephalosporinases, which degrade penicillins, third-generation cephalosporins, and aztreonam. Resistance to Pseudomonas aeruginosa developed in as many as 25% of patients when imipenem was used as monotherapy
- *Indications:* Because of its remarkably broad antimicrobial spectrum, imipenem may be useful as empiric therapy for severe nosocomial pneumonias. It is particularly useful in patients with pneumonias and complications in whom regimens have failed, or in patients in whom antimicrobial resistance to more conventional β-lactams is likely. Because of its expense, CNS toxicity, and potential for selection of resistant organisms, imipenem is not indicated for CAP or uncomplicated nosocomial infections susceptible to other β-lactams

Meropenem is a new carbapenem currently being evaluated in clinical trials in the United States, and has an extraordinarily broad spectrum of activity. It appears to be slightly less active than imipenem against gram-positive organisms but may be slightly more active against gram-negative organisms; anaerobic activity is comparable. As with imipenem, Xanthomonas maltophilia is usually resistant. Meropenem may have some advantages over imipenem; e.g., meropenem carries no definite risk of seizures, induction of β-lactamases is less, and it is stable to human renal dehydropeptidases, thus not requiring the concomitant administration of an enzyme inhibitor.

Monobactams

Aztreonam (Azactam). Aztreonam is the first of a generation of monobactams within the β-lactam group. Elimination of the second carbon ring leaves the β-lactam ring as a monocyclic compound. Although aztreonam is a β-lactam, the cleavage of the second member of the β-lactam ring makes this agent structurally dissimilar from other β-lactams, such as penicillin, cephalosporins, and imipenem/cilastin. Thus, aztreonam may be used safely in patients who are allergic to penicillins or cephalosporins because cross-reactivity with these agents does not occur

- _Antimicrobial spectrum:_ Aztreonam is highly active against aerobic GNB, including most strains of P. aeruginosa, and is stable against β-lactamases; however, it has no significant activity against gram-positive organisms or anaerobes. Aztreonam may provide synergy with aminoglycosides; also, synergy may be achieved with aztreonam and other β-lactams in >40% of isolates
- _Toxicity:_ Uncommon (<1% rash, <2% serious diarrhea)
- _Dosage:_ 1–2 g q 8 h (lower doses of 1 g q 12 h may be adequate provided the organism is susceptible with a low MIC (<1 μg/l). Dosage must be ↓ in the presence of impaired renal function
- _Indications:_ Aztreonam has a greater role in nosocomial infections in which aerobic GNB are suspected or documented. In combination with agents with gram-positive activity, such as clindamycin, vancomycin, or a β-lactam, it provides exceptional broad-spectrum activity—however, as empiric therapy for serious nosocomial pneumonia. The use of aztreonam may eliminate the need for an aminoglycoside in this context. Aztreonam has minimal activity against common pathogens implicated in bronchitis and CAP, such as S. pneumoniae and M. catarrhalis, and should not be used as empiric therapy in these conditions

Aminoglycosides

These include gentamicin (Garamycin), tobramycin (Nebcin), and amikacin (Amikin). The use of aminoglycosides in the treatment of pneumonia is controversial. Several factors argue against the use of these agents: their high toxicity (nephrotoxicity/ototoxicity); their low penetration into bronchial secretions and lung tissue; their inactivation at low pH (conditions that may prevail in infected lung parenchyma); and the availability of alternative broad-spectrum agents with gram-negative activity and less toxicity (e.g., β-lactams, quinolones). Despite these arguments, aminoglycosides may be useful as adjunct therapy (combined with a broad-spectrum antimicrobial agent, such as β-lactams or quinolones), primarily to achieve synergistic killing

- _Antimicrobial spectrum:_ Exceptionally broad spectrum against aerobic GNB; no significant activity against anaerobes. May confer synergistic killing against certain gram-positive organisms, such as enterococci and staphylococci, in combination with β-lactams
- _Toxicity:_ Nephrotoxicity and ototoxicity are most important. Synergistic toxicity may occur when aminoglycoside is combined with other nephrotoxic agents, such as vancomycin. Risk factors associated with enhanced nephrotoxicity include old age, prior aminoglycoside use, and pre-existing renal disease. The toxicity of tobramycin and gentamicin are comparable; both agents may be slightly more nephrotoxic than amikacin and netilmicin. Netilmicin shows the least ototoxicity. Peak and trough serum levels are mandatory to limit toxicity. Peak levels >6 μg/ml are required for optimal microbiocidal activity; however, trough levels >2 μg/ml (2 mg/l) correlate with excessive toxicity
- _Dosage:_ 3–5 mg/kg/day IV, or I.M. in divided doses q 8 h for gentamicin/tobramycin; 15 mg/kg/day for amikacin. (Two- to threefold higher

doses are required in patients with cystic fibrosis because of the rapid clearance of aminoglycosides in this patient population.) Dose adjustment may be required (need peak and trough serum levels). Higher serum levels are achieved with single daily dosing, thus suggesting that bactericidal activity may be enhanced. Single dosing would be cost-saving because less pharmacy and nursing time would be required. Single-dose regimens, however, have not been studied in humans; thus, the safety and efficacy of this practice have not been established

- *Indications:* Aminoglycosides are inadequate as single agents for pulmonary infections. The addition of an aminoglycoside to a broad-spectrum antimicrobial should be considered in the following circumstances to provide synergistic killing: as initial empiric therapy for serious sepsis or nosocomial pneumonias caused by suspected or proven gram-negative enteric bacteria; as therapy for pneumonia caused by highly virulent pathogens, such as Pseudomonas spp, Enterobacter spp, Serratia, and Acinetobacter spp (continue aminoglycoside for duration of therapy); and to treat infections caused by enterococci (combine with penicillin or vancomycin)

Macrolides

The macrolides represent a class of antimicrobials characterized by substituted 14-, 15-, or 16-member rings. Macrolides penetrate into tissues better than do β-lactams. Erythromycin (a 14-member macrolide) has been the only antibiotic of this class in clinical use in the United States for the past 2 decades. Several newer 14-member macrolides with a spectrum of activity similar to that of erythromycin but with more resistance to acid hydrolysis have been synthesized; these include roxithromycin, clarithromycin, dirithromycin, erythromycylamine, and flurithromycin. Clarithromycin (Biaxin) is the only one of these newer macrolides currently available in the United States.

Erythromycin is active against S. pneumoniae, M. catarrhalis, mycoplasma, and Legionella spp, and has been used extensively for community-acquired bronchitis and pneumonia. Penicillins and cephalosporins, however, have a much broader spectrum of activity and are the preferred agents for most CAP. Erythromycin is not consistently reliable against H. influenzae, has no significant activity against GNB, and is less active than penicillins against streptococci, staphylococci, and anaerobes. Thus, erythromycin should be reserved primarily for CAP in young healthy adults who are at low risk for resistant pathogens or in patients in whom Mycoplasma, Chlamydia, or Legionella spp are suspected

- *Mechanism of action:* Interferes with microbial protein synthesis at the ribosomal level (binds to 50S ribosome subunit)
- *Antimicrobial spectrum:* Effective against S. pneumoniae, other streptococci (except enterococcus), and M. catarrhalis; not reliable against S. aureus or S. epidermidis (10–40% of strains are resistant). Only 40–70% of H. influenzae are susceptible. Anaerobic coverage is modest (10–20% of oral anaerobes and 30–40% of B. fragilis are resistant). No significant gram-negative activity. Excellent against Legionella and Mycoplasma spp; less active than tetracyclines against Chlamydia spp
- *Toxicity:* GI side effects (principally nausea, epigastric distress, diarrhea, and vomiting) are common (>20%) and limit its usefulness. IV erythromycin is intensely irritating to veins and may cause phlebitis. Hepatotoxicity (cholestatic hepatitis) is a rare complication (primarily with the estolate form) that usually resolves with cessation of therapy

- *Dosage:* 500–1,000 mg q 6 h IV; 250–500 mg q 6 h po. The active component is the erythromycin base. Oral forms include an acid-resistant enteric coated tablet, erythromycin stearate (a salt), erythromycin ethylsuccinate (an ester), and erythromycin estolate (an ester salt). These salts and esters confer more stability against gastric acids than does the parent compound. Erythromycin lactobionate and erythromycin gluceptate are available for IV use (oral absorption is not consistently reliable). IV administration is recommended as initial therapy for serious infections (e.g., Legionella spp); oral therapy may be substituted once a clinical response has occurred
- *Indications:* Erythromycin provides excellent coverage against common pathogens acquired in the community, including S. pneumoniae, Legionella, Chlamydia, and Mycoplasma spp, and may be used as first-line therapy among young, previously healthy adults with CAP in whom potentially resistant pathogens, such as S. aureus and enteric GNB, are rarely problematic. In view of its limited spectrum of activity against GNB and marginal activity against H. influenzae, however, erythromycin is not adequate as monotherapy for CAP in patients at risk for infections with these pathogens (e.g., age >55, ethanol abuse, cigarette smoking, or any pre-existing underlying disease). Erythromycin has no role in the treatment of nosocomial pneumonias, except as adjunctive therapy when Legionella spp are suspected

Clarithromycin (Biaxin) is the first of the newer macrolides to be introduced into the United States. Clarithromycin retains the antimicrobial activity of erythromycin, but also extends its spectrum to include H. influenzae and some Enterobacteriaceae. Clarithromycin is as effective as cefaclor (Ceclor), cefuroxime axetil (Ceftin), and cefixime (Suprax) for mild to moderate lower respiratory tract infections (bronchitis, pneumonia)

- *Toxicity:* Much less than erythromycin; significant GI symptoms complicate its use in only 3–6% of cases
- *Dosage:* 250–500 mg bid for 7–14 days

Azalides

The addition of a nitrogen atom to the macrolide ring (resulting in a 15-member ring) results in compounds (azalides) that are far more resistant to acid hydrolysis than are macrolides. Azalides have greater penetration into tissues, a larger volume of distribution, and a longer half-life (>2 days) compared to macrolides, β-lactams, or quinolone antibiotics. Azithromycin is the first azalide to be developed for clinical use, although several other agents are currently being studied.

Azithromycin (Zithromax). Azithromycin is a promising agent that extends the spectrum of erythromycin to cover H. influenzae and some Enterobacteriaceae and has few side effects. It has only recently become available in the United States and additional studies are required to determine its position for empiric therapy of CAP

- *Mechanism of action:* Inhibits protein synthesis at 50S ribosomal level
- *Antimicrobial spectrum:* Azithromycin is highly active (comparable to erythromycin) against Chlamydia, Mycoplasma, and Legionella spp. It is bactericidal against S. pneumoniae and erythromycin-sensitive strains of streptococci and staphylococci, but is less active than erythromycin against these organisms. Azithromycin has no activity against erythromycin-resistant strains of streptococci or staphylococci; MRSA and enterococci are usually resistant. Activity against

anaerobes is slightly superior to that of erythromycin. Most oral anaerobes, such as peptococci, peptostreptococci, and Bacteroides melaninogenicus, are readily inhibited; activity against B. fragilis is marginal. Azithromycin is much more active against GNB than are the 14-member-ring macrolides. Azithromycin is bactericidal against H. influenzae, Neisseria spp, and M. catarrhalis. Activity against Enterobacteriaceae is inconsistent, but some strains of E. coli, Klebsiella, Enterobacter, and Citrobacter spp are susceptible. Most isolates of Serratia or Acinetobacter spp are resistant; activity is insignificant against Pseudomonas spp or Xanthomonas maltophilia

- *Toxicity:* Minor, primarily GI
- *Dosage:* 500 mg initial dose, then 250 mg once daily for 2–5 days
- *Distinguishing features:* Azithromycin is more acid stable and better absorbed following oral administration than is erythromycin. It also has a much longer biologic half-life. A unique property of azithromycin is its ability to be concentrated in phagocytes and tissues; phagocytes continue to concentrate azithromycin intracellularly for as many as 24 h. The preferential distribution of the drug in tissues and its slow release result in high concentrations of active drug at sites of infection for prolonged periods despite low serum concentrations. Levels of azithromycin in sputum, bronchial mucosa, and alveolar macrophages may exceed the MIC for most common respiratory pathogens for 2–4 days following a single 500-mg oral dose
- *Indications:* In view of its excellent activity against common respiratory pathogens (S. pneumoniae, H. influenzae, M. catarrhalis, chlamydia, mycoplasma, legionella), prolonged half-life (permitting once-daily dosing), and low incidence of side effects, azithromycin may be a logical agent for CAP among nonimmunocompromised hosts in whom the risk of serious gram-negative pathogens is low. Data evaluating azithromycin for moderately severe or severe pneumonias are limited. Studies in Europe and the United States, however, have shown oral azithromycin to be superior or equivalent to amoxicillin or cefaclor for the treatment of sinus and lower respiratory tract (primarily bronchitis) infections. The role of azithromycin as empiric therapy for CAP in moderately ill patients at risk for gram-negative pathogens (e.g., patients with ethanol abuse, diabetes mellitus, age >65 years, residence in chronic care facility, COPD, and serious underlying diseases) needs to be studied. Currently, cefuroxime or ceftriaxone are preferred in this context. Azithromycin is not appropriate treatment for nosocomial pneumonia

Tetracyclines

Tetracyclines, derived from Streptomyces spp were isolated in the early 1950s. Substitutions on the hydronaphthacene 4-ringed nucleus differentiate the derivatives tetracycline hydrochloride, oxytetracycline, chlortetracycline, doxycycline, and minocycline. Tetracyclines (particularly doxycycline) are inexpensive and relatively effective agents for uncomplicated bronchitis, but have a limited role as therapeutic agents for pneumonia

- *Mechanism of action:* Bind to 30S subunit of bacterial ribosomes
- *Antimicrobial spectrum:* Tetracyclines are active against S. pneumoniae, modest against other Streptococcus spp, and generally not adequate for S. aureus or enterococci. Anaerobic activity is modest (B. fragilis spp are resistant); marginal against H. influenzae; and not active against most enteric GNB. It is the drug of choice for Chlamydia and Rickettsia spp; acceptable for Mycoplasma and Legionella spp

- *Toxicity:* GI (nausea, emesis, GI distress) common; photosensitivity (doxycycline or minocycline); discoloration of teeth or depression of bone growth in infants and children; vertigo. Outdated tetracyclines may cause renal tubular acidosis. Fatal hepatotoxicity has been described but is rare
- *Dosage:* 250–500 mg po qid for tetracycline, oxytetracycline, and chlortetracycline; doxycycline and minocycline 100 mg bid (po or IV). Food binds the drug and impairs absorption; tetracyclines need to be taken on empty stomach. This effect is less problematic with doxycycline and minocycline
- *Distinguishing features:* Doxycycline (Vibramycin) has a prolonged half-life (permitting twice-daily dosing) and is less affected by food; activity is as good as that of other tetracyclines, and it is the preferred agent
- *Indications:* Tetracyclines are the drug of choice for pulmonary infections caused by Chlamydia and Mycoplasma spp and are acceptable alternatives to erythromycin for legionella infections

Fluoroquinolones

Fluoroquinolones are derivatives of nalidixic acid and include ciprofloxacin (Cipro); norfloxacin (Noroxin), ofloxacin (floxin), lomefloxacin (Maxaquin), enoxacin, and perfloxacin, the last 2 not being available in the United States. Norfloxacin is recommended only for urinary sepsis, whereas both ciprofloxacin and ofloxacin may have important roles in the treatment of lower respiratory tract infections, including serious gram-negative bacillary pneumonias. Lomefloxacin (Maxaquin), a fluoroquinolone released in 1992, has only marginal activity against S. pneumoniae and is less active than ciprofloxacin or ofloxacin against GNB (particularly P. aeruginosa)

- *Antimicrobial spectrum:* Excellent potency against aerobic GNB, including most Enterobacteriaceae, H. influenzae, Neisseria spp, M. catarrhalis, and Pseudomonas aeruginosa. Less active against P. cepacia or Xanthomonas maltophilia. Good activity against S. aureus and S. epidermidis, but less active against streptococci (including S. pneumoniae). Minimal activity against anaerobes
- *Distinguishing features:* Fluoroquinolones (with the exception of norfloxacin) exceed most other antibiotics in their ability to penetrate the lower respiratory tract. Ciprofloxacin and ofloxacin penetrate into the bronchial lining and achieve high concentrations in the lung, bronchial mucosa, and sputum; concentrations in the lung typically exceed serum concentrations. The concentration of quinolones in macrophages and polymorphonuclear leukocytes may enhance clinical efficacy
- *Mechanism of action:* Antagonizes bacterial DNA gyrase (interferes with DNA replication)
- *Antimicrobial resistance:* Resistance can be mediated by mutations affecting DNA gyrase, drug permeability, or both; plasmid-mediated resistance has not been observed. Resistance to Pseudomonas aeruginosa may require multiple mutations, whereas a single-step mutation may be sufficient to induce resistance against S. aureus

Ciprofloxacin (Cipro). Ciprofloxacin was released in the United States in 1987 as the first oral antibiotic with activity against Pseudomonas aeruginosa. It has excellent activity against common respiratory pathogens implicated in CAP, such as H. influenzae, M. catarrhalis, chlamydia, and legionella. Oral or IV ciprofloxacin has been associated with cure rates >80% in community-, nursing home-, and hospital-acquired pneumonias. Significant gaps in the spectrum of ciprofloxacin exist, however. Despite its excellent gram-negative activity, ciprofloxacin has only modest activity against S. pneumoniae, other gram-positive organisms, and anaerobes. Ciprofloxacin is less than optimal therapy for infections caused by S. pneumoniae. Thus, it is not generally recommended as first-line therapy for CAP nor should it be used for anaerobic or aspiration pneumonias. IV ciprofloxacin appears comparable to broad-spectrum β-lactams, including ceftazidime, for hospital-acquired pneumonias or sepsis in neutropenic patients, and may be suitable for suspected or documented gram-negative bacillary infections. Unrestricted use of ciprofloxacin, however, may lead to ↑ antimicrobial resistance; thus, alternative agents (penicillins and cephalosporins) are preferred as first-line therapy

- *Antimicrobial spectrum:* Exceptionally broad activity against aerobic gram-negative organisms (including Pseudomonas aeruginosa, H. influenzae, and Enterobacteriaceae. Excellent against S. aureus, including MRSA. Marginal activity against S. pneumoniae and group A streptococci. Poor anaerobic activity. Excellent against chlamydia, Legionella spp, and M. catarrhalis
- *Toxicity:* Uncommon; GI symptoms most common (3–6%); colitis rare. CNS effects (headache, dizziness, sleep disturbance) occur in 1–2%; rash in 0.5–2%. Do not use in pregnancy because fetal deaths and skeletal abnormalities have been noted in animals in utero
- *Dosage:* 200–400 mg IV q 12 h; po, 500–750 mg bid
- *Indications:* Because oral bioavailability is excellent, oral ciprofloxacin may be adequate for nursing home-acquired or hospital-acquired pneumonias provided the pathogen is susceptible and S. pneumoniae has been reasonably excluded. More importantly, oral ciprofloxacin may be substituted in hospitalized patients receiving more expensive parenteral agents, such as β-lactams, for documented infections caused by susceptible pathogens. The substitution of an effective oral agent may markedly reduce drug costs and shorten the hospital stay. IV ciprofloxacin IV (400 mg q 12 h) combined with an aminoglycoside is a reasonable option for the treatment of nosocomial pneumonia in patients unable to tolerate β-lactams or with organisms resistant to β-lactams. Antimicrobial resistance, particularly among S. aureus and Pseudomonas aeruginosa, may develop quickly when ciprofloxacin is used alone. Thus, when ciprofloxacin is used for serious nosocomial pneumonias, P. aeruginosa infections, or sepsis in neutropenic patients, it is advisable to combine this agent with an aminoglycoside. Ciprofloxacin is not recommended as first-line empiric therapy for nosocomial pneumonia because β-lactams are usually efficacious. (Ciprofloxacin is not suitable for infections caused by streptococci or anaerobes.)
- *Antimicrobial resistance:* Although ciprofloxacin remains highly active against aerobic GNB, and has broad-spectrum activity, data from Europe suggest that increasingly drug-resistant strains of Pseudomonas aeruginosa and S. aureus have been associated with the liberal use of ciprofloxacin. Emergence of resistance may be particularly common for infections in which many organisms are present, such as in cystic fibrosis, or for infections in sequestered areas where tissue penetration of the antibiotic may be inadequate, such as osteomyelitis. Within 3 years of the introduction of the drug to the United States, 4–6% of strains of Pseudomonas aeruginosa and S. aureus were resistant; higher rates of resistance (10–15%) have been observed in some institutions. This potential for rapid induction of antimicrobial resis-

tance has led to concerns about using ciprofloxacin as first-line therapy. Whether combining ciprofloxacin with an additional antibiotic limits or reduces the emergence of resistance is not known; however, combination therapy appears ineffective in limiting resistance against Pseudomonas aeruginosa in patients with cystic fibrosis. Notwithstanding these concerns, ciprofloxacin remains an excellent drug, particularly for the treatment of gram-negative pneumonia with pathogens displaying broad resistance to other antimicrobials

Ofloxacin (Floxin). Ofloxacin represents an attractive agent for empiric treatment of CAP because its spectrum covers most common respiratory pathogens, including streptococci, staphylococci, H. influenzae, Enterobacteriaceae, Chlamydia, Mycoplasma, and Legionella. In a recent multicenter trial, Sanders and associates reported that oral ofloxacin (400 mg q 12 h) was as effective as parenteral antibiotic therapy (specific antimicrobial agents were selected by individual investigators) for patients hospitalized for CAP. Among 69 patients receiving oral ofloxacin, 56 were cured and 13 were improved. In that study, patients with neutropenia, rapidly fatal illnesses, or severe renal failure were excluded

- *Antimicrobial spectrum:* Similar to that of ciprofloxacin. Excellent activity against H. influenzae (both ampicillin-sensitive and ampicillin-resistant strains), Neisseria, E. coli, M. catarrhalis, and most Enterobacteriaceae. Less active in vitro against Pseudomonas aeruginosa as compared to ciprofloxacin; studies in vivo in cystic fibrosis exacerbations suggest both agents may be comparable. Modest gram-positive activity; less active than penicillins against streptococci, including S. pneumoniae (comparable to ciprothoxacin). Moderate activity against staphylococci (including S. epidermidis and MRSA). Anaerobic activity fair to poor. Active against Chlamydia, Mycoplasma, and Legionella spp
- *Toxicity:* Similar to that of ciprofloxacin; few serious adverse effects. Unlike ciprofloxacin, no effect on theophylline
- *Dosage:* Oral 400 mg q 12 h (98% bioavailability); IV 400 mg q 12 h
- *Antimicrobial resistance:* As with other fluoroquinolones, development of resistance, particularly by Pseudomonas aeruginosa and S. aureus, may be problematic with ofloxacin. Susceptibility to ofloxacin, however, has been demonstrated in some strains exhibiting high-grade resistance to ciprofloxacin

Other Agents

Chloramphenicol (Chloromycetin). The recognition that aplastic anemia and the "grey baby syndrome" were complications arising from its use led to a dramatic decline in prescriptions for this agent in the 1960s. Currently, chloramphenicol should be restricted to infections resistant to alternative agents

- *Mechanism of action:* Binds to 50S subunit of the 70S bacterial ribosome (blocks the attachment of aminotransfer RNA to the ribosomes)
- *Antimicrobial spectrum:* Broad-spectrum agent, but other antimicrobials preferred for common pathogens. Excellent activity against unusual pathogens that exhibit resistance to most antimicrobials (e.g., Rickettsia, Pseudomonas pseudomallei, P. cepacia, and Salmonella typhi)
- *Toxicity:* Aplastic anemia (<1:20,000 cases); dose-related myelosuppression; hemolytic anemia; grey baby syndrome in infants; reversible neurologic dysfunction

- *Dosage:* 100 mg/kg po or IV
- *Indications:* Chloramphenicol is rarely used unless alternative agents are contraindicated because of allergies or antimicrobial resistance (e.g., Rickettsia, Salmonella typhi, Pseudomonas cepacia, and some strains of P. pseudomallei)

Trimethoprim/Sulfamethoxazole (Bactrim, Septra, Co-trimoxazole). Formulated as a fixed ratio of 1:5 TMP/SMZ, this agent has primarily been used for the treatment of opportunistic organisms (principally Pneumocystis carinii and Nocardia spp), but also has a wide spectrum of activity against gram-positive and gram-negative organisms. TMP/SMZ is equal to or superior to ampicillin for the treatment of acute and chronic bronchitis; even with prolonged use, emergence of resistance has been uncommon

- *Mechanism of action:* TMP and SMZ interfere with bacterial cell replication by inhibiting sequential enzymes involved in the formation of tetrahydrofolic acid. TMP inhibits dihydrofolate reductase; SMZ competitively inhibits synthesis of dihydrofolic acid from paraaminobenzoic acid. The inhibition of differing enzyme steps improves antimicrobial activity and confers synergistic killing
- *Antimicrobial spectrum:* Active against >99% of S. pneumoniae and M. catarrhalis; excellent activity against most gram-positive organisms, including streptococci and staphylococci (including MRSA); not adequate against group A streptococci or enterococci. Active against >80% of strains of H. influenzae (including ampicillin-resistant strains). Anaerobic activity is limited; most isolates, including Bacteroides spp, are susceptible in vitro, but clinical efficacy has not been established. TMP/SMX has excellent activity against Enterobacteriaceae, and emergence of resistance has been rare. Consistently high activity against E. coli, Proteus mirabilis; active against most strains of P. vulgaris, Klebsiella, and Serratia spp; Pseudomonas aeruginosa is usually resistant. TMP/SMX is usually active against P. cepacia, P. pseudomallei, Xanthomonas maltophilia, Citrobacter, Enterobacter cloacae, and Acinetobacter spp (pathogens that are often resistant to third-generation cephalosporins). Excellent activity against Legionella spp in vitro and in animal models of legionellosis; data in man are lacking, however
- *Toxicity:* Skin rash (3%) (usually minor); exfoliative dermatitis (Stevens-Johnson syndrome) or erythema multiforme rare (<1:10,000); excessive fluid when administered IV in high doses; nausea, GI distress (3–10%); diarrhea (<1%); may contribute to marrow toxicity in patients with hematologic neoplasia or underlying marrow disorder; substantial ↑ in incidence and severity of side effects in patients with AIDS
- *Dosage:* Regular strength tablets (80 mg TMP; 400 mg SMZ) or double strength (160/800); for parenteral use, 1 ampoule (5 ml) contains 80 mg TMP and 400 mg SMX/ml. Doses of 20 mg/kg/day for TMP component in 4 divided doses for Pneumocystis carinii; lower doses q 8–12 h may be adequate for bacterial infections
- *Indications:* TMP/SMZ is a reasonable option for both CAP and nosocomial pneumonias in patients with hypersensitivity reactions to penicillins or β-lactams. TMP/SMZ is less expensive than third-generation cephalosporins or antipseudomonal penicillins, and may be given orally following a favorable response to parenteral therapy (60–75% bioavailable). Despite an excellent in vitro susceptibility profile, clinical experience with TMP/SMX in the treatment of pneumonia has been limited. TMP/SMX, however, has been successfully used in nosocomial infections caused by staphylococci (including MRSA) and in

serious gram-negative infections caused by Enterobacteriaceae, Serratia marcescens, and Acinetobacter spp

Clindamycin (Cleocin, Dalacin [UK and Canada]). Clindamycin is a derivative of lincomycin, which has outstanding anaerobic activity and excellent activity against most aerobic gram-positive cocci (with the exception of MRSA). Because of its lack of activity against GNB, clindamycin has no role as monotherapy for empiric therapy of polymicrobial or nosocomial pneumonia

- *Mechanism of action:* Binds to 50S subunit of bacterial ribosomes and suppresses intracellular protein synthesis. Clindamycin, erythromycin, and chloramphenicol act at the same site and thus antagonize each other
- *Antimicrobial spectrum:* Highly active against anaerobes, including Fusobacterium spp, peptostreptococci, peptococci, clostridia, and Bacteroides spp (including B. fragilis); excellent activity against S. pneumoniae, most streptococci, and methicillin-sensitive S. aureus; enterococci, and MRSA are resistant. No significant activity against aerobic gram-negative rods. Does not cover Mycoplasma, Chlamydia, or Legionella spp
- *Toxicity:* Skin rash (5–10%); diarrhea (2–10%); pseudomembranous colitis no more common with clindamycin than with many other antibiotics commonly prescribed; metallic taste in mouth with parenteral administration (4%)
- *Dosage:* 150–450 mg tid (po); maximal IV dose 900 mg q 8 h, but 600 mg q 8 h is probably adequate even for serious infections; dose must be ↓ in renal failure
- *Indications:* Primary therapy for community-acquired anaerobic lung abscess or aspiration pneumonia (penicillin G is an alternative, but clindamycin may be more efficacious). Combination of clindamycin with aztreonam may provide outstanding empiric therapy for nosocomial pneumonia in patients allergic to β-lactams in whom penicillins, cephalosporins, and imipenem are contraindicated

Vancomycin (Vancocin). Vancomycin, a complex glycopeptide initially isolated from Streptomyces orientales, has been in use since 1956 primarily for treatment of staphylococcal infections. The use of vancomycin declined following the introduction of methicillin, but interest in this agent has surged over the past decade concomitant with an ↑ incidence of awareness of methicillin-resistant staphylococci, the increasing prevalence of gram-positive infections among patients with granulocytopenic cancer, and its efficacy against Clostridium difficile colitis

- *Mechanism of action:* Multiple mechanisms of action include inhibition of bacterial cell wall synthesis (interferes with glycopeptide synthesis); occurs at an earlier step than penicillins; interferes with RNA synthesis; alters permeability of bacterial cell membrane
- *Antimicrobial spectrum:* Vancomycin is exceptionally active against aerobic gram-positive cocci but has a narrow spectrum. It is bactericidal against aerobic gram-positive organisms (S. epidermidis and S. aureus, including MRSA), diphtheroids (e.g., Corynebacteria), streptococci, pneumococci, and clostridia, but is only bacteriostatic against enterococci. No significant activity against gram-negative organisms, anaerobes, Mycoplasma, Chlamydia, or Legionella spp
- *Toxicity:* Phlebitis (>10% in some series); maculopapular or erythematous rash (4–5%); hearing loss, particularly with high serum levels; "red man's syndrome" (erythematous flushing of the torso, neck, and face associated with pruritus, hypotension, and rarely cardiac arrest

caused by histamine release). Nephrotoxicity rare, but may occur when administered concomitantly with aminoglycoside

- *Dosage:* Loading dose 15 mg/kg; then 500–1,000 mg IV q 12 h. Administer slowly over 60 min; more rapid infusion rates may be associated with red man's syndrome, pain, or hypotension. Substantial dose reductions required in presence of renal failure; in this situation, serum levels are required to assure therapeutic levels and reduce toxicity (peak levels: aim for serum concentrations of 20–40 μg/ml 2 h post completion of infusion; trough levels, 5–10 μg/ml). I.M. route not available. Oral administration does not provide adequate tissue or serum levels
- *Indications:* Vancomycin should be restricted to proven or suspected infections caused by gram-positive organisms resistant to more conventional agents, such as penicillins. Because of its narrow spectrum, vancomycin is not adequate as single-agent empiric therapy for pneumonia. Vancomycin is bactericidal against MRSA and other gram-positive organisms that exhibit resistance to penicillins (e.g., pathogenic Corynebacterium spp, S. epidermidis) and is the drug of choice for these pathogens. Effective against infections caused by enterococci but need to combine with gentamicin for bactericidal activity
- Special Considerations: Antimicrobial resistance to vancomycin rarely (if ever) develops during therapy; no cross-resistance occurs between vancomycin and unrelated antibiotics. Thus, vancomycin remains exceptionally reliable against traditionally susceptible organisms (gram-positive cocci) even with widespread use

Suggested Reading

Craven DE, Barber TW, Steger KA, Montecalvo MA: Nosocomial pneumonia in the 1990s: Update of epidemiology and risk factors. Semin Respir Infect *5*:157, 1990.

Fang GD, Fine M, Orloff J, et al.: New and emerging etiologies for community-acquired pneumonia with implications for therapy. A prospective multicenter study of 359 cases. Medicine *69*: 307, 1990.

Farr BM, Sloman AJ, Fisch MJ: Predicting death in patients hospitalized for community acquired pneumonia. Ann Intern Med *115*: 428, 1991.

Grayston JT, Campbell LA, Kuo CC, et al.: A new respiratory tract pathogen: Chlamydia pneumoniae strain TWAR. J Infect Dis *161*: 618–625, 1990.

Lynch JP, III, Toews GB: Bacterial pneumonia. *In* Khan M Gabriel, Cardiac and Pulmonary Management. Philadelphia, Lea & Febiger, 1993.

Marrie TJ, Durant H, Yates L: Community-acquired pneumonia requiring hospitalization: 5-year prospective study. Rev Infect Dis *11*:586, 1989.

Sanders WE, Morris JF, Alessi PK, et al.: Oral ofloxacin for the treatment of acute bacterial pneumonia: Use of a nontraditional protocol to compare experimental therapy with usual care in a multicenter clinical trial. Am J Med *91*:261, 1991.

Schaberg DR, Culver DH, Gaynes RP: Major trends in the microbial etiology of nosocomial infection. Am J Med *91* (suppl 3B): 72S, 1991.

Fungal, Mycobacterial, and Viral Pulmonary Infections

18

Galen B. Toews and Joseph P. Lynch, III

PNEUMOCYSTIS CARINII

- P. carinii is a unicellular eucaryote whose exact taxonomic position is unclear. Recent studies suggest that P. carinii may well be a fungal organism rather than a protozoan
- P. carinii is likely acquired by inhalation of an airborne particle at an early age. Its fungal nature raises the possibility that unidentified stage(s) (spores) or environmental sources may be importantly involved in its epidemiology. Most children develop antibody to P. carinii by the age of 4 years. P. carinii might be spread through contact with infected persons or other environmental foci. These transmitted organisms could then be the source of a new infection or complicate a pre-existent latent infection in the immunocompromised host. The possibility of person-to-person spread of P. carinii is suggested by outbreaks of pneumocystis pneumonia among malnourished infants, in hospitals caring for immunosuppressed patients, and in elderly patients
- The major predisposing conditions are characterized by impaired cellular immunity and include AIDS, primary immunodeficiency diseases, the use of intensive cytotoxic chemotherapeutic agents for malignant tumors, the use of corticosteroids, the use of immunosuppression in transplant recipients, protein malnutrition, prematurity, and patients with adult T-cell leukemia. The risk of P. carinii in patients with HIV infection correlates with the number of CD4 cells. P. carinii pneumonia occurs almost exclusively in patients whose CD4 counts are <200 cells/mm^3 and particularly in those whose counts are <100 cells/mm^3. An HIV-infected individual with a CD4 count >700 cells/mm^3 has only a 3.8% chance of developing P. carinii pneumonia within a 3-year period. A patient whose CD4 count is 200–350 cells/mm^3 has a risk over this same period of 23%
- The presentation of pneumocystis pneumonia in HIV-infected patients is different from its presentation in those with other forms of immunodeficiency. In oncologic patients, its presentation is usually that of a rapidly progressive disease with fever, tachypnea, dyspnea with nonproductive or mildly productive cough, and crepitations (crackles). Severe hypoxemia usually develops within 5–10 days of initial manifestations. In HIV-infected patients, the onset of symptoms is usually more insidious, with nonspecific symptoms, such as a low-grade fever, mild cough, dyspnea on exertion, fatigue, and weight loss, being present for weeks to months before pulmonary symptoms become sufficiently bothersome to prompt medical intervention. Certain

features have been shown to be of value in predicting the clinical course of AIDS-related P. carinii pneumonia. Duration of symptoms does not correlate with prognosis; however, a normal chest x ray at the time of admission is a good prognostic sign. A wide alveolar-arterial gradient, a low PaO_2 (<50 or 60 mm Hg), and a respiratory rate ≥30 have all been associated with a poor prognosis. If an initial PaO_2 is <50 or 60 mm Hg, the mortality rate approaches 50%. Mortality of untreated P. carinii pneumonia approaches 100%

- The examination of expectorated sputum in P. carinii pneumonia not associated with AIDS rarely yields the diagnosis, but detection of organisms in AIDS-associated P. carinii pneumonia may be more readily accomplished because of the larger numbers of organisms present. Examination of the sputum obtained by hypertonic saline nebulization yields a diagnostic sensitivity of ≤78%. The use of monoclonal antibodies can ↑ the sensitivity of the procedure to >90%. Although a negative induced sputum is not sensitive enough to exclude the diagnosis, the patients with positive sputum are spared the need for bronchoscopic procedures. If sputum or nonbronchoscopic lavage is negative, FB is the procedure of choice. BAL alone or with transbronchial biopsy can make the diagnosis rapidly in nearly all cases of HIV-associated P. carinii pneumonia

Treatment

- Two antibiotic regimens are available: TMP/SMX and parenteral pentamidine isethionate. The efficacies of these 2 regimens in the therapy of AIDS-associated P. carinii pneumonia appear to be generally comparable, although TMP/SMX is preferable because of its lower incidence of severe side effects
- In moderate to severe disease, TMP/SMX should be given IV (in divided doses) at a total daily dose of 20 mg trimethoprim and 100 mg sulfamethoxazole/kg body weight. In mild cases, oral administration is preferable. Peak sulfamethoxazole levels should be monitored, especially when the drug is given orally, to assure adequate serum levels (100–150 μg/ml). Additionally, the frequency of adverse reaction is lessened if sulfamethoxazole levels are <200 μg/ml
- Most clinicians prefer to treat episodes of AIDS-associated P. carinii pneumonia for 21 days. Response rates range from 60 to 80%. Ninety-day survival rates after P. carinii pneumonia are similar in patients with and without AIDS, but relapse is more frequent in the AIDS-related group, occurring in ≥20–40% of surviving patients. The incidence of side effects from either drug is quite high: >60% in most series
- Dapsone is another antifolate that can be utilized for treatment of P. carinii. Dapsone alone is not as effective as conventional therapy or dapsone plus trimethoprim. Dapsone plus trimethoprim may be as effective, better tolerated, and associated with fewer side effects than conventional agents. Dapsone plus trimethoprim may, therefore, be an acceptable alternative to TMP/SMX or pentamidine in some patients
- Trimetrexate, an inhibitor of dihydrofolate reductase that is 1,000-fold more potent than trimethoprim, induces a response rate of 77–92% when administered by IV infusion. A major drawback of trimetrexate therapy thus far has been the high relapse rate (≤60%) when this drug is used as a single agent
- Deterioration in respiratory function, need for mechanical ventilation, and death can all be ↓ significantly by the use of corticosteroids. Early adjunctive corticosteroid therapy should be utilized in individu-

als with an alveolar-arterial O_2 difference >35 mm Hg or a PaO_2 <70 mm Hg on room air at the time therapy is initiated. Adjunctive corticosteroids should be started as early as possible and no later than within 72 h of initiating specific antimicrobial therapy for P. carinii pneumonia. No data are available regarding the efficacy of adjunctive steroids for patients who fail to respond after >3 days of antimicrobial therapy, and, accordingly, no recommendations regarding salvage therapy can be made. Although the optimal steroid regimen has not been determined, the regimen recommended is prednisone 40 mg bid (days 1–5), prednisone 20 mg bid (days 6–10), and prednisone 20 mg qd (days 11–21). Clinical relapse may occur following abrupt, simultaneous discontinuation of corticosteroids and specific microbial therapy

PREFERRED THERAPY

TMP/SMX. Trimethoprim, 20 mg/kg/day IV or po in 3 or 4 doses for 21 days. For patients with $PaO_2 \leq 70$ mm Hg or A-a gradient ≥ 33 mm Hg. Prednisone, 40 mg po bid, days 1–5; 20 mg po bid, days 6–10; 20 mg po qd, days 11–21. *Alternate Therapy:* Pentamidine, 3–4 mg/kg, IV qd for 21 days. Trimethoprim, 5 mg/kg po q 6 h for 21 days + dapsone, 100 mg po qd for 21 days.

Prophylaxis is required in patients with P. carinii pneumonia because approximately 60% of AIDS patients relapse within 1 year of their first episode of pneumonia. *Preferred Therapy:* TMP/SMX, 1 double-strength tablet qd. Prophylaxis when CD4 count <200 cells/mm^3; secondary prophylaxis for all patients with a history of P. carinii pneumonia. *Alternate Therapy:* Aerosolized pentamidine, 300 mg q 4 weeks using the Respirgard II nebulizer.

SPECIFIC DRUGS

Trimethoprim-sulfamethoxazole. This agent blocks folate metabolism at 2 sites. TMP inhibits dihydrofolate reductase and dihydrofolic synthetase. TMP has at least a 2,000-fold greater affinity for microbial than mammalian dihydrofolate reductase. SMX interferes with dihydrofolic synthetase, an enzyme found only in microbes. Peak serum levels occur at 1–3 h, and the serum half-life is 12–13 h. Common adverse reactions that necessitate discontinuance of the drug include a rash with exfoliation or mucositus, severe neutropenia, thrombocytopenia, or hepatitis. Less severe adverse reactions include nausea, vomiting, and hyponatremia.

Pentamidine is an aromatic diamidine whose mechanism of action is unknown. Pentamidine interferes with folate metabolism, oxidative phosphorylation, nucleic acid replication, and anaerobic glycolysis. Peak serum levels occur within 1 h, and the half-life of the drug is 6–10 h. The tissue half-life of pentamidine may be as long as 30 days in the lung. Parenteral administration is necessary because GI absorption is poor. The drug is best administered IV over a period of 60–90 min in 250 ml of 5% dextrose. I.M. administration should be avoided because of SQ abscess formation at the injection site. Adverse reactions to pentamidine include hypoglycemia, azotemia, neutropenia, chemical hepatitis, nausea with vomiting, and cardiac arrhythmias. Pentamidine may induce damage to β cells in the pancreas and may result in diabetes mellitus. Although cardiac arrhythmias are rare, they are difficult to manage because of the long tissue half-life of pentamidine.

Dapsone-Trimethoprim is another antifolate combination that inhibits purine synthesis. Each drug in this combination interferes with the metabolism of the other; thus, an optimal dosage regimen is not known. Adverse effects include mild to severe nausea, vomiting, and a rash. Hyperkalemia, methemoglobinemia, elevated liver enzyme neutropenia, and thrombocytopenia also occur.

Trimetrexate is a potent inhibitor of mammalian and protozoal dihydrofolate reductase. This agent is lipid soluble and easily enters both mammalian cells and P. carinii. Folinic acid (leucovorin), which is not lipid soluble, is actively transported into mammalian cells but not into P. carinii. Folinic acid must be administered to protect host tissues from toxic antifolate effects.

FUNGAL DISEASE

Aspergillus

- Aspergillus spp (A. fumigatus, A. flavus, A. niger) are ubiquitous in the environment, and infection with these septated fungi may occur via environmental exposures or endogenous reactivation of latent spores in susceptible (immunocompromised) hosts. Host defenses against Aspergillus spp involve both granulocytes (PMNs) and mononuclear phagocytes; abrogation of both lines of defenses appears necessary to predispose to clinical disease. Thus, invasive aspergillosis occurs in patients with severe aberrations in *both* cellular immunity and granulocyte number or function. Infection most commonly occurs by endogenous spread in granulocytopenic patients previously colonized with Aspergillus spp
- Aspergillus spp may cause a wide spectrum of pulmonary disease, including ABPA, mycetoma (fungal ball), chronic necrotizing aspergillosis, and invasive aspergillosis. More recently, locally invasive aspergillosis involving the tracheobronchial tree in immunocompromised hosts has been described. ABPA represents a hypersensitivity response to Aspergillus antigens in asthmatic patients, and is revealed by blood and tissue eosinophilia, wheezing, pulmonary infiltrates, high serum IgE, and positive immediate skin tests to Aspergillus. Corticosteroids (to ablate the exaggerated antigenic response) are the mainstay of therapy. This syndrome does not result in systemic dissemination and does not require antifungal therapy. Aspergillus spp may also infect pre-existing pulmonary cavities in patients with chronic granulomatous or obstructive lung disease, thereby resulting in the formation of a distinct mass or fungal ball (i.e. aspergilloma or mycetoma). A crescent, with an intracavitary mass of hyphae, may be observed on chest x rays or CT scans. Hemoptysis may result from erosion of the fungal hyphae into pulmonary vessels; specific antifungal therapy is of no value in this context. Surgical resection should be accomplished when feasible, although in many patients severe impairment in pulmonary function may contraindicate surgery
- The diagnosis of invasive pulmonary aspergillosis is difficult, as only 10–30% of sputum cultures are positive in this context. Further, isolation of Aspergillus spp from sputum or tracheobronchial secretions suggests, but does not *prove*, the presence of invasive disease. Isolation of Aspergillus spp from sputum or BAL has been associated with invasive disease in only 30–80% of patients at risk; in the remaining cases,

positive cultures simply have represented asymptomatic colonization. Blood cultures are invariably negative. Serologic studies for aspergillar antigens using immunodiffusion and CIE techniques are of no practical value. A *definitive* diagnosis of invasive aspergillosis requires demonstration of the typical septated hyphal forms within tissue. The fungal elements may be identified on hematoxylin-eosin stains, but silver-methenamine stains more clearly reveal the organisms.

Preferred therapy: Amphotericin B (plus 5-fluorocytosine when possible); restoration of immune function (or reverse underlying disease); surgical resection or drainage may be required as *adjunctive* therapy; itraconazole (200 mg bid po) appears to be comparable to amphotericin B and is much less toxic. (Ketoconazole, miconazole, and fluconazole are not recommended.)

Blastomycosis

- Blastomycosis is produced by the soil-dwelling dimorphic fungus Blastomyces dermatitidis. The western border of the endemic area extends from the Canadian province of Manitoba south to east Texas and Louisiana. The endemic area extends eastward across the midwest and southern United States, overlapping the endemic area for histoplasmosis. The organism presumably grows in nitrogen-enriched soil
- Blastomycosis enters the host via the lung. After inhalation of the conidia, the yeast form of the fungus multiplies and induces a neutrophilic inflammatory response. The development of cell-mediated immunity activates macrophages. B. dermatitidis may disseminate to skin, bones, genitourinary tract, and meninges
- Most exposed individuals are believed to be asymptomatic. Symptomatic blastomycosis usually presents with cough with purulent sputum production, fever, chills, myalgias, and arthralgias. Chest roentgenographic abnormalities include lower lobe infiltrates, nodules, and pleural disease. Skin is the most frequent extrapulmonary site of involvement, and SQ ulcerative nodules are commonly seen
- Identification of the organism by culture or histopathologic observation is the only reliable means of diagnosing blastomycosis. A doubly refractile yeast (8–20 μm) with a wide bud is a characteristic finding on 10% KOH, digested sputum, or pus. The PAS or silver stain may help identify the organism

Preferred therapy: Ketoconazole, 400 mg/day for 6 months; if new foci develop in first month, ↑ dose to 600–800 mg/day. Alternate Therapy: Amphotericin B, 0.4 mg/kg/day for 42 days, then 0.8 mg/kg/day for 28 doses. Total dose, 2 g.

Coccidioidomycosis

- Coccidioidomycosis is an illness caused by Coccidioides immitis, a dimorphic fungus that grows in the soil as a mold and in tissues as an endosporulating spherule. The endemic area includes the southwestern United States, including California, Nevada, Arizona, New Mexico, and Texas. Windy conditions and disruption of the soil lead to contaminated air. Outdoor recreational activities, excavation, and agriculture all contribute to aerosol formation
- Arthrospores enter the host via the lung, where they settle in alveoli and germinate to produce the giant spherule (50–100 μ). Spherules stimulate both a granulocytic and mononuclear inflammatory re-

sponse and sensitize T cells. Cell-mediated immunity develops and successfully localizes most infection. Certain groups of patients are at high risk, including blacks, Filipinos, diabetic patients, immunosuppressed patients, transplant patients, and patients with AIDS

- Primary pulmonary coccidioidomycosis produces an influenza-like illness similar to that seen with other fungal diseases. Common symptoms include cough, fever, and chest pain. Headache and sore throat occur commonly. A rash is noted in approximately 50% of patients, whereas erythema nodosum and erythema multiforme occur less frequently. When the infective dose is high, the patient may be toxic with high fever, and ARDS may develop. The most common radiographic manifestation of primary coccidioidomycosis is patchy infiltrates, ranging in size from segmental to lobar infiltrates
- The diagnosis of coccidioidomycosis depends on the identification of C. immitis within the body tissues or fluids. Histologic demonstration of spherules is acceptable in lieu of positive culture. Large quantities of CSF may be required for positive results. Serologic diagnosis may aid in indirectly identifying the infecting organism and may provide some assistance in determining the severity and extent of disease. The CF test is the serologic gold standard. Titers of 1:8–1:16 are common in pulmonary infection, and a titer of ≥1:32 or a rising titer suggests dissemination. If the CF test is used to guide treatment, the test must be performed in a reference laboratory and specimens must be tested together to ensure comparable results. Because the results of serologic tests in patients with AIDS may be falsely negative, biopsy or culture results are of primary importance in these patients

Preferred therapy: Primary coccidioidomycosis: No therapy. Symptomatic primary coccidioidomycosis in immunosuppressed patients or patients at high risk (diabetic patients, blacks, Filipinos, pregnant women): Ketoconazole, 400 mg/day for 6 months. Pulmonary and extrapulmonary: Ketoconazole, 400 mg/day for 6 months. Coccidioidal meningitis: Amphotericin B IV 0.4 mg/kg/day for 42 days, then 0.8 mg/kg/day for 28 doses (total dose ≥2.5 g) plus amphotericin B intrathecally, 0.1–0.3 mg via an intraventricular reservoir until CSF is normal. AIDS patients: Amphotericin B IV 0.4 mg/kg/day for 42 days, then 0.8 mg/kg/day for 28 doses (total dose ≥2.5 g).

Cryptococcosis

- Cryptococcosis is an invasive disease caused by C. neoformans, a ubiquitous encapsulated yeast with worldwide distribution. C. neoformans has been widely identified in nature, particularly in soil, in the excreta of birds, in animals, and on fruits
- C. neoformans is inhaled either as a small yeast (<10 μm) or a basidiospore. Under the influence of high CO_2 tensions in the lung, the organism forms a prominent polysaccharide capsule. The initial pulmonary host defenses against this organism involve complement, polymorphonuclear leukocytes, and macrophages. Cryptococci are found both within and outside phagocytic cells in the lung. C. neoformans is readily differentiated from other fungi by the presence of a polysaccharide capsule, which is likely important because of its antiphagocytic properties. The importance of cell-mediated immunity in this infection cannot be denied, and in fact, early recognition of its importance led to the mistaken assumption that cell-mediated immunity was the only protective immune response. Cell-mediated immunity develops over 2–4 weeks and involves both CD4 and CD8 lymphocytes. Following the development of cell-mediated immunity,

macrophages are activated and intracellular and possibly extracellular killing of C. neoformans occurs. Antibody to cryptococcal polysaccharide neutralizes its protective effect, but cryptococcal polysaccharide is not strongly antigenic, and antibody may not be formed sufficiently early to provide protective effects

- Direct human-to-human or animal-to-human infection is not known to occur. Certain factors that predispose to infection include AIDS, Hodgkin's disease, chronic lymphocytic leukemia, other lymphomas, organ transplantation, sarcoidosis, diabetes, treatment with corticosteroids, and cytotoxic chemotherapy. In approximately 50% of patients, no abnormality in host defenses or predisposing conditions are noted
- C. neoformans can induce a broad spectrum of pulmonary disease. Patients may present with chronic cough and fever. Chest pain is also a common symptom. Pulmonary involvement may be subacute or chronic, and in the extreme instances with severe immune depression, patients can develop ARDS. The radiographic presentations of cryptococcal lung disease may be any type of infiltrate, a nodule, or a pleural effusion. The radiologic presentation of cryptococcal lung disease may mimic other mycoses, tuberculosis, bacterial infections, and infections with other opportunists, such as Pneumocystis carinii and Aspergillus. Although the lung is the portal of entry, the usual clinical presentation is that of disseminated disease, particularly meningitis. Meningitis may be asymptomatic or include some acute symptoms, such as low-grade fever, headache, meningismus, nausea, vomiting, and papilledema. CSF shows modest pleocytosis (10–30 cells/mm^3), and cellular reaction is characteristically lymphocytic
- Definitive diagnosis is made by visualizing the organism or culturing the organism from body fluid or body tissues. C. neoformans can usually be isolated from sputum, BAL fluid, or lung biopsy specimen in 4–7 days. Histopathologic study of tissue or cytologic examination of fluids demonstrates encapsulated yeasts with stains, such as methenamine silver, Alcian blue, or mucicarmine. Normal individuals may harbor Cryptococci as part of their normal respiratory tract flora. Accordingly, recovery of the organism does not define infection. Serologic studies may help to document cryptococcal infection. Although no antibody test is commercially available, an excellent latex agglutination antigen test can reliably detect circulating cryptococcal polysaccharide antigen in serum or in CSF. Most patients with infection limited to the lung have no detectable polysaccharide antigens circulating in the serum. If antigen is found in the serum, one should seriously consider the possibility of a disseminated infection. A lumbar puncture should be performed on any patient, including asymptomatic patients and patients without underlying disease, from whose respiratory tract C. neoformans has been isolated. Diagnosis of cryptococcal meningitis depends on the demonstration of Cryptococci in the CNS, antigen detection, or culture. The cryptococcal latex agglutination test has remarkable sensitivity and specificity and allows rapid detection of cryptococcal antigen when controlled for the presence of rheumatoid factor. A false-positive rate of as high as 9% may be seen in the presence of rheumatoid factor. The diagnosis of cryptococcal meningitis is sometimes difficult, and repeated lumbar punctures may be required to make the diagnosis. In patients with AIDS-associated cryptococcosis, abnormalities in CSF protein, glucose, and leukocyte count are frequently minimal or totally absent. In most instances, however, many organisms are easily identified on india ink smears. Titers of cryptococcal antigen in both CSF and serum obtained from patients with

AIDS are enormously elevated. Titers as high as 1:2,000,000 have been reported in patients with AIDS

Preferred therapy: Pulmonary disease: Amphotericin B, 0.4–0.5 mg/kg/day for 6 weeks. Pulmonary disease only, immunosuppressed patient: Amphotericin B, 0.4 mg/kg/day for 42 days, then 0.8 mg/kg/day for 28 doses (total dose, 2 g). Meningitis: Amphotericin B, 0.4 mg/kg/day for 42 days, then 0.8 mg/kg/day for 28 doses (total dose, 2.5 g) plus flucytosine, 25–37.5 mg/kg po q 6 h for 6 weeks; AIDS patients: Amphotericin B, 0.4 mg/kg/day for 42 days, then 0.8 mg/kg/day for 28 doses (total dose, 2.5 g) plus flucytosine, 25–37.5 mg/kg po q 6 h for 6 weeks. Chronic suppressive therapy for all patients with AIDS: Fluconazole, 200 mg po qd indefinitely. Alternate Therapy: Nonmeningeal cryptococcosis: Fluconazole, 400 mg on first day, then 200 mg/day for undetermined duration.

Histoplasmosis

- The Mississippi and Ohio River areas are endemic areas of histoplasmosis. The organism exists in large quantities in soil that has been mixed with the excreta of chickens, starlings, and pigeons. Cleaning chicken houses and cutting or bulldozing trees in which birds have roosted often results in the inhalation of many spores that lead to human infections. The overall incidence of histoplasmin sensitivity in the United States is about 22%, but almost all individuals <18 years of age are positive in certain areas of the Mississippi and Ohio River Valleys
- Human infection with H. capsulatum almost always results from inhalation of microconidia of H. capsulatum into the alveoli of the lung, where germination leads to conversion into the yeast form. Multiplication of the organism occurs in the lung, and early fungemia spreads organisms to lymph nodes, liver, and spleen. The initial inflammatory response is an infiltration of polymorphonuclear leukocytes, which is followed by the appearance of mononuclear phagocytes. The fungus is ingested by mononuclear phagocytes, but is not destroyed. The fungus multiplies intracellularly for 2–3 weeks until cell-mediated immunity develops, thereby activating macrophages and enabling macrophages to kill the fungal organism
- H. capsulatum produces a wide spectrum of clinical syndromes. Acute primary histoplasmosis occurs in individuals previously unexposed to H. capsulatum and is asymptomatic or produces symptoms that are so minimal that medical attention is not sought. When present, symptoms are influenza-like, with fever, malaise, headache, nonproductive cough, and roentgenographic infiltrates. Erythema nodosum and erythema multiforme are skin lesions that may occur during acute histoplasmosis. In most instances primary infections resolve completely, but in some patients, the infection becomes progressive. Chronic histoplasmosis most frequently occurs in patients with underlying COPD. Pulmonary infiltrates may wax and wane, or cavitation may occur. In patients without cavitation, 80% resolve, but in those patients with cavitation, only 20% resolve spontaneously. Symptoms of chronic pulmonary histoplasmosis are chronic sputum production, fever, weight loss, and hemoptysis. Five-year mortality rates may approach 50% in untreated patients
- Disseminated histoplasmosis is a multisystem disease that may appear as a mild chronic disease or acute life-threatening disease. Acute life-threatening disease occurs in patients with deficiencies in cell-mediated immunity, whereas chronic disease is found in adults without previous identifiable deficiencies in whom cell-mediated immunity

fails to develop or is inadequate. The clinical manifestations include fever, interstitial pneumonia, hepatosplenomegaly, adrenal involvement, oropharyngeal ulcers, and meningitis. Anemia, leukopenia, and thrombocytopenia may be found. Histoplasmomas and pulmonary nodules occur when concentric layers of necrosis and fibrosis surround an area of old histoplasmosis. These lesions calcify sequentially to form a target lesion and are of no physiologic significance

- Histoplasmosis is a formidable illness in patients with AIDS. Histoplasmosis may mimic sepsis in individuals with diffuse pneumonia and may present a picture similar to that of ARDS. Alternatively, progressive histoplasmosis may present with hepatosplenomegaly, lymphadenopathy, leukopenia, thrombocytopenia, anemia, chorioretinitis, meningoencephalitis, pancreatic or renal lesions, endocarditis, adrenal or thyroid lesions, prostatitis, testicular lesions, or as oral mucosal, cutaneous, or GI ulcerations. Fever of unknown origin in these patients may also be caused by H. capsulatum. Blood cultures are frequently positive, and organisms may be present in sufficient numbers to be visualized on smears of leukocyte buffy coats
- A definitive diagnosis of histoplasmosis can be made only by demonstrating the presence of H. capsulatum in tissue specimens or secretions either by culturing the organism or by visualizing the organism in histopathologic materials. Growth may occur after as early as a few days or may require ≤6 weeks. In patients with diffuse diseases, the blood or bone marrow should be cultured and the organism should be searched for with PAS or silver stains. A variety of quantitative serologic tests may be utilized in diagnosis. CF tests are positive 3–6 weeks after exposure and may remain positive for years. A fourfold ↑ in paired sera or a titer >1:32 is suggestive of infection with H. capsulatum. CF titers are usually low in chronic histoplasmosis. CF tests of >1:8 in CSF suggests H. capsulatum meningitis. Immunodiffusion studies measure precipitating antibodies to the M and H antigens. The H band is specific for active infection, but is present less often than the M band

Preferred therapy: Acute histoplasmosis: Seldom requires treatment; ketoconazole, 400 mg/day for 1 month, if symptomatic. Pulmonary disease, localized disease, disseminated disease in immunocompetent patients: Ketoconazole, 400 mg/day for 6 months. All disease in immunocompromised patients, including patients with AIDS: amphotericin B, 0.4 mg/kg/day for 42 days, then 0.8 mg/kg/day for 28 doses (total dose, ≥2.5 g). Patients with AIDS: Should receive ketoconazole, 400 mg/day, indefinitely following amphotericin B.

Mucormycosis (Mucoraceae)

- Mucormycosis refers to deep mycotic infection caused by nonseptated fungi belonging to the order Mucorales within the species Zygomycetes
- The major forms of mucoraceous infections include rhinocerebral, pulmonary, GI, disseminated, and cutaneous. Pulmonary or disseminated mucormycosis typically affects patients with malignant hematologic disorders, profound granulocytopenia, or global impairment in host defenses. These fungi (Phycomyces, Mucor) have a predilection to invade the vasculature; ischemia, infarction, and severe (even fatal) hemorrhage may occur in this context. Pulmonary mucormycosis may occur as a disease limited to the lung or in the context of widespread disseminated disease. Chest x rays may demonstrate patchy bronchopneumonia, nodular infiltrates, consolidation, or cavities. Hyphae

may penetrate bronchial walls and invade pulmonary blood vessels, thereby leading to thrombosis, distal hemorrhagic infarction, and (rarely) pseudoaneurysm formation. Massive, fatal hemoptysis may result from erosion of the mucoraceous process through a pulmonary artery

- Sputum cultures are positive in only 10–40% of invasive infections; blood cultures are uniformly negative. No useful serologic or skin test exists. Thus, invasive techniques (e.g., bronchoscopy, percutaneous needle aspiration biopsy) are usually required to substantiate the diagnosis. A *definitive diagnosis requires demonstration of the typical fungal hyphae in tissue specimens or on culture*

Preferred therapy: Amphotericin B combined with surgical resection or débridement of involved tissue.

Specific Drugs

Amphotericin B is an antimycotic polyene antibiotic obtained from a strain of Streptomyces nodosus. The polyene group of antibiotics exists as a chemical and biologic subdivision of macrolides. The prime site of action of amphotericin B is the cell membrane where the polyene binds to sterols, chiefly ergosterol, to produce defects in membrane function. The binding is irreversible, and the membrane is made more permeable after specific attachment. The size of the defect induced in the membrane varies, depending on the molecular structure of the polyene. The alteration in cell permeability allows small molecules, notably K and glucose, to leak out. The polyene does not penetrate past the cell membrane and has no known effect on intermediary metabolism or DNA synthesis. Passage of intracellular molecules into the extracellular space is believed to arrest the growth of the organism or cause death of the cell. Yeast, animal cells, and artificial membranes appear to have a similar common pathway of injury. The involvement of amphotericin B with mammalian membranes may account for some side effects noted with this agent. Additionally, the defects in membrane permeability may permit entry of other antifungal agents, such as flucytosine, that might impede fungal growth by interfering with nucleic acid synthesis. Conversely, ketoconazole, which also interferes with ergosterol synthesis, reduces binding sites on the membrane and, therefore, interferes with and reduces activity of amphotericin B in experimental animals and in vitro.

Amphotericin B is associated with significant toxicity and, accordingly, requires careful monitoring. A test dose, 1 mg, in 500 ml of 5% dextrose and H_2O should be infused over 3–4 h, and the patient should be observed for the presence of an anaphylactic reaction. If the test dose is tolerated, the patient should then be infused with a daily dose of 10 mg, increasing the daily dose 10 mg each day until 50 mg/day is reached. A daily dose is continued until a clinical response is evident (often within 1 week). Subsequent doses then can be given on an every-other-day basis. Dosage should be adjusted to the requirements of each patient, because individual tolerance to amphotericin B varies. Amphotericin B should then be administered IV over 4–6 h on an every-other-day basis. The use of this regimen would require approximately 18 weeks to complete a 2-g course of therapy.

Unpleasant reactions to amphotericin B are virtually universal. Fever, shaking chills, nausea, vomiting, anorexia, and headache are frequent complaints. Pretreatment with aspirin, diphenhydramine, or hydrocortisone (20–50 mg) may be helpful. Local phlebitis and thrombophlebitis may occur at the injection site. Heparin, 500 U, may ↓ the phlebitis associated with IV delivery. Acute reactions tend to improve as the treatment course progresses.

The patient should be monitored carefully for adverse reactions, some of which are dangerous. Abnormal renal function, including azotemia, hypokalemia, hypomagnesemia, renal tubular acidosis, and nephrocalcinosis, are often observed. Normocytic, normochromic anemia may also result. Serum creatinine, BUN, electrolytes, magnesium, and a CBC should be evaluated weekly during amphotericin B therapy. Serum creatinine ↑ in almost all subjects, and no adjustment in dose is required until the creatinine level reaches 2.5 mg/dl (221 μmol/l). Improvement in renal function usually occurs with interruption of therapy, but permanent impairment can occur with cumulative doses >3 g. Other nephrotoxic antibiotics and chemotherapeutic agents should not be given concomitantly unless absolutely required.

In summary, amphotericin B is considered the gold standard of antifungal therapy, especially for systemic mycoses. Amphotericin B has several significant drawbacks, including:

- The necessity of IV administration
- Poor penetration to CSF
- Intolerance by many patients because of unpleasant side effects
- Significant toxicity to bone marrow and kidneys

Ketoconazole is well absorbed orally, with peak serum levels occurring 1–6 h after ingestion. Metabolism and excretion of ketoconazole occur by hepatobiliary mechanisms; little active drug is excreted in the urine. Ketoconazole requires gastric acidity for dissolution and absorption. The data on the effect of food on the absorption of ketoconazole are conflicting. Cimetidine and antacids that impair absorption should be withheld until 2 h after the administration of a dose of ketoconazole. Many physicians prefer to administer the drug just prior to a meal. Oral ketoconazole possesses some undesirable properties:

- A low, but real, potential for hepatotoxicity
- Dose-related inhibition of testosterone and adrenal corticosteroid synthesis
- Adverse interactions with other drugs, especially rifampin and cyclosporin

Symptomatic hepatic toxicity has been reported to occur in 1 in 10,000–12,000 treatment courses. Two deaths attributable to ketoconazole-induced hepatitis were reported in 1 series. Suppression of testosterone may be accompanied by ↓ sperm counts, ↓ libido, impotence, and gynecomastia. These effects of ketoconazole are reversible when the drug is withdrawn. Ketoconazole also blunts the response to ACTH stimulation. This effect on steroid synthesis appears to be the result of P450 enzyme inhibition, thereby leading to ↓ steroid synthesis. Additionally, ketoconazole has been shown to block glucocorticoid receptor sites by competitive binding. Hypoadrenalism is rare.

Ketoconazole may enhance the anticoagulant effect of coumarin-like drugs. Keotconazole ↑ blood levels of cyclosporin A; accordingly, blood levels of cyclosporin A should be monitored if the 2 drugs are given concomitantly. Concomitant administration of ketoconazole with phenytoin may alter the metabolism of 1 or both drugs. Both ketoconazole and phenytoin should be monitored if both drugs are given concurrently. Because severe hypoglycemia has been reported in patients concomitantly receiving oral miconazole and oral hypoglycemic agents, the potential interaction of ketoconazole and oral hypoglycemic agents should be monitored.

Fluconazole is a H_2O-soluble triazole whose mode of action is inhibition of the demethylase enzyme that is involved in the synthesis of ergosterol. Oral absorption is rapid and nearly complete within 2 h. Oral absorption of fluconazole is more uniform than that of ketoconazole. Elimination of the drug is predominantly renal, and dose modification is required in moderate or severe renal insufficiency. Fluconazole has good penetration into CSF. Numerous studies have shown that CSF levels of fluconazole are 60–80% of simultaneous serum concentrations, even in the presence of uninflamed meninges. Because of its high level of penetration into CSF, high volume of distribution to body tissues, good absorption after oral dosing, and long half-life, fluconazole is an attractive alternative to IV amphotericin B for the treatment of fungal meningitis.

Oral fluconazole is generally well tolerated. Inhibition of testicular and adrenal steroidogenesis has not been seen at the doses studied. The frequency of GI complaints and hepatic toxicity is lower than that found with ketoconazole. Fluconazole interferes with phenytoin, cyclosporin, and warfarin. Drug levels of these agents should be monitored when given concomitantly with fluconazole.

Itraconazole is the most H_2O soluble of the azole drugs. Like fluconazole, it appears to be less toxic than ketoconazole. Despite relatively poor penetration of itraconazole into CSF, animal models and limited human data suggest that this drug is more effective than ketoconazole for therapy of meningitis. This drug has only recently become available in the United States. However, several ongoing, noncomparative clinical trials suggest that itraconazole is at least as effective as oral ketoconazole for therapy of non-life-threatening forms of histoplasmosis, blastomycosis, and coccidioidomycosis. Studies of in vitro murine models and limited human studies suggest that itraconazole may be effective therapy for aspergillosis.

Flucytosine is a fluorinated pyrimidine analog that was initially synthesized as an antileukemic agent. Flucytosine has a narrow spectrum of activity and is never used alone because secondary resistance develops quickly. Flucytosine is a small molecule that rapidly distributes to all tissues, including CSF. The kidneys secrete >90% of the drug unchanged. Flucytosine exerts its antifungal effect in fungi that possess cytosine deaminase. This enzyme metabolizes the drug to 5-fluorouracil, an antimetabolite that is incorporated into fungal RNA and interferes with protein synthesis. Antifungal activity might also be mediated by effects on DNA synthesis. Cytosine permease is required for entrance of flucytosine into the cell. Resistant fungi either lack the deaminase or have ↓ cytosine permease activity.

Flucytosine is usually used in combination with amphotericin B, which causes changes in fungal cell wall permeability and may therefore enhance the entrance of flucytosine into the cell. Alternatively, other authors have suggested that amphotericin B impedes entrance of flucytosine into the cell and that the 2 drugs interact in a sequential rather than a synergistic fashion.

Toxicity of flucytosine includes leukopenia and thrombocytopenia, which occur in ≤5% of patients and may be life threatening. Cytopenias are most common in patients with impaired renal function and correlate with high serum concentrations, usually >100 μg/ml. Flucytosine should be given in the usual single dose (37.5 mg/kg) bid if the creatinine clearance is 20–40 ml/min and once daily if it is 10–20 ml/min. Direct measurements of blood levels are necessary to prevent toxicity for all patients with ↓ renal function at the beginning of treatment and for all patients receiving concomitant amphotericin B if their serum creatinine is increasing.

TUBERCULOSIS

Although the number of cases of tuberculosis reported annually in the United States declined steadily from 1953 (84,304) to 1984 (22,255), this trend was dramatically reversed when the number of cases rose by 3% in 1986 and by 5% in 1989 (23,495). This resurgence of tuberculosis is largely related to the HIV epidemic

- Mycobacteria are aerobic, nonmotile, curved or straight rods that are occasionally branched. They are free-living saprophytes that form part of the natural ecology of the soil. M. tuberculosis is the major cause of human disease and depends on host transmission for its survival
- Transmission of infection with M. tuberculosis is primarily from person to person by aerosolization of microdroplets (1–5 μm) that usually contain ≤3 tubercle bacilli. Droplets of this size reach the alveoli, where macrophages ingest the organisms and process and present mycobacterial antigens to T-cells. In naive hosts, macrophages have a limited ability to kill the organism, which proliferates within and outside macrophages. Specific immune responses develop following presentation of antigens to T-cells. Sensitized T-lymphocytes secrete lymphokines, which activate macrophages, thereby greatly enhancing their capacity to ingest and kill mycobacteria. The time required for the generation of a specific immune response is unknown but probably requires approximately 6 weeks. During the interval between inhalation of the aerosol and the development of T-cell immunity, a clinically silent bacillemia, which seeds the lung as well as other organs in the host, usually occurs. With the development of cell-mediated immunity, the majority of organisms are killed throughout the body, although few dormant bacilli remain in most hosts. Clinically apparent tuberculosis develops in approximately 10% of infected patients either soon after infection (primary infection) or years later (reactivation tuberculosis). Both of these consequences are thought to be the result of defects in T-cell or macrophage function or both
- Infection of the naive host usually produces a subclinical syndrome whose only manifestation is the development of a positive PPD. Occasionally fever, nonproductive cough, or shortness of breath may occur. Chest x rays show an infiltrate in the apical or posterior segment of the upper lobes or in the middle or lower lobes. Alternatively, primary tuberculosis may present with a pleural effusion with pleurisy but no parenchymal infiltrate. The patient frequently complains of pleuritic chest pain, nonproductive cough, fever, chills, sweats, and dyspnea. The finding of a unilateral exudative pleural effusion in a patient with a positive PPD is highly suggestive of this diagnosis. When untreated, a high percentage of these patients develop active tuberculosis within 5 years
- Progressive primary tuberculosis results from a failure to develop cell-mediated immunity. Its appearance is usually cryptic, with unexplained fever being common. Alternatively, a clinical syndrome of low-grade fever, night sweats, fatigability, loss of appetite, cough, hemoptysis, and the development of cavitary lung lesions may occur. This syndrome is differentiated from reactivation tuberculosis only by documentation of the natural history of the disease

- Reactivation tuberculosis is the most common manifestation of infection with M. tuberculosis. Cavitary disease involving the posterior segments of the upper lobes or the apical segments of the lower lobes is common. Symptoms include night sweats, chills, fatigue, fever, and hemoptysis
- Approximately 15% of cases of tuberculosis are extrapulmonary. Lymphatic tuberculosis is the most common form of extrapulmonary tuberculosis. In patients >12 years of age, 95% of lymphadenitis in the context of tuberculous infection is caused by M. tuberculosis. Genitourinary tuberculosis usually produces symptoms and signs of a urinary tract infection. Vertebral tuberculosis is a major source of morbidity because of resultant kyphosis and spinal cord abnormalities. The patient typically appears after weeks to months of back pain, fever, and weight loss. Tuberculous meningitis is a dreaded complication of tuberculosis. Fever, weight loss, and malaise predate CNS involvement in many patients, and most patients have CNS symptoms for <2 weeks. Other sites of extrapulmonary tuberculosis include tuberculous peritonitis, involvement of the distal ileum, and involvement of the skin
- The diagnosis of tuberculosis requires the isolation of M. tuberculosis from the infected host. A presumptive diagnosis may be made if acid-fast bacilli are noted in specimens or tissues obtained from patients. At least 3 samples of sputum obtained from the lower respiratory tract should be evaluated. Culture of M. tuberculosis requires 3–6 weeks for growth. If sputum cultures are negative, bronchoscopy with transbronchial biopsy can be performed. At present, evaluation of tissue or body fluids for mycobacterial RNA or DNA does not offer improved sensitivity. The role of polymerase chain reaction amplification of mycobacterial DNA is uncertain
- The tuberculin skin test is a useful diagnostic and epidemiologic tool. Concepts concerning the cutoff point for a positive test undergo continuous revision. The cut-off point of 5 mm has been proposed for HIV-infected patients, household contacts, or patients whose chest x ray suggests prior tuberculosis. The cutoff point of 10 mm has been proposed for patients with recent skin test conversion and for patients with predisposing conditions. The cutoff point of 15 mm may be appropriate in otherwise healthy individuals with no known contact with an active case
- The incidence of tuberculosis in patients with AIDS is almost 500 times the incidence in the general population. The risk of tuberculosis varies with the prevalence of infection with mycobacteria in the specific patient at risk. Foreign-born patients, IV drug abusers, and male homosexuals have the highest risk. Infection with tuberculosis usually precedes the diagnosis of AIDS. Extrapulmonary tuberculosis in patients with HIV infection has been an AIDS-defining condition since 1987. Among patients with relatively well-preserved immune function, findings on chest x ray are similar to those of reactivation tuberculosis in immunocompetent patients and include cavitation and upper lobe infiltrates. In severely immunocompromised patients with HIV infection, findings on chest x ray are typically those of primary tuberculosis and include hilar adenopathy, pleural effusions, and/or a miliary pattern. Lymphadenitis, meningitis, brain abscess, and bone, pericardial, peritoneal, and gastric involvement are the main outcomes of extrapulmonary tuberculosis. Blood cultures are positive in 50% of patients

Treatment

Antituberculous chemotherapy is based on 3 basic principles:

- Treatment should always include 2 drugs to which the organisms are susceptible
- The duration of treatment must continue for a sufficient period of time (at present, 6 months is the minimal duration)
- Promoting and monitoring compliance are central for treatment to be successful

Tuberculous chemotherapy can be successful only if the clinical and social management of patients and their contacts are considered.

Initial Treatment Regimen

The American Thoracic Society and Centers for Disease Control recommend a 6-month regimen consisting of a 2-month period of daily isoniazid (5 mg/kg, ≤300 mg), rifampin (10 mg/kg, ≤600 mg), and pyrazinamide (20–35 mg/kg, ≤2 g), followed by 4 months of twice weekly isoniazid (20–40 mg/kg, ≤90 mg) along with rifampin (10 mg/kg, ≤600 mg). Ethambutol should be included in the initial phase when isoniazid resistance is suspected. A 9-month regimen consisting of isoniazid and rifampin is also highly successful. When resistance to isoniazid is documented, rifampin and ethambutol, perhaps supplemented initially by pyrazinamide, should be given for >12 months. Although little data exist regarding treatment for extrapulmonary tuberculosis, the above 9-month regimen is known to be effective. Regimens of 6 months are probably as effective in extrapulmonary disease as in pulmonary disease, but data are not presently available. Longer therapy may be necessary for lymphadenitis and bone and joint tuberculosis.

Patients treated for tuberculosis should have baseline measurements of hepatic enzymes, bilirubin, serum creatinine or BUN, and serum uric acid, and a CBC. All patients should be monitored clinically at least monthly during therapy and should be specifically questioned regarding symptoms suggestive of drug toxicity. Symptoms of concern include nausea and vomiting, fatigue or weakness of >3 days' duration, dark urine, icterus, rash, paresthesias and/or fever of >3 days' duration, and right upper quadrant tenderness. Routine laboratory monitoring for subclinical drug toxicity is not necessary.

The response to antituberculous chemotherapy should be monitored and is best evaluated with examinations of sputum. Sputum should be cultured monthly until sputum conversion is documented, or at a minimum, sputum should be obtained after 3 months of therapy, at which point >90% of patients should have converted to negative. If patients have not converted by the end of 3 months of therapy, serious consideration should be given to administering the treatment under direct observation. Patients whose sputum is negative after 3 months of treatment should have sputum smear and culture performed at the completion of therapy. Patients who have completed a 9-month course of isoniazid/rifampin and who have had a prompt bacteriologic response do not require further follow-up treatment. Patients who have completed a 6-month regimen should have follow-up evaluations 6 and 12 months after completion of therapy.

Patients whose sputum has not converted after 5–6 months of treatment are considered treatment failures. Susceptibility of the organism should be determined on the patient's current regimen. The regimen should be adjusted in accordance with the susceptibility tests, and treatment should be administered under direct observation. Patients whose organisms are susceptible to treatment at the outset of treatment and who relapse after the completion of an approved regimen usually relapse with organisms that remain susceptible to isoniazid and rifampin. Reinstitution of the isoniazid-rifampin previously used is recommended for these patients.

Preventive Therapy

Preventive therapy with isoniazid is useful in infected patients judged at high risk of progression to disease. Priorities for preventive therapy must compare the risk of developing tuberculosis to the risk of isoniazid toxicity. Preventive therapy is recommended for:

- Household members and other close associates of persons with potentially infectious tuberculosis
- Newly infected persons
- Persons with past tuberculosis
- Persons with significant reaction to tuberculin skin tests and abnormal chest x rays
- Persons with significant reactions to tuberculin skin tests who have special clinical conditions, such as silicosis, diabetes mellitus, prolonged therapy with adrenal corticosteroids, immunosuppressive therapy, such hematologic and reticuloendothelial disease as leukemia or Hodgkin's disease, AIDS, ESRD, and conditions associated with rapid weight loss and chronic undernutrition
- Persons with tuberculin skin test reactions who are <35 years of age and have none of the previously mentioned risk factors

Isoniazid (300 mg/day for adults, 10–14 mg/kg/day for children not to exceed 300 mg/day) is used alone for preventive therapy. Isoniazid has been given for 12 months in most clinical trials, but good evidence suggests that 6 months of preventive therapy confers a nearly comparable degree of protection. Household contacts have a 2–4% risk of developing active disease in the first year. Young children and adolescents may have twice the adult risk. Accordingly, all persons in contact with a patient with tuberculin skin test of 5 mm or more should be treated with isoniazid. Preventive therapy for 3 months is prudent even if the skin test is negative. Initially, nonreactive household members should all undergo repeated skin testing after 3 months. If negative, isoniazid can be discontinued in children who have received 3 months of therapy. If positive, isoniazid should be continued. Patients receiving preventive therapy should be monitored in person or by phone at monthly intervals. The symptoms suggestive of toxic side effects mentioned earlier should be specifically sought.

Patients with HIV Infection

More prolonged treatment is recommended in patients with HIV infection because the efficacy of standard therapy in such patients is uncertain. Isoniazid, rifampin, and pyrazinamide are given daily for 2 months, followed by isoniazid and rifampin for 7 months, or for 6 months after cultures are negative, whichever is longer. If patients are intolerant to rifampin, several investigators suggest isoniazid, pyrazinamide, and ethambutol for 18–24 months, or for 12 months after cultures are negative, whichever is longer.

Of HIV-infected patients with positive tuberculin skin tests, 8% are diagnosed with tuberculosis each year. Accordingly, chemoprophylaxis for patients coinfected with HIV and M. tuberculosis is a critical public health priority. The initial evaluations of all patients with HIV infection should include the intradermal administration of 5 tuberculin U of PPD tuberculin and ≥2 companion antigens, such as Candida, mumps, or tetanus toxoid. A 5-mm cutoff point is considered positive in patients with HIV infection because their delayed hypersensitivity response is ↓. Patients with a positive PPD should receive chemoprophylaxis regardless of age, unless a specific contraindication exists. Chemoprophylaxis should be administered to anergic HIV-seropositive patients with a documented history of a positive tuberculin skin test and who have not received treatment, to those with abnormalities on chest x ray suggestive of previously untreated tuberculosis, and to those in close contact with patients with tuberculosis. Persons with skin test results of ≥5 mm who refuse serologic testing for HIV but are suspected of having HIV infection should be considered candidates for preventive therapy regardless of age. The duration of chemoprophylaxis in confirmed or presumed HIV-infected patients is 12 months.

Preferred Therapy: Active Tuberculosis

NONIMMUNOCOMPROMISED HOST

- 6-month regimens are effective
- First 2 months: Isoniazid 5 mg/kg/day, max 300 mg/day; rifampin 10 mg/kg/day, max 600 mg/day; and pyrazinamide 25 mg/kg/day, max 2 g/day
- Final 4 months: Isoniazid qd (as above) or twice weekly, 15 mg/kg/day, max 900 mg/day; and rifampin qd (as above) or twice weekly, 10 mg/kg/day, max 600 mg/day
- Patients with positive sputum at 6 months are considered treatment failures

AIDS

- First 2 months: Isoniazid 5 mg/kg/day, max 300 mg/day; rifampin 10 mg/kg/day, max 600 mg/day; and pyrazinamide, 25 mg/kg/day, max 2 g/day
- Final 7 months: Isoniazid qd (as above) or twice weekly, 15 mg/kg/day, max 900 mg/day; and rifampin qd (as above) or twice weekly, 10 mg/kg/day, max 600 mg/day

EXTRAPULMONARY

- 9-month and probably 6-month regimens are effective

Preferred Therapy: Infection without Disease (+PPD)

NONIMMUNOCOMPROMISED HOST

- Isoniazid 5 mg/kg/day, max 300 mg/day for 6–12 months
- Results with 6 months (65%) nearly as good as with 12 months (75%) in reducing disease

AIDS

- Isoniazid 5 mg/kg/day, max 300 mg/day for 12 months
- All persons with PPD >5 mm should be treated regardless of age

Specific Drugs

Isoniazid is the most widely used of the antituberculosis agents. This bactericidal, nontoxic, easily administered, inexpensive agent is an ideal drug. Oral administration (3–5 mg/kg) produces a peak concentration of approximately 5 μg/ml 1–2 h after administration. Most strains of M. tuberculosis are inhibited by concentrations of 0.05–0.20 μg/ml.

Hepatitis is the major toxic effect of isoniazid. The rate of hepatitis ↑ directly with ↑ in age to 65 years. The incidence of hepatitis is <1% in patients under age 35 and is approximately 2% in patients over age 50. Peripheral neuropathy caused by interference with metabolism of pyridoxine is also associated with isoniazid administration. In patients with diabetes, uremia, alcoholism, and malnutrition, pyridoxine, 10–25 mg/day, should be given with isoniazid. The interaction of isoniazid and phenytoin ↑ the serum concentration of both drugs, and accordingly, serum levels of phenytoin should be monitored.

Rifampin is bactericidal for M. tuberculosis. It is rapidly absorbed from the GI tract. Oral administration produces peak concentrations of 6–7 mg/ml 1–2 h after ingestion. Most M. tuberculosis is inhibited in vitro by concentrations of 0.5 μg/ml. Rifampin is 75% protein bound but penetrates well into tissues and cells. Penetration through noninflamed meninges is poor, but therapeutic concentrations are achieved in CSF when the meninges are inflamed.

Adverse reactions to rifampin include hepatitis, GI upset, skin eruptions, and rarely thrombocytopenia. The rate of these reactions is variable, but hepatitis occurs in approximately 3% of patients being treated with isoniazid and rifampin for 6 months. Twice-weekly administration of higher doses of rifampin is associated with an influenza-like syndrome, hemolytic anemia, acute renal failure, and thrombocytopenia. Rifampin is excreted in urine, tears, sweat, and other body fluids, and colors them orange. Patients should be advised of possible prominent discoloration of soft contact lenses. Rifampin may accelerate clearance of methadone, coumadin derivatives, glucocorticoids, estrogens, oral hypoglycemic agents, digitalis, anticonvulsants, ketoconazole, and cyclosporin.

Pyrazinamide is bactericidal for M. tuberculosis in an acid environment. The drug is particularly active against organisms in macrophages, presumably because of the acid environment within the cell. Administration of the drug in doses of 20–25 mg/kg results in serum concentrations of 30–50 μg/ml 2 h after ingestion. At a pH of 5.5, the minimal inhibitory concentration of pyrazinamide for M. tuberculosis is 20 μg/ml. Penetration of the drug into cells and tissues seems to be good, although data are limited. The most important adverse reaction to pyrazinamide is liver injury, but apparently a significant ↑ in hepatotoxicity does not occur when pyrazinamide is added to a regimen of isoniazid and rifampin during the initial 2 months of therapy.

Ethambutol in usual doses has a bacteriostatic effect on M. tuberculosis. Following administration of 15 mg/kg, peak concentrations of 4 μg/ml are noted 2–4 h after ingestion. Inhibitory concentrations for this drug range from 1 to 5 μg/ml. CSF concentrations are low even in the presence of meningeal inflammation.

Retrobulbar neuritis is the most frequent and serious adverse effect of ethambutol. This complication occurs in <1% of patients at a daily dose of 15 mg/kg. Symptoms include central scotomata, blurred vision, and red-green color blindness.

Streptomycin is bactericidal in an alkaline environment. Streptomycin must be given parenterally. Following administration of 15 mg/kg, the peak concentration in serum is 40 μg/ml 1 h after an I.M. dose. The drug should be used in ↓ dosage and with extreme caution in patients with renal insufficiency. Streptomycin enters the CSF only in the presence of meningeal inflammation.

The most common adverse effect of streptomycin is ototoxicity. Vertigo is more common, but hearing loss may also occur. Nephrotoxicity occasionally occurs, and patients with pre-existing renal insufficiency or who are simultaneously using other nephrotoxic drugs are at ↑ risk. A total dose of >120 g should not be given. Ototoxicity and nephrotoxicity are more common in persons >60 years of age, and streptomycin should be avoided, if possible, in this group.

VIRAL INFECTIONS

Infections with DNA viruses (CMV, herpes simplex, varicella zoster, adenovirus) occur with ↑ frequency in immunocompromised hosts, and may give rise to serious pneumonias in this context.

Cytomegalovirus

- CMV is the most important cause of severe viral infections in immunocompromised patients. CMV rarely causes clinical infections in normal hosts; however, serum antibodies are present in 45–80% of normal adults, thus suggesting that asymptomatic infection occurs commonly. Serious CMV infections are almost exclusively confined to severely immunocompromised hosts (typically patients with AIDS or organ transplant recipients); other groups at risk include patients on high-dose corticosteroid or immunosuppressive therapy or patients with malignant hematologic disease receiving intensive chemotherapy. CMV is the most common pathogen complicating both bone marrow and solid organ transplantation. Serious pneumonia have been noted among heart-lung and lung transplant recipients
- The manifestations of CMV infections are diverse. Asymptomatic viral shedding (viruria, viremia) is frequent among organ transplant recipients; however, disseminated disease or fulminant CMV pneumonitis may be fatal. The most common manifestation of CMV infection in immunocompromised patients is an atypical mononucleosis syndrome with fever, circulating atypical lymphocytes in peripheral blood, anemia, leukopenia, and abnormal liver function tests. Pneumonia occurs in 10–20% of infected patients, but higher rates (>50%) have been noted in lung transplant recipients receiving positive donor organs. Diffuse interstitial or alveolar infiltrates on chest x ray are characteristic of CMV pneumonitis; however, focal infiltrates mimicking bacterial pneumonia may be observed. A miliary pattern on chest x ray reflects hematogeneous spread, and is often associated with a

more fulminant course. Large nodular infiltrates or cavities, which are virtually never seen with primary CMV pneumonitis, suggest alternative diagnoses. More than 80% of patients with CMV pneumonitis are viremic, which usually antedates the development of pulmonary infection by 7–14 days. CMV infections are confined to a relatively well-defined time period post organ transplantation. Virtually all infections occur 30–120 days post transplantation, with a mean of 40–55 days. Infections before day 21 or after 6 months are rare

- The diagnosis of CMV pneumonitis can be established by demonstrating the typical large CMV-infected cells containing intranuclear inclusions (an "owl's eye" appearance) and multiple smaller cytoplasmic inclusion bodies in lung tissue or cytologic specimens. These basophilic intranuclear inclusions can be demonstrated readily by hematoxylin-eosin, Wright's, Giemsa, or Papanicolaou's stains. Conventional viral cultures are positive in 70–90% of confirmed cases, but may take 2–6 weeks to grow. More recently, several new techniques have been employed to substantiate the diagnosis in a more timely fashion. IF studies using monoclonal antibodies against CMV antigens (shell vial cultures) enable a rapid diagnosis (within 24 h) of CMV-infected cells in BAL fluid, blood, urine, or tissue, with diagnostic accuracy ≥ that of conventional cytologic and cultural techniques

Preferred Therapy: Ganciclovir (DHPG) initial dose of 10 mg/kg/day in 2 divided doses for 21 days, followed by 5 mg/kg/day for period of risk (as long as 90–120 days for organ transplant recipients). High-dose (3,200 mg/day) acyclovir may substitute for 5 mg/kg/day ganciclovir for longterm prophylaxis among patients who have received initial induction therapy with 10 mg/kg/day ganciclovir for 21 days. Alternate Therapy: Foscarnet sodium (60 mg/kg q 8 h for 21 days, followed by maintenance 90 mg/kg once daily 5 days/week). IV may be used for cases refractory to ganciclovir or experiencing side effects for ganciclovir.

Herpes Simplex Virus

- Primary herpes simplex pneumonitis may rarely accompany serious mucocutaneous herpes simplex infections in immunocompromised hosts; in >80–90% of patients, herpetic lesions involving the lip or oropharynx precede or occur simultaneously with the pulmonary lesion. Individuals at greatest risk are children with acute leukemia and organ transplant recipients. Herpetic infections involving the lower respiratory tract have been associated with a wide gamut of clinical manifestations. Mild extension of HSV from the oropharynx may result in a mild tracheobronchitis; more fulminant hemorrhagic pneumonitis has also been described, but is rare. In severe cases, bronchoscopy may demonstrate punctate ulcerations of tracheal or bronchial mucosa, edema, and thick pseudomembranes within the tracheobronchial tree. With fulminant HSV pneumonitis, pulmonary edema and hemorrhage may ensue. Radiographic findings are diverse; both focal pneumonia and diffuse interstitial infiltrates have been described. Cavitation does not occur. Bacterial or fungal superinfection complicates HSV pneumonitis in ≤50% of patients and may contribute to mortality
- Herpes simplex may be demonstrated by cytologic methods or cultures of BAL fluid or lung biopsies; eosinophilic intranuclear inclusions and multinucleated (syncytial) giant cells may be detected in infected tissue. Distinction of colonization from clinical HSV pneumonitis is diffi-

cult, however. In many patients, HSV colonizes the lower respiratory tract as a saphrophyte while other pathogens are present concomitantly. In documented HSV pneumonitis, mortality may be >80% in severely ill, immunocompromised patients; however, concomitant infections and host factors may contribute to this observed high mortality

Preferred Therapy: IV acyclovir 250 mg/m^2 q 8 h for 7–10 days (reduce level of immunosuppression when possible)

Adenovirus

- Adenovirus may give rise to lower or upper respiratory tract infections in both normal and compromised hosts; fatal, hemorrhagic pneumonia may occur. Adenovirus is a rare opportunist, but has been associated with frequent pulmonary and hepatic involvement and a high mortality in immunocompromised hosts. Adenovirus is isolated from approximately 5% of bone marrow transplant recipients. Pneumonia caused by adenovirus is characterized histologically by interstitial infiltrates and necrosis, sloughing of bronchial mucosa, pulmonary edema, and alveolar hemorrhage
- Chest x rays typically demonstrate diffuse interstitial or alveolar infiltrates; unilateral involvement has also been described. CNS involvement with diffuse meningoencephalitis and progressive hepatic necrosis is a rare complication. Unfortunately, no specific therapy is available

Suggested Reading

Toews G, Lynch JP III: Fungal, mycobacterial, and viral pulmonary infections. *In* Khan M Gabriel, Cardiac and Pulmonary Management. Philadelphia, Lea & Febiger, 1993.

19 Acid-Base Disorders

Paul L. Marino and David Nierman

RULE-BASED ACID-BASE INTERPRETATIONS

Acid-base regulation is a well-defined process that allows for a highly organized approach to identifying acid-base disorders. A "rule-based" method is used in the acid-base interpretations in this chapter. This method creates predictions based on the observed behavior of acid-base regulation, and these predictions are used as statements or instructions (rules) that identify acid-base abnormalities. Rules create rigid guidelines that reduce uncertainty and simplify the problem-solving process; these attributes can improve the accuracy of acid-base interpretations.

Acid-Base Relationships

The principal features of acid-base regulation are defined by the chemical relationship between pH, CO_2, and bicarbonate ions in the extracellular fluid. This relationship is expressed below, using the partial pressure of carbon dioxide (PCO_2) and the concentration of bicarbonate ions [HCO_3] and hydrogen ions H^+ in circulating blood.

$$(\text{mEq/l})\ H^+ = 24 \times (PCO_2/[HCO_3])$$

This relationship defines the PCO_2/HCO_3 ratio as the principal factor in determining the acid-base properties of extracellular fluid. As such, the PCO_2/HCO_3 ratio can be used to describe the different types of acid-base disorders (see Table 19–1). The "primary" acid-base disorders are defined by the component of the PCO_2/HCO_3 ratio that is altered either initially or by the greatest magnitude; i.e., the "respiratory" acid-base disorders indicate a primary change in PCO_2, and the "metabolic" acid-base disorders identify HCO_3 as the primary abnormality. "Secondary" or compensatory adjustments are identified as a ↓ in the magnitude of change in PCO_2/HCO_3 produced by the primary acid-base disorder.

Compensatory Changes

The goal of acid-base regulation is to reduce or eliminate the change in pH (i.e., change in PCO_2/HCO_3 ratio) produced by an acid-base disturbance. This is accomplished by compensatory adjustments to primary acid-base changes, and these adjustments are aimed at reducing the change in the PCO_2/HCO_3 ratio produced by the primary disturbance. For example, a ↑ in PCO_2 (primary respiratory acidosis) must be accompanied by a ↑ in HCO_3 (compensatory metabolic alkalosis) to limit the change in the PCO_2/HCO_3 ratio caused by the change in PCO_2. In other words, compensatory responses to primary respiratory acid-base disorders will involve changes in serum bicarbonate levels in the same direction as the PCO_2 changes. These adjustments in serum bicarbonate are

Table 19–1
Expected Compensatory Responses

PRIMARY DISORDER	EXPECTED RESPONSE
Metabolic Acidosis	Expected $PCO_2 = 1.5 \times HCO_3^- + 0.8\ (+2)$
Metabolic Alkalosis	Expected $PCO_2 = 0.7 \times HCO_3^- + 20\ (+1.5)$
Respiratory Acidosis	$\Delta pH/\Delta PCO_2 =$ 0.008 (Acute) 0.003 (Chronic)
Respiratory Alkalosis	$\Delta pH/\Delta PCO_2 =$ 0.008 (Acute) 0.017 (Chronic)

produced in the kidneys and represent changes in urinary bicarbonate excretion. These renal adjustments require 3–5 days for completion, thus creating a period of "partial compensation." Table 19–1 shows the changes in pH associated with partial and full compensation. Note that the compensatory changes are not enough to maintain constant pH; i.e., compensation differs from correction.

Compensation for primary metabolic acid-base disorders involves a change in ventilation that changes the arterial PCO_2 in the same direction as the original change in serum bicarbonate level. These responses are mediated by chemoreceptors that respond to changes in pH and modulate the activity of the respiratory centers in the lower brain stem. Metabolic acidosis produces a ↑ in ventilation and a ↓ in PCO_2, while metabolic alkalosis depresses ventilation and raises the PCO_2. Table 19–1 shows the expected changes in PCO_2 in each type of metabolic acid-base disorder. Note that there is no period of partial compensation; i.e., the respiratory response is fully developed at onset.

Rules for Acid-Base Disorders

The equations in Table 19–1 define the changes expected in the different types of acid-base disorders. These relationships have been used to generate the following rules.

Rule 1. A primary metabolic disorder is present if:

A. The pH and PCO_2 change in the same direction, or
B. The pH is abnormal but the PCO_2 is normal.

Rule 2. In primary metabolic disorders, a secondary disturbance is identified by a difference between the PCO_2 expected from respiratory compensation and the PCO_2 measured in arterial blood.

A. For Primary Metabolic Acidosis, Expected $PCO_2 = 1.5(HCO_3) + 8(\pm 2)$
*B. For Primary Metabolic Alkalosis, Expected $PCO_2 = 0.7(HCO_3) + 20(\pm 1.5)$

Measured $PCO_2 >$ Expected $PCO_2 =$ Associated Respiratory Acidosis

Measured $PCO_2 <$ Expected $PCO_2 =$ Associated Respiratory Alkalosis

* The respiratory response to metabolic alkalosis can be variable and unpredictable, creating some concern about the validity of the expected PCO_2 in metabolic alkalosis. Several equations are available for predicting the PCO_2 in metabolic alkalosis; this one was selected because it is currently the most popular. The accuracy of this relationship when the HCO_3 >40 mEq/l is not known.

Rule 3. A primary respiratory disorder is present if the pH and PCO_2 change in opposite directions.

Rule 4. In primary respiratory disorders, the relative changes in pH and PCO_2 will determine the extent of compensation and identify secondary metabolic disturbances, using the following guidelines:

A. For Respiratory Acidosis:

pH/PCO_2	Disorder
>0.008	Associated metabolic acidosis
0.008	Acute uncompensated acidosis
0.002–0.008	Partially compensated acidosis
<0.002	Associated metabolic alkalosis

B. For Respiratory Acidosis:

pH/PCO_2	Disorder
>0.008	Associated metabolic acidosis
0.008	Acute uncompensated acidosis
0.002–0.008	Partially compensated acidosis
<0.002	Associated metabolic alkalosis

Rule 5. A mixed metabolic-respiratory disorder is present if the pH is normal and the PCO_2 is abnormal.

Acid-Base Interpretations

The rules in the previous section are now applied to acid-base interpretations, and the flow diagrams for this approach are shown in Figures 19–1 and 19–2. These interpretations are based on the relationships

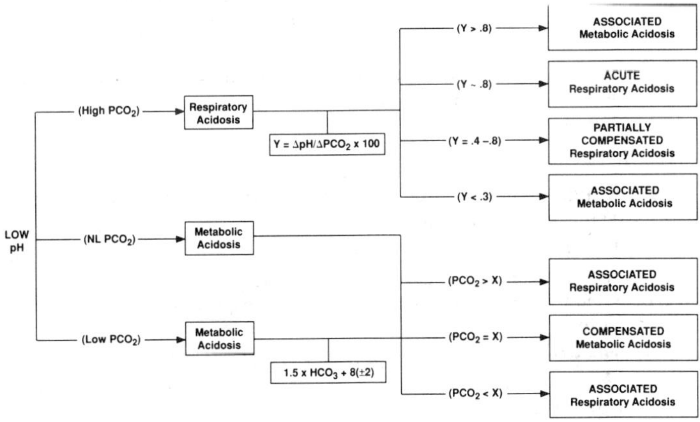

Figure 19–1. Flow diagram for acid-base interpretation when arterial pH is below normal. (See text for explanation.) From: Marino PL: The ICU Book. Philadelphia, Lea & Febiger, 1991.

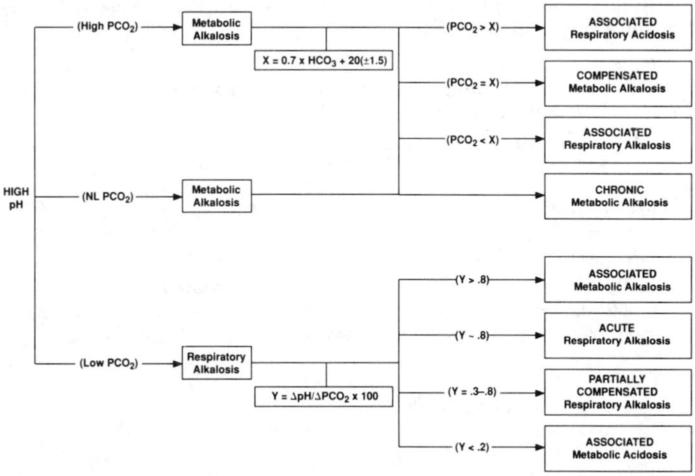

Figure 19–2. Flow diagram for acid-base interpretation when arterial pH is above normal. (See text for explanation.) From: Marino PL: The ICU Book, Philadelphia, Lea & Febiger, 1991.

between pH and PCO_2, and are organized according to the change in pH. The normal ranges for acid-base parameters in arterial blood are as follows: pH = 7.36–7.44; PCO_2 = 36–44 mmHg; HCO_3 = 22–26 mEq/l.

If pH is LOW:

A. A low or normal PCO_2 indicates a primary metabolic acidosis (see Rules 1A and 1B).

The equation in Rule 2A ($PCO_2 = 1.5[HCO_3] + 8[\pm 2]$) is then used to to identify an associated respiratory disorder.

B. A high PCO_2 indicates a primary respiratory acidosis (see Rule 3).

The change in the pH/PCO_2 ratio is then used to determine the degree of compensation and to identify an associated metabolic disorder (see Rule 4).

If pH is HIGH:

A. A high or normal PCO_2 indicates a primary metabolic acidosis (see Rules 1A and 1B).

The equation ($PCO_2 = 0.7[HCO_3] + 20[\pm 1.5]$) in Rule 2B is then used to identify an associated respiratory disorder.

B. A low PCO_2 indicates a primary respiratory alkalosis (see Rule 3).

The pH/PCO_2 ratio is then used to determine the degree of compensation and to identify an associated metabolic disorder (see Rule 4B).

If pH is NORMAL:

A. A high PCO_2 indicates a mixed respiratory acidosis-metabolic alkalosis (see Rule 5).

B. A low PCO_2 indicates a mixed respiratory alkalosis-metabolic acidosis (see Rule 5).
C. A normal PCO_2 may indicate normal acid-base status but does not rule out combined metabolic acidosis-metabolic alkalosis. In this situation, the anion gap can prove to be valuable.

RESPIRATORY ACIDOSIS

Respiratory acidosis, defined as a ↑ PCO_2, results from alveolar hypoventilation. Physiologically, there will be either ↓ total minute ventilation V_E (e.g., narcotic overdose or neuromuscular weakness) or ↑ physiologic dead space (e.g., ↑ V_D/V_T ratio as in COPD) (Table 19–2). Distinguishing the underlying physiology becomes important when deciding upon diagnosis and treatment. To differentiate these 2 physiologic causes, the Arterial-alveolar (A-a) gradient can be calculated on room air ($FIO_2 = 0.21$) using the shortened alveolar gas equation:

$$PAO_2 = 150\text{-}PCO_2/0.8$$

$$\text{A-a gradient} = PAO_2\text{-}PaO_2$$

If the ↑ PCO_2 is from a ↓ minute ventilation, the A-a gradient will be normal. However, if it is from ventilation-perfusion abnormalities, the A-a gradient should be ↑.

RESPIRATORY ALKALOSIS

Respiratory alkalosis, defined as a ↓ PCO_2, occurs as a result of ↑ alveolar ventilation from hyperventilation (Table 19–3).

METABOLIC ACIDOSIS

Metabolic acidosis is defined as a primary ↓ in plasma bicarbonate and is caused either by the accumulation of fixed exogenous inorganic or

Table 19–2
Respiratory Acidosis

Central nervous system depression:
- Narcotics, sedatives, head trauma, CNS infections, CVAs, cerebral ischemia, obesity-hypoventilation syndrome

Spinal cord and peripheral nerve disease:
- Guillain-Barré syndrome, myasthenia gravis, botulism

Musculoskeletal disorders:
- Kyphoscoliosis, flail chest, bilateral phrenic nerve damage, polymyositis

Pleural disease:
- Massive pleural effusion, pneumothorax

Intrinsic lung disease:
- COPD, advanced ARDS, large pulmonary emboli, severe pneumonia, severe pulmonary edema, stage IV asthma

Table 19–3
Respiratory Alkalosis

Central nervous system disease or stimulants:
Anxiety (voluntary hyperventilation), fever, pain, third trimester pregnancy, salicylates, progesterone, sepsis, liver cirrhosis, brain trauma, infection, CVAs, tumors
Thoracic disease:
Small to moderate pleural effusion, pneumothorax
Intrinsic lung disease:
Interstitial fibrosis, pneumonia, mild pulmonary edema, stages I + II asthma

endogenous organic acids or loss of HCO_3^- buffer, as in diarrhea. Acidemia refers to a plasma pH that is ↓. Interpretation of a metabolic acidosis follows a straightforward algorithm (Fig. 19–3).

Anion Gap

First, decide whether there is a normal or ↑ anion gap (Fig. 19–4). The anion gap, calculated by ($Na^+ - [Cl^- + HCO_3^-]$), is normally 12 ± 4

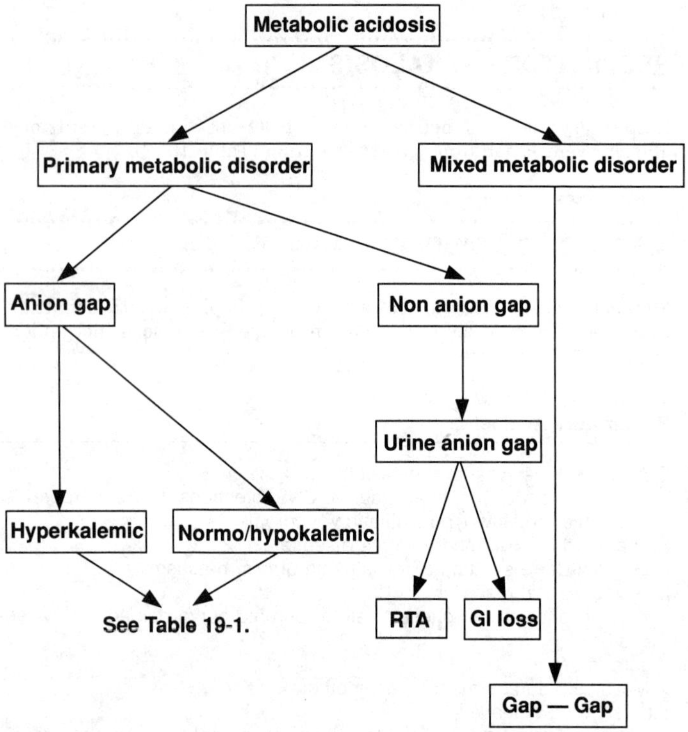

Figure 19–3. Diagnostic evaluation of metabolic acidosis.

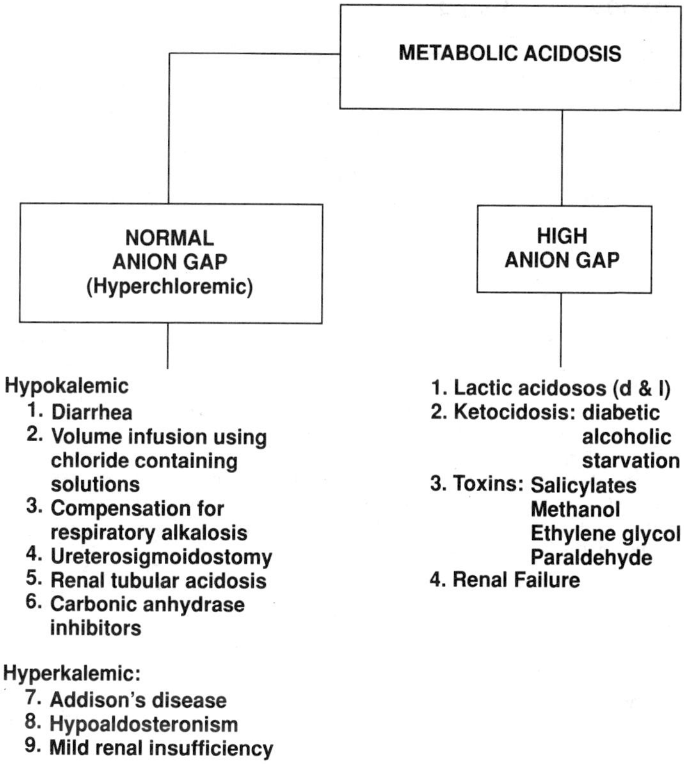

Figure 19–4. Classification of metabolic acidosis.

mEq (mmol)/l and is composed of negatively charged proteins (largely albumin), phosphate, sulfate, and other organic anions. When a fixed acid donates a proton (H^+) to the serum, the bicarbonate should ↓ 1 mEq/l for every 1 mEq/l of H^+ added. Therefore, the anion gap should ↑ by the same amount, and a ↑ in the anion gap almost always indicates acid accumulation. In contrast, if bicarbonate is lost in the urine or stool, the kidneys will hold on to chloride to compensate, thereby maintaining the total negative equivalency and keeping the calculated anion gap normal.

Recently, the sensitivity of the anion gap in stratifying metabolic acidoses has been questioned. The main problem is which value to choose as the upper limit of normal. Most laboratories currently use ion-selective electrodes to measure Na^+, K^+, and Cl^-. This technology frequently gives higher Cl^- levels and lower Na^+ levels than older photometric or colorimetric assays, yielding a consistently smaller normal anion gap. Using this new technology, the upper limit of normal for the anion gap is often ≤6 mmol/l and practically always ≤11 mmol/l. However, even when using 11 as the upper limit of normal, 29% of surgical ICU patients with elevated lactate levels were not identified. The anion gap was least sensitive for patients with mildly elevated lactate levels between 2.5 and 4.9 mmol/l.

Hypoalbuminemia

The serum albumin contributes about half (11 mEq/l out of a total of 23 mEq/l) of the total unmeasured anion pool. Assuming normal serum electrolytes, a 50% ↓ in serum albumin will reduce the calculated anion gap by 5–6 mEq/l; this should be added to the calculated number when deciding in which category to place the acidosis. Since hypoalbuminemia is very common in ICU patients, this correction should be kept in mind whenever the calculation is made, as this may help recategorize a previously unsuspected elevated anion gap acidosis.

Urinary Anion Gap

The next step in interpretation is to further subcategorize these 2 broad groups. Normal anion gap acidoses are subdivided into hypokalemic and hyperkalemic groups (Fig. 19–4). In patients with a normal anion gap and hypokalemic hyperchloremic acidosis, the urinary anion gap can help differentiate a renal tubular acidosis from GI bicarbonate loss (Fig. 19–4). The major unmeasured cation in the urine is ammonium, which is the excretable form of titratable acid. When urine acidification is deranged and the kidneys are unable to excrete acid, the urine anion gap becomes more positive. Measuring the urinary anion gap requires a spot urine for Na^+, K^+, Cl^-, and pH.

$$\text{Urinary Anion Gap: Total Anions} = \text{Total Cations}$$

$$UA + Cl^- = Na^+ + K^+ + UC$$

$$\text{Anion gap: } UA - UC = (Na^+ + K^+) - Cl^-$$

Urine anion gap	Urine pH	Diagnosis
Negative	<5.5	Normal
Positive	>5.5	RTA
Negative	>5.5	Diarrhea

Ratio of Anion Gap Excess to Decrease in Serum Bicarbonate

The final step in analysis is to look at the ratio of anion gap excess to the ↓ in serum bicarbonate, referred to as the "gap-gap" ratio (Fig. 19–5).

"Gap-gap ratio": AG Excess/HCO_3 Deficit = [AG – 12/24 – HCO_3].

This ratio has the following 3 uses

- To determine whether there is a mixed metabolic acidosis, which is a common occurrence in the ICU. When an organic acid such as lactic acid is added to blood, there will be an equal drop in HCO_3 for every mEq acid added to the anion gap, and the gap-gap ratio will remain 1. When there is a hyperchloremic acidosis from loss of HCO_3, the numerator remains low as the denominator ↑ and the ratio will approach zero. When there is a mixed metabolic acidosis, the ratio will fall to between 0 and 1
- To follow responses to treatment in diabetic ketoacidosis. Prior to treatment, when serum ketones are elevated and serum bicarbonate is low, the gap-gap ratio will be high. Once treatment has begun with fluids and insulin, the ketone level drops, but the serum HCO_3 may remain low because of the dilutional effect of IV fluids. Although this

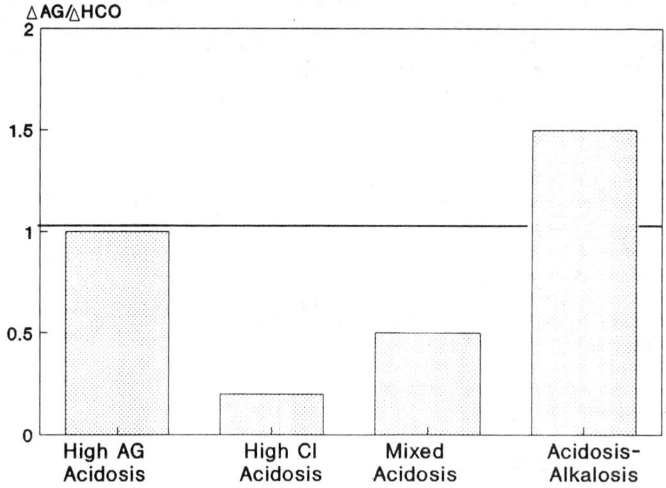

Figure 19–5. The gap–gap ratio.

low HCO_3 may be incorrectly interpreted as an inadequate response to treatment, the drop in gap-gap ratio actually indicates that the ketones are being cleared and that the acidosis is changing from a high gap acidosis to a low one

- To evaluate the presence of a mixed metabolic acidosis and alkalosis. In the presence of a high anion gap acidosis, adding alkali will make the gap-gap ratio >1

LACTIC ACIDOSIS

Lactic acidosis is a common cause of acute metabolic acidosis in critically ill patients and usually results from inadequate tissue oxygenation.

Lactate is produced within all cells in the body by the conversion of pyruvate to lactate, a reaction catalyzed by the enzyme LDH. Cellular levels of lactate are mainly determined by mitochondrial function; therefore, states of impaired mitochondrial function (such as cellular hypoxia) will cause cellular levels of lactate to ↑, which will then be added to the circulation. Hyperlactatemia is not synonymous with lactic acidosis. In situations such as beriberi or Reye's syndrome, lactate accumulation without an acidosis can occur (formerly referred to as Type B1 Lactic Acidosis). Although all cells except RBCs are capable of extracting lactate from the circulation, most is removed by the liver and kidneys and converted back to pyruvate via LDH for either gluconeogenesis or energy production. A normal liver is capable of increasing lactate clearance to 10 times the baseline.

Normal serum lactate levels are ≤2 mEq/l (normal arterial blood is <1.5 mmol/l, and normal venous blood is <2.0 mM/l). Increased production by the tissues and/or ↓ clearance of lactate by the liver will result in ↑ serum levels.

Cardiogenic shock and septic shock are common states in which the O_2 supply may be inadequate to meet the needs of the tissues. Although there may not be frank hypotension (a common criterion used to indicate systemic shock), elevated lactate levels with acidosis in these settings still imply shock at a cellular level. In any case of clinical shock, an elevated lactate level carries a poor prognosis.

When discussing inadequate O_2 supply-demand ratios, it is worthwhile to review the determinants of O_2 delivery ($\dot{D}O_2$):

$$\dot{D}O_2 = (\text{Cardiac output}) \times ([\text{Hb}][\text{saturation}][1.34] + [\text{Pa}O_2][0.003]).$$

Lack of adequate cardiac output resulting in a peripheral low flow state is the most important contributor to the development of lactic acidosis. Although hypoxemia (a low PaO_2) is commonly listed as a cause of lactic acidosis, patients with respiratory insufficiency have been shown to tolerate an arterial PO_2 as low as 22 mmHg without developing an acidosis.

Thiamine Deficiency

Thiamine causes ↑ lactates by reducing the mitochondrial oxidation of pyruvate. Pyruvate, instead of being converted to acetyl CoA, is diverted into the production of lactate. In patients with elevated lactate levels out of proportion with the degree of clinical hemodynamic instability, serum thiamine levels should be checked while empiric thiamine is given.

LACTIC ALKALOSIS

Severe alkalosis (pH >7.6) can cause ↑ lactate production by RBCs, probably by enhancing certain pH-dependent enzymes in the glycolytic pathway. In normal flow states, the liver is usually able to handle the ↑ lactate production. However, in low flow states where hepatic clearance is ↓, serum lactate levels may climb, particularly with exogenous alkali therapy.

Diagnosis

Intensivists should have a low threshold for obtaining serum lactate levels. Although the patient with a high anion gap acidosis in circulatory shock will clearly have an elevated lactate level, so might the patient with a relatively normal anion gap and only mildly lowered bicarbonate. There are no distinctive clinically significant features that suggest l-lactic acidosis, and levels elevated only slightly to 2.5 mmol/l already have a marked ↑ in mortality. In any patient suspected of having inadequate tissue O_2 supply, lactate levels are essential for diagnosis and management.

Arterial blood will reflect both production and clearance of lactate, whereas blood drawn from a peripheral vein will only reflect regional production. Excellent correlation has been shown between arterial blood and either superior vena cava or PA blood (mixed venous), and these sites can be used. The blood sample should either be placed immediately on ice or drawn into a vacuum tube containing a glycolytic inhibitor such as sodium fluoride to limit further lactate production by the RBCs.

KETOACIDOSIS

Ketoacidosis is characterized by the metabolism of free fatty acids by the liver with the generation of acetoacetate, β-hydroxybutyric acid, and acetone. In order for ketoacidosis to occur, there are 2 requirements. First, there must be ↑ delivery of free fatty acids from the peripheral adipose tissue to the liver, a process primarily induced by relative or absolute insulin deficiency. Next, the liver must channel these fatty acids into ketone bodies rather than through the normal pathway of triglyceride synthesis, a process apparently induced by a ↑ in the ratio of glucagon to insulin in portal blood.

There are 3 ketoacidoses

- *Diabetic ketoacidosis:* The result of either an absolute or relative insulinopenia. Concentrations of free fatty acids may reach 2–4 times that of a normal fasting state, which drives ketone production and results in a metabolic acidosis. Treatment of diabetic ketoacidosis consists of 2 simultaneous goals—the correction of the ketoacidosis by adequate exogenous insulin and the correction of fluid and electrolyte deficits
- *Alcoholic ketoacidosis:* Usually arises in alcoholics who abstain from alcohol ≥1 days prior to presentation and requires 3 simultaneous factors to occur. First, low caloric intake leads to ↓ liver glycogen stores and ↓ insulin. Next, dehydration ↓ renal clearance of ketone bodies. Finally, oxidation of ethanol impairs hepatic gluconeogenesis and ↑ the NADH:NAD ratio, which results in the conversion of acetoacetate to β-hydroxybutyrate. Alcoholic ketoacidosis usually resolves within 24 h with infusion of saline and glucose and does not require additional insulin
- *Starvation ketoacidosis:* Occurs from the mobilization of fatty acids from peripheral tissues and is usually mild. In prolonged fasting, serum insulin levels, although low, are present and are enough to prevent free fatty acid levels in plasma from continuing to ↑

Diagnosis

Diagnosis of a ketoacidosis is made by a positive nitroprusside test. This colorimetric reaction, in which either a nitroprusside tablet or stick turns purple, only measures serum acetoacetate at levels >3 mEq/l but not β-hydroxybutyric acid. Acetoacetate and β-hydroxybutyric acid exist in equilibrium with each other, with their interconversion catalyzed by the enzyme β-hydroxybutyrate dehydrogenase.

Acetoacetate + NADH + H^+ BHBDH β-Hydroxybutyrate + NAD^+

Tissue hypoxia can lead to ↓ availability of intracellular NADH. This will ↑ the ratio of NADH/NAD^+, which drives the above reaction to the right. Since the nitroprusside reaction does not occur with β-hydroxybutyrate, it is possible to have a severe ketoacidosis and hypoxia yet a negative or trace positive nitroprusside test.

TREATMENT

Should a Metabolic Acidosis be Treated?

Metabolic acidosis has established detrimental effects, especially on cardiovascular function. Myocardial dysfunction, a ↓ threshold for VF, direct arterial vasodilation, indirect sympathetic-mediated vasoconstriction, and direct venous vasoconstriction can occur in vivo. In addition, metabolic acidosis can cause marked ↑ in pulmonary vascular resistance resulting in ↑ right heart afterload. Finally, although mild acidosis causes tachycardia secondary to catecholamine release, as the acidosis worsens, bradycardia occurs. Despite all this, it is not clear if these are clinically applicable. Acidemia causes catecholamine release, and the vasodilation may counteract the drop in cardiac output. Additionally, patients with diabetic ketoacidosis can tolerate pH levels as low as 7.0 without cardiovascular compromise.

There are data that suggest that elevated blood lactate can have harmful negative inotropic effects independent of pH. Increased intracellular lactate suppresses the activity of glyceraldehyde 3-phosphate dehydrogenase, thereby inhibiting glycolysis and limiting myofibril ATP production.

Although avoiding the detrimental effects of a severe acidosis may be desirable, there is no clear consensus concerning when or how to treat. Any treatment decision must be made firmly in the context of what is causing the acidosis, whether the accumulation is of inorganic or organic acids and whether it is a primary process as with poisonings or a reflection of other pathology, as in lactic acidosis or ketoacidosis. Appearance of lactic acidosis in a critically ill patient usually indicates inadequate O_2 delivery to meet the metabolic O_2 demand of the tissues. Therefore, the focus of treatment should not be on exogenous bicarbonate replacement but on aggressive correction of $\dot{V}O_2/\dot{D}O_2$ imbalances.

Is Bicarbonate Beneficial?

A debate has raged for years over the use of sodium bicarbonate to correct lactic acidosis. Bicarbonate therapy can produce a number of harmful effects, including hyperosmolarity, hypercapnia, and aggravation of intracellular acidosis, hypotension, and ionized hypocalcemia. In hypoxic dogs, bicarbonate therapy has been shown to worsen lactic acidosis. Most importantly, the use of bicarbonate has never been shown to improve either hemodynamics in critically ill patients with lactic acidosis or their outcome.

When lactic acid is buffered by sodium bicarbonate, CO_2 is generated by the following process:

$$\text{Lactate}^{-}\text{H}^{+} + \text{NaHCO}_3 \rightarrow \text{Na}^{+}\text{lactate-} + \text{H}_2\text{O} + \text{CO}_2.$$

In shock situations where microvasculature circulation ↓ or in other settings where ventilation is fixed (e.g., the patient has been deliberately paralyzed), CO_2 will accumulate in the tissues, rapidly pass into cells, and cause an intracellular acidosis, with harmful effects. A clear example of this has been shown in cardiac arrest. Closed cardiac massage can, at most, generate 20–25% of normal cardiac output. Arterial blood drawn at this time will reveal a normal to low $PaCO_2$ (depending on the effectiveness of ventilation). Mixed venous blood drawn simultaneously will show a markedly elevated PCO_2, reflecting tissue respiratory acidosis. Exogenous bicarbonate is converted to CO_2 in the tissues, adds to venous acidosis and worsen the situation.

Other alkalinizing agents have been developed that do not cause this undesirable CO_2 production

- *Carbicarb:* (Table 19–4) Carbicarb, which consists of 1/3 M Na_2CO_3 and 1/3 M $NaHCO_3$ and has the same alkalinity as bicarbonate, has been found to raise blood pH without raising $PaCO_2$. Clinical experi-

Table 19–4
Alkali Solutions

	CARBICARB	$NaHCO_3$
Na^+	1,000	1,000 (mmol/L)
HCO_3	333	1,000
CO_3^{2-}	333	0
PCO_2	3	over 200 (mm Hg)
pH 25 C°	9.6	8.0
Osmolality	1,667	2,000 (mOsm/kg)

From: Sun JH, Filley GF, Hord K: Carbicarb: An effective substitute for $NaHCO_3$ for the treatment of acidosis. Surgery, *102*:835, 1987.

ence with carbicarb is limited at present, but the preliminary results are encouraging

- *Dichloroacetate:* Sodium dichloroacetate stimulates pyruvate dehydrogenase and diverts pyruvate away from lactate production toward mitochondrial oxygenation. Although DCA has been shown to ↓ serum lactate levels, this has not translated into improved clinical outcome

If bicarbonate is to be used, the standard recommendation is to keep the serum pH >7.2. To calculate the approximate amount to give, the space of distribution is approximately 0.5% of body weight, but this may be twice as large with severe acidosis. With a normal $PaCO_2$, a goal of a serum bicarbonate of 15 mEq/l should be sufficient.

$$HCO_3 \text{ deficit} = 0.5 \times \text{wt (kg)} \times (\text{desired } HCO_3 - \text{serum } HCO_3)$$

One half of the calculated deficit is given IV bolus and the rest is added to hyponatremic solution and run over 4–6 h. Periodic determinations of acid-base balance are necessary to titrate therapy.

The treatment for lactic acidosis resulting from cellular hypoxia is correction of the cellular hypoxia. There should be aggressive attempts to ↑ flow to the tissues, using invasive hemodynamic monitoring. The $\dot{V}O_2$, the $\dot{D}O_2$, and the extraction ratio are closely followed. A lower than normal extraction ratio in the setting of lactic acidosis implies that the peripheral tissues are unable to remove the required O_2 from the circulation, probably because of an endothelial defect. This is a poor sign. If the extraction ratio is normal or high with a ↓ $\dot{D}O_2$, the next step is to ↑ delivery. First, volume load with colloid or crystalloid and follow the above parameters. If the $\dot{D}O_2$ remains low despite volume loading, add inotropic agents. If possible, avoid using PRBCs because of concerns about increasing viscosity and sludging at the microvascular level.

The use of exogenous alkalinizing agents for a lactic acidosis is a temporizing measure and is doomed to failure unless the cause of the acidosis is resolved.

METABOLIC ALKALOSIS

Metabolic alkalosis is the most common acid-base disorder in hospitalized patients. The hallmark of a metabolic alkalosis is a serum bicarbonate that is > expected for the patient's PCO_2. While a drop of pH to

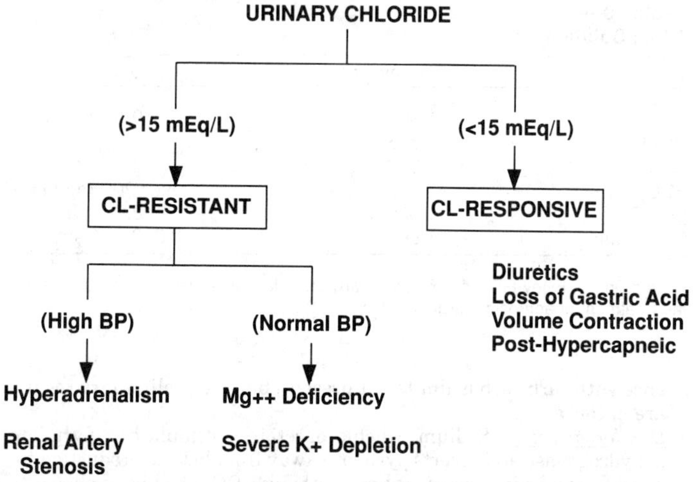

Figure 19–6. Classification of metabolic alkalosis.

7.0–7.2 may be tolerated by many patients without adverse effects, a pH >7.55 has an associated mortality of 40% in the critically ill. Overall, the most common causes of metabolic alkalosis in the ICU are loss of gastric juice protons and chloride through either NG suction or vomiting and renal retention of bicarbonate secondary to hypovolemia and chloride depletion.

Metabolic alkalosis can be categorized into 3 broad groups for both diagnosis and treatment strategies. Differentiating these 2 groups requires a spot urinary chloride (Fig. 19–6)

- *Chloride-responsive:* Urinary chloride <15 mEq/l. Chloride is the only nonbicarbonate anion that contributes to ECF volume. Therefore, in conditions such as the following, where chloride is depleted, the kidney holds on to bicarbonate as compensation to maintain the total anion equivalency.
    - (a) Gastric acid loss: Will cause depletion of both H^+ and Cl^- ions.
    - (b) Diuretics: Cause loss of K^+, Mg^{++}, and most importantly, Cl^-. By contributing to a ↑ in renal acid excretion, diuretics lead to a disproportionate loss of fluid rich in Cl^- and a transcellular shift of hydrogen ions. Some of this can be prevented by either using or adding K-sparing diuretics such as triamterene or spironolactone.
    - (c) Extracellular volume contraction
    - (d) Post hypercapneic
- *Chloride-resistant:* Urinary chloride >15 mEq/l. The chloride-resistant alkaloses are usually mild and hypervolemic, and treatment is directed toward the underlying disorder. These alkaloses are generated and maintained by the kidneys and result from either a chloride-reabsorptive defect (i.e., Bartter's syndrome) or from a hypermineralocorticoid state (i.e., Hyperaldosteronism, Cushing's syndrome)
- *Alkali administration:* Exogenous bicarbonate administration rarely causes a metabolic alkalosis, secondary to the kidneys' tremendous ability to excrete excess bicarbonate

Treatment

Most of the metabolic alkalosis encountered in the ICU, and practically all of the serious alkaloses (HCO_3 >40) belong in the hypovolemic chloride-responsive group. Therefore, initial treatment strategies first involve chloride replacement using either NaCl, KCl, HCl, or combinations of these 3

- <u>NaCl:</u> Patients who are volume depleted generally respond well to treatment with 0.9% NaCl. The chloride deficit is calculated by the following equation:

$$\text{Cl Deficit (mEq)} = 0.27 \times \text{Wt (kg)} \times (100 - \text{Present Cl})$$

 Since a liter of normal saline contains 154 mEq of Cl^-, the volume of NaCl needed is:

$$\text{Normal Saline Replacement (mEqs)} = \text{Cl Deficit}/154$$

- <u>KCl:</u> Because of the prohibitive amount of K^+ that would be needed, KCl alone is not adequate to provide adequate chloride replacement. If hypokalemia is present, however, it must be corrected, because hypokalemia will sustain the metabolic alkalosis even after the calculated Cl^- deficit has been replaced. Correction of hypokalemia has a crucial role in the treatment of metabolic alkalosis
- <u>HCl:</u> In severe alkalosis, dilute HCl may be necessary. HCl must be administered through a central line to avoid its sclerosing actions, glass bottles must be used, and the IV tubing must be changed frequently. The solution that is used is 0.1 N HCl, which contains 100 mEq H^+/l. To calculate the amount needed, the following equations are used:

$$H^+ \text{ Deficit (mEq)} = 0.5 \times \text{Wt (kg)} \times (\text{Present } HCO_3 - \text{Desired } HCO_3)$$

$$\text{Volume (l) of 0.1N HCl} = H^+ \text{ Deficit}/100$$

$$\text{Infusion Rate} = 0.2 \text{ mEq/kg/hr}$$

 Arginine HCl, lysine HCl, and NH_4Cl are solutions that were previously used but are no longer commercially available

 Drug therapy has a role when there is a chloride-responsive metabolic alkalosis in normovolemic or hypervolemic patients. Neither Diamox nor H_2 blockers will correct a preexisting alkalosis

- <u>*Acetazolamide:*</u> Diamox (250–1,000 mg/day in divided doses), a carbonic anhydrase inhibitor, blocks bicarbonate resorption in the proximal tubule and may be useful when extracellular volume is high. Unfortunately, Diamox may also cause additional K^+ and volume depletion, which as mentioned above, can perpetuate an alkalosis
- <u>*H_2 Blockers:*</u> Can be used to prevent H^+ loss with loss of gastric juice and may have a particular role in normovolemic chronic renal failure patients. It is important to first check the gastric secretions to identify the presence of acid. The treatment goal is to keep the pH >5. Because of concerns about gastric superinfection, aspiration, and translocation of bacteria through the gut, the use of H_2 blockers in the ICU should be avoided

A final option for a severe metabolic alkalosis in patients with renal failure is hemodialysis with a high-chloride, low-acetate bath. If the patient has a high-volume status, another alternative is to use CAVH with simultaneous IV chloride replacement.

Suggested Reading

Marino PL, Nierman D: Acid-base disorders. *In* Khan M Gabriel, Cardiac and Pulmonary Management. Philadelphia, Lea & Febiger, 1993.

Acute Respiratory Failure and Adult Respiratory Distress Syndrome

20

Amy O'Brien-Ladner and
Susan K. Pingleton

ACUTE RESPIRATORY FAILURE

Diagnosis

ARF is diagnosed by abnormalities in ABGs. Clinically, it can be obvious in a patient who is apneic secondary to drug overdose or head trauma; however, in other instances during early phases of respiratory failure, a high level of clinical suspicion is necessary in the diagnosis of ARF. Measuring arterial gas tensions (P_aO_2, P_aCO_2) and pH is most useful in evaluating the severity of respiratory dysfunction and failure. Two types of abnormalities are found when ABGs are evaluated

- Hypoxia is defined as $P_aO_2 < 50$ mm Hg on room air, or FiO_2 (0.21). The most common mechanisms by which reductions in P_aO_2 are produced include: Alveolar hypoventilation ($P_aCO_2 > 40$ mm Hg), ventilation-perfusion mismatching, and/or right-to-left intrapulmonary or intracardiac shunting of blood

Hypoxemia, which is caused primarily by hypoventilation, suggests that the lung is normal and that the only necessary therapeutic goal is to ↑ ventilation. This type of hypoxemia is characterized by normal alveolar-to-arterial difference ($P_AO_2 - P_aO_2$), which is determined using the alveolar gas equation. P_AO_2 is calculated by a simple equation

$$P_AO_2 = ([\text{barometric pressure} - \text{water vapor pressure}][FiO_2]) - (P_aCO_2/0.8)$$

$$770 \text{ mm Hg} = \text{barometric pressure at sea level}$$

$$47 \text{ mm Hg} = \text{water vapor pressure}$$

$$FiO_2 = O_2 \text{ concentration}$$

$$0.8 = \text{respiratory quotient}$$

$$P_AO_2 - P_aO_2 = (770 - 47)FiO_2 \frac{P_aCO_2}{0.8} - P_aO_2$$

P_aO_2 is determined from actual ABG samples. This value is subtracted from the calculation of P_AO_2 value. For example, on room air with a normal P_aO_2 of 90 mm Hg and P_aCO_2 of 40 mm Hg, the $P_AO_2 - P_aO_2$ difference can be determined by inserting the values.

$$= (770 - 47)0.21 - \left(90 + \frac{40}{0.8}\right)$$

$$= 10$$ (normal range 5–15, up to 20 at age 70) (see p. 349).

Another example of ARF secondary to hypoventilation is exemplified by: a P_aO_2 of 60 mm Hg and a P_aCO_2 of 70 mm Hg. Calculated P_AO_2 is 68 mm Hg; P_aO_2 gradient difference is 8 mm Hg, a normal value. In this instance of ARF, the normal A-a gradient suggests that the mechanism of hypoxia is hypoventilation and not abnormal lung structure. Hypoventilation can cause ↑ alveolar arterial O_2 gradients when severe.

ARF often occurs with an ↑ A-a gradient. For example, in a patient with pneumonia, a P_aO_2 of 55 mm Hg and a P_aCO_2 of 35 mm Hg would result in an A-a gradient >60 mm Hg, suggesting significant lung dysfunction. Mechanisms of hypoxemia with a widened P_AO_2-P_aO_2 gradient include ventilation-perfusion mismatch and shunting. Shunted blood is blood that traverses the capillary beds and never "sees" alveolar air. When hypoxemia resulting from ventilation-perfusion mismatch occurs, ventilation is inappropriate to the level of alveolar capillary perfusion or vice versa. The distinction between ventilation-perfusion mismatch and shunting can be made by measuring the response of the hypoxic patient to the administration of 100% O_2. Normal arterial oxygenation will ↑ to values of nearly 600 mm Hg if the hypoxemia is due purely to ventilation-perfusion mismatching. With shunt, however, arterial O_2 tension is markedly ↓ in relation to the magnitude of shunt flow. This is because shunted blood has no capacity to be oxygenated, despite high levels of inspired O_2 tension. Figure 20–1 shows the relationship between P_aO_2 and FiO_2 with different shunt fractions. Figure 20–2 demonstrates the effect of increasing amounts of mismatch of ventilation to perfusion on P_aO_2 with different FiO_2 values.

It is important to determine the mechanism of hypoxemia in ARF because the approach to treatment varies considerably depending on which mechanism has caused the hypoxemia. Small amounts of supplemental O_2 can ↑ the P_aO_2 with ventilation-perfusion mismatching. However, when shunting is the mechanism of hypoxemia, high levels of inspired O_2 and even mechanical ventilation are required

- Hypercapnia is defined as elevation of CO_2 tension, P_aCO_2 >50 mm Hg on room air. Hypercapnia is caused by alveolar hypoventilation. It can occur secondary to: ↑ in production of CO_2, ↓ in ventilation, and/or ↑ in wasted ventilation or dead space

Most commonly, hypercapnia results from ↓ ventilation caused by the lung, either from disease (e.g., COPD) or suppressed ventilatory drive. The calculation of dead space requires knowledge of the P_aCO_2 tension and the partial pressure of CO_2 in mixed expired air. Dead space is commonly expressed as a fraction of V_T; normal values for the V_D/V_T ratio are 0.3:0.35.

Acute hypercapnic respiratory failure can result in respiratory acidosis, which is characterized by a ↑ in P_aCO_2. The relationship between P_aCO_2 and plasma bicarbonate concentrations determines the arterial pH. However, the relationship between P_aCO_2 and arterial pH varies while the P_aCO_2 becomes elevated. The acuity or chronicity of CO_2 elevation can be inferred by examining the relationship between P_aCO_2, arterial pH, and serum HCO_3^-. Acute ↑ in P_aCO_2 are accompanied by small ↑ in bicarbonate, and arterial pH changes in a nearly linear fashion. For every 1 mm Hg change in P_aCO_2, there is approximately a 0.008 pH unit change in the opposite direction. For example, an acute ↑ in P_aCO_2 40–60 mm Hg would be expected to cause a ↓ in arterial pH to 7.25 (see Chap. 19).

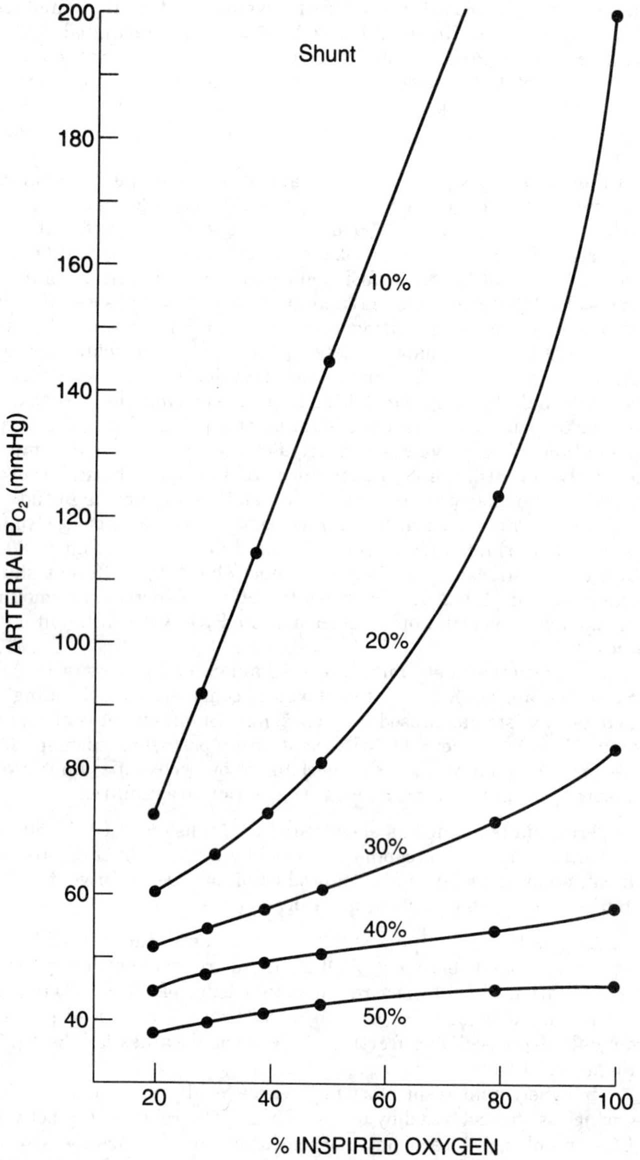

Figure 20–1. The relationship between inspired oxygen concentration and arterial PO_2 for lungs with varying degrees of shunt. The increase in PO_2 is small for lungs with large shunts. Reproduced with permission: Dantzker DR: Gas exchange in the adult respiratory distress syndrome. Clin Chest Med, *3*:57, 1982.

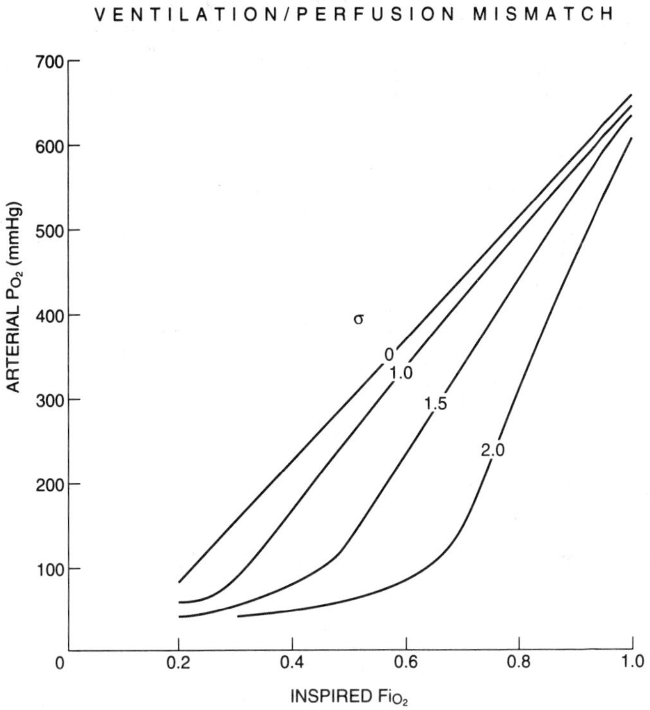

Figure 20–2. The relationship of P_aO_2 to FiO_2 with increasing amounts of ventilation to perfusion mismatching (0 = standard deviation of log normal distribution of ventilation and perfusion). Note that even with marked mismatching, the P_aO_2 increases to nearly normal values with a very high FiO_2. From: West JR: Pulmonary Pathophysiology: The Essentials. Baltimore, Williams & Wilkins, 1977.

Clinical Evaluation

- Clinical signs of hypoxia include confusion, restlessness, impaired coordination, coma, and death. Physiologic parameters suggesting hypoxia include tachycardia, hypertension, and tachypnea. During progressive hypoxemia, physiologic parameters may change to include bradycardia, hypotension, cardiac arrhythmias, vasoconstriction, and cyanosis. Cyanosis requires 5 g/dl of reduced Hb in the circulation
- Signs and symptoms of hypercapnia depend on the time during which the P_aCO_2 becomes elevated. When the P_aCO_2 ↑ rapidly, clinical symptoms include primarily CNS disturbances such as apprehension, confusion, sedation, and coma. Physiologic parameters during acute hypercarbia include vasodilation causing headache, engorged retinal vessels, encephalopathy, asterixis, and perspiration. Tachycardia and hypertension secondary to ↑ catecholamine levels may also be present. If CO_2 retention progresses over several days to weeks, the kidneys allow for compensation by the retention of bicarbonate. In this instance, even with P_aCO_2 >80, the clinical and physiologic parameters may be nonapparent or very mild and the patient usually maintains a near-normal pH

- The respiratory rate, although influenced by a number of factors, may serve as an indicator of the severity of respiratory distress and can be used to monitor response to therapy. Severely tachypneic patients will be able to speak only a few words at a time. Retraction of the sternum and the supraclavicular, supersternal, and intercostal spaces indicates a ↑ work of breathing. In COPD, these findings correlate with the severity of airway obstruction. In asthma, the ↓ in arterial systolic BP that occurs with inspiration (pulsus paradoxus) also correlates with the severity of airway obstruction
- Examination of the lung does not always provide specific information concerning the severity of respiratory dysfunction. The following is notable: In severe airway obstruction, airflow may be ↓ and inadequate to produce flow rates required for wheezing. Secondly, asymmetry of breath sounds is important in the evaluation of respiratory distress. The absence of sounds on 1 side may suggest pneumothorax, which is especially important to mechanically ventilated patients because of the greater likelihood of a tension pneumothorax

Categories of Acute Respiratory Failure

The treatment of ARF depends on the underlying mechanism causing respiratory failure.

ACUTE RESPIRATORY FAILURE WITH NORMAL LUNG FUNCTION

Hypoventilation, a ↓ amount of air entering the lungs and reaching the alveoli, is manifest by excess amounts of arterial CO_2, as reflected by an elevated P_aCO_2 tension in ABGs. In normal lungs, the ability to oxygenate blood is not as dependent on alveolar ventilation as on the removal of CO_2. Thus, hypoxia does not manifest itself unless the degree of hypoventilation is extreme. In this type of ARF, lung structure and function may be normal. What is abnormal is the function of the respiratory muscles, thoracic cage, or respiratory center, which is responsible for the respiratory drive. The causes of ARF in normal lungs would include

- Thoracic cage abnormalities such as flail chest or kyphoscoliosis
- Upper airway obstruction such as laryngeal edema or epiglottitis
- Diseases of the brain stem, cerebral vascular accident, trauma
- Respiratory center depression (narcotics or general anesthesia)
- Neurologic disease (polio, amyotrophic lateral sclerosis)
- Hypoventilation of obesity (Pickwickian Syndrome)
- Diseases of muscles (muscular dystrophy, polymyositis)
- Sleep apnea, sudden infant death syndrome, botulism, heavy metal intoxication, organic phosphate poisoning

Characteristically, patients who develop ARF because of neurologic compromise have a FVC <4–5 ml/kg body weight, a progressive inability to handle oral secretions, and a cough. An FVC of <1 l in this situation indicates the need for consideration of mechanical ventilation. This leaves the patient at risk for lobar atelectasis and pneumonia, which may result in hypoxia and elevated A-a gradient.

ACUTE RESPIRATORY FAILURE WITH ABNORMAL LUNG FUNCTION

ARF is most frequently caused by abnormal lung function. Two types of ARF occur: either hypoxemic and hypercapnic respiratory failure, or simple hypoxemic respiratory failure without aberrancy in CO_2 elimination.

Chronic Obstructive Pulmonary Disease. The primary diagnosis of patients with hypoxemic hypercapnic respiratory failure is usually COPD. High work loads placed on the respiratory muscles secondary to abnormal lung mechanics of the chronically obstructed airway cause early respiratory muscle fatigue. Since the primary gas exchange problem is hypoventilation (assuming pneumonia and/or pulmonary edema are not present), hypoxemia responds well to supplemental O_2 administration. However, because ventilatory drive in severe COPD may be dependent on a low O_2 level, increasing hypoventilation can occur with the removal of hypoxemia by aggressive supplemental O_2 use. Adequate oxygenation is a primary goal, and the concern of increasing hypercapnia should not inhibit the use of O_2, but careful observation of ABGs is necessary.

Conditions that can precipitate ARF in the patient with COPD are multiple

- Infection, either upper or lower airway (acute bronchitis, pneumonia)
- Cardiac arrhythmia
- CHF
- Pulmonary embolus
- Pneumothorax
- Pleural effusion
- Rib fracture
- Metabolic derangement such as hypophosphatemia, hypocalcemia, hypokalemia, and metabolic alkalosis
- Medicine noncompliance
- Medicine toxicity such as theophylline
- Sedative agents such as benzodiazepenes or barbiturates

Interventional considerations in the COPD patient with hypercapnic respiratory failure should include several modalities

- Management within a critical care or hospital unit with close observation
- Supplemental O_2 with a P_aO_2 goal of approximately 60 mm Hg
- Bronchodilators (β agonists, aerosolized anticholinergics, oral or IV aminophylline)
- IV steroids

As in all cases of ARF, consideration of intervention with general diagnostic tests and support is important

- Antibiotics for possible upper or lower respiratory infections
- Capacity for the institution of mechanical ventilation
- Analysis of electrolytes and blood count
- X-ray analysis to rule out pneumothorax or large pleural effusion
- ECG to rule out cardiac arrhythmias such as AF and multifocal atrial tachycardia
- Consideration of CHF and the use of diuretics for preload ↓ and vasodilators for afterload ↓

Asthma. The hallmark of respiratory failure in asthma is marked obstruction of airflow (see Chap. 16).

ACUTE RESPIRATORY FAILURE IN PATIENTS WITH HYPOXEMIA AND NORMOCAPNIA OR HYPOCAPNIA

The causes of ARF in patients with primarily hypoxic respiratory failure are those processes involving the pulmonary vascular bed, the lung interstition, or the alveoli of the lung. These disorders are primarily manifest by a ↓ in diffusion and not alveolar hypoventilation. Thus, hypercapnia is rarely found. However, any process involving the lung parenchyma, given enough time and severity, may result in ↑ P_aCO_2. Causes of ARF involving the parenchyma of the lung include

- Pneumonia (bacterial, viral, or fungal)
- ARDS or noncardiogenic pulmonary edema
- Cardiogenic pulmonary edema; interstitial lung diseases
- Autoimmune lung diseases (idiopathic pulmonary fibrosis, SLE, scleroderma, rheumatoid arthritis, Wegener's granulomatosis, Goodpasture's disease), pulmonary emboli

Diagnostic Tests

- The chest x ray will verify alveolar infiltrate in an area in which crackles were auscultated and may reveal a concomitant disorder—such as pleural effusion, pneumothorax, bilateral infiltrates, and/or atelectasis—that was not evident on physical examination. Entities evident radiographically that complicate the diagnosis and course of ARF include: Atelectasis, pneumothorax, nosocomial pneumonia, pleural effusion, and enlarging cardiac silhouette. The ECG may demonstrate P. pulmonale, right heart hypertrophy, and right axis. Ischemia or infarction in the setting of ARF has an ominous prognosis
- Pulmonary function studies may be helpful in early ARF, especially in the face of asthma or COPD. In this setting, spirometry may indicate ↓ FEV_1 and ↓ FVC. In patients with COPD, the comparison of baseline spirometry with that during an acute exacerbation can help determine the severity of the episode. In the setting of ARF with airway obstruction, the patient's ability to cooperate and, thus, the validity of pulmonary function studies is quite marginal. Serial measurement of the vital capacity is required in patients with normal lungs and pulmonary function impairment secondary to neuromuscular disease. Monitoring the patient's vital capacity serially is a sensitive indicator of the progression of ARF in these patients. A vital capacity of >1 l is considered adequate pulmonary function. If the patient's weakness progresses, such that the vital capacity is <1 l, ventilatory support should be strongly considered
- Bedside PA catheterization for measurement of PCWP helps distinguish cardiogenic pulmonary edema from noncardiogenic pulmonary edema or ARDS

Management

Supplemental oxygen. The patient's need for O_2 should not be underestimated. The decision to use mechanical ventilation with endotracheal intubation or an external O_2 delivery depends on 3 factors

- The amount of O_2 needed
- The level of patient cooperation
- The potential consequence of failure to provide O_2 if the external device is malpositioned

A variety of external O_2 delivery systems are available. Nasal prongs are the simplest and most comfortable. However, the FiO_2 provided cannot be quantitated reliably and humidification is poor. Open face masks or tents provide a high flow of well-humidified gas with a moderately reliable FiO_2 set by a Venturi device. Tight-fitting masks with a nonrebreathing valve and reservoir bag can be used to provide even higher concentrations of O_2, perhaps an FiO_2 of 0.7–0.8 for short periods. These masks can be quite uncomfortable and require a high level of patient cooperation. Another version of O_2 delivery involves the CPAP, in which a constant pressure is delivered throughout inspiration and expiration. The use of this device in ARF is unpredictable in patients who are experiencing airway obstruction and elevated P_aCO_2. Investigations now demonstrate some early success with CPAP during exacerbation of COPD. Mechanical ventilation delivered by face mask has been reported and is usually reserved for the patient with chronic respiratory failure in decline as an alternative to endotracheal intubation.

Ventilatory assist devices and mechanical ventilation. Indications for endotracheal intubation are difficult to define. Certainly, the level of hypoxemia and hypercapnia are taken into account. However, other objective criteria such as patient awareness, ability to cooperate, and level of fatigue, as well as course over a period of several hours may be as important in the decision to intubate. Regardless of the situation, intubation should be performed on a semi-elective basis rather than emergently; close patient monitoring is required to assess the effect of therapy in a patient course. Endotracheal tubes may be passed through the nose or the mouth. The mouth allows for a larger diameter tube, which is not as comfortable for the patient. Oral intubation requires more sedation, while the spontaneously ventilating awake patient may be nasally intubated.

Immediately after the tube is placed, either by direct laryngoscopy or blindly nasally, the lungs should be auscultated to determine if air is entering both lungs. Because of the anatomical advantage at the main carina, the endotracheal tube will often enter the right main stem bronchus. Position should be confirmed by chest x ray or bronchoscope. The tube should be secured by taping or another measure to avoid malposition and extubation. All endotracheal tubes should be fitted with a low pressure cuff to avoid tracheal mucosal injury. Overinflation of the cuff should be avoided, since this may cause pressure necrosis of adjacent tracheal mucosa.

There is no absolute time limit for endotracheal intubation beyond which tracheostomy is indicated. The institution of tracheostomy depends on the prognosis of the patient, previous failure to wean from mechanical ventilation, patient comfort, and rehabilitation. It is not unreasonable to consider tracheostomy after 14–21 days of mechanical ventilation.

Airway maintenance in the nonintubated and intubated patient with reactive airways generally requires aerosolized β agonists, anticholinergics, and possibly IV corticosteroids. In mechanically ventilated patients, the use of aerosolized bronchodilators is routine. Careful attention to suctioning of secretions is also a high priority in the mechanically ventilated patient. This is especially true during the period of weaning.

Infection is a common cause of ARF in patients with chronic lung disease. Cultures of sputum, blood, and urine should be routinely acquired. Careful identification of infection risks, especially factors leading to an immunocompromised state (e.g., diabetes, renal failure), must also be entertained and a broader spectrum of antibiotics used in this patient group. In the immunocompromised patient, bronchoscopy for acquisition of alveolar samples by bronchial alveolar lavage and PSB can be helpful in identifying causative agents of uncommon processes.

Nosocomial pneumonia is a common complication of patients treated in an ICU. The patient with mechanical ventilated needs is more susceptible. Unfortunately, current clinical parameters for diagnosis of pneumonia in the ICU are inadequate. Radiographic infiltrates, transient fevers, and elevated WBCs are not specific indicators of pneumonia in the ICU. Thus, different mechanisms for acquiring cultures have been developed. Bronchoscopy via an endotracheal tube is a low-risk procedure in the intubated patient. Samples from alveolar spaces can be taken via protective specimen brush in areas involved in infiltrates. Significant growth in culture of an agent suggests pneumonia; quantitative cultures are necessary if results are to be useful. These methods of diagnosing pneumonia in the ICU are necessary not only to adequately treat pneumonia but also to avoid the consequences of prolonged broad spectrum antibiotic use in the ICU. These consequences include infection with more virulent strains of bacteria as well as ↑ mortality (see Chap. 17).

Nutrition. It is generally accepted that the involvement of the gut in feeding is more advantageous than TPN in the ICU patient. Patients in ARF are often unable to maintain adequate caloric intake secondary to respiratory distress, anorexia, endotracheal intubation, and/or higher caloric needs. Nutritional needs should be defined, and adequate total calories, protein, carbohydrates, and fats should be prescribed. The goal of nutritional support in a patient with ARF is maintenance of total body mass and the avoidance of protein catabolism and lost muscle mass, especially regarding muscle strength.

Prophylaxis for gastrointestinal bleeding. The use of H_2 blockers and antacids has been routine in ICUs. The rationale has included the protection of the gastric mucosa during a period of nonfeeding and a subsequent ↓ in gastric stress ulceration and GI bleeding. This has come under some scrutiny in the last few years, and there is evidence that the use of antacids may be associated with ↑ nosocomial pneumonia due to gastric colonization with gram-negative bacilli. There is no clear evidence that H_2 blockade alone or sucralfate has been associated with a ↑ incidence of nosocomial pneumonia. Further studies with H_2 blockers are needed.

Open lung biopsy. The acquisition of lung tissue is indicated in the setting of ARF when x-ray infiltrates are present, but the etiology for the parenchymal process cannot be identified by nonsurgical techniques including BAL and transbronchial biopsy, cultures, VQ scans or associated systemic processes. Open lung biopsy can be obtained with relatively low risk and supplies invaluable information regarding the etiology and prognosis in ARF.

ADULT RESPIRATORY DISTRESS SYNDROME

ARDS, or noncardiogenic pulmonary edema, is a form of ARF occurring in a wide variety of medical, surgical, obstetric and gynecologic, and trauma patients. A complex inflammatory cascade follows a severe systemic or pulmonary injury and results in a constellation of findings, including severe hypoxemia, diffuse infiltrates on chest x ray, and ↓ respiratory compliance. Several diagnostic characteristics of ARDS can be identified

- Acute lung injury as evidenced by diffuse alveolar damage, including interstitial and alveolar edema and hyaline membranes

- The lack of elevated left heart filling pressures by PA catheter measurement, which documents noncardiogenic pulmonary edema
- Association with previously identified clinical disorders or inciting factors
- Association with progressive multiple organ systems dysfunction or failure

Lung Injury in ARDS

Murray and Matthay recommend evaluation of 4 parameters of lung injury to define ARDS: the chest x ray, the hypoxemia score, compliance, and the need for PEEP

- The chest x ray: Radiographically, ARDS can be a patchy process; however, it often progresses to include all 5 lobes of the lungs. Usually, the chest x ray in ARDS demonstrates a diffuse 5-lobe alveolar infiltrate. The chest x ray is also important in identifying potential reversible processes that may be remedied by simple therapy, including pleural effusions, cardiogenic pulmonary edema, and pneumothorax. The chest x ray also is important to monitor during a course of ARDS. Many complications of ARDS treatment with mechanical ventilation and associated high peak inspiratory pressures may be apparent by chest x ray: interstitial air, pneumothorax, pneumomediastinum, SQ emphysema. Other processes that occur with lung parenchyma after significant injury can also be reflected in the chest x ray: cavitation, consolidation, atelectasis, pneumatocele formation
- Hypoxemia score = P_aO_2/FiO_2: The hypoxemia score is defined as the ratio of arterial O_2 tension divided by the inspired O_2 concentration. It is a reflection of the severity of the disease process and, therefore, the difficulty in oxygenating the patient. The information gained from the P_AO_2-P_aO_2 difference equation is similar, in that it reflects the severity of gas exchange dysfunction; however, the hypoxemia score is simpler to calculate and does not take CO_2 into account. An example: a patient with P_aO_2 of 67 mm Hg on a ventilator delivering an FiO_2 of 0.6 has a P_aO_2/FiO_2 ratio of 112. A range of <100 (severe injury) to >300 (minimal to no injury) is observed
- Compliance: This is defined as the ratio of V_T delivered by the pressure required to deliver that volume. In a ventilated patient, it is calculated by dividing the V_T over the plateau airway pressure minus the PEEP. Compliance reflects the "flexibility" of the interstitium. Initially in ARDS, a compliance can be near normal, but with progression of disease, compliance decreases and the classic "stiff" lung results. The progression of a decline in compliance prognostically is an ominous factor. An example: A 65-kg patient is delivered a 750-ml V_T breath by mechanical ventilation. The pressure after the breath is delivered and airflow has stopped is 50 cm H_2O; PEEP is 5 cm H_2O. The compliance of this patient would be 750 ml/50 to 5 ml of H_2O = 17 ml/cm H_2O. Normal compliance is >40 ml/cm H_2O
- PEEP: PEEP is end expiratory pressure that is positive instead of the normal negative end expiratory pressure. PEEP is begun in patients requiring mechanical ventilation who have failed to oxygenate adequately with conventional ventilation. Thus, the addition of added pressure support at the end expiratory phase is made to recruit distal alveoli that have been lost secondary to collapse and/or filling with an inflammatory exudate. PEEP can be a very helpful modality in improving oxygenation; however, its association with pulmonary barotrauma such as pneumothorax can be a serious problem

Associated Disorders

ARDS is characteristically associated with a wide variety of clinical disorders that result in lung insult and subsequent acute lung injury. Unfortunately, the associated entities are often multiple, and the risk of ARDS ↑ with the number of clinical disorders that occur in each patient.

Despite the heterogeneity of associated clinical disorders, the time course from any insult to the development of ARDS is <24 h in most patients and often <12 h in patients with sepsis-related ARDS. The importance of the earliest hours of ARDS is the clarification and possible intervention of whichever mechanism is responsible for the development of the lung injury

- Sepsis is the most common disorder associated with the development of ARDS. It is difficult to establish the true incidence of sepsis in associated ARDS since there has been a lack of consensus on the definition of sepsis. In general, definitions now cover a range of disease severity
- Bacteremia indicates positive blood cultures for bacteria, pathogenic virus, fungi, Rickettsia, or mycobacteria
- Sepsis suggests clinical evidence of infection and signs of a systemic response to the infection such as tachypnea, tachycardia, and hyperthermia or hypothermia. Blood cultures demonstrating bacteremia are not required
- Sepsis syndrome includes parameters of sepsis plus evidence of altered organ perfusion. For example: P_aO_2/FiO_2 no higher than 280, lactate level at the upper limit of normal, oliguria, and altered mental status
- Early septic shock includes the above description plus hypotension (systolic BP <90 mm Hg) for <1 h, which responds to fluids or pharmacologic intervention
- Refractory septic shock includes hypotension for >1 h despite adequate volume and vasopressors (dopamine >6 μg/kg/min administered for 1 h)

Despite the presence of clinical sepsis, the site of infection is not always clear. In clinical sepsis, associated with ARDS, postmortem examination has shown that if the site of infection is unclear and the blood cultures are positive, the source is often the abdomen. If blood cultures are negative but septic physiology has been present, the source is most commonly the lung.

Infection is the most common cause of ARDS in nonsurvivors. Adequate antibiotic treatment does not favorably influence survival in this patient group. Overall, survival in ARDS associated with sepsis is estimated to be approximately 20–40%. Sepsis is also the most common cause of early and late deaths in patients with ARDS

- Aspiration of gastric contents is another important cause of ARDS. Prognosis depends on the degree of injury. In witnessed episodes of aspiration, prognosis is correlated with the O_2 requirements of the patient at 1 h
- Major trauma such as that secondary to motor vehicle accidents and crush injuries may develop ARDS on a multifactorial basis. Examples include lung contusion, hypotension, transfusion, sepsis, and fat emboli (long bone fractures)
- Overdose of various pharmacological agents is associated with ARDS. Common agents include aspirin, narcotics, tricyclic antidepressants, and barbiturates. Often, the exact disorders causing the ARDS is not clear because these patients may also be hypotensive, aspirate, and/or have direct lung injury caused by the ingested drug

- Cardiopulmonary bypass is another important clinical condition associated with acute lung injury and ARDS. This procedure, commonly used for CABS or open heart surgery, has the best prognosis of any entities associated with ARDS. The survival rate approaches 100%
- In contrast, ARDS associated with bone marrow transplantation or hepatic failure has an approximately 0% survival rate
- Early death in ARDS secondary to the respiratory tract occurs in approximately 10% of patients. Only 20% of patients surviving 1 week of ARDS will die secondary to respiratory failure. The clinical disorders associated with ARDS clearly affect survival and must be identified for a realistic assessment of prognosis and appropriate intervention

Pathophysiology

The pathologic features of the lung in ARDS derive from severe injury to the alveolar capillary unit. Because of the injury, the capillary "leaks" with extravasation of intravascular fluid into the alveolus, thus the term "permeability pulmonary edema." This process is at least partly responsible for the resultant hypoxia. The histologic appearance of this damage can be divided into 3 phases

- Exudative phase of edema and hemorrhage
- Proliferative phase of organization and repair
- Fibrotic phase of end-stage fibrosis

The source of injury to the alveolus may enter from its vascular bed, as in sepsis, and fat emboli or from within the lung, as in aspiration and pneumonia. It must be emphasized that the course and prognosis of ARDS depend on the mechanism by which it occurred.

The mediation of inflammation has recently been proposed to involve the circulating and tissue macrophages because of their ability to produce and release the newly described class of peptide mediators termed "cytokines." Because ARDS involves intense inflammation in the lung, no review of this is now possible without a brief discussion of cytokines, which refers to cell-derived peptide molecules that cause a target cell to alter ≥1 of its functional activities. Multiple cytokines have been implicated in the pathogenesis of ARDS, including the following

- TNF is produced by the alveolar macrophage and circulating monocyte. TNF can cause fever, neutrophil sequestration in the lung, and hemorrhage and edema of many organs, including the kidney, gut, and lung. Antibodies to TNF attenuate its effects during ARDS and sepsis in animal models
- IL-1 is a cytokine produced by the alveolar macrophage and circulating monocyte. It has many characteristics clinically similar to TNF. Injected into animal models, it can reproduce the septic physiology in end-organ changes

The most important modification of the ARDS concept in recent years is the recognition that there are significant extrapulmonary components to this syndrome. Dysfunction and failure of the renal, hepatic, cardiovascular, GI, and central nervous systems can also occur.

Systemic physiologic derangements occur in ARDS. For reasons that are not entirely clear, the uptake of O_2 at the cellular level depends on delivery of O_2 to tissues at nearly all levels of O_2 uptake in patients with ARDS. Normally, O_2 uptake is independent of O_2 delivery as long as a certain threshold is reached. Two basic changes in physiology allow for this derangement in O_2 delivery and uptake

- Altered blood flow distribution: Oxygenated blood bypasses nutrient capillary beds, often redistributing portions of the cardiac output to lower O_2 extraction tissues
- Endothelial and/or parenchymal cell injury: Edema with ↑ diffusion distances and/or ↓ in capillary surface area may account for the inability of O_2 to leave the circulation. When injured, the endothelium and other cells within the parenchyma are potent inflammatory mediators that may impair basic protective responses of normal physiology such as the maintenance of BPs or shunting of blood to vital organs

These may account for at least part of the multisystem injury in ARDS. In simple terms, the scenario may occur in 3 phases

- Initially, multisystemic interactions between neutrophils and endothelial cells occur. This results in microvascular injury and involves endothelium throughout the vascular bed. The lung has more dramatic consequences, because the intact permeability barrier is a unique prerequisite for respiratory "success." At this point, only clinical signs of ARDS may be present
- Secondly, recurrent or sustained injury, possibly by endotoxemia, is probably necessary for endothelial dysfunction to progress to extrapulmonary organ dysfunction
- In the terminal phase, overt multisystem failure occurs

It is recognized that the high likelihood of association of nonpulmonary organ failure and death in ARDS occurs after secondary multi-organ failure, and not necessarily respiratory failure. The incidence of organ involvement with ARDS has been estimated

- Renal: 40–55%
- Hepatic: 12–95%
- CNS: 7–30%
- GI: 7–30%
- Hematologic: 0–26%
- Cardiac: 0–23%

Prevention and Treatment of ARDS

As sepsis is the most common cause of ARDS, prevention tactics are geared toward blunting the inflammatory response. Unfortunately, although current strategies are promising, they are in the preliminary stages of therapeutic application

- Antiendotoxin therapy is aimed at removing or inactivating LPS. This toxic bacterial component of the gram-negative bacterial cell wall is a potent inducer of systemic cytokine release, including TNF and IL-1. Ziegler and associates demonstrated a significant advantage in the outcome of patients with gram-negative sepsis by using polyclonal antibody to the cell wall of J5 strain E. coli. Preliminary reports using monoclonal antiendotoxin antibodies have demonstrated ↓ mortality from the septic syndrome if overt shock had not developed by the time therapy was initiated. Unfortunately, antiendotoxin therapy would be effective only in gram-negative sepsis
- Anti-inflammatory is aimed at a variety of pathways throughout the immune cascade. Corticosteroid treatment in sepsis has been disappointing in that it has no benefit in prevention of ARDS or multisystem dysfunction. In fact, steroids may ↑ the mortality by increasing the incidence of serious secondary infections. Prostaglandin E1 has antiinflammatory properties, and initial reports in trauma patients demonstrated that it may improve survival in patients with ARDS.

However, follow-up reports now suggest no effect in the outcome of ARDS patients. NSAIDs such as ibuprofen may benefit hemodynamics and ventilation. However, the assessment of its role in attenuation of ARDS and multisystem dysfunction is incomplete

- Antibodies to various cytokines or their receptors are in early stages of investigation. Blocking or neutralizing the TNF response may have therapeutic potential. However, a brief half-life in the circulation may narrow the window of opportunity. The advantage of cytokine blockade is that it would be effective in both gram-positive and gram-negative sepsis. For example, levels of TNF are as high in patients with gram-positive sepsis as in those with gram-negative sepsis. However, the potential of dysfunctional inflammatory response is of concern and there are no clear data suggesting the routine use of anti-TNF antibodies
- Support efforts have improved the ARDS mortality rate of 95% when the entity was first described in 1967 to a current mortality rate of 40–60%. This is probably attributable to the improvement of ventilatory and hemodynamic support as well as the improvement of antibiotics and nutritional awareness

Mechanical Ventilation

A few points concerning the mechanical ventilation of patients with ARDS should be made. (See earlier discussion of ARF.)

- Of all forms of ARF, ARDS often requires mechanical ventilation because support with high tidal volumes re-expands atelectatic and partially fluid-filled alveoli. PEEP is especially helpful in recruiting alveoli for ventilation. This helps reduce the fraction of inspired O_2 required and may avoid O_2 toxicity
- One of the most difficult problems in managing patients with ARDS is determining the optimal level of PEEP. While PEEP is used to improve oxygenation and avoid toxic levels of O_2, it may also ↓ cardiac output and tissue-O_2 delivery. While evaluating the level of PEEP that improves oxygenation but does not compromise cardiac output significantly, the use of the PA catheter is quite helpful
- Data suggest that O_2 concentrations in the range of $\leq$50–60% are unlikely to contribute in a major way to progressive, acute lung injury. Thus, a reasonable goal is to adjust the level of PEEP to achieve an FiO_2 of around 60%
- Patients with ARDS may not tolerate the addition of PEEP secondary to the relative ↓ in preload that is caused by ↑ thoracic pressures. Volume expansion may improve the tolerance of PEEP
- Patients requiring mechanical ventilation and high levels of PEEP often require muscle paralysis. Paralysis alleviates added resistance to ventilation that may be manifest by muscle tone in the thoracic cage. If the patient is paralyzed, a sedative and/or anxiolytic agent must be used as well

Other modalities involving mechanical ventilation, such as inverse ratio ventilation, jet ventilation, and high-frequency ventilation, have been used in patients with ARDS with varying success. No modality has proven predictably superior to conventional ventilation with PEEP. Extracorporeal membrane oxygenation for patients with severe ARDS also has not improved mortality. Currently, several centers are experimenting with extracorporeal CO_2 removal, although the preliminary data is not promising.

Hemodynamic Monitoring

In the early phases of ARDS, hemodynamic monitoring of pulmonary vascular pressures may be helpful

- Measurement of PA wedge pressures can help confirm the cause of pulmonary edema as noncardiogenic
- It has been shown that some patients with primary acute lung injury have coexistent modest elevations of PA wedge pressures. The use of diuretics may be particularly helpful in these patients, although recently there has been some concern that patients who are at risk for multisystem dysfunction may actually benefit from full-volume expansion and even supernormal cardiac output. Because the patient with ARDS often has associated systemic hypotension, a PA catheter can be quite helpful in guiding IV fluid, transfusion, and plasma expander therapy

Nosocomial Pneumonia

- Diagnosis of nosocomial pneumonia in a ventilated ARDS patient with infiltrate is difficult. Clinical criteria of pneumonia (fever, leukocytosis, radiographic infiltrate, and purulent sputum) raise the clinical suspicion for pneumonia but are inadequate for a diagnosis in the clinical setting. Recently, quantitative culture of the lower airway by a protected specimen brush or BAL with or without bronchoscopy have been shown to be more sensitive and specific than routine tracheal aspirate cultures
- Therapy of nosocomial pneumonia requires identification of a potential pathology (usually gram-negative organism) and administration of appropriate antibiotics. Mortality is high in nosocomial pneumonia in ARDS, even with the appropriate antibiotics, suggesting that the basic disease process may be more important in ultimate outcome than choosing the right antibiotic. (See Chap. 17.)
- Efforts to avoid gastric and/or nasopharyngeal colonization have included aerosolized antibiotics and selective gut decontamination, as well as preformed antibody. However, these studies are in investigational stages and are not currently recommended
- The use of SQ heparin therapy in the ICU for prophylaxis against pulmonary emboli is generally accepted. The patient requiring mechanical ventilation of ARDS is often paralyzed. The opportunity for venous stasis in deeper thigh and pelvic veins with embolization to the PA is a concern
- Dopamine is particularly useful as an agent to ↑ renal bloodflow if the patient is at risk for multi-organ system dysfunction. However, dopamine may cause a mild ↑ in PCWP. For the patient who has difficulty oxygenating, an alternative is required. Dobutamine is the preferred agent, especially in the setting of lower-limit cardiac indices (see Chap. 4)

The course of ARDS can often be long and complicated, necessitating intense patient and family support. This dimension of patient care should not be lost in the confusion of the complicated therapy required for these patients.

Suggested Reading

Murray JF, Matthay MA, Luce JM, et al.: An expanded definition of the adult respiratory distress syndrome. Am Rev Respir Dis *138*: 720, 1988.

O'Brien-Ladner A, Pingleton SK: Acute respiratory failure and adult respiratory distress syndrome. *In* Khan M Gabriel, Cardiac and Pulmonary Management. Philadelphia, Lea & Febiger, 1993.
Pingleton SK, Harmon G: Nutritional management of acute respiratory failure. JAMA *257*: 3094, 1987.
Pingleton SK: Complications of acute respiratory failure: State of the art review. Am Rev Respir Dis *137*: 1463, 1987.
Bone RC: A new therapy for the adult respiratory distress syndrome. N Engl J Med *328*:431, 1993.

Pleural Diseases, Pleural Effusions

21

Richard W. Light

Anytime a patient with an abnormal chest x ray is evaluated, the possibility of a pleural effusion should be considered. Increased densities on the chest x ray are frequently attributed to parenchymal infiltrates, although they actually represent pleural fluid. The earliest radiologic sign of a pleural effusion is blunting of the posterior costophrenic sulcus on lateral x ray. If this angle is blunted, bilateral decubitus chest x rays should be obtained to ascertain whether free pleural fluid is present. The presence of pleural fluid can be documented by 1 of the following

- Bilateral decubitus x rays of the chest
- CT scan of the chest
- Ultrasonic examination of the chest

Physiology of Pleural Fluid Formation

Fluid can enter the pleural space from

- Capillaries in the parietal pleura
- Capillaries in the visceral pleura
- Interstitial spaces of the lung

Pleural fluid accumulates when the rate of fluid formation > the rate of fluid absorption. This situation can be caused by either a ↑ rate of formation or a ↓ rate of absorption. Rate of formation is normally 0.01 ml/kg/hr, whereas capacity for absorption is 0.20 ml/kg/hr

- Absorption is almost exclusively via the lymphatics in the parietal pleura
- Lymphatics in the visceral pleura do not communicate with the pleural space; little fluid exits the pleural space via capillaries

Fluid entry into the pleural space from the capillaries follows Starling's equation. The following factors ↑ the rate of pleural fluid formation from the capillaries

- Increased hydrostatic pressure in the capillaries in either the visceral or the parietal pleura
- Decreased pressure in the pleural space
- Decreased oncotic pressure in the blood
- Increased oncotic pressure in the pleural fluid

The rate of fluid entry into the pleural space from the interstitial spaces of the lungs ↑ when interstitial fluid is ↑; the lymphatics that normally drain the lung become disrupted, such as occurs with lung transplantation.

Symptoms of pleural effusion: Dyspnea on exertion; chest tightness; pleuritic chest pain. Signs of pleural effusion: Dullness to percussion absent tactile fremitus ↓ breath sounds.

APPROACH TO PATIENTS WITH PLEURAL EFFUSION

Pleural effusions can occur as complications of many different diseases (Table 21–1). The vigor with which various diagnoses are pursued depends on the likelihood that the individual has that particular disease. Rough estimates as to the incidence of the most common causes of pleural effusions are provided in Table 21–2.

When a patient has a pleural effusion that measures >10 mm on the decubitus x ray, a diagnostic thoracentesis usually should be performed. If the patient has obvious CHF, consideration can be given to postponing the thoracentesis until the CHF is treated. The characteristics of pleural fluid change little with diuresis over several days. If, however, such a patient is febrile or has pleuritic chest pain, or if the effusions are not of comparable size on both sides, a thoracentesis should be performed without delay.

Performing a Diagnostic Thoracentesis

This procedure is usually performed while the patient sits upright. A table should be available for the patient to rest his arms upon. The patient's back should remain relatively vertical, for if the patient leans forward too far, the lowest part of the hemithorax may move anteriorly and no fluid will remain posteriorly. Insert the needle posteriorly where the ribs are easily palpable and where the fluid gravitates. Make the first attempt 1 interspace below the level where the tactile fremitus is lost. Most unsuccessful thoracentesis procedures result from attempting to perform the thoracentesis at a level that is too low. Insertion of the needle at a low level is dangerous because the spleen or liver may be lacerated. Evaluate with ultrasound if fluid is not obtained after 2 or 3 attempts

- Thoroughly cleanse the skin over the site
- Anesthetize the skin with lidocaine using a short 25-gauge needle
- Anesthetize the periosteum of the underlying rib and the parietal pleura by performing the following steps with a 22-gauge needle 1.5 inches long. Move the needle up and over the rib with frequent injections of small amounts (about 0.1 ml) of lidocaine. Once superior to the rib, slowly advance the needle toward the pleural space, with aspiration followed by the injection of 0.1–0.2 ml lidocaine q 1–2 mm. Once pleural fluid is obtained through the anesthetizing needle, withdraw the needle
- Withdraw the fluid by using a second 22-gauge needle attached to a 50- to 60-ml syringe that contains 0.5–1.0 ml heparin. Slowly insert the needle along the same tract with constant aspiration until pleural fluid is obtained. Continue aspiration until the syringe is filled
- Withdraw the needle

If >60 ml of pleural fluid is to be removed, a plastic catheter rather than a sharp needle should be utilized. Complications of thoracentesis include: Pneumothorax, which occurs in 10% of patients (20% of these patients require a chest tube); infection of the pleural space; hemothorax from laceration of an intercostal artery or vein, the spleen, or the liver; seeding of the needle tract with tumor cells; vasovagal reaction with bradycardia and hypotension.

Table 21–1
Differential Diagnosis of Pleural Effusions

I. TRANSUDATIVE PLEURAL EFFUSIONS
   A. Congestive heart failure
   B. Cirrhosis
   C. Peritoneal dialysis
   D. Nephrotic syndrome
   E. Superior vena cava obstruction
   F. Fontan procedure
   G. Urinothorax
   H. Myxedema
   I. Pulmonary emboli

II. EXUDATIVE PLEURAL EFFUSIONS
   A. Neoplastic diseases
      1. Metastatic disease
      2. Mesothelioma
   B. Infectious diseases
      1. Bacterial infections
      2. Tuberculosis
      3. Fungal infections
      4. Viral infections
      5. Parasitic infections
   C. Pulmonary embolization
   D. Gastrointestinal diseases
      1. Acute pancreatitis
      2. Chronic pancreatic pleural effusion
      3. Esophageal perforation
      4. Intra-abdominal abscesses
      5. Diaphragmatic hernia
      6. Postabdominal surgery
      7. Endoscopic variceal sclerotherapy
   E. Collagen vascular diseases
      1. Rheumatoid pleuritis
      2. Lupus erythematosus
      3. Churg-Strauss syndrome
      4. Familial mediterranean fever
      5. Immunoblastic lymphadenopathy
   F. Drug-induced pleural disease
      1. Nitrofurantoin
      2. Dantrolene
      3. Methysergide
      4. Bromocriptine
      5. Procarbazine
      6. Amiodarone
   G. Asbestos exposure
   H. Postcardiac injury syndrome
   I. Pericardial disease
   J. Postcoronary artery bypass surgery
   K. Uremia
   L. Yellow nail syndrome
   M. Sarcoidosis
   N. Trapped lung
   O. Meigs' syndrome

Table 21–2
Approximate Annual Incidence of Various Types of Pleural Effusions in the United States

CAUSES	INCIDENCE (REPORTED CASES)
Congestive heart failure	500,000
Pneumonia (Bacterial)	300,000
Malignant disease	200,000
Lung	60,000
Breast	50,000
Lymphoma	40,000
Other	50,000
Pulmonary embolization	150,000
Viral disease	100,000
Cirrhosis with ascites	50,000
Gastrointestinal disease	25,000
Collagen vascular disease	6,000
Asbestos exposure	2,000
Mesothelioma	1,500
Tuberculosis	1,000

Separating Transudative from Exudative Pleural Effusions

The first question to be answered with a diagnostic thoracentesis is whether the patient has a transudative or an exudative pleural effusion. An exudative effusion results from disease of the pleural surfaces; a transudative effusion results from alterations in the systemic factors that influence the formation and reabsorption of pleural fluid.

This differentiation can be made by simultaneous analysis of the protein and LDH levels in the pleural fluid and in the serum. Exudative pleural effusions meet ≥1 of the following criteria, whereas transudative pleural effusions meet none

- Ratio of pleural fluid to serum protein >0.5
- Ratio of pleural fluid to serum LDH >0.6
- Absolute level of pleural fluid LDH >2/3 upper normal limit for serum

If none of the above criteria is met, the patient has a transudative pleural effusion, and the pleura itself can be ignored while the CHF, cirrhosis, or nephrosis is treated. Remember, however, that transudative pleural effusion can result from pulmonary embolization.

If a transudative pleural effusion is probable, the most cost-effective use of the laboratory is initially to measure only the pleural fluid protein and LDH levels. Other diagnostic tests, such as cytology, cell count, and differential, amylase, glucose, and cultures, are obtained only if the patient is proved to have an exudative pleural effusion.

TRANSUDATIVE PLEURAL EFFUSIONS

CHF is the disease most responsible for pleural effusions. The accumulation of pleural fluid in patients with CHF appears to be related more to LV than to RV failure. LV failure leads to ↑ interstitial fluid, which then traverses the visceral pleura to enter the pleural space. In animal experiments, approximately 25% of pulmonary edema fluid moves directly from the lung into the pleural space. Patients with pleural effusions secondary to CHF usually have other signs and symptoms (see Chap. 5).

Hepatic hydrothorax. Pleural effusions sometimes develop in patients with cirrhosis, particularly if ascites is present. The incidence of pleural effusion is approximately 6% in patients with cirrhosis and ascites, but is <1% in patients with cirrhosis with hypoalbuminemia but without ascites. The predominant mechanism is the movement of the ascitic fluid directly from the peritoneal cavity through the diaphragm into the pleural space. Small pores in diaphragm have been demonstrated.

The pleural effusion with hepatic hydrothorax tends to be large because of the large reservoir of fluid in the peritoneal cavity that can flow directly into the pleural space with its lower pressure. Usually tense ascites is present, but occasionally the ascites is subclinical. A large effusion may produce severe dyspnea. The pleural effusions are usually right sided (67%), but may be left sided (16%) or bilateral (17%).

In a patient with cirrhosis, tense ascites, and a pleural effusion, the diagnosis is easy

- Both a paracentesis and a thoracentesis should be performed to ascertain that both fluids are transudates. The pleural fluid protein level, although usually slightly higher than the ascitic fluid protein level, is still <3.0 g/dl
- Patients with hepatic hydrothoraces are prone to develop bacterial infections of the pleural space
- Primary treatment is geared toward treatment of the ascites because the hydrothorax is an extension of the peritoneal fluid. A low-salt diet is recommended and diuretics should be administered judiciously. Serial therapeutic thoracenteses are not indicated because the pleural fluid rapidly reaccumulates and the thoracenteses deplete the patient of body protein

If the pleural effusion persists despite optimal therapy directed toward the ascites, 3 therapeutic options, none of which is ideal, are available

- Tube thoracostomy followed by the injection of a sclerosing agent; however, electrolyte depletion can lead to death
- Implantation of a peritoneal-to-venous shunt; however, these shunts frequently do not control the effusion
- Thoracotomy with surgical repair of the diaphragmatic leak; however, thoracotomy is a major surgical procedure

Peritoneal dialysis. Large pleural effusions occasionally complicate peritoneal dialysis

- Dialysate appears to move directly through the diaphragm
- Incidence is 10% in those on continuous ambulatory peritoneal dialysis
- The effusion is almost always on the right side
- The pleural fluid has biochemical characteristics between those of the dialysate and of the serum
- Treat with chemical pleurodesis combined with a short period of small-volume, intermittent peritoneal dialysis

Nephrotic syndrome. Pleural effusion occurs in approximately 20% of patients with nephrotic syndrome

- Effusions are usually bilateral transudates because of the low oncotic pressure in the serum

- Pulmonary embolus must be ruled out in this situation because emboli are common in patients with nephrotic syndrome
- Primary treatment is aimed at treating the nephrotic syndrome, but chemical pleurodesis occasionally may be performed

Superior vena caval syndrome. Pleural effusions are not present in most patients with superior vena caval obstruction. Pleural effusions do occur in neonates with superior vena caval thrombosis, however.

Fontan procedure. This procedure is used to treat infants and children with hypoplastic right ventricles. The right ventricle is bypassed with an anastomosis between the superior vena cava, the right atrium, or the inferior vena cava and the PA. Almost all patients develop postoperative bilateral pleural effusions, which are frequently large and clinically significant. With refractory effusions, consider chemical pleurodesis or a pleuroperitoneal shunt.

Urinothorax. Pleural fluid can accumulate in the presence of retroperitoneal urinary leakage secondary to urinary obstruction, trauma, or retroperitoneal inflammatory or malignant processes

- Effusion develops within hours of the precipitating event
- Pleural fluid looks and smells like urine
- Diagnosis is confirmed by demonstrating a higher creatinine level in the pleural fluid than in the serum
- Effusion resolves once urinary tract obstruction is relieved

Myxedema. Pleural effusions occasionally occur as a complication of myxedema: Incidence is probably <5%. Pleural fluid may have biochemical characteristics of either a transudate or an exudate.

Miscellaneous causes of transudative pleural effusions. About 20% of the pleural effusions secondary to pulmonary embolism are transudative. Although pleural effusions secondary to Meigs' syndrome and sarcoidosis have been described as transudative, this is probably not the case.

EXUDATIVE PLEURAL EFFUSIONS

Pneumonia, malignant disorders, and pulmonary embolization account for most exudative pleural effusions (see Table 21–2).

Tests on Pleural Fluid

The following tests should be performed on the pleural fluid from a patient with an exudative pleural effusion of unknown origin: Glucose level, amylase level, LDH level, differential cell count, microbiologic studies, and cytology. In selected patients, other tests on the pleural fluid, such as the pH, ANA level, ADA level, rheumatoid factor level, and lipid analysis, may be of value.

Appearance. The gross appearance of the pleural fluid should always be described and its odor noted

- Bloody fluid: Obtain hematocrit. If hematocrit is >50% that of peripheral blood, hemothorax is present and tube thoracostomy should be considered
- Cloudy fluid: Centrifuge fluid. If supernatant is clear, the initial cloud-

iness was caused by cells or debris. If supernatant is cloudy, the initial cloudiness was caused by high lipid levels and the patient has chylothorax or pseudochylothorax

- Putrid odor indicates bacterial infection (probably anaerobic) of the pleural space
- Urine-like odor strongly suggests urinothorax

Glucose. Measurements of the pleural fluid glucose level are indicated, because a ↓ level (<60 mg/dl [3.4 mmol/l]) narrows the diagnostic possibilities to the following 7 conditions: Parapneumonic effusion, malignant effusion, tuberculous effusion, rheumatoid effusion, hemothorax, Churg-Strauss syndrome, and paragonimiasis.

Amylase. Measurement of the pleural fluid amylase level is indicated because a ↑ level (above the upper normal limit of serum) indicates that the patient has 1 of the following 3 diseases: Esophageal perforation (important to establish diagnosis early because mortality is high if not properly treated), pancreatic disease (patients with chronic pancreatic pleural effusions often appear to have cancer), or pleural malignancy (salivary-type amylase in this situation).

LDH. The pleural fluid LDH level is not used in the differential diagnosis of exudative pleural effusion. Nevertheless, a pleural fluid LDH level should be measured every time a diagnostic thoracentesis is performed because it is a good indicator of the degree of inflammation in the pleural space. Increasing levels with serial thoracenteses indicate that the degree of inflammation is worsening and that the diagnosis should be pursued more aggressively.

White blood cell count and differential. The absolute pleural fluid white blood cell count has limited utility

- Counts >10,000/mm^3 are most common with parapneumonic effusions, but are also seen with pancreatitis, pulmonary embolism, collagen vascular disease, malignant disorders, and tuberculosis
- The differential cell count on the pleural fluid is of more utility than is the absolute cell count
- Presence of predominantly polymorphonuclear leukocytes indicates an acute disease process, such as pneumonia, pulmonary embolization, pancreatitis, intra-abdominal abscess, or early tuberculosis
- Presence of predominantly mononuclear cells indicates a chronic disease process, such as malignant disease, tuberculosis, or a resolving acute process
- Presence of predominantly small lymphocytes indicates that the patient probably has tuberculosis or a malignant disease
- Presence of >10% eosinophils usually indicates that the patient has had either blood or air in the pleural space. If neither air nor blood is present in the pleural space, several unusual diagnoses should be considered: Benign asbestos pleural effusions, pleural effusions caused by drug reactions, paragonimiasis, or the Churg-Strauss syndrome. Diagnosis is never determined for approximately 20% of exudative pleural effusions, and, interestingly, pleural fluid eosinophilia is found in approximately 40% of these effusions
- The presence of >5% mesothelial cells in the pleural fluid basically rules out a diagnosis of pleural tuberculosis

Cytology. Pleural fluid cytology is useful in establishing the diagnosis of malignant pleural effusion

- Cytologic results are positive in 40–90% of malignant pleural effusions and depend on the type of tumor (difficult with lymphomas), the amount of fluid submitted (more fluid, higher yield), and the skill of the cytologist

- Immunohistochemical tests using monoclonal antibodies are complementary to cytology
- Flow cytometry can demonstrate abnormal numbers of chromosomes in approximately 2/3 of patients with malignant pleural effusions. The number of chromosomes is normal in benign cells
- Diagnosis of malignancy can be facilitated via electron microscopy

Culture and bacteriologic stains. The following pleural fluid cultures should be obtained on patients with undiagnosed exudative pleural effusions: Aerobic and anaerobic bacterial cultures plus a Gram's stain; mycobacterial cultures; fungal cultures and fungi.

pH. The pleural fluid pH is most useful in determining whether chest tubes should be inserted in patients with parapneumonic effusions

- If the pleural fluid pH is <7.00, tube thoracostomy should be instituted
- If the pleural fluid pH is >7.20, the patient probably does not require tube thoracostomy

The ↓ of pleural fluid pH to <7.20 can occur with 9 other conditions

- Systemic acidosis (pleural fluid pH approximates blood pH normally)
- Esophageal rupture (caused by concurrent infection)
- Rheumatoid pleuritis
- Tuberculous pleuritis
- Malignant pleural disease (if tumor burden is large)
- Hemothorax
- Paragonimiasis
- The Churg-Strauss syndrome (the patient also has asthma)
- Urinothorax (protein and LDH levels may be low)

When the pleural fluid pH is used as a diagnostic test, the pleural fluid must be measured with the same care as arterial pH

- The fluid should be collected anaerobically in a heparinized syringe
- The fluid should be placed in ice between collection and analysis
- The analysis should be performed with a blood gas machine

Immunologic studies. Patients with SLE or rheumatoid arthritis may have a pleural effusion during the course of their disease

- The best screening test for lupus pleuritis is the pleural fluid ANA titer. With lupus pleuritis, the pleural fluid ANA titer is ≥1:160 or ≥ the serum titer. The test is both sensitive and specific
- Only patients with rheumatoid pleuritis have a pleural fluid rheumatoid factor titer ≥1:320 or ≥ the serum titer

Other diagnostic tests. Several other tests are useful at times in the differential diagnosis of pleural effusions

- Pleural fluid ADA levels: Levels >70 U/l are virtually diagnostic of tuberculous pleuritis, whereas levels <40 U/l virtually rule out this diagnosis
- Pleural fluid lipid analysis: A pleural fluid triglyceride level >110 mg/dl is diagnostic of chylothorax. With pseudochylothorax, the pleural fluid cholesterol level is elevated
- Perform lipoprotein analysis of the pleural fluid in confusing cases. The demonstration of chylomicrons in the pleural fluid establishes the diagnosis of chylothorax
- Measurements that have not been unequivocally demonstrated to be of value in the differential diagnosis of pleural effusions are

carcinoembryonic antigen, hyaluronic acid, lysozyme, alkaline and acid phosphatase

Invasive Tests for Undiagnosed Exudative Effusions

In most patients, the cause of the pleural effusion is apparent after the initial clinical assessment and a diagnostic thoracentesis. If the diagnosis is not apparent, the following invasive tests might be considered: Needle biopsy of the pleura, pleuroscopy, bronchoscopy, and open biopsy of the pleura. Because pulmonary embolism is 1 of the leading causes of pleural effusion, this diagnosis should be considered in all patients with an undiagnosed pleural effusion (see Chap. 22). A diagnosis is never established for approximately 20% of the exudative pleural effusions that resolve spontaneously leaving no residua. Three factors should influence the vigor with which one pursues the diagnosis in patients with undiagnosed exudative effusions

- The symptoms and clinical course of the patient: If the symptoms are minimal or improving, a less aggressive approach is indicated
- The trend of the pleural fluid LDH level: If the pleural fluid LDH tends to ↑ with serial thoracenteses, a more aggressive approach is indicated because the process is getting worse
- The attitude of the patient: If the patient is desperate to know why a pleural effusion has developed, an aggressive approach should be taken

Needle biopsy. With special needles, small specimens of the parietal pleura can be obtained relatively noninvasively

- Useful mainly to establish the diagnosis of malignant or tuberculous pleural effusion
- The initial biopsy is positive for granulomas in 50–80% of patients with pleural tuberculosis. The demonstration of granulomas on the pleural biopsy is virtually diagnostic of tuberculous pleuritis. Culture of a portion of the pleural biopsy specimen for mycobacteria ↑ the diagnostic yield
- The initial biopsy is positive in about 40% of patients with malignant pleural disease
- Overall, the yield from pleural fluid cytology is higher than that obtained by needle biopsy
- When malignant disease is strongly suspected, pleural biopsy should be performed only if initial cytology is nondiagnostic

Pleuroscopy. With this procedure, also called thoracoscopy, a rigid scope or a fiberoptic scope is introduced through the chest wall into the pleural space after a pneumothorax has been induced on the side of the pleural effusion

- Excellent results are obtained when the procedure is done by experienced personnel
- In this country, only a few physicians are well trained in pleuroscopy
- This procedure is nearly as invasive as open pleural biopsy
- Diagnoses of benign disease are rarely made
- The open biopsy procedure is generally preferable unless personnel experienced in pleuroscopy are available

Bronchoscopy. The procedure is recommended for undiagnosed pleural effusions in the following situations

- Parenchymal infiltrate is apparent on chest x ray or CT scan

- Presence of hemoptysis
- Diagnostic yield should exceed 70% in these 2 situations

Open biopsy. Thoracotomy with direct biopsy of the pleura is the most invasive procedure used to diagnose pleural effusion

- Open biopsy provides the best visualization of the pleura and the best biopsy specimens
- The procedure does not provide a definitive diagnosis in a substantial percentage of patients
- Open biopsy should be done in conjunction with pleural abrasion to prevent recurrence

MALIGNANT PLEURAL EFFUSIONS

The annual incidence of malignant pleural effusions is approximately 200,000 in the United States. The 3 tumors that cause approximately 75% of all malignant pleural effusions are lung carcinoma (30%), breast carcinoma (25%), and tumors of the lymphoma group (20%). The initial step in the development of pleural metastases is the embolization of the tumor to the lung and/or visceral pleura: Parietal pleura is involved via secondary seeding from the visceral pleura or the pleural fluid. Direct mechanisms include the following

- Pleural metastases can ↑ the permeability of the pleural surfaces so more fluid is formed
- Lymphatic involvement can lead to ↓ pleural fluid clearance
- The thoracic duct can be interrupted, thereby leading to a chylothorax
- Bronchial obstruction can lead to markedly ↓ pleural pressure and a pleural effusion
- Pericardial involvement with a malignant tumor is frequently associated with the accumulation of pleural fluid

Indirect mechanisms

- Hypoproteinemia can ↓ the serum oncotic pressure and lead to pleural effusion
- Patients with a malignant disorder have a higher incidence of pulmonary embolism, which may cause a pleural effusion
- The postobstructive pneumonia secondary to bronchogenic carcinoma may cause a parapneumonic effusion
- The therapy for the tumor (radiation or chemotherapy) may itself cause the effusion

The most common symptom reported by patients with malignant pleural effusions is dyspnea, which occurs in about 50% of patients

- Only about 25% of patients with malignant pleural effusions have chest pain. The pain is usually dull and aching rather than pleuritic in nature
- Symptoms attributable to the tumor itself are frequent, e.g., weight loss in 32%, malaise in 21%, and anorexia in 14%
- The pleural fluid is an exudate
- The ratio of pleural fluid to serum protein level is <0.5 in about 20% of patients with pleural malignancy, but the LDH ratio is >0.60, or the absolute pleural fluid LDH meets exudative criteria in this 20%
- The fluid may be serous or bloody
- The predominant cells can be lymphocytes, other mononuclear cells, or polymorphonuclear leukocytes

- Pleural fluid eosinophilia is uncommon
- The pleural fluid glucose level is reduced to <60 mg/dl in 15–20% of malignant pleural effusions, thereby indicating that the patient has a high tumor burden. Mean survival is <2 months. (The pleural fluid pH is also reduced in most patients with a low glucose malignant pleural effusion)

The diagnosis of a malignant pleural effusion is established by demonstrating malignant cells in the pleural fluid or in the pleura itself

- Diagnosis is most commonly established with pleural fluid cytology, which is positive in approximately 60% of patients
- Needle biopsy of pleura is positive in 40% of patients
- Immunohistochemical tests using monoclonal antibodies directed against various antigens are useful in differentiating malignant from benign pleural effusions and adenocarcinomas from mesotheliomas
- Chromosomal abnormalities demonstrated by flow cytometry are highly suggestive of malignant disease
- Pleuroscopy effectively establishes the diagnosis, as does open biopsy

Treatment

The initial step is to identify the location of the primary tumor

- The clinician must determine whether the tumor is of a type that is responsive to chemotherapy. Small-cell lung carcinoma, lymphomas, leukemias, and rarely germ-cell tumors may have an associated pleural effusion and respond to chemotherapy
- Obliteration of the pleural space via a pleurodesis, or removal of fluid via a pleuroperitoneal shunt, should be considered if the patient is symptomatic (dyspnea at rest or during exercise) from the presence of the pleural fluid and the dyspnea is relieved with a therapeutic thoracentesis
- Pleurodesis should not be attempted if the mediastinum is shifted toward the side of the effusion
- Tetracycline, the most commonly used sclerosing agent for the past decade, is no longer available. The following 5 agents are reasonable alternatives: minocycline 300 mg intrapleurally; doxycycline 500 mg intrapleurally; bleomycin 60 IU intrapleurally (cost exceeds $700); Mitoxantrone hydrochloride (Novantrone) 30 mg intrapleurally (cost exceeds $600); and talc (an excellent sclerosing agent but must be used in conjunction with pleuroscopy or open biopsy)
- The goal of a chemical pleurodesis is obliteration of the pleural space so that room is not available for the pleural fluid to reaccumulate
- Intense inflammatory response results in fusion of the visceral and parietal pleurae and obliteration of the intervening space
- A chest tube should be inserted
- Systemic sedation and local anesthesia (4 mg/kg lidocaine) should be given because the procedure at times is painful
- The sclerosing agent should be injected only if the underlying lung has expanded
- After injection, the patient is repositioned frequently and the chest tube is clamped for 1–2 h
- Suction is maintained for ≥48 h and until the pleural drainage is <150 ml/day

Pleurodesis effectively controls the pleural effusions in 80–90% of properly selected patients. Most failures occur because of poor patient selection; either the mediastinum is shifted toward the side of the pleural effusion or the lung does not expand after the chest tube is inserted.

PARAPNEUMONIC EFFUSIONS AND BACTERIAL INFECTIONS OF THE PLEURAL SPACE

A parapneumonic effusion is any pleural effusion associated with bacterial pneumonia, lung abscess, or bronchiectasis. Parapneumonic effusions are probably the most common exudative pleural effusions in the United States. Approximately 40% of the 1.2 million individuals who develop a bacterial pneumonia in the United States each year have a pleural effusion.

The subcategories of parapneumonic effusions are

- Complicated parapneumonic effusions, which require tube thoracostomy for their resolution
- An empyema, which is an exudative effusion on which the Gram's stain of the pleural fluid is positive

The evolution of a parapneumonic effusion can be divided into 3 stages that represent a continuous spectrum

- The exudative stage is the first stage and is characterized by the collection of sterile fluid in the pleural space. The pleural fluid in this stage is an exudate with primarily polymorphonuclear leukocytes, a normal glucose level, and a normal pH level. Appropriate antibiotic therapy effects resolution of both the pneumonic process and the pleural disease
- The fibropurulent stage is the next stage and is characterized by infection with the offending bacteria of the previously sterile pleural fluid. The pH and glucose levels of the pleural fluid become progressively lower while the LDH level of the pleural fluid becomes progressively higher. As this stage progresses, the pleural space becomes loculated as the result of the formation of fibrin membranes
- The organization stage is the final stage and is characterized by fibroblasts growing into the exudate from both the visceral and the parietal pleural surfaces to produce an inelastic membrane called the pleural peel. This peel encases the lung and renders it nearly functionless

Prior to the antibiotic era, S. pneumoniae or hemolytic streptococci were responsible for most empyemas. At present, anaerobic organisms, aerobic organisms, and mixed infections with aerobes and anaerobes each account for about 1/3 of culture-positive parapneumonic effusions.

The clinical picture depends on whether organisms are aerobic or anaerobic

- If aerobic, an acute febrile illness with chest pain, sputum production, and leukocytosis ensues
- If anaerobic, a subacute illness with weight loss, anemia, and leukocytosis ensues. Most patients also have a history of an episode of unconsciousness or some other factor that predisposes them to aspiration and anaerobic pneumonia

The possibility of a parapneumonic effusion should be considered whenever a patient with a bacterial pneumonia is initially evaluated

- Obtain bilateral decubitus chest x rays if either of the posterior costophrenic angles is blunted on the lateral chest x ray or if either diaphragm is not visible throughout its length
- Semiquantitate the amount of pleural fluid by measuring the distance between the inside of the chest wall and the outside of the lung. If the thickness of the fluid is <10 mm, the effusion is not clinically significant and a thoracentesis is not indicated. If the thickness of

the fluid is >10 mm, a diagnostic thoracentesis should be performed immediately

Treatment

One can identify a complicated parapneumonic effusion only by examining the pleural fluid. A diagnostic thoracentesis should be performed as soon as the presence of a significant amount of pleural fluid is demonstrated

- Aliquots of the pleural fluid should be sent for measurement of the pleural fluid glucose, LDH, amylase and protein levels, pH, a differential and total white blood cell count, Gram's stain, and aerobic and anaerobic bacterial cultures
- Usually the fluid also is submitted for mycobacterial and fungal smears and cultures, as well as for cytologic studies

At the time of the initial evaluation, the pleural effusion of some patients with parapneumonic effusions is already loculated

- Ultrasonic examinations of the pleural space are quite effective in distinguishing loculated fluid from pneumonic infiltrates
- Perform thoracentesis with ultrasonic guidance
- Loculated fluid by itself is not an indication for tube thoracostomy

The decision whether to initiate tube drainage of the pleural space must be made and an appropriate antibiotic must be selected

- Individuals who require tube thoracostomy must be identified immediately. A delay of even 24 h ↑ morbidity and mortality
- Indications for chest tube insertion are the presence of gross pus in the pleural space, organisms on the pleural fluid Gram's stain, pleural fluid glucose <60 mg/dl, and pleural fluid pH <7.00

Even when none of these criteria is met, tube thoracostomy should still be considered if the pleural fluid pH is <7.20 or if the pleural fluid LDH is >1,000 IU/l

- In borderline cases, serial thoracenteses at 12- to 24-hour intervals are quite useful in deciding whether to place chest tubes. If the pleural fluid LDH tends to ↓ and the pleural fluid pH and glucose levels tend to ↑ with serial thoracenteses, the patient is improving and tube thoracostomy is not indicated. Alternatively, if the LDH is ↑ and the pH and glucose levels are ↓, tube thoracostomy should be performed without delay

A relatively large chest tube should be utilized (small tubes are likely to become obstructed with fibrin and debris)

- Position tube in the most dependent part of the effusion
- Leave tube in place until the volume of the pleural drainage is <50 ml/24 hr and until the draining fluid becomes clear yellow
- If no clinical and radiologic improvement occur within 24 h, either the pleural drainage is unsatisfactory or the patient is receiving the wrong antibiotic: Review culture results
- If drainage is inadequate, check position of chest tube and consider facilitating drainage with intrapleural SK or urokinase

Certain factors can help to predict whether closed tube drainage will be sufficient therapy for a complicated parapneumonic effusion. In general, when a patient has a purulent empyema that is loculated, chest tubes alone usually are not sufficient therapy. The following scheme is a useful classification of complicated parapneumonic effusions

- Class I, low pH pleural effusion: Pleural fluid pH is <7.20, but pleural fluid cultures are negative. Tube thoracostomy by itself is usually successful
- Class II, classic empyema: Pleural fluid cultures are positive, but no loculations. Patient may need thrombolytic therapy in addition to chest tubes
- Class III, complicated empyema: Multiple loculations on chest x ray, initially or subsequently, or trapped lung. Almost all patients require thrombolytic therapy and many require decortication or open drainage procedure

TUBERCULOUS PLEURAL EFFUSIONS

In many parts of the world, the most common cause of an exudative pleural effusion is tuberculosis. Such pleural effusions, however, are relatively rare in the United States, with an annual incidence of 1,000 cases.

Tuberculous pleural effusions are thought to result when a subpleural caseous focus in the lung ruptures into the pleural space

- Delayed hypersensitivity is responsible for pleural effusion
- Tuberculous pleuritis can appear as an acute or a chronic illness. The acute presentation is characterized by cough and chest pain; the chronic presentation is characterized by low-grade fever, weakness, and weight loss
- The effusion is almost always unilateral and is usually small to moderate in size, although at times it may be massive. One-third of patients have concurrent parenchymal infiltrates
- When untreated, the effusion resolves, but most patients subsequently develop tuberculosis
- Pleural fluid is an exudate with predominantly small lymphocytes
- The diagnosis is established by needle biopsy of the pleura demonstrating granuloma or positive mycobacterial cultures of the pleural fluid or pleural biopsy specimen. Elevated levels of ADA or gamma interferon in the pleural fluid are suggestive of the diagnosis
- Appropriate therapy is the administration of 2 antituberculous drugs for 9 months. All patients with an undiagnosed exudative pleural effusion and a positive PPD should be treated (see Chapter 18.)

PLEURAL EFFUSIONS IN PATIENTS WITH AIDS

- Pleural effusions are uncommon in patients with AIDS
- The most common cause is Kaposi's sarcoma. Diagnosis is difficult, and open biopsy usually is required
- Parapneumonic effusions are the second most common cause, followed by tuberculosis, cryptococcosis, and lymphoma
- Effusions are unusual with Pneumocystis carinii infection
- Patients with AIDS and pleural effusion should undergo diagnostic thoracentesis. If no diagnosis, a needle biopsy of pleura is performed if fluid is exudative. If still no diagnosis, one should consider treatment for tuberculosis. If the patient is symptomatic, a pleuroperitoneal

shunt should be implanted or chemical pleurodesis should be attempted

PLEURAL EFFUSIONS CAUSED BY PULMONARY EMBOLIZATION

Although pulmonary embolism is 1 of the most common causes of pleural effusion (Table 21–2), it is frequently not considered in the differential diagnosis of pleural effusion

- Effusion may be either a transudate or an exudate with any cell type. Pleural fluid may or may not be bloody
- Patients have usual symptoms of pulmonary embolization
- Parenchymal infiltrate is also apparent in 50% of patients
- The initial diagnostic study is usually a perfusion lung scan. If the perfusion scan is abnormal, a ventilation lung scan should be obtained. (See Fig. 22–1). If doubt still exists after these tests, a pulmonary arteriogram should be performed (see Chap. 22)
- The treatment is the same as that for any patient with a pulmonary embolus. If effusion enlarges during treatment, thoracentesis should be repeated to rule out infection or hemothorax

PLEURAL EFFUSIONS CAUSED BY DISEASES OF THE GI TRACT

Several different GI diseases may have an associated pleural effusion.

Pancreatitis. Approximately 20% of patients with acute pancreatitis have an exudative pleural effusion

- The effusion probably results from diaphragmatic inflammation
- Occasionally chest symptoms dominate the clinical picture
- The pleural fluid is an exudate with predominantly polymorphonuclear leukocytes and an elevated amylase
- The effusion does not alter the treatment plan for a patient with acute pancreatitis

Chronic pancreatic pleural effusion. The possibility of a chronic pancreatic pleural effusion should be considered in all patients who seem to have a malignant pleural effusion but in whom the pleural fluid cytologic results are negative

- Results from a sinus tract leading from the pancreas through the aortic or esophageal hiatus into the mediastinum
- Clinical picture is dominated by chest symptoms such as dyspnea, cough, and chest pain
- Effusion is usually very large and recurs rapidly after a therapeutic thoracentesis
- Markedly elevated pleural fluid amylase level is key to the diagnosis
- Usually therapy requires abdominal exploration with ligation or excision of the sinus tract and drainage or partial resection of the pancreas

Esophageal perforation. This diagnosis should be considered in all acutely ill patients with exudative pleural effusions, because if this condition is not treated rapidly and appropriately, the mortality approaches 100%

- Usually follows instrumentation of esophagus, but may occur spontaneously
- Severe symptoms result from intense infection of the mediastinum
- Pleural fluid amylase level is a good screening test. The amylase level is markedly elevated because saliva, with its high amylase content, enters the mediastinum through a hole in the esophagus. The diagnosis is confirmed with contrast studies of the esophagus
- The treatment of choice for esophageal perforation is exploration of the mediastinum with primary repair of the esophageal tear and drainage of the pleural space and mediastinum

Intra-abdominal abscess. Approximately 80% of subphrenic abscesses, 40% of pancreatic abscesses, 30% of splenic abscesses, and 20% of intrahepatic abscesses have an accompanying pleural effusion

- Effusion results from diaphragmatic irritation
- The possibility of an abscess should be considered strongly in any patient with an undiagnosed exudative pleural effusion containing predominantly polymorphonuclear leukocytes when pulmonary parenchymal infiltrates are absent
- The diagnosis of intra-abdominal abscess is best established with abdominal CT scanning
- Treatment consists of drainage of the abscess

PLEURAL DISEASE CAUSED BY COLLAGEN VASCULAR DISEASES

Rheumatoid pleuritis. Approximately 5% of patients with rheumatoid arthritis develop a pleural effusion in the course of their disease

- The pleural effusion usually develops only after the arthritis has been present for several years
- Most patients are male, >35 years, and have SQ nodules
- The pleural fluid is characterized by a glucose level <30 mg/dl, an LDH level >700 IU/l, a pH <7.20, and a rheumatoid factor titer >1: 320
- No treatment has proved effective for rheumatoid pleuritis

Lupus pleuritis. The incidence of pleural effusion with either systemic or drug-induced lupus erythematosus is about 40%

- Arthritis or arthralgias are usually present before effusion develops
- Almost all patients with lupus pleuritis have pleuritic chest pain, and most are also febrile
- Many different drugs have been incriminated for producing drug-induced lupus erythematosus. Hydralazine, procainamide, isoniazid, phenytoin, and chlorpromazine are most commonly indicted. The presenting signs, symptoms, and radiographic abnormalities are similar to those of spontaneous lupus
- The pleural fluid is an exudate that may have predominantly polymorphonuclear leukocytes or lymphocytes. The pleural fluid glucose level is usually >60 mg/dl, the LDH level is <500 IU/l, and the pH is >7.20
- Measurement of the level of ANA in the pleural fluid is the best test

for lupus pleuritis. With lupus, the ANA titer is ≥1:160 or the pleural fluid to serum ANA ratio is ≥1
- Oral corticosteroids are effective therapy for lupus pleuritis

PLEURAL EFFUSIONS CAUSED BY DRUG REACTIONS

Administration of the following drugs has been associated with the development of a pleural effusion

- Nitrofurantoin, the urinary antiseptic
- Dantrolene, the muscle relaxant
- Methysergide, the antimigraine drug
- Bromocriptine, the anti-Parkinson's drug
- Procarbazine, the antineoplastic drug
- Amiodarone, the antiarrhythmic drug

Individuals with drug-induced pleural effusions may appear with acute, subacute, or chronic illnesses: Concomitant pulmonary infiltrates are sometimes present. Characteristics of fluid are poorly described, but it is frequently eosinophilic.

Suggested Reading

Light RW: Pleural Diseases. Philadelphia, Lea & Febiger, 1991.
Light RW: Pleural Diseases, Pleural Effusions. *In* Khan M Gabriel, Cardiac and Pulmonary Management. Philadelphia, Lea & Febiger, 1993.

Pulmonary Embolism

22

M. Gabriel Khan and Lucy B. Palmer

PATHOGENESIS

Pulmonary emboli arise from a number of sites, but the primary sources are the deep iliofemoral and thigh veins. Other sites include the pelvic veins and, less commonly, the right atrium and ventricle. The calf veins do not give rise to significant emboli but may extend upward in about 15% of cases. Risk factors include any processes that ↑ venous stasis, damage the intima of the venous system, or cause a hypercoagulable state. Certain clinical conditions present particularly high risk for pulmonary embolism. Patients with these conditions must be considered for prophylactic measures and a diagnostic workup must be initiated promptly if there are any symptoms of pulmonary embolism. High-risk clinical conditions include the following: History of thromboembolic disease; prolonged anesthesia associated with surgery; surgery or injury to the lower extremities or pelvis; bed rest; pregnancy (particularly postpartum) or use of estrogen-containing compounds; CHF; malignancy; obesity; and hypercoagulable diathesis (protein C, S, or antithrombin III deficiency). The latter condition comprises <15% of cases of DVT.

PATHOPHYSIOLOGY

The effects of pulmonary emboli on gas exchange are multifold

- ↑ in dead space
- Bronchoconstriction in the area of the embolus
- Hyperventilation
- Hypoxemia

Hypoxemia has been attributed to multiple causes, including ↑ shunt (both intrapulmonary and intracardiac, in cases of patent foramen ovale), widening of the A-V O_2 difference caused by acute changes in cardiac output secondary to right heart failure, ↑ perfusion to low V/Q units secondary to elevated pulmonary pressures, and atelectasis associated with the loss of surfactant.

Hemodynamic effects of pulmonary emboli depend not only on the size of the embolus but on the patient's baseline cardiopulmonary status. Normal individuals can tolerate an embolic event of substantial size without significant changes in PA pressures. Pulmonary hypertension may occur when ≥30% of the vascular bed is obstructed. But in patients with significant underlying pulmonary vascular disease, smaller emboli can result in cor pulmonale if acute elevations of the mean pulmonary arterial pressure are >40 mm Hg. Pulmonary hypertension appears to be due not only to ↓ cross-sectional area of the vascular bed but to PA constriction, which may result from hypoxemia and neural and humoral factors. In a patient with no preexisting cardiopulmonary disease, shock is caused by obstruction of >50% of the pulmonary circulation.

PROGNOSIS

The prognosis for patients with pulmonary embolism is usually excellent if they survive the first hour and the diagnosis is made. The degree and rate of resolution are most abnormal in patients with underlying cardiopulmonary disease. Recurrent thromboembolism is uncommon in patients with an acute presentation of pulmonary embolism if treated appropriately. The rate of resolution has been examined using hemodynamic, angiographic, and scan abnormalities

- Hemodynamic improvement may be minimal the first week after a large embolus
- Most scans and angiograms will show significant improvement in 3 weeks
- Complete angiographic resolution can occasionally occur as soon as 7 days after the embolic event
- There will be minimal further resolution after 2–3 months
- With underlying cardiopulmonary disease, complete resolution may never occur

DIAGNOSIS

The diagnosis of pulmonary embolism should be strongly considered in patients who manifest ≥1 of the following clinical patterns.

Acute Unexplained Dyspnea

Patients present with tachypnea and possibly tachycardia; the chest x ray and ECG are usually normal; patients frequently have sustained a large embolus or have underlying cardiopulmonary disease.

Pulmonary Hemorrhage and/or Infarction

Patients usually have sustained, submassive embolus. Most will have pleuritic chest pain, dyspnea, hemoptysis, and chest x-ray infiltrate. At least 3 out of 4 of these findings are usually present. Other common findings, including fever, occasional friction rub, mild wheeze, and/or crepitations, may be detected on auscultation. Leukocytosis may also occur, but there is a conspicuous absence of band cells that are virtually always present in patients with a bacterial pneumonia, which is frequently the main differential diagnosis.

A small pleural effusion with blunting of the costophrenic-angle and pleural-based consolidation are frequent. Large effusions with bronchial breathing, which may persist for some weeks, occasionally occur. The effusion is often blood-tinged or frankly hemorrhagic and has the qualities of an exudate; however, ≤20% of cases yield a transudative pattern. When an exudative effusion is present, a pH <7.2 suggests infection. When requesting pH of the pleural aspirate, it is crucial to use the same technique for collecting and transporting the pleural aspirate as is used for ABG analysis (see Chap. 21).

As lung parenchyma is oxygenated by the airways as well as by the pulmonary and bronchial circulation, infarction usually occurs when there is damage to 2 of the 3 supplies. Therefore, pulmonary infarction occurs more commonly in patients with underlying cardiopulmonary disease. After an infarct, the necrosis of intra-alveolar septae with dense hemorrhage undergoes slow resolution with fibrosis and scar formation, as opposed to complete resolution in patients with no underlying disease.

Acute Cor Pulmonale and Cardiogenic Shock

Massive emboli cause obstruction or large filling defects in ≥2 lobar arteries. If >70% of the pulmonary vascular cross-sectional area is obstructed, this results in acute pulmonary hypertension >40–45 mm Hg. Acute right ventricular dilation and failure supervene, but BP may be temporarily preserved because of a ↑ in systemic vascular resistance caused by adrenergic reflexes. Over 1/2 of deaths due to thromboembolic disease result from massive pulmonary embolism, which is responsible for the majority of deaths that occur within the first hour after the onset of symptoms. The mortality rate of patients with massive pulmonary embolism and shock is approximately 33%. Symptoms and signs include the following

- Presyncope or syncope
- Abrupt unexplained severe dyspnea and signs that may simulate an acute exacerbation of COPD
- Oppressive central chest pain (usually nonpleuritic)
- Marked apprehension
- Clouding of consciousness
- Cold, clammy skin
- Signs of cardiogenic shock
- Intensified pulmonic component of the second heart sound, accompanied by wide physiologic splitting of the second heart sound due to prolonged right ventricular ejection

Chronic Cor Pulmonale in Patients with Recurrent Pulmonary Embolism or an Undetermined Cause

While most pulmonary emboli resolve over weeks, residual obstruction persists in a small group of patients, resulting in pulmonary hypertension and cor pulmonale. This may be secondary to persistent major vessel obstruction or to recurrent small emboli or possible in situ thrombosis. In patients with major vessel obstruction, the diagnosis is often not made at the time of the initial embolic event. Clinical features include the following

- Patients present with increasing dyspnea and fatigue, as well as signs of right ventricular failure. These symptoms appear to be due to pulmonary hypertension, which causes further vessel damage
- The perfusion scan may reveal large bilateral perfusion defects without ventilation abnormality

- Right heart catheterization and pulmonary angiography are required for diagnosis

APPROACH TO DIAGNOSIS

Certain symptoms and signs, while nonspecific, are quite sensitive and, when combined with significant risk factors (Tables 22–1, 22–2, and 22–3), ↑ the likelihood of pulmonary embolism. Tables 22–1 and 22–2 show the most commonly demonstrated signs and symptoms in the NHLBI PIOPED, a large multicenter study examining the accuracy of lung scans compared to pulmonary angiography

- Dyspnea and pleuritic pain are the most common symptoms
- Tachypnea and crepitations are the most common findings on physical examination

Combining the results of clinical diagnosis and lung scanning can greatly ↑ the accuracy of diagnosis in certain settings and help direct decision making as soon as the result of the lung scan is available (Fig. 22–1). This was demonstrated in PIOPED. When a clinical impression of high probability of pulmonary embolism was combined with a high-probability scan, the condition was present in 96% of the cases. Conversely, if both scan and clinical impression were low probability for embolism, the diagnosis was correctly excluded in 96% of the cases. For example, if a patient presents with sudden pleuritic pain and becomes hypoxemic on the fifth postoperative day and the chest x ray shows a small area of atelectasis, the diagnosis of pulmonary embolism is likely. If the scan is high probability, it is not necessary for the workup to proceed. This is a logical approach, but unfortunately, it does not embrace many scenarios that may be encountered, and the assignment of high probability and low probability to clinical assessment is still quite subjective. In PIOPED, the majority of assessments were intermediate, with 20–79% likelihood of pulmonary embolism.

Table 22–1
Symptoms: No Preexisting Cardiac or Pulmonary Disease

	PULMONARY EMBOLISM N = 117 NUMBER (%)	NO PULMONARY EMBOLISM N = 248 NUMBER (%)
Dyspnea	85 (73)	178 (72)
Pleuritic pain	77 (66)	146 (59)
Cough	43 (37)	89 (36)
Leg swelling	33 (28)	55 (22)
Leg pain	30 (26)	60 (24)
Hemoptysis	15 (13)	20 (8)
Palpitations	12 (10)	44 (18)
Wheezing	10 (9)	28 (11)
Angina-like pain	5 (4)	15 (6)

No significant differences were seen.
Reproduced with permission from Stein PD, Terrin ML, Hales CA, et al.: Clinical, laboratory, roentgenographic and electrocardiographic findings in patients with acute pulmonary embolism and no pre-existing cardiac or pulmonary disease. Chest, *100*:600, 1991.

Table 22–2
Signs of Acute Pulmonary Embolism: No Preexisting Cardiac or Pulmonary Disease

	PULMONARY EMBOLISM N = 117 NUMBER (%)	NO PULMONARY EMBOLISM N = 248 NUMBER (%)
Tachypnea (20/min)	82 (70)	169 (68)
Crackles	60 (51)	98 (40)*
Tachycardia (> 100 min)	35 (30)	59 (24)
Fourth heart sound	28 (24)	34 (14)*
Increased P_2	27 (23)	33 (13)*
Deep venous thrombosis	13 (11)	27 (11)
Diaphoresis	13 (11)	20 (8)
Temperature > 38.5	8 (7)	29 (12)
Wheezes	6 (5)	21 (8)
Homan's sign	5 (4)	6 (2)
Right ventricular lift	5 (4)	6 (2)
Pleural friction rub	3 (3)	6 (2)
Third heart sound	3 (3)	11 (4)
Cyanosis	1 (1)	5 (2)

* $p < 0.05$

Reproduced with permission from Stein PD, Terrin ML, Hales CA, et al.: Clinical, laboratory, roentgenographic and electrocardiographic findings in patients with acute pulmonary embolism and no pre-existing cardiac or pulmonary disease. Chest, *100*:600, 1991.

Table 22–3
Risk Groups for Thromboembolism

RISK GROUP	INCIDENCE OF VENOUS THROMBOSIS (%)	INCIDENCE OF FATAL PE (%)
Medical patients	15	1
General and gynecologic surgery	15–20	1
Neurologic surgery	15–20	1
Urologic surgery	15–20	5
Total knee replacement	40–70	5
Hip replacement	40–70	1–2
Hip fracture	40–70	1–5

Data from Hyers T, Hull R, Weg J: 2nd American College of Chest Physicians Conference on Antithrombotic Therapy, Antithrombotic Therapy for Venous Thromboembolic Disease. Chest, *95*:37S, 1989.

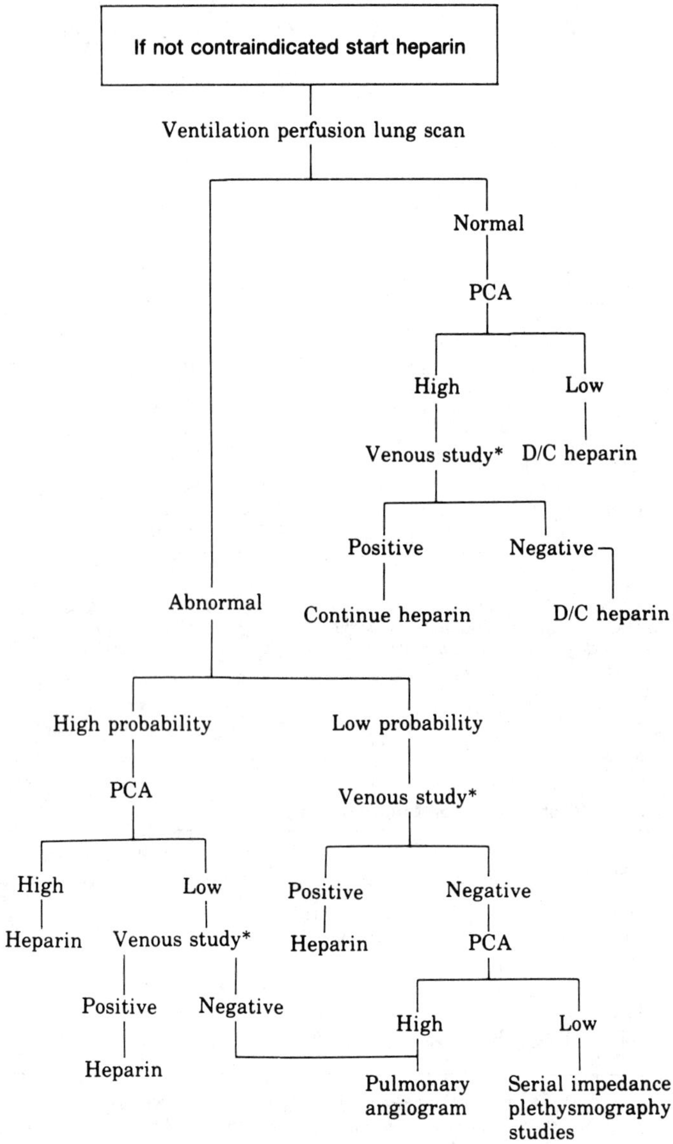

PCA = Probability from clinical assessment
D/C = Discontinue
* Venous study = Venogram, or impedance plethysmography

FIGURE 22–1. Algorithm for the management of suspected pulmonary embolism.

STANDARD LABORATORY TESTS

CBC and blood chemistries are nonspecific. As mentioned above, leukocytosis may be present with absence of bands. LDH may be ↑ in approximately 60% of cases; however, it may be a nonspecific and delayed finding.

Chest X Ray

Numerous radiographic abnormalities have been described. None of them, however, are specific or sensitive

- Atelectasis
- Pleural effusion
- Elevated hemidiaphragm
- Pleural-based consolidation (Hampton's hump)
- PA enlargement
- Abrupt vessel cutoff (knuckle sign)
- Area of hyperlucency: Oligemia (Westermark's sign)
- Dilation of azygos vein
- Enlargement of any chamber of the heart

Arterial Blood Gas

The most common abnormalities of the ABG include

- Hypoxemia: P_aO_2 <80 mm or < age predicted is present in >70% of cases but is nonspecific. Importantly, >30% of patients with proven pulmonary embolism have a P_aO_2 >80 mm Hg, on room air, especially if the blood sample is drawn several hours after the event. The alveolar–arterial (A–a) gradient is >20 mm Hg in ≤86% of patients with proven pulmonary embolism, but as with hypoxemia this is nondiagnostic
- Respiratory alkalosis: This is a common finding and usually will be present even in patients with COPD and CO_2 retention. CO_2 retention from pulmonary emboli is seen only in the setting of massive emboli

Swan-Ganz Catheter

Many patients who present with severe hypoxemia while in the ICU setting may have a Swan-Ganz catheter in place. Elevated PA pressures and the inability to obtain a good wedge tracing may suggest a massive embolus. If the embolus is massive and sufficient to cause right ventricular failure and ↓ cardiac output, PA pressures may be only moderately elevated.

Electrocardiogram

- Sinus tachycardia is common but too nonspecific to assist in diagnosis
- A pattern of acute cor pulmonale: S1 Q3 T3 (T wave inversion in 3) with lead 2 following the pattern in lead 1 rather than lead 3; a finding that is unlike inferior infarction
- S1 S2 S3
- Right axis deviation

- Right ventricular strain pattern: Inverted T waves V_1 to V_3 with more prominent S waves in V_5, V_6 due to right ventricular dilation
- Transient RBBB
- Nonspecific ST segment or T wave inversion (in ≤33% of patients)
- ST segment depression V_4 to V_6 (may be due to poor coronary perfusion in patients with CHD)

These findings are uncommon and nonspecific but may occur suddenly; their transient appearance ↑ the likelihood of pulmonary embolism. Patterns of acute right heart strain should raise the concern of a large embolic event.

Lung Scan

The first-line investigation for patients with suspected pulmonary embolism is a V/Q scan, except for patients with acute cor pulmonale pattern and/or cardiogenic shock, in whom emergency pulmonary angiography is essential. It must be emphasized that the lung scan may not be useful in many patients with underlying cardiopulmonary disease who will have an indeterminate scan. The PIOPED study did reveal, however, that the specificity of a high-probability scan in patients with prior cardiopulmonary disease was similar to patients with no underlying disease (97% versus 98%). Many radiologists request a scan prior to angiographic study to guide their injection and permit a selective study if appropriate. The perfusion scan should be performed first because a normal scan will usually negate the need for further workup. The following rules govern the properly interpreted lung scan report. (Table 22–4 shows definition of scans in PIOPED study.)

NORMAL SCANS

A normal scan associated with a normal chest x ray usually indicates the absence of pulmonary embolism. Although some investigations have revealed a 2–4% incidence of positive pulmonary angiograms, it has been shown that patients with normal scans who have negative studies of their lower extremities for venous thrombosis have an excellent prognosis without anticoagulation. In this setting, it is likely that a clot undetected by a scan is not clinically significant.

NONDIAGNOSTIC LUNG SCANS

Recent data from large multicenter studies suggest that nondiagnostic lung scans should include all scans other than normal and high-probability scans. Previously, scans have been rated in compartments of likelihood of pulmonary embolus. With the exception of high-probability and normal scans, these terms are frequently misleading and may be dangerous because of the high frequency of low-probability scans in patients with angiographic pulmonary embolism. Both PIOPED and a large series by Hull have shown that pulmonary emboli may be present in 25–40% of patients with low-probability scans (Table 22–5).

HIGH-PROBABILITY SCANS

These scans reveal multiple segmental perfusion defects with ventilation mismatch. These scans are specific but lack sensitivity, which can be as low as 40%. In the PIOPED study, sensitivity of these scans was

Table 22–4
PIOPED Central Scan Interpretation Categories and Criteria

HIGH PROBABILITY

≥ Two large (>75% of a segment) segmental perfusion defects without corresponding ventilation or x-ray abnormalities.

≥ Two moderate segmental (≥25% and≤75% of a segment) perfusion defects without matching ventilation or chest x-ray abnormalities and one large mismatched segmental defect.

≥ Four moderate segmental perfusion defects without ventilation or chest x-ray abnormalities.

INTERMEDIATE PROBABILITY (INDETERMINATE)

Not falling into normal, very low, low, or high probability categories.

Borderline high or boderline low.

Difficult to categorize as low or high.

LOW PROBABILITY

Nonsegmental perfusion defects (e.g., very small effusion causing blunting of the costophrenic angle, cardiomegaly, enlarged aorta, hila and mediastinum, and elevated diaphragm).

Single moderate mismatched segmental perfusion defect with normal chest x-ray.

Any perfusion defect with a substantially larger chest x-ray abnormality.

Large or moderate segmental perfusion defects involving no more than four segments in one lung and no more than three segments in one lung region with matching ventilation defects either equal to or larger in size and chest x-ray either normal or with abnormalities substantially smaller than perfusion defects.

> Three small segmental perfusion defects (<25% of a segment) with a normal chest x-ray.

VERY LOW PROBABILITY

≥ Three small segmental perfusion defects with a normal chest x-ray.

NORMAL

No perfusion defects present.

Perfusion outlines exactly the shape of the lungs as seen on the chest x-ray (hilar and aortic impressions may be seen, chest x-ray and/or ventilation study may be abnormal).

Reproduced from: The PIOPED Investigators: Value of the ventilation/perfusion scan in acute pulmonary embolism. JAMA, *263*:2755, 1990.

97%, but only 102 of 251 patients (41%) with positive angiograms had high-probability scans. Similarly, in an investigation by Hull, only 52 of 98 (41%) with pulmonary embolism by angiogram had high-probability scans.

Venography and Impedance Plethysmography

Above-the-knee DVT is present in 70–90% of patients with angiographic pulmonary embolism. Thus, evaluation of the lower extremities is often warranted in decision making in patients suspected of having pulmonary embolism. Femoral venography remains the gold standard against which other methods are measured, but there are sufficient data to support the use of IPG for the diagnosis of acute venous thrombosis of <7

Table 22–5
Lung Scan and the Incidence of Pulmonary Embolus

	PULMONARY EMBOLISM PRESENT*	
LUNG SCAN REPORT	REF. 5	REF. 11
Normal	2%	4%
High probability	57%	88%
Nondiagnostic	42%	16–33%

* Differences between these two large clinical studies are most likely due to different definitions of subgroups of scans.
Ref. 5—Hull RD, Raskob GE: Low probability lung scan findings: A need for change. Ann Int Med, *174*:142, 1991.
Ref. 11—PIOPED Investigators: Value of the ventilation-perfusion scan in acute pulmonary embolism. JAMA, *263*:2753, 1990.

days' duration, as it will detect 95% of clots involving the popliteal vein or above. Duplex scanning is a sensitive technique for DVT but is not a good test in asymptomatic individuals. DVT and its management are discussed in Chapter 11.

Pulmonary Angiography

Pulmonary angiography is performed to confirm or exclude the diagnosis of pulmonary embolism in the following situations

- Nondiagnostic lung scan with a negative femoral venogram or IPG and remaining suspicion of pulmonary embolism
- As an emergency procedure for diagnostic confirmation prior to embolectomy in patients with acute cor pulmonale pattern and/or cardiogenic shock. In this setting, lung scan is not indicated
- High-probability scan in a patient with a history of pulmonary emboli (these scans have less specificity in this group)
- High-probability scan with a high risk of bleeding

Risks of the procedure include

- Allergic reaction to contrast material. The procedure can be carried out, if strongly warranted, using premedication with corticosteroids and antihistamine with epinephrine standby
- Cardiac perforation (occurs in ≤0.3%, but is virtually nonexistent in experienced hands)
- Arrhythmias (usually easily controlled)
- Depression of myocardial contractility may precipitate CHF within mins to 1 h of the procedure in patients with LV dysfunction. Also, a large volume of contrast material is required and imposes an osmotic load; thus, IV furosemide may be required
- Pulmonary hypertension may be exacerbated by the procedure, but selective injections are often possible and are well tolerated
- The morbidity rate is 2–4%; the mortality rate is <0.2%

THERAPY

Heparin (5,000–10,000 U) is given as an IV bolus if there is no contraindication to anticoagulant therapy. The bolus is followed immediately by an infusion of heparin 1,000 U/h. PTT is done 6 h later and the infusion adjusted to maintain the PTT 1.5–2 times the patient control level. Heparin is usually continued for 7–10 days, and coumadin is started between the first and fifth day. See Chapter 11 for instructions on heparin infusion guidelines and coumadin therapy. For submassive pulmonary embolism however, coumadin can be commenced on the first or second night and heparin is discontinued when the PT is in the therapeutic range of 1.3–1.5 times the control or INR 2–3. This approximately 5-day course of IV heparin can result in considerable savings for patients and hospitals. Coumadin is continued for 3–6 months. In some patients with ongoing risk factors, prolonged therapy may be required.

Thrombolytic therapy is of value to restore circulation in patients with hemodynamic compromise in the setting of massive emboli or shock. SK, urokinase, and tPA are the 3 agents currently available. Despite their ability to accelerate the early rate of resolution, there has been no proven benefit in longterm morbidity or mortality compared to heparin therapy alone. The unknown benefits must be weighed against the significant bleeding risks associated with the use of these agents. Despite early speculation that tPA might be associated with less bleeding, early investigations have not shown this to be true.

The current indication for thrombolytic agent use is massive pulmonary embolism and hemodynamic compromise. Dosage: The 2 most commonly used agents are SK and urokinase

- SK: 250,000 U/30 min IV, then infusion of 100,000 U for 12–24 h followed by IV heparin
- Urokinase: 4,400 IU/kg for 12 h followed by IV heparin

After 3 h of treatment with either agent, testing should be done to ensure a "lytic state." This can be monitored with a number of tests, including euglobulin lysis time, fibrinogen level, fibrinogen degradation products, PT or PTT. This testing is not used to adjust dosing but to determine whether systemic fibrinolysis has been achieved. If it has not, then the patient may need to be rebolused. See Chapter 3 for contraindications and further discussion of thrombolytic agents.

Pulmonary embolectomy. This is a controversial treatment reserved for patients with massive embolism and hypotension who have not responded to conventional therapy. The mortality is approximately 50%, which most likely reflects the severity of the process being treated (frequently these patients have already arrested and are requiring CPR). This option is a viable one in only a few institutions. When pulmonary embolectomy is performed, the patient must also have placement of a vena caval filter.

Inferior vena cava barrier. This useful intervention prevents the migration of large clots. Currently, the ideal method is transvenous insertion of a filter device that permits blood flow to prevent occlusion and longterm complications. There are a variety of types and sizes of devices available, and these vary from institution to institution. *Indications include*

- Patients recovering from life-threatening pulmonary embolism to prevent further massive embolism
- Contraindication for anticoagulants
- Recurrent emboli during adequate anticoagulation
- Patients undergoing pulmonary embolectomy

Suggested Reading

Hull RD, Raskob GE: Low-probability lung scan findings: A need for change. Ann Intern Med *174*:142, 1991.

Palmer LB, Khan M Gabriel: Pulmonary Embolism. *In* Khan M Gabriel, Cardiac and Pulmonary Management. Philadelphia, Lea & Febiger, 1993.

PIOPED Investigators: Value of the ventilation-perfusion scan in acute pulmonary embolism. JAMA *263*:2753, 1990.

Stein PD, Athanasoulis C, Alavi A, et al.: Complications and validity of pulmonary angiography in acute pulmonary embolism. Circulation *85*:462, 1992.

Gastrointestinal Bleeding 23

Irving Waxman and Sanjiv Chopra

The initial approach to the bleeding patient depends on the site, extent, and rate of bleeding

- Maintaining adequate intravascular volume and hemodynamic stability while localizing the bleeding site and providing adequate therapy is the mainstay of successful management
- Clinical predictors of ↑ mortality include age >60 years, multiple serious underlying illnesses, recurrent bleeding, bleeding requiring ≥5 units of blood, and red-colored stool with NG aspirate at presentation
- Initial evaluation aims to assess patient's intravascular volume and rate of bleeding, and tailor degree of resuscitating efforts

Patient's appearance: Decreased mental status, diaphoresis, pallor, or complaints of light headedness, thirst, and nausea are usually associated with significant blood loss (>500 ml), except in the elderly, where smaller volumes may lead to same signs and symptoms.

Initial exam: Aimed at assessing volume status

- Orthostatic hypotension manifested by a drop in systolic BP of >10 mm Hg or ↑ in HR of >20 beats/min is associated with moderate blood loss (10–20% of circulatory volume)
- Supine hypotension indicates severe blood loss (>20% of circulatory volume)
- Hypovolemic shock: manifested by hypotension, tachycardia, and multi-organ failure, i.e., oliguria, confusion, myocardial ischemia. Exam will reveal pallor, cool skin, delayed capillary filling due to peripheral vasoconstriction. Type and cross for 3–6 U of packed RBCs should be done as well as initial CBC, platelets, prothrombin time, PTT, and serum chemistries, as well as an ECG

Resuscitation

- Two large-bore IV (14–16 gauge) should be placed for rapid volume infusion. This is usually quicker and with less morbidity than placing central vein catheters
- Rate of fluid infusion will depend on patient's hemodynamic status. 0.9% saline or Ringer lactate are adequate starting solutions while blood is available from the blood bank
- Blood transfusion: aim to keep hematocrit around 30% or until patient is hemodynamically stable. In actively bleeding patients where >5 U of packed RBCs have been transfused; fresh frozen plasma (FFP) should be given to correct for dilution of clotting factors

Further evaluation: Once patient is stable, attention is focused on determining the source of bleeding

- A pertinent concise history together with a careful physical exam will usually suggest the source. Look for peptic symptoms, past history of ulcer disease, alcohol or NSAID use, vascular surgery (aorto-enteric fistula), and nausea and vomiting antedating bleeding (Mallory-Weiss tear)

- Hematemesis is the vomiting of blood. The color of vomited blood will depend on the rate of bleeding and the contact time with HCl. HCl and pepsin will degrade Hb, causing dark brown fluid (coffee grounds)
- Inspection of the stool: *Melena*, described as black, sticky, or tarry stool, is present when bleeding source is proximal to the cecum. Approximately 100 ml of blood are necessary to produce melenic stools. If bleeding ceases, melena can be present for ≤3 days and stool may present with occult blood for up to a week. *Maroon stool* is usually seen when bleeding site is located at the distal ileum or proximal colon. *Hematochezia*, or passage of bright red blood per rectum, usually indicates a distal colonic or anorectal pathology, but can also be seen in very rapid UGI bleeding
- NG aspirate: When a UGI source of bleeding is suspected and no hematemesis is present, NG aspirate is mandatory. In patients with a history of hematemesis, the NG aspirate helps to assess the presence of continuous bleeding. There is a 16% false negative rate for NG aspiration in patients with endoscopically proven UGI bleeding. Therefore, a negative aspirate does not completely rule out an upper source. This may be due to coiling of the NG tube in the stomach or esophagus, or pylorospasm in patients with active duodenal ulcer bleeding. After the diagnostic aspirate is performed, the NG tube should be removed unless persistent vomiting or signs of gastric outlet obstruction are present, given that the continuous presence of an NG tube may lead to mucosal trauma and gastro-esophageal reflux
- It is important to recognize other manifestations of GI bleeding. Pulmonary complaints are not uncommon, specially in the patient with altered mental status, and protection of the airway by endotracheal intubation may be necessary to prevent recurrent aspiration. The hematocrit is not a good indicator of acute GI bleeding, given that it takes hours to equilibrate. The BUN is elevated >30 mg/dl in ≤75% of patients with UGI bleeding due to resorption of nitrogen products from the proximal small bowel

UPPER GASTROINTESTINAL BLEEDING

The 4 most common causes of UGI hemorrhage are: peptic ulcer, erosive gastritis, variceal bleeding, and Mallory-Weiss tear. These account for ≥90% of UGI bleeds.

Diagnosis

The diagnostic approach to the patient varies depending on clinical stability, rate of bleeding, and procedural expertise

- UGI endoscopy has largely supplanted barium studies of the GI tract in the evaluation of GI bleeding. Not only does it accurately identify the source of bleeding (90% accuracy), it also offers therapeutic options for hemostasis
- Barium studies may identify the source of hemorrhage but suffer from the following drawbacks: They may not identify mucosal lesions (Mallory-Weiss tear, erosive gastritis); the identified lesion may not be the

actual source of bleeding; and the presence of barium may hamper future endoscopic or angiographic examination

- Arteriography: In the presence of continuous bleeding and a negative endoscopic exam, or with massive hemorrhage (blood loss of ≥0.5 ml/min), selective angiography may localize the site. In addition to identifying the site, it can also offer therapeutic options like intra-arterial, continuous vasopressin infusion in patients with Mallory-Weiss tear or gastric ulcer. Additionally, embolization into the selective bleeding vessel may be undertaken

Peptic ulcers. They are the most common cause of UGI bleeding, but 85% will stop bleeding spontaneously

- Therapeutic endoscopy: in large meta-analysis studies, has been shown to ↓ hospital stay, blood requirements, and emergency surgery. Modalities include injection therapy, bipolar electrocoagulation, laser therapy, and heater probe, all of which have similar success rates
- Surgery: mainly indicated for patients with intractable or recurrent bleeding. Surgical consultation should be obtained early in the patient's course
- Selective Angiography: should be considered in patients who are not good surgical candidates and who have failed endoscopic therapy. Intra-arterial vasopressin infusion is successful in about 60–70% of peptic ulcers. Careful monitoring for evidence of ischemic organ damage (i.e., myocardial, mesenteric) should be done. Selective embolization is also an alternative

Variceal bleeding. Characteristically abrupt and massive. In the Western world, it is usually secondary to alcoholic cirrhosis via portal hypertension. Although a history of cirrhosis or chronic liver disease suggests the possibility of varices as the cause of bleeding, ≤50% of patients may have another source. Therefore, accurate identification of the source of bleeding is essential. After the patient is stabilized, early endoscopy should be performed to confirm the diagnosis. Admission to an ICU should be considered, and in patients with compromised mental status and active bleeding, endotracheal intubation for airway protection may be necessary.

Therapy

- Endoscopic sclerotherapy or rubber band ligation can achieve adequate hemostasis in ≤90% of patients. Sclerotherapy consists of injecting a sclerosing agent, such as sodium tetradecol into or around the varix, producing an inflammatory reaction that leads to thrombosis and eventually fibrosis of the vessel. Although significant rebleeding occurs, it usually responds to repeat treatment. Rubber band ligation is just as effective, and preliminary data suggest fewer complications
- IV vasopressin is effective in ≤60% of patients. *Dosage:* Starting dose 0.4 U/min (100 U of vasopressin in 250 ccs of D5W). Increments should be started at a dose of 0.3 U/min for 30 min and, if ineffective, ↑ at approximately 30- to 60-min intervals to a max of 0.9 U/min. Once hemostasis is achieved, the infusion rate should be reduced. Because of its vasoconstrictive properties, common side effects include myocardial ischemia, arrhythmias, bowel ischemia, and even cardiac arrest. Patients should be monitored in an ICU setting, and extreme caution should be taken in patients with known atherosclerotic disease or coronary artery disease. Concomitant nitroglycerin infusion has been shown to ↓ side effects and may improve efficacy of vasopressin ther-

apy. Infusion is started at 5 μ/min and ↑ by 5 μ/min q 3–5 min, titrated to a systolic BP of 100 mm/Hg. Sublingual NTG (0.6 mg q 30 min for 6 h) as well as nitropaste have also been used successfully
- Balloon tamponade: The use of this method should be undertaken only with the aid of personnel experienced in this procedure. The reported success for controlling bleeding varies from 40–90%. Major complications of balloon tamponade include aspiration, esophageal necrosis and rupture, and airway obstruction. Because of the high risk of rebleeding and the serious nature of the complications, it should be viewed as a temporizing measure in patients who continue to bleed in spite of routine therapy and IV vasopressin, while waiting for more definitive therapy either endoscopic or surgical
- Emergent Shunt Surgery: either with a porto-caval shunt or a distal spleno-renal shunt, is very effective in controlling variceal bleeding but is associated with significant hospital mortality (12–50%) and postoperative hepatic encephalopathy. Elective shunt surgery should be considered in patients with good hepatic function (as measured by the child's classification) who fail sclerotherapy, are noncompliant, or cannot return for follow-up visits
- Other therapies include the transjugular intrahepatic porto-systemic shunt procedure, which involves creating a shunt via a transjugular approach between a hepatic and a portal vein. Preliminary results indicate that the technique is safe and effective. Orthoptic liver transplantation restores normal circulation and prevents further variceal bleeding, but few patients are candidates for this procedure

Mallory Weiss Tear. Vertical mucosal tear at the gastro-esophageal junction. A history of repeated vomiting prior to hematemesis is a common symptom; its absence, however, does not exclude this diagnosis. Most bleeds are self-limited. In patients with persistent bleeding, endoscopic hemostasis or selective angiography are excellent therapeutic options. Surgery should be reserved for intractable bleeding, which is very rare.

LOWER GASTROINTESTINAL BLEEDING

- The most common etiologies for lower GI bleeding include anorectal pathology (hemorrhoids, fissures, rectal trauma), angiodysplasia, diverticulosis, and neoplasms
- Lower GI bleeding will stop spontaneously in ≤80% of cases
- Initially, patients should be stabilized as described earlier
- The patient's history is the most important diagnostic tool and can often lead to the source of bleeding. Blood mixed with stool, or coating or streaking of the stool, is usually from or distal to the sigmoid colon. Blood only seen in the toilet paper suggests anal canal pathology. A UGI source should always be suspected in the presence of massive hematochezia

Diagnosis

- Digital exam, anoscopy, and sigmoidoscopy should be performed in every patient with rectal bleeding. These will identify a bleeding source or will document bleeding coming from above the range of the instrument

- Radiolabeled Erythrocyte Scanning will detect blood loss of 0.1 ml/min and should be used in patients with mild persistent bleeding who are hemodynamically stable. If a source is localized, the therapeutic option (angiographic therapy, colonoscopy, surgery) will depend on the clinical condition. If no source is found, a colonoscopy should be performed
- Angiography detects bleeding lesions with blood loss of 0.5 ml/min. It should be the test of choice in a patient with rapid lower-GI bleeding or who is hemodynamically unstable. If an actively bleeding site is detected, infusion of vasopressin, or embolization with a substance like gel foam, can be performed successfully to obtain hemostasis
- Colonoscopy is indicated in patients who have ceased bleeding or who have a mild and hemodynamically stable GI bleed. In addition to localizing a specific colonic lesion, therapeutic interventions with electrocautery or laser therapy are possible

Suggested Reading

Silverstein FE, et al. The national ASGE survey on upper gastrointestinal bleeding. Gastrointest. Endosc. *27*:73, 1981.

Proceedings of the Consensus conference on Therapeutic endoscopy in bleeding ulcers. March 6-8, 1989. Gastrointest. Endosc (1990 Sep-Oct) *36*(Suppl): S1-65.

Jensen DM, et al. Diagnosis and Treatment of severe hematochezia. The role of urgent colonoscopy after purge. Gastroenterology 1988; *95*: 1569.

Gastrointestinal Diseases

24

Sanjiv Chopra and Irving Waxman

PEPTIC ULCER DISEASE

Peptic ulcer disease (UD) is a common malady that affects millions of people in all parts of the world. It is estimated that 10% of Americans will develop peptic UD at some point in life.

The term "peptic ulcer" can refer to either gastric or duodenal ulcers, duodenal being more common than gastric. It is used to define a breach in the mucosa that extends through the muscularis mucosa into the submucosa or deeper. The term "peptic" signifies that proteolysis by pepsin is important in the development of this lesion. (In contrast, an erosion is defined as a superficial hole that extends into the mucosa but does not penetrate the muscularis mucosa. Erosions are frequently encountered in patients taking aspirin or NSAIDs, or in the setting of stress gastritis, a condition commonly present in patients in the intensive care, burn, or trauma unit.)

Etiology

The important factors related to peptic UD include heredity, gastric acid hypersecretion, the use of NSAIDs, smoking, and Heliocobacter pylori

- The risk of ulcer is 2- to 2.5-fold in 1st° relatives and appears to be site specific. Approximately 40% of patients with duodenal ulcers have ≥1 family member with the disease. The likelihood of concordance for peptic ulcers is greater for identical than for fraternal twins. Inherited disorders in which peptic UD is often present include multiple endocrine neoplasia, Type I syndrome (MEN type 1) and familial systemic mastocytosis, alpha$_1$, antitrypsin deficiency, and "stiff skin syndrome"
- An accepted dictum attributed to a Dr. Schwartz in 1910 states: "No acid, no ulcer." A certain level of acid secretion is indeed necessary for duodenal UD to develop. In most patients with duodenal UD, acid secretion is normal or ↑. However, with the exception of hypersecretory states such as gastrinoma or G-cell hyperplasia, the secretion of acid alone does not appear to be a sufficient cause of peptic UD. Most patients with gastric ulcer have normal or ↓ acid secretion. Gastric ulcers almost always occur in the non-acid-secreting mucosa
- NSAIDs. These drugs produce both gastritis and peptic ulceration. The major damage is felt to be secondary to inhibition of endogenous prostaglandin production. The risk of gastric ulcer and duodenal ulcer is ↑ tenfold in individuals taking 1 g of aspirin on a daily basis. Gastric ulcer is also more likely in patients who take NSAIDs, occurring in 2–4% per patient-year. More importantly, NSAIDs are associated with ulcer complications, notably perforation and bleeding

- Smoking. Individuals who smoke are more likely than nonsmokers to develop ulcers. In addition, ulcers appear to heal more slowly in smokers and to recur sooner. Cigarette smoking ↑ the likelihood that surgical treatment will be required for peptic UD, and aggravates the operative risk. Physiologic effects related to smoking include a ↑ in the rate of gastric emptying, a ↓ in pancreatic bicarbonate secretion, and a ↓ in gastric mucosal blood flow and prostaglandin synthesis
- H. pylori is a gram negative, microaerophilic, S-shaped rod that has been proven to cause active antral gastritis in humans. This organism evokes both a local response (IgA and IgM antibodies to H. pylori are present in the gastric juice) and a systemic one (IgG and IgA antibodies to H. pylori are present in the serum). H. pylori is found in the antrum of >95% of patients with duodenal UD and about 75% of those with gastric UD. This organism is also found in 50% of patients with non-ulcer dyspepsia and in approximately 20% of normal volunteers. It is estimated that <5% of individuals harboring H. pylori develop peptic ulceration. H. pylori is associated with hypergastrinemia that reverses when the H. pylori is eradicated. Several recent studies have demonstrated that eradication of H. pylori leads to a significant ↓ in the recurrence of symptomatic UD.

In summary, peptic UD can be viewed as occurring in 1 of 3 kinds of settings:

a) Acid hypersecretion (Patients with gastrinoma, g-cell hyperplasia, and some patients with duodenal ulcer disease)
b) The use NSAIDs
c) In association with Helicobacter pylori.

Clinical Features

According to classic teaching, ulcer pain is epigastric; gnawing; relieved by foods, antacids or H_2 blockers; and recurs 2–3 h after eating. Although it may interrupt sleep, the pain is virtually never present when the patient first awakens, unless the patient has gastric outlet obstruction. However, ulcer pain may bear no relationship to meals, may occur within an hour of eating, and may actually worsen after eating. Moreover, while 90% of ulcer patients report nocturnal pain relieved by antacids or H_2 blockers, >30% of patients with chronic abdominal pain *not* due to an ulcer also report this feature. It is usually not possible to distinguish between duodenal ulcer and gastric ulcer based on symptoms, and it should be noted that the disappearance of symptoms does not always signal that the ulcer crater has disappeared.

Duodenal UD is rare before the age of 15. Symptoms most commonly occur between the ages of 25 and 60. Gastric ulcer usually appears between 40 and 65.

Sites of chronic peptic UD include the duodenal bulb and stomach. Sometimes ulcers occur in the postbulbar duodenum. In such patients, one should exclude acid hypersecretory states such as Zollinger-Ellison syndrome (gastrinoma) and antral G-cell hyperplasia. Peptic ulcers may also occur in the ileum in patients with Meckel's diverticulum, and in the jejunum in patients after a gastrojejunostomy. Peptic ulcers occurring in the esophagus are most unusual, with the exception of ulcerations that occur in acquired columnar epithelium, a condition referred to as Barrett's esophagus.

COMPLICATIONS

The major complications of peptic UD are: hemorrhage (20%), perforation (5–10%), and gastric outlet obstruction (5%). In general, complica-

Table 24–1
Bleeding Peptic Ulcer

ENDOSCOPIC APPEARANCE	INCIDENCE (%)	REBLEEDING RISK (%)
Active spurting	5–10	80–90
Visible vessel	25	40–50
Overlying clot	15	30
Flat spots	15–20	5
Clean base	35	0–5

tions are more frequent in patients with gastric ulcers. It is not possible on clinical grounds to predict accurately which patients will develop these complications, although NSAIDs ↑ the risk for ulcer complications, notably perforation and bleeding.

DIAGNOSIS

Investigative studies in peptic UD include UGI series, endoscopy, assessment of acid secretion, and measurement of serum gastrin.

A UGI series is accurate in detecting ulcers in 85% of cases. The distinction between benign and malignant gastric ulcers can be ascertained in 90% of patients, based on radiographic criteria. However, endoscopy is necessary in most cases of gastric UD in order to obtain adequate specimens for biopsy and brush cytology.

Endoscopy should be performed in patients with persistent dyspepsia despite a normal UGI series. In patients who have undergone gastric surgery, the UGI series is notoriously unable to distinguish surgical deformity from active PUD. Endoscopy is also indicated in patients with UGI bleeding. (See Chapter 23.) This procedure can detect active spurting from an ulcer crater or a "visible vessel"—2 findings which portend rebleeding and the need for active intervention such as endoscopic hemostasis or surgery (Table 24–1).

Therapy

Medical treatment is intended to relieve pain, accelerate healing of the ulcer crater, and prevent complications and recurrences. A few general comments are noteworthy

- Special diets offer no advantage. Patients are instructed to eat 3 meals a day and food of their own choosing. Acid secretion is the same whether coffee is decaffeinated or regular since the critical factor is an increment in serum gastrin associated with the peptide present in the roasted grain from which the coffee is made. Patients should be advised to quit smoking cigarettes and to avoid taking salicylate-containing drugs or NSAIDs
- Patients with duodenal UD or ulcer disease should be treated for 4–6 weeks with an antacid, a histamine H_2 receptor antagonist, or sucralfate. Those with benign gastric ulcers should be treated for 8–12 weeks with either an antacid or an H_2 receptor antagonist. Additionally, it is important to ensure that gastric ulcers heal completely and to document this fact by repeat endoscopy

Antacids. Antacids are superior to placebo and comparable to H_2 receptor antagonists in healing duodenal ulcers. Liquids are more potent than tablets. The dose is 30–60 ml 1 and 3 h after meals, and as needed. Side effects include constipation (aluminum-containing antacids), diarrhea (magnesium-containing antacids), and acid rebound (Ca-containing antacids). In some cases the Na+ load of the antacids may be clinically significant.

Cimetidine. This histamine H_2 receptor antagonist inhibits basal acid secretion by 80–95%, and meal-stimulated acid secretion by 60%. The dose is 400 mg bid, or 800 mg at bedtime. Although this drug has been used by millions of patients, toxic effects are rare. One potentially significant side effect is its ability to interact with other drugs by virtue of its inhibition of the cytochrome p-450 mixed oxidase system. Occasionally mental confusion has been noted, particularly in elderly patients with liver disease or renal insufficiency.

Ranitidine. Ranitidine is more potent and has a longer duration of action than cimetidine. The oral dose is 150 mg bid or 300 mg at bedtime. Side effects are probably less common with ranitidine—notably, there is no interaction with hepatic microsomes, no bone marrow suppression, no antiandrogen effect, and less CNS toxicity.

Famotidine. This drug is 32 times more potent than cimetidine and 9 times more potent than ranitidine. Although it appears to be safe, clinical experience has been less extensive than with the 2 mentioned above. The oral dose is 40 mg at bedtime.

Anticholinergics. These drugs ↓ basal acid secretion by 50–60% and meal-stimulated acid secretion by 30–35%. Dry mouth, urinary retention, blurred vision, and mental confusion are the most common side effects of the commonly prescribed anticholinergics. Hence, these drugs are not used as first-line therapy for peptic UD. Pirenzipine, a new muscarinic M_1 receptor antagonist, selectively inhibits acid secretion and appears to be a promising drug.

Sucralfate. This is a basic aluminum salt of sucrose octasulfate. At a pH of ≤4.0 it becomes a viscous gel that tenaciously adheres to ulcerated mucosa. Sucralfate neutralizes acid, binds bile salts, and inhibits peptic activity. In addition, it offers cytoprotection by releasing endogenous prostaglandins. It is as effective as H_2 receptor antagonists in the treatment of duodenal ulcer. The dose is 1 g qid, or 2 g bid. Side effects include constipation and the potential to bind to other orally administered drugs.

Prostaglandins. Misoprostol, a prostaglandin E analog, is used for prophylaxis of NSAID-induced gastropathy. Prostaglandins have both antisecretory and cytoprotective properties. The dose is 200 μg qid for prevention of NSAID-induced ulcers. Side effects include diarrhea and uterine contraction. This drug should not be used in women of child-bearing age.

Omeprazole (Hydrogen Potassium ATPase (Proton Pump) Inhibitor. This highly potent agent virtually abolishes gastric acid secretion. It is the drug of choice in patients with gastrinoma (Zollinger-Ellison syndrome) or severe gastroesophageal reflux disease (GERD). It has been approved for short-term treatment of duodenal ulcer disease. Concerns about toxicity include the development of anacidity and hypergastrinemia, which may predispose to GI infections and promote hyperplasia of enterochromaffin-like cells and gastric carcinoids respectively.

Maintenance Therapy. Patients with frequent ulcer recurrence may benefit from maintenance therapy. It is possible that eradication of H.

pylori with triple therapy (bismuth, amoxicillin, metronidazole) will obviate the need for maintenance therapy with H_2 blockers or sucralfate.

Surgical Treatment. Surgery is indicated for complications such as persistent or recurrent GI bleeding, obstruction, or perforation. In patients with nonhealing UD prior to surgery, a concerted effort should be made to exclude surreptitious use of aspirin or NSAIDs. In addition, gastrinoma should be excluded.

Surgical procedures include subtotal gastrectomy, vagotomy with antrectomy, vagotomy with pyloroplasty, vagotomy with gastrojejunostomy, and superselective (parietal cell) vagotomy. Postoperative complications include early satiety, bilious vomiting, diarrhea, malabsorption, dumping, anemia, osteoporosis, and osteomalacia.

Ulcers occurring in the jejunum after a Billroth II anastomosis can be due to incomplete vagotomy, an acid hypersecretory state such as Zollinger-Ellison syndrome, the retained antrum syndrome, or ingestion of NSAIDs.

Zollinger-Ellison Syndrome

The classic triad consists of severe peptic UD, gastric acid hypersecretion, and a non-β-cell tumor of the pancreas. The term "gastrinoma" is preferred. Fewer than 0.1% of patients with duodenal UD will have gastrinoma. Some patients are diagnosed at an early stage with abdominal pain (about 80%) and diarrhea (about 30%). In 20% of patients the syndrome is associated with the MEN type I syndrome.

Diagnosis is based on evidence of acid hypersecretion and an elevated serum gastrin. Other rare causes of acid hypersecretion and hypergastrinemia include the retained antrum syndrome and antral G-cell hyperplasia. The secretin test is positive in patients with gastrinoma. A positive test is defined as an increment in serum gastrin of >200 pg/ml above baseline following IV administration of secretin. Radiologic clues on a UGI series include prominent gastric folds, evidence of acid hypersecretion (a "wet-looking stomach"), postbulbar ulcers, and multiple ulcers.

Candidates for surgical resection can be identified by

- Excluding those with the MEN type I syndrome
- Performing abdominal CT or MRI to exclude hepatic metastases
- Performing selective venous sampling or intraoperative ultrasound to localize the tumor

Removal of the gastrinoma is successful in 10% of patients. Associated hyperparathyroidism should be treated. If no tumor is found at the time of exploratory laparotomy, parietal cell vagotomy may be considered. This procedure can significantly facilitate medical control of the acid hypersecretion. The drug of choice is Omeprazole at the starting dose of 60 mg per day. Omeprazole results in control of acid hypersecretion, healing of ulcers, and resolution of the diarrhea and steatorrhea.

DIARRHEA

The human GI tract handles about 9 liters of fluid on a daily basis. Most of the fluid is absorbed in the small bowel; only 1–1.5 liters enter the colon, where most of it is absorbed, leaving 100–150 ml of fluid to be excreted in the feces. When the water content of the stool is >150 ml or the total weight of the stool is >250 g, the bowel secretion is usually perceived by the patient as diarrhea.

Mechanisms of Diarrhea

- Secretory: large volume (>1 L q 24 h; persists during fasting)
- Osmotic: volume >1 L/d; diarrhea abates when the patient fasts or no longer ingests the poorly absorbed solute; positive osmotic gap in stool (stool osmolality-stool ($Na^+ + K^+$) x 2 = >50 mOsm) in patients with carbohydrate malabsorption, the stool is often acidic (pH 5–6; normal pH is 7.0)
- Dysmotility: volume may vary, usually associated with systemic disorder
- Exudative: <1 L q/d; if longstanding, hypoalbuminemia and anemia can be present; tenesmus and urgency are present with rectal bleeding
- Malabsorptive (see below)

COMMON ETIOLOGIES

- Secretory: infectious (enterotoxin-mediated like Cholera, E. coli, Bacillus cereus); neuroendocrine tumors (gastrin, vasoactive intestinal peptide); miscellaneous (bile salt malabsorption)
- Osmotic: lactase deficiency; magnesium-containing drugs; sorbitol ingestion (chewing gum diarrhea)
- Exudative: infectious, IBD
- Dysmotility: rapid transit time like hyperthyroidism, carcinoid, pyloroplasty, irritable bowel syndrome; delayed transit time, scleroderma, amyloidosis
- Malabsorption: lymphatic obstruction, pancreative disorders, mucosal disease

Usually >1 pathophysiologic process is involved (see Chapter 26)

Acute Diarrhea

- Acute diarrhea: <3 weeks
- Etiology: INFECTIONS: viral; bacterial, parasitic. DRUGS: antacids, antibiotics, alcohol, digitalis, quinidine, propranolol, colchicine, lactulose, laxatives
- Evaluation: complete history, including recent travel (see Chapter 26); recent antibiotic therapy
- Management: correction of fluid and electrolyte disturbances; treatment of specific underlying disease if warranted; antidiarrheal agents

SPECIFIC ETIOLOGIC AGENTS

Bacterial and Viral Infections. Most patients with infectious diarrhea have a mild, self-limited course. It usually does not require stool culture or specific treatment. The presence of high fever (>103° C), systemic illness, tenesmus, bloody diarrhea, or dehydration warrant further diagnostic studies and treatment. Infectious diarrhea is classified into

- Toxigenic (enterotoxin mediated), i.e., Escherichia Coli, Vibrio cholera, Bacillus cereus, Aereomonas spp

- Invasive (organism penetrates mucosal barrier), i.e., Shigella, Campylobacter, Salmonella, Yersinia

Parasitic Infections. Amebiasis is caused by Entamoeba histolytica. Manifestations range from asymptomatic carrier to fulminant colitis. Diagnosis is made by coproparasitoscopic examination of 3–6 fresh stool specimens. Recommended treatment is: asymptomatic Intestinal Infection: Iodoquinol 650 mg po tid for 20 days; Mild to Moderate Intestinal Disease: Metronidazole 750 mg po tid for 10 days or paromomycin 25–35 mg/kg/d in 3 doses for 7+ days. Iodoquinol 650 mg po tid for 20 days

Giardiasis is caused by Giardia lamblia. Manifestations range from mild diarrhea to malabsorption and steatorrhea. Diagnosis can be made by stool examination, but as many as 50% of stool specimens may not contain the parasite, requiring mucosal biopsy or duodenal aspiration. Treatment of choice is quinacrine 100 mg po tid for 7 days or metronidazole 250 mg po tid for a week.

Chronic Diarrhea

Need to differentiate between functional and organic categories according to 4 features: weight loss, bloody diarrhea, nocturnal diarrhea, and incontinence. The presence of any of these suggests an organic source. In addition, the history may suggest the etiology: the presence of tenesmus or urgency would place the process in the distal colon. Periumbilical pain and bulky and large-volume stools suggest a small bowel source. A history of greasy or oily stools, or of stools that stick to the bowl, requiring repeated flushings, may suggest steatorrhea and point to the small bowel or pancreas as the cause of the problem. Surreptitious laxative abuse should be kept in mind in the differential diagnosis of chronic unexplained diarrhea; alkalization of the stool with sodium hydroxide is a simple way to confirm the presence of phenolphthalein-containing laxatives (by turning the sample to a pink or red color).

Clinical Management. Request fecal leukocytes; stool cultures and ova and parasites; stool specimen for anal/rectal swab. An etiologic agent will be identified in 50% of cases. If no etiology is found, consider colonoscopy, upper endoscopy, and small bowel biopsy, which may raise the yield to 80%.

Therapy. Supportive therapy includes correction of fluid and electrolyte disturbances, antidiarrheal agents, treatment of specific pathogens, and in refractory cases using somatostatin analogs.

Diarrhea in AIDS

Diarrhea is very common (>50%) in patients with AIDS. Three clinical syndromes can be described

- Enteritis (crampy periumbilical abdominal pain, weight loss, large-volume diarrhea, and/or steatorrhea): cryptosporidiosis, Isospora belli, microsporidiosis, Mycobacterium avium-intracellulare complex, M. tuberculosis, Salmonella, Shigella, Campylobacter, Giardia, CMV, KS, lymphoma, idiopathic (HIV enteropathy)
- Proctocolitis (small-volume diarrhea, lower quadrant abdominal pain): Campylobacter, Shigella, Salmonella, Amebiasis, C-difficile, Chlamydia (LGV), CMV, Blastocystis hominis
- Proctitis (tenesmus, hematochezia, small-volume diarrhea): Herpes

simplex virus, N. Gonorrhea, Chlamydia, CMV, T. pallidum, lymphoma, trauma

Malabsorption

Characterized by weight loss and steatorrhea. May be generalized or highly selective.

PHYSIOPATHOLOGIC MECHANISMS

- Impaired intraluminal digestion: pancreatic disorders like chronic pancreatitis, pancreatic cancer, biliary obstruction
- Altered mucosal absorption: celiac sprue, abetalipoproteinemia
- Impaired transport from the mucosa to systemic circulation: lymphatic obstruction

DIAGNOSIS AND WORK-UP

- Initial laboratory studies should try to establish the presence of malabsorption. A quick screening test for fat malabsorption is a qualitative fecal fat test, or Sudan III stain. In the presence of moderate steatorrhea (>15 g/d of stool fat), the test has a sensitivity and specificity of 90–95%. The gold standard remains a 72-hour collection of stool for fecal fat analysis after the patient has been on a 100 g fat/d diet for 48 h. Massive steatorrhea (80–100 g fat/d in stool) is highly suspicious for pancreatic insufficiency. A D-xylose absorption test helps rule out small intestine disease. If the D-xylose absorption is abnormal, a small bowel biopsy either via endoscopy or by a suction tube (Rubin tube) is indicated. A small bowel aspirate to rule out the presence of Giardia should be done simultaneously. Serum Ca^{++} and magnesium should be measured as well as CBC, PT, vitamin B_{12} and folate, which may be abnormal in malabsorptive states
- Determination of the physiopathologic category will help tailor further work-up
- By far the most common causes of malabsorption in the Western world include: pancreatic insufficiency, bacterial overgrowth in association with GI surgery or dysmotility disorders (blind loop syndrome, ileal resection, small bowel diverticulosis, scleroderma), giardiasis, and lactose intolerance. A history and physical exam may provide clues (ingestion of unfiltered water, surgical history or abdominal scars, dietary history, etc.)
- Treatment is aimed at correcting specific disorders and nutrient deficiencies

INFLAMMATORY BOWEL DISEASE

Ulcerative Colitis

Ulcerative colitis is a recurrent inflammatory process of unknown etiology involving the mucosa and submucosa of the colon. The disease may be limited to the rectum, involve the left side of the colon, or extend in a continuous fashion to the cecum. Most cases start between the ages of 15 and 40; nevertheless, IBD in the elderly is well described. Clinical features include diarrhea with watery stools, rectal bleeding, and abdominal pain. Clinical presentation is variable. The disease is characterized by periods of remission and exacerbation. It is classified, according to symptoms, into mild, moderate, and severe. Patients with mild IBD usually have distal colonic/rectal involvement, often with mild diarrhea or insidious rectal bleeding, tenesmus, and mild cramping. Patients with moderate symptoms usually have ≤10 bowel movements a day, frequent bleeding, mild anemia, and abdominal pain. Patients with severe or fulminant symptoms usually have pancolitis, >10 bowel movements a day, bleeding requiring transfusion, severe abdominal pain, and fever.

DIAGNOSIS

After routine stool cultures have ruled out infectious processes, flexible sigmoidoscopy and biopsy readily establish the diagnosis, given that the disease *always* affects the rectum. Mucosal change includes edema, friability, loss of vascular pattern to macro-ulceration, and pseudopolyps.

THERAPY

Sulfasalazine. Efficacious in approximately 80% of patients with mild to moderate IBD. Also has a prophylactic role in patients in remission; 75% of patients maintained on sulfasalazine stay in remission for ≤3 years.

Sulfasalazine consists of sulfapyridine linked to 5-ASA by an azo bond. Intestinal bacteria cleave the bond, releasing 2 metabolites. Sulfapyridine is largely absorbed, metabolized by the liver, and excreted in the urine. The 5-ASA is mostly unabsorbed, stays in contact with the diseased mucosa, and is excreted in the feces. Most of the drug's side effects—such as headaches, nausea, and allergic reactions—can be traced to the sulfa moiety. *Dosage:* Starting dose is 0.5 mg po bid advancing as tolerated ≤2–4 g in 4 divided doses. Optimum maintenance dose is 2 g/d. *Side Effects*: ≤1/3 of patients may develop side effects. Headaches, nausea, malaise, and abdominal pain are the most common and are dose related. Idiosyncratic reactions include hemolytic anemia, aplastic anemia, hepatitis, pulmonary dysfunction, agranulocytosis, skin rash, fever, and occasionally Steven-Johnson syndrome. The drug should not be restarted in patients with hypersensitivity reactions.

Mesalamine: Mild to moderate colitis. *Dosage:* 1.2–2.4 g/d in 3 divided doses. Mesalamine enemas also available for distal colitis.

Olsalazine: Maintenance of remission. *Dosage:* 1–2 g po qd in 2 divided doses. Although these newer agents are as efficacious as sulfasalazines, and have fewer side effects, they are more costly.

Glucocorticoids: Successful in treating moderate to severe disease. Disease limited to the rectum and distal colon can be treated with glucocorticoid enemas (100 mg hydrocortisone Qhs, or 20 mg of methylprednisolone qd) for several weeks. More extensive disease should be treated with oral prednisone in doses of 40–60 mg qd. In patients responding promptly, withdrawal should be gradual at rates not exceeding a 5-mg ↓ q 3–7 days. If no improvement appears after 2–3 weeks of oral steroids, parenteral therapy should be considered. In the severely ill patient, hydrocortisone 50–100 mg IV q 6 h or prednisolone 100 mg in divided doses or by continuous infusion is recommended. Failure to improve after 2 weeks of therapy should indicate colectomy.

Azathioprine: Has a limited role in ulcerative colitis. Should be considered in patients who are refractory to conventional medical therapy and not surgical candidates. May also be used to ↓ the glucocorticoids maintenance dose in patients who cannot undergo surgery. The effects may not be apparent for ≤3 months. *Dosage:* 1.5 mg/kg/d orally with frequent CBC follow-up.

Antidiarrheals: Agents like diphenoxylate, loperamide, and tincture of opium must be used cautiously in patients with chronic IBD since they may precipitate ileus and even toxic megacolon in patients with active disease. Their use is contraindicated during an exacerbation.

Nutrition: No specific diet has been shown to help in this disorder: A low-roughage diet may provide symptomatic relief by decreasing stool weight. Lactose intolerance should be considered as possibly contributing to the symptoms. TPN is indicated to improve and maintain nutritional status but has not been shown to affect the cause of the disease for patients with disease so severe they require hospitalization.

Total Colectomy: Surgery is indicated in patients with refractory disease or complications (perforation, high-grade dysplasia, or severe toxic megacolon).

COMPLICATIONS

Toxic megacolon occurs in ≤10% of patients with ulcerative colitis. Clinical presentation is characterized by fever, abdominal pain, distention, and malaise. Physical exam reveals an ill-appearing patient with fever, dehydration, tachycardia, hypoactive bowel sounds, abdominal distention, and localized or diffuse rebound tenderness. Leukocytosis, anemia, and hypoalbuminemia are common laboratory findings. On plain abdominal radiography, dilation (usually by >7 cm) of the mid-transverse colon diameter is the most conspicuous finding.

TREATMENT

- Careful correction of fluid and electrolyte deficits. Particular attention should be paid to hypokalemia. 100 meq of KCl may be needed during the first 24 h
- Blood transfusions should be given to correct anemia and hypovolemia in the presence of colonic bleeding
- Nasogastric suction to prevent further bowel distention should be instituted
- IV glucocorticosteroids such as hydrocortisone 100 mg IV q 6 h should be started
- Parenteral antibiotics to cover for intra-abdominal sepsis should be administered
- Anticholinergics and opiates should be withdrawn
- Early surgical consultation is mandatory
- Total colectomy should be considered for patients who deteriorate or fail to improve within 48 h after aggressive medical therapy has been instituted

Colonic Cancer: Patients with ulcerative colitis have 10 times the risk for adenocarcinoma of the colon depending on the duration, extent, and severity of their IBD. The highest risk is in those with pancolitis and those who have had the disease for >10 years. Colonoscopy with biopsy surveillance for dysplasia is indicated. In patients in whom high-grade dysplasia or carcinoma is found, colectomy is indicated.

Crohn's Disease

May affect any portion of the GI tract. About 1/3 of patients have only small intestine involvement, with most of these cases occurring in the distal ileum; 20% may have only colonic involvement. In contrast to ulcerative colitis, Crohn's disease is a transmural process in which the inflammatory reaction extends through all layers of the bowel wall. On the serosal surface, mesenteric fat becomes hyperemic and edematous and encases the bowel wall ("creeping fat").

CLINICAL MANIFESTATIONS

- Diarrhea
- Crampy abdominal pain
- GI bleeding—in rare instances, massive
- Small bowel obstruction due to strictures
- Fistulas: enterovesical (pneumaturia), entero-cutaneous, and ano-rectal
- Bowel perforation

DIAGNOSIS

- Colonoscopy: very useful when Crohn's colitis is suspected. Findings include focal segmental colitis with aphthoid ulcerations in between normal mucosa
- Small bowel x rays: Remain the mainstay in the diagnosis of Crohn's disease of the small intestine. Radiologic features include nodularity, ulceration, stricture formation, and separation of bowel loops (due to small bowel thickening). In biopsy specimens, granulomas can be found in ≤30% of cases

TREATMENT

Sulfasalazine: In doses of ≤1 g po qid, is effective in mild to moderate disease, including colonic or ileocolic disease. Not helpful in ileal disease per se. No role for maintenance therapy.

Mesalamine: Can be used in mild to moderate Crohn's disease, but no advantage over sulfasalazine has been reported. Dosage: 1.2–2.4 g po qd in 3 divided doses.

6-Mercaptopurine: May be used in patients refractory to steroids or for steroid-sparing effect. Serious side effects include bone marrow suppression and pancreatitis. Careful follow-up CBCs are mandatory.

Glucocorticoids: Prednisone is beneficial in acute exacerbations. Dose is 20–40 mg po qd. In severe disease, IV glucocorticoids should be used, i.e., hydrocortisone 50–100 mg IV q 6 h.

Antibacterials: Metronidazole 250 mg po tid or ciprofloxacin have been shown to be effective in colonic disease and should be considered in patients intolerant of other agents.

Antidiarrheals: Can be used for mild exacerbation.

Nutrition: Specific replacement of B_{12} or folate may be necessary in patients with extensive ileal disease. Oxalate nephrolithiasis can be a problem; therefore, a low-oxalate diet is indicated.

Surgery: Reserved for complications such as obstruction, fistulae, perforations, or abscess.

COMPLICATIONS

- Intestinal Obstruction: May occur at a strictured segment. Treatment is supportive and consists of nasogastric suction, IV fluid replacement, and IV corticosteroids aimed at decreasing edema. Avoidance of seeds and indigestible foods (nuts, popcorn) should be recommended
- Fistulae: Medical management includes TPN, metronidazole (Flagyl), and perhaps 6-MP, which some studies have suggested may be useful although recurrences are high. Surgical evaluation should be obtained
- Perianal disease: Flagyl 250 mg po or IV tid may be useful

Pseudomembranous Colitis

Syndrome characterized by fever, diarrhea, and abdominal cramping that develops within 10 weeks of antibiotic therapy. Most of the cases are associated with Clostridium difficile.

CLINICAL MANIFESTATIONS

- Nonbloody diarrhea, but blood may be present in ≤10% of cases; fever; leukocytosis; fecal leukocytes in 50% of cases; rebound tenderness in 10–20% of cases; although usually left-sided, 10% of cases may involve the right colon

DIAGNOSIS

- Proctosigmoidoscopy: pseudomembranes seen in 85–90% of cases. Positive C-difficile toxin in ≤90% of cases

TREATMENT

- Vancomycin 125 mg po q 6 h for 7 days
- Metronidazole 250 mg po q 6 h for 7 days
- IV metronidazole 500 mg q 6 h should be given to patients with ileus or where questionable oral absorption is suspected
- Relapses usually respond to repeated courses of the above agents

Diverticular Disease

Diverticula is herniation of colonic mucosa and submucosa through the bowel wall. It is thought to be due to ↓ in dietary fiber, which causes ↓ transit time, ↓ stool bulk, ↑ straining at stool, and ↑ colonic segmentation, which ↑ intracolonic pressure. In Western countries, 5% of the population is affected by age 40, increasing linearly to 50% by age 80.

CLINICAL MANIFESTATIONS

- Asymptomatic diverticulosis
- Spastic diverticular disease (constipation, left lower quadrant pain, postprandial distention; no fever or peritoneal signs present)
- Diverticulitis (left lower quadrant pain, fever, leukocytosis; may have sign of peritoneal irritation)
- Diverticular bleeding
- Complications: abscess formation, perforation, fistulae to bladder or skin

TREATMENT

For spastic diverticular disease, management includes reassurance of the patient and ↑ dietary fiber. Metamucil 2 tsp bid may be required for complete relief of constipation. Antispasmodic drugs like dicyclomine 20 mg po qid can be used for painful episodes. For very mild diverticulitis, a clear liquid diet with an oral antibiotic (ampicillin, tetracycline, or a cephalosporin) may be given. Standard therapy for acute diverticulitis consists of bowel rest with NPO. If abdominal distention is present, consider nasogastric suction. Antibiotic therapy to cover intra-abdominal sepsis is indicated.

GALLSTONES

Epidemiology

- It is estimated that 20 million Americans have gallstones and that 1 million new cases develop each year. Gallstones can be divided according to composition into cholesterol and pigment stones. Cholesterol stones, which account for 80–90% of gallstones, are mostly radiolucent, solitary, tan or clay-colored, and larger than pigment stones, which are multiple, small, and black or brown. Chemical dissolution therapy is only effective on cholesterol stones
- Risk factors for cholesterol gallstones: female gender, pregnancy, estrogen therapy, age, ileal disorders, obesity, and gallbladder stasis (patient receiving TPN or somatostatin)
- Risk factors for pigment gallstones: hemolytic disorders, cirrhosis

Clinical Presentation

- Asymptomatic: Prophylactic cholecystectomy is recommended only for children and patients with sickle cell disease
- Biliary pain: Recurrent right upper quadrant or epigastric pain is steady, lasts several hours, and self-resolves. Irradiates to right scapula or right shoulder
- Acute cholecystitis: severe abdominal pain, nausea, vomiting, fever, leukocytosis
- Choledocholithiasis: present with biliary pain. Can be associated with cholangitis (infection of the bile ducts) or gallstone pancreatitis

Diagnosis

- Ultrasonography can detect stones >1–2 mm in size
- Oral cholecystography
- Nuclear cholesyntigraphy: permits rapid evaluation of gallbladder function when cholecystitis is suspected

Treatment

Cholecystectomy is the best treatment for recurrent symptomatic cholelithiasis and acute cholecystitis. It can be performed in standard fashion or via a laparoscope. No studies comparing both techniques are available, but shorter hospital stay and rapid recovery time has made laparoscopic cholecystectomy very popular.

ORAL DISSOLUTION THERAPY

- This is an alternative option. Ursodeochycolic acid 300 mg po bid or in combination with chenodeoxycholic acid 375 mg qd for symptomatic cholelithiasis can achieve complete dissolution of small cholesterol stones in patients who refuse or are not candidates for surgery. Dissolution rate is 1 mm per month. Recurrence after dissolution is approximately 43% after 4 years
- Indications and criteria for treatment: radiolucent stones, patent cystic duct, stones <2 cm in diameter, and floating stones. Not indicated for the management of acute cholecystitis or complicated biliary disease (choledocholithiasis or gallstone pancreatitis)
- *Side Effects:* diarrhea, reversible elevation of aminotransaminases
- Contact dissolution therapy requires percutaneous catheter into the gallbladder or an endoscopically placed nasobiliary catheter
- Methyl-tert-butyl: Instillation can achieve dissolution in 24 h. If contact with duodenum is severe, mucosal irritation can be seen. Recurrence is a significant problem
- Extracorporeal biliary lithotripsy: uses focused high-amplitude sound waves to fragment stones. Experience with this technique is limited and, in available series, only 25–30% of referred patients were suitable candidates. Longterm concomitant oral dissolution therapy may be required, and the abnormal gallbladder remains in place
- Choledocholithiasis: Endoscopic retrograde cholangiopancreatography (ERCP) with sphincterotomy and stone removal is an extremely valuable alternative to open common bile duct exploration for treatment of symptomatic choledocholithiasis (cholangitis or gallstone pancreatitis). In a recent study of patients with cholangitis and bile duct stones, emergency endoscopic biliary drainage was associated with less morbidity and mortality than immediate surgery

PANCREATITIS

Acute Pancreatitis

- Conditions associated with pancreatitis include: alcoholism, gallstones, drugs (e.g., Azathioprine, thiazides, valproic acid, and pentamidine), hyperlipemia, hypercalcemia, and trauma

- Clinical manifestations: severe unremitting epigastric pain that frequently radiates to the back and is usually accompanied by nausea and vomiting
- Physical exam in patients with mild pancreatitis reveals epigastric tenderness and guarding. Bowel sounds are hypoactive or absent. In severe disease, signs of vascular collapse may be present, with tachycardia and hypertension. A mass may be palpable in the epigastrium. Tachypnea may be present secondary to pulmonary complications from pancreatitis (pleural effusion, ARDS). Mild fever (37.5–38.5° C) is commonly seen

DIAGNOSIS

- Serum amylase elevation twofold or more
- Elevation of serum lipase helpful in patients who present late in the clinical course (remains elevated longer than amylase) or when diagnosis unclear
- Dynamic CT scan is very useful in confirming diagnosis and evaluating complications

MANAGEMENT

- Mainly supportive. Specific therapy treats complications
- Narcotic analgesics: Meperidine is the most commonly used agent that has no significant effect on the sphincter of Oddi
- Patient should be kept NPO until pain and nausea resolve. Nasogastric suction is indicated in patients with recurrent vomiting or symptomatic abdominal distention from an ileus
- Aggressive fluid resuscitation with lactate ringer or normal saline with careful monitoring of input/output
- Antibiotics have no proven role in the management of acute pancreatitis
- Serum Ca^{++}, Mg, glucose, triglycerides, and hematocrit should be monitored and corrected as necessary
- Patients with prolonged bowel rest should be started on TPN

COMPLICATIONS

- Infection: infected phlegmon or abscess is suspected when high, spiking fever with an elevated WBC occurs ≥7 days into the course of the illness. A CT scan of the pancreas with a "skinny needle" aspiration of peripancreatic fluid collection, may show bacteria on Gram's stain which suggests the diagnosis. Treatment includes surgical damage and in very selected cases percutaneous damage via CT-guided catheter placement with parenteral broad-spectrum antibiotics
- Pseudocysts: Should be suspected in the presence of persistent pain or hyperamylasemia. Most acute pseudocysts will subside spontaneously within several weeks. Large (>5 cm) pseudocysts that persist for >6 weeks should be treated surgically or percutaneously, as they may become infected or bleed
- Pulmonary complications: Include pleural effusions, atelectasis, or ARDS in the severely ill patient
- Renal insufficiency: May be due to prerenal azotemia or ATN. Careful monitoring of fluid balance, serum creatinine, and BUN are necessary. Occasionally patients require peritoneal dialysis or hemodialysis support

- Surgery: Indicated in complicated pancreatitis, i.e., abscess, hemorrhagic pancreatitis, or persistent pseudocyst
- Endoscopic therapy: In patients with gallstone pancreatitis, ERCP with sphincterotomy may have a role in removing obstructing gallstones and decompressing the biliary tree

Chronic Pancreatitis

- Alcohol is the leading cause of chronic pancreatitis. Other conditions include hereditary pancreatitis, cystic fibrosis, hemochromatosis, and tropical obstructive pancreatitis (India, Southern Africa, Indonesia)
- Clinical manifestation includes chronic pain and exocrine and endocrine insufficiency manifested by diabetes, steatorrhea, and weight loss. It should be suspected in any patient with abdominal pain, diabetes, steatorrhea, or jaundice

DIAGNOSIS

- ≤30% of patients have pancreatic calcifications on plain abdominal x rays
- Stool sample for Sudan III staining
- Bentiromide test: after an overnight fast, 500 mg of *N*-benzoyl-L-tryosila-para-aminobenzoic acid (NBT-PABA) is given and a 6-hour urine collection performed. If the PABA ↑ in the urine is <50%, the probability of severe pancreatic insufficiency is significant
- CT scan may reveal pancreatic calcification, ductal dilation, or the presence of pseudocysts
- ERCP may show specific roentgenographic changes of chronic pancreatitis and can help in differentiating pancreatitis from pancreatic cancer

MANAGEMENT

- Pain: Narcotics are frequently needed. Large meals, fatty foods, and alcohol should be avoided. The role of pancreatic enzymes in pain management remains controversial. Celiac plexus block may give initial relief in ≤70% of patients, but by 6 months only 50% continue to show benefit
- Surgery should be reserved until no other modalities are available. Drainage procedures are indicated when dilated ducts are present, and they can relieve pain in ≤70% of cases. The role of pancreatic resection in patients without ductal dilation is more controversial
- Exocrine insufficiency: Treatment consists of a low-fat diet (<50 g/d) and oral pancreatic supplement. A variety of agents is available; a nonenteric coated medication with a total lipase content of 20,000–40,000 U per meal is adequate. Enzyme replacements should be taken 30 mins before the meal and at bedtime. If no improvement occurs, 650 mg of sodium bicarbonate or an H_2 receptor antagonist can be given before meals to prevent degradation by gastric acid. If switching to an enteric coated preparation, the bicarbonate or H_2 receptor antagonist should be discontinued
- Endocrine insufficiency: Pancreatic diabetes usually requires insulin therapy

Suggested Reading

Calleja GA, Barkin JS: Acute pancreatitis. Med Clin North Am. *77*: 1037, 1993.

Chopra S: Peptic ulcer disease. *In* Chopra S, May RJ (eds.), Pathophysiology of Gastrointestinal Disease. Little Brown and Company, Boston, 1989, pp 71–96.

Graham DY, Lew GM, Klein PD, et al.: Effect of treatment of helicobacter pylori infection on long-term recurrence of gastric or duodenal ulcer. Ann Intern Med *116*:705, 1992.

Griffing MR, Piper HM, Daugherty JR, et al.: Non-steroidal anti-inflammatory drug use—an increased risk for peptic ulcer disease in elderly persons. Ann Intern Med *114*:257, 1991.

Hanauer SB: Medical therapy of ulcerative colitis. Lancet *342*:412, 1993.

Hentschel E, Brandstatter G, Dragosics B, et al.: Effect of ranitidine and amoxicillin on the eradication of Helicobacter pylori and the recurrence of duodenal ulcer. N Engl J Med *328*:308, 1993.

Johnston DE, Kaplan MM: Pathogenesis and treatment of gallstones. N Engl J Med *328*:412, 1993.

Marshall JB: Acute pancreatitis. A review with emphasis on new developments. Arch Intern Med *153*:1185, 1993.

NIH Consensus Conference: Gallstones and laparoscopic cholescystotomy. JAMA *269*:1018, 1993.

Peppercorn, MA: Advances in the drug therapy for inflammatory bowel disease. Ann Intern Med *112*:50, 1990.

Liver Disorders

25

Sanjiv Chopra and Irving Waxman

Because specific therapy of liver diseases involves mainly management of their complications, most of this chapter focuses on that. *The second part of the chapter deals with the now commonly encountered hepatobiliary manifestations of AIDS.*

Complications of severe liver disease can be dramatic and life threatening. They are most frequently encountered in patients with cirrhosis of the liver. The complications are listed in Table 25–1.

VARICEAL BLEEDING

Variceal bleeding is most often encountered in patients with cirrhosis of the liver and significant portal hypertension, defined as: Elevation in the portal pressure >22 mm Hg when measured directly during surgery, a portal pressure that > that of the IVC by >8 mm Hg when measured by the percutaneous transhepatic route, or a wedged hepatic venous pressure that > that of the IVC by >5 mm of mercury. This gradient, referred to as the portal vein pressure gradient, is >10 mm Hg in patients with clinically significant portal hypertension. Esophageal varices are demonstrable in 50–75% of patients with cirrhosis of the liver. Rupture of varices is likely to occur in patients with large varices; with cirrhosis of the liver, Grade Child's B or C; and who at the time of endoscopy have cherry red spots or red wale markings on the varices.

Portal hypertension is classified as presinusoidal, sinusoidal, or postsinusoidal. Presinusoidal causes of portal hypertension include portal vein thrombosis, splenic vein thrombosis, schistosomiasis, congenital hepatic fibrosis, sarcoidosis, and myeloid metaplasia. Cirrhosis of the liver and severe chronic active hepatitis are examples of sinusoidal portal hypertension. Examples of postsinusoidal portal hypertension include

Table 25–1
Complications of Liver Disease

1. Variceal bleeding
2. Hepatic encephalopathy
3. Ascites
4. Spontaneous bacterial peritonitis
5. Hepatorenal syndrome
6. Altered hemostasis
7. Disorders of pulmonary function
8. Abnormalities of the endocrine system
9. Increased susceptibility to a variety of infections
10. Primary hepatocellular carcinoma

veno-occlusive disease, Budd-Chiari syndrome, constrictive pericarditis, and CHF.

Bleeding from esophageal varices is often dramatic. It may manifest as hematemesis or melena. The diagnosis of variceal bleeding is best established by endoscopy. Approximately 30% of patients with advanced alcoholic cirrhosis and variceal bleeding succumb during the initial hospital stay.

Management of patients with variceal bleeding is best done in an ICU. The major aim is to stop the acute variceal bleeding. Steps to prevent recurrent variceal bleeding also need to be taken.

- Patients should receive appropriate blood and, if necessary, fresh frozen plasma replacement
- If the bleeding is torrential, a bolus of 20 units of IV vasopressin in 100 ml of 5% dextrose should be given IV over a 10-minute period. Vasopressin infusion results in cessation of bleeding in a significant number of patients, but its utility is limited by a high rate of rebleeding and failure to show improvement in the rate of survival
- Another agent that may be useful is somatostatin, 50–250 micrograms as a bolus and 250 ug/h as an IV infusion
- Balloon tamponade, endoscopic sclerotherapy, rubber band ligation, and emergency shunt procedures are discussed in Chapter 23

ASCITES

Ascites refers to the accumulation of serous fluid within the abdominal cavity. Important causes of ascites are listed in Table 25–2.

Ascites and edema in patients with liver disease occur as a result of avid Na^+ retention by the kidney, ↑ splanchnic lymph flow, elevated hydrostatic pressure in the hepatic sinusoids or portal vein, and ↓ plasma oncotic pressure.

Major hypotheses for the formation of ascites include the following

- In the underfill hypothesis the primary event is portal hypertension. The ↑ physical force drives fluid into the abdominal cavity, resulting in redistribution of the plasma volume. Although the total volume is

Table 25–2
Important Causes of Ascites

1. Cirrhosis of the liver.
2. Metastatic peritoneal carcinomatosis.
3. Congestive heart failure and constrictive pericarditis.
4. Tuberculosis peritonitis.
5. Fungal peritonitis.
6. Pancreatic ascites.
7. Budd-Chiari syndrome and veno-occlusive disease.
8. Nephrogenic ascites.
9. Myxedema ascites.
10. Bile ascites.
11. Peritoneal mesothelioma.
12. Pseudomyxoma peritonei.
13. Eosinophilic gastroenteritis.
14. Meig's syndrome

↑, the effective circulating volume—that is, the component of circulating plasma volume that stimulates volume receptors—decreases. As a result, "the kidneys believe their owner is underfilled," leading to avid Na^+ and water retention by the kidneys and further aggravation of the existing fluid derangement. Na+ retention is mediated by the hormone aldosterone (the renin angiotensin aldosterone system is stimulated)

- In the overflow hypothesis, the primary event is believed to be inappropriately ↑ Na^+ retention by the kidneys. Vasomotor derangements (A-V shunting and ↓ peripheral resistance) commonly occur in patients with cirrhosis, thus initiating this primary event. The result is ↓ renal blood flow. Na^+ retention by the kidneys leads to expansion of the plasma volume, which is preferentially sequestered in the peritoneal cavity secondary to ↑ hydrostatic pressure and ↓ oncotic pressure within the portal venous bed and hepatic sinusoids
- In the peripheral arterial vasodilation hypothesis, cirrhotics have peripheral arterial vasodilation because of the presence of A-V fistulas in the dermal and pulmonary circulation and the splanchnic vascular bed. This leads to a ↓ "effective" plasma volume and activation of compensatory hormonal systems (renin, angiotensin, aldosterone, vasopressin), with resultant Na^+ retention by the kidneys
- It has recently been proposed that NO acts as an endogenous vasodilator mediating the hyperdynamic circulation of cirrhosis. The trigger for NO release is bacterial endotoxin

Systemic endotoxemia occurs because of portosystemic shunts and is commonly present in patients with cirrhosis.

Clinical Features

Ascites may be first noticed by the patient, a friend, or a physician. Its presence can be detected on physical examination by demonstrating shifting dullness and/or a positive fluid wave. Patients with tense ascites may have an everted umbilicus. In patients in whom it is not certain on clinical examination whether ascites is present, ultrasonic examination should be performed prior to a diagnostic paracentesis. Patients with ascites may on occasion have pleural effusions and striking penile, scrotal, and peripheral edema. Ascites is present in virtually all patients having spontaneous bacterial peritonitis, hepatorenal syndrome, Budd-Chiari syndrome, and veno-occlusive disease.

Complications of ascites include abdominal discomfort, respiratory embarrassment, rupture of umbilical hernia, and spontaneous bacterial peritonitis.

Analysis of Ascitic Fluid

Traditionally the fluid is characterized as a transudate or exudate based on its protein content. Patients with a protein concentration >2.5 g/dl are considered to have exudative ascites. Common causes of exudative ascitic fluid include metastatic peritoneal carcinomatosis, tuberculous peritonitis, pancreatic ascites, Budd-Chiari syndrome, myxedema ascites, and peritoneal mesothelioma. About 10% of patients with uncomplicated cirrhosis of the liver may have ascitic fluids classifiable as exudative based on the above criteria. Additionally, patients with CHF may have exudative ascitic fluid (based on protein content). Causes of transudative ascites include cirrhosis of the liver, alcoholic hepatitis, chronic active hepatitis, and nephrotic syndrome. Hemorrhagic or bloody ascites occurs in patients with malignant disease (notably hepatoma), Budd-Chiari syndrome, tuberculous peritonitis, or trauma. Chylous ascites refers to the presence of grossly milky, creamy, or turbid peritoneal fluid and an elevated triglyceride >200 mg/dl. Causes of chylous ascites in children include malignancy and congenital abnormalities of the lymphatic system. Trauma and tuberculosis are other causes. The protein concentration of chylous ascites ranges from <2 g/dl to >6 g/dl. Pancreatic ascites refers to the accumulation of ascitic fluid in a patient with complicated pancreatitis such as a ruptured pancreatic duct or a leaking pseudocyst. The ascitic fluid amylase is always elevated. Recently it has been proposed that ascitic fluid be classified based on serum-ascites albumin concentration gradient (SAAG). SAAG = [Δ serum albumin]–[Ascitic fluid albumin]. If the SAAG is ≥1.1 g/dl, the patient has portal hypertension with greater than 90% accuracy.

Management of Ascites

- In rare instances treatment aimed at correcting the underlying pathophysiologic abnormalities results in the cure of ascites. Examples include tuberculous peritonitis, pancreatitis ascites, and Budd-Chiari syndrome due to the presence of a web in the inferior vena cava
- Bed rest and dietary Na^+ restriction. Na^+ intake should be restricted to 500 mg–1 g of Na^+
- Spironolactone, 300–1,000 mg per day is the recommended diuretic. This is superior to furosemide in initiating diuresis in patients with cirrhosis and ascites, although furosemide or hydrochlorothiazide should be added if high-dose spironolactone therapy is not effective
- Large-volume paracentesis. Up to 5 l of fluid may be removed slowly while patients are clinically monitored. Paracentesis should be followed by IV infusion of 40 g of albumin, particularly if there is no peripheral edema or if renal function is marginal
- Peritovenous shunts (Levine or Denver shunts) may be useful in 5% of patients with ascites refractory to all medical therapy. Complications include disseminated intervascular coagulation, shunt occlusion, fever, and a unique form of small bowel obstruction
- Portosystemic Shunts. Side-to-side portocaval shunts decompress both the splanchnic and hepatic sinusoidal bed
- Liver transplantation

Spontaneous Bacterial Peritonitis

- SBP may be defined as bacterial peritonitis that occurs in patients with ascites in the absence of demonstrable causes of peritonitis such as intra-abdominal abscesses or bowel perforation. It occurs in 10–25% of hospitalized patients with ascites. The unifying feature of the type of ascites susceptible to SBP is a low protein concentration of ascitic fluid (characteristically <1 g/dl). Patients are at risk for developing SBP because of defects in reticuloendothelial system function, defects in neutrophil function, complement deficiency, and opsinization impairment
- All cirrhotic patients with ascites and evidence of any clinical deterioration (which may be subtle and include mild worsening of hepatic encephalopathy, low-grade fever, leukocytosis, hypotension, hypothermia, low back pain, or refractoriness to diuretics) should undergo a diagnostic paracentesis
- The diagnosis can be made when the ascitic fluid contains >250 polymorphonuclear leukocytes. The highest yield on ascitic fluid cultures is derived by obtaining 10 ml of ascitic fluid and inoculating it at the bedside into blood culture bottles

- The most common organisms include E. coli, pneumococcus, and streptococcus. Polymicrobial organisms and anaerobes are encountered very infrequently, and their presence should raise the suspicion that the patient has secondary bacterial peritonitis due to an intra-abdominal process
- The distinguishing features of spontaneous bacterial peritonitis and secondary bacterial peritonitis include the initial ascitic fluid white count and protein concentrations. In patients who have an exudative fluid or an initial ascitic fluid WBC >10,000, the assumption can be made that they have bacterial peritonitis secondary to an intra-abdominal abscess or perforation. CT scans, barium contrast studies, and surgical consultation are required in such patients

Treatment of SBP

Empiric antibiotic therapy with the third-generation cephalosporin (cefotaxime or ceftriaxone) should be instituted in suspected cases. Aminoglycosides should not be used, as they may result in precipitation of renal failure and confusion with hepatorenal syndrome. Cefotaxime, 2 g IV q 8 h for a total of 7–10 days is frequently effective. (See Chapter 26.)

Mortality is 30–40%. Poor prognostic factors include a serum bilirubin >8 mg/dl, serum albumin <2.5 g/dl, serum creatinine >2.1 mg/dl, hepatic encephalopathy, and development of hepatorenal syndrome. Recurrence of SBP is common in patients surviving an episode. SBP is an expression of severe end-stage liver disease, and patients should be evaluated for liver transplantation.

HEPATORENAL SYNDROME

- This dreaded complication occurs in patients with end-stage liver disease. It is defined as unexplained renal failure occurring in patients with liver or biliary tract disease in the absence of clinical, pathologic, or anatomic evidence of other known causes of renal failure. Its pathogenesis is unknown. Pathologic abnormalities in the kidneys are trivial and inconstant. Postmortem angiography shows striking reversal of the pronounced corticomedullary shunting of blood in the kidney
- Recovery from hepatorenal syndrome can occur after successful orthotopic liver transplantation. Kidneys from patients with hepatorenal syndrome have functioned normally when transplanted into patients with end-stage kidney disease and normal hepatic function. All this points to the fact that the nature of renal failure is indeed functional
- Hepatorenal syndrome is almost invariably encountered in patients who have already been admitted to a hospital with severe end-stage liver disease, are suffering a number of complications, and are being subjected to a variety of treatments. Thus, in some patients it appears that hepatorenal syndrome is precipitated by GI bleeding, paracentesis, excessive diuretic use, infection, or medication. Aminoglycosides and NSAIDs should be avoided in patients with severe liver disease

Diagnosis

- Most patients with hepatorenal syndrome have severe hepatocellular disease with characteristic abnormalities in hepatic synthetic func-

tion such as prolongation of the prothrombin time and a low serum albumin. Hyperbilirubinemia is common. The serum ALT and AST levels are variably elevated. Hyponatremia is common, and partially compensated respiratory alkalosis is frequently encountered. The BUN and creatinine values are elevated in the mild to moderate range
- The salient urinary analysis findings include a normal urine sediment, a urine osmolality that is ≥100 mOsm >plasma osmolality, a urine to plasma creatinine >30:1, and a daily urine Na^+ excretion of <10 meq (urine Na^+ is frequently <3 meq/liter and often 0 meq/liter). These findings are not specific for hepatorenal syndrome and can be identical to those seen in patients with prerenal azotemia

Management

- Avoid making the diagnosis, which is a way of saying that the physician should look for causes of "pseudohepatorenal syndrome." Exclude hypovolemia, obstructive uropathy, urinary tract infection, and electrolyte imbalances
- Discontinue any potentially offending drugs, such as aminoglycosides, NSAIDs, or lactulose
- Trial of volume expansion. Ideally, salt-poor albumin should be infused under carefully monitored conditions with the use of a Swan-Ganz catheter with measurements of PCWP as a guide
- Appropriate nutritional support
- There is no proven therapy for hepatorenal syndrome, with the exception of liver transplantation
- Although scattered anecdotal reports suggest that portocaval shunting, peritoneovenous shunting, and TIPS may result in reversal of hepatorenal syndrome, they are as of yet of unproven efficacy

HEPATIC ENCEPHALOPATHY

Hepatic encephalopathy can be defined as a neuropsychiatric syndrome characterized by intellectual deterioration, altered state of consciousness, and personality changes in a patient with severe liver diseases and/or portosystemic shunting. It can occur in 2 major settings

- acute fulminant hepatic failure, and
- portosystemic encephalopathy and variant syndromes

Pathogenesis

The diffuse nature of the neurologic process and its potential for restoration to complete normality suggest that metabolic factors are operative. The diseased liver is unable to detoxify a toxin or a number of toxins, which then affects cerebral function, resulting in encephalopathy. The inability to detoxify is due to severe hepatocellular injury. Alternatively, although liver function is intact, the putative toxin(s) bypasses the liver because of shunting. The various putative toxins include ammonia, mercaptines, short-chain fatty acids, and gamma aminobutyric acid.

The diagnosis of hepatic encephalopathy is based on a constellation of findings that include the following

- The obligatory presence of liver disease and/or portosystemic shunting

Table 25–3
Causes of Hepatic Encephalopathy, and their Mechanism

CAUSE	PRESUMED MECHANISM
Gastrointestinal bleeding	Substrate for increased production of ammonia and other nitrogenous toxins. 100 ml of blood = 15–20 g protein. Contribution of ammonia in stored blood. Hypovolemia: Decreased hepatic, cerebral and renal perfusion.
Sedatives and tranquilizers	Hypoxia from depression of respiratory center. Direct depressant effect on brain.
Constipation	Increased production and absorption of toxins (eg ammonia) due to increased contact time between nitrogenous substances in gut and intestinal bacteria. Straining leads to increased portal pressure and may induce variceal rupture.
Uremia (spontaneous or diuretic)	Increased enterohepatic circulation of urea nitrogen with increased ammonia production. Direct depressant effect of uremia. Increased renal vein ammonia output if alkalosis present. Hypovolemia (overvigorous diuresis) leads to decreased vital organ perfusion
Infection	Increased tissue metabolism, leading to increased endogenous nitrogenous load and increased ammonia production. Hypoxemia, hyperthermia augment ammonia toxicity.
Excess dietary protein	Increased substrate for ammonia production.

- Abnormal mental state (confusion, restlessness, reversal of sleep rhythm)
- Abnormal neuromuscular state (asterixis)
- Variably present clinical features (fetor hepaticus, hyperventilation)
- Characteristic pathologic findings (elevations in arterial ammonia and an abnormal EEG)
- A favorable response to appropriate therapy in most patients

Hepatic encephalopathy should be a clinical diagnosis and can be easily made by the astute clinician. If the patient has evidence of liver disease by either physical examination or laboratory features and has any of the above-mentioned features, the diagnosis should be made and therapy instituted. Obtaining an EEG or arterial pneumonia is not usually necessary.

The precipitating causes of hepatic encephalopathy and their presumed mechanism are shown in Table 25–3. They are nitrogenous or non-nitrogenous. Examples of the former include dietary protein, constipation, GI bleeding, uremia, and infection. Non-nitrogenous precipitants include sedative drugs, hepatocellular injury, and infection.

Treatment

- Identify and correct precipitating factors
- Dietary protein restriction is instituted for patients with Stage 1 and

2 encephalopathy. For patients with Stage 3 or 4 encephalopathy, protein intake is withheld and then reinstituted in slow increments (10–20 grams per day) every 3–5 days as the patient's condition improves (Table 25–4). Some patients better tolerate vegetable proteins
- Cleansing the bowel is important. Lactulose is administered in a daily dose of 60–120 ml in divided amounts to promote 2 or 3 soft stools daily. In patients with coma, lactulose may be given as an enema of 300 ml in 700 ml of water. **Caution:** Lactulose can precipitate or worsen hepatorenal syndrome (see p. 432). In refractory cases, neomycin, 1 g po may be given bid
- Experimental agents that appear promising include benzodiazepine receptor antagonists such as Flumazenil

HEPATOBILIARY MANIFESTATIONS OF AIDS

Hepatobiliary disorders are frequently encountered in patients with AIDS. This phenomenon is undoubtedly a reflection of the profound immunosuppression present in these patients and leads to the ↑ propensity for a multitude of opportunistic infections and neoplasms. In addition, the epi demiologic risks for AIDS, such as homosexuality and IV drug abuse, expose the patient to a variety of infectious processes that can occur prior to the onset of AIDS. Laboratory assessment of hepatic function discloses abnormalities in the vast majority of patients. At times the hepatic or biliary disorder is asymptomatic or trivial in its significance, while in other instances it is the cause of significant morbidity and even mortality.

Hepatitis B

- Markers of hepatitis B virus (HBV) infection are very common in patients with AIDS. Serologic evidence of past or current HBV infection is present in 80–95% of patients. Most of these markers reflect previous (80%) rather than active (10–20%) infection
- Patients with established HIV infection who subsequently become infected with HBV have a substantially ↑ risk of becoming chronic HBV carriers compared with HIV seronegative controls. However, despite active HBV replication, patients have minimal biochemical and histologic signs of inflammation
- The immunologic impairment secondary to HIV infection appears to be responsible for the attenuated clinical course of acute and chronic HBV infection seen in these patients
- Fulminant viral hepatitis B in a patient with AIDS has been reported in the setting of hepatitis Delta virus coinfection
- In a recent study, the prevalence of HBsAg was > twice as great (10.7% vs. 4.7%; $p<0.02$) in patients with AIDS compared to HIV positive patients without AIDS. However, survival of HBsAg positive patients was similar to that of HBsAg negative patients. These findings support the notion that patients with the more advanced immunosuppression characteristic of AIDS are more likely to have reactivation of latent HBV infection, are less likely to clear HBV infection after exposure, or both. However, survival was not influenced in either group by the presence of hepatitis B surface antigen

Table 25–4
Stages of Hepatic Encephalopathy

STAGE	MENTAL STATE	ASTERIXIS	EEG	% MORTALITY*
I	Loss of affect, depression, altered sleep pattern	(±)	Normal	20
II	Confusion, disorientation, drowsiness	(+)	Abnormal	60
III	Stuporous, incoherent but arousable	(+)	Abnormal	60
IV	Not arousable, decerebrate/decorticate posturing	Not testable	Abnormal	80

* Applicable to patients with massive hepatic necrosis. Age of patient is important prognostic indicator. Mortality rate higher in patients over 40 years of age.

Hepatitis C

- HCV infection is common in patients who are HIV positive. In about 15% of HIV positive patients, the HCV antibody is positive. Of these patients, 50% have hepatitis C viremia
- Recent studies suggest that there is a tendency for HIV positive patients to have higher levels of viremia
- Severe liver disease with rapid progression to cirrhosis and liver failure has been noted in some patients with both HIV and HCV antibody positivity
- There is limited data on the efficacy of alphainterferon in the treatment of such patients. In a recently published study, 4 of 12 patients had a complete response, while 3 of 12 had a near-complete response. However a sustained response, that is, persistently normal LFTs after cessation of interferon treatment, was only seen in a single patient

Other Infections

- Approximately 30–50% of liver biopsies performed in patients with AIDS will yield evidence of an infectious organism. Infections may be multiple
- MAI, CMV, Mycobacterium tuberculosis, Pneumocystis carinii, Histoplasmosis, Cryptococcosis, Leishmaniasis, Coccidiomycosis and Microsporidiosis have all been reported
- MAI is often associated with a substantial elevation of the serum alkaline phosphatase (mean 750 IU/l) and a normal serum bilirubin. Pathologically there may be granulomas which are often poorly formed. Occasionally the cultures will be positive with no tissue evidence of infection. This has been seen with MAI and TB
- Hepatosplenomegaly is commonly present in patients with MAI infections. 80% of MAI-infected individuals have liver involvement at autopsy. Currently recommended regimens for the treatment of MAI include a combination of Amikacin, Rifampin (or Rifabutin), Ethambutol and Ciprofloxacin

Peliosis Hepatis

- Sinusoidal dilation, perisinusoidal fibrosis and peliosis hepatis are frequently encountered in patients with AIDS
- The lesion consists of multiple, small, blood-filled cystic spaces in the liver without zonal predominance
- Patients frequently have hepatomegaly and splenomegaly
- On average the serum ALT and AST are twice the upper limit of normal, and the serum alkaline phosphatase is 5 times the upper limit of normal. The serum bilirubin is normal or slightly elevated
- Both peliosis hepatis and cutaneous bacillary angiomatosis have been reported in patients with HIV infection
- Recent evidence suggests that peliosis hepatis is due to a Rickettsia-like organism closely related to R. quintana. Patients may respond favorably to Erythromycin

Tumors

- Neoplastic lesions are present in 10–20% of liver biopsies
- KS is a frequent finding at autopsy but is rarely seen at liver biopsy.

Lymphomas both of the Hodgkin's and non-Hodgkin's variety also frequently involve the liver

- Patients with non-Hodgkin's lymphoma involving the liver have a marked elevation of the serum alkaline phosphatase (mean 900 IU/l) and a mild elevation of the serum bilirubin (4 mg/dl)
- Primary bile duct lymphoma has also been described

Acalculous Cholecystitis

Disorders of the biliary system noted in patients with AIDS are listed in Table 25–5.

The triad of right upper quadrant abdominal pain, fever, and an elevated serum alkaline phosphatase is present in a number of syndromes which on occasion overlap.

- The range of symptoms includes mild right upper quadrant pain, evaluation of which may reveal thickening of the gallbladder wall on sonographic examination, as well as fulminant gangrenous cholecystitis
- Acalculous cholecystitis has been associated with CMV, Cryptosporidiosis, Candida, Campylobacter, and Serratia
- Both acute and chronic changes may be present at the time of histologic examination. The gallbladder mucosa is often hemorrhagic, with focal punctuate ulcers and exudates. Severe necrotizing inflammation can be present in patients with acalculous cholecystitis secondary to CMV. The characteristic inclusions can be seen in epithelial and endothelial cells

Sclerosing Cholangitis

- Patients may be asymptomatic or have mild symptoms. On occasion patients can have severe right upper quadrant or epigastric pain with nausea and vomiting
- It may be complicated by acute polymicrobial cholangitis and sepsis
- Some patients have accompanying papillary stenosis
- Sclerosing cholangitis has been reported in patients with CMV, Cryptosporidiosis, MAI, and Microsporidia
- ERCP reveals the characteristic picture with strictures, dilation, and ulcerations of the biliary tree
- Endoscopic sphincterotomy has resulted in symptomatic improvement in some patients. Rapid drainage of contrast material can be achieved with successful sphincterotomy. Although the serum alkaline phos-

Table 25–5
Biliary System in AIDS

1. Acalculous cholecystitis
2. Sclerosing cholangitis
3. Papillary stenosis
4. Bile duct lymphoma

phatase will decline in some patients, in others it will continue to rise and may reflect intrahepatic disease that is not benefited by endoscopic sphincterotomy or coinfection with intrahepatic MAI

Papillary Stenosis

- Patients with papillary stenosis have a similar clinical presentation to those with sclerosing cholangitis
- ERCP reveals stenosis of the distal common bile duct that may extend to the intraduodenal segment
- Biopsies of the ampulla have revealed the characteristic CMV inclusions in some patients
- Some patients have both sclerosing cholangitis and papillary stenosis
- Patients may benefit by the endoscopic placement of a biliary stent or from a sphincterotomy. These procedures may need to be repeated

SUMMARY

Hepatobiliary abnormalities are common in patients with AIDS. Patients may be asymptomatic or have severe and disabling symptoms. The liver may be the site for a multitude of infections that are often part of a disseminated process. In addition, neoplastic lesions such as KS and lymphoma are frequently present. An intriguing lesion is peliosis hepatis, which was seen in the past with another chronic wasting disorder, namely, tuberculosis, as well as with the use of androgenic anabolic steroids. However, the peliosis hepatis noted in patients with AIDS appears to be uniquely associated with the presence of a Rickettsia-like organism. The spectrum of extrahepatic biliary involvement encountered in patients with AIDS includes acalculous cholecystitis, sclerosing cholangitis, and ampullary stenosis.

In approaching these patients, the differential diagnosis of abnormalities of liver function tests should be noted. It is worth remembering that there is no specific pattern of biochemical abnormality that points to a particular disease process. However, marked elevations of the serum alkaline phosphatase with mild to modest hyperbilirubinemia or a markedly elevated serum LDH should suggest the possibility of lymphoma. Radiographic studies such as HIDA scan, ultrasonography, and CT, may provide important clues favoring a diagnosis of acalculous cholecystitis or sclerosing cholangitis with or without ampullary stenosis. Fundoscopic examination (looking for CMV retinitis), blood cultures, and bone marrow examination may be helpful in suggesting a diagnosis. If these tests point to a specific diagnosis, treatment can then be initiated. Often the liver function test abnormalities will improve or resolve and one can infer that the same process that was occurring elsewhere in the body was also affecting the liver. In patients with unexplained abnormal elevations of liver function test and symptoms, a liver biopsy should be performed. The diagnosis may offer important prognostic insight. On occasion, therapy can result in substantial palliation of the patient's symptoms. Liver biopsy may be accompanied by an ↑ bleeding risk in patients with AIDS; prior to performing this procedure, or an endoscopic sphincterotomy, it is prudent to check the routine coagulation parameters as well as a bleeding time.

Finally, in addition to the wide spectrum of hepatobiliary and pancreatic disorders mentioned above, it should be remembered that a number of medicines, including trimethoprim-sulfamethoxazole, Zidovudine, and 2[1], 3[1] Dideoxyinisine (ddI) have been reported to cause significant hepatotoxicity.

Suggested Reading

Arora S, Fawaz KA: Complications of severe liver disease. *In* Chopra S and May RJ (eds), Pathophysiology of Gastrointestinal Diseases. Boston, Little Brown and Company, 1989, pp 431–462.

Chopra S: Disorders of the Liver. Philadelphia, Lea and Febiger, 1988.

Stark ME, Szurszewski JH: Role of nitric oxide in gastrointestinal and hepatic function and disease. Gastroenterology *103*:1928–1949, 1992.

Lichtenstein DR, Makadon HJ, Chopra S: Fulminant hepatitis B and delta virus co-infection in AIDS. Am J Gastroenterol *87*:1643–1647, 1992.

Kavin H, Jonas B, Chowdhury L, Kabins S: Acalculous cholecystitis and cytomegalovirus infection in the Acquired Immune Deficiency Syndrome. Ann Intern Med *104*:53–54,1986.

Beaugerie L, Deilhac M-F, Deluol A-M, et al.: Cholangiopathy associated with microsporidia infection of the common bile duct mucosa in a patient with HIV infection. Ann Intern Med *117*:401–402,1992.

Boyer N, Marcellin P, Degott C, et al.: Recombinant interferon-alpha for chronic hepatitis C in patients positive for antibody to human immunodeficiency virus. J Inf Dis *165*:723–726,1992.

Infectious Diseases

26

John G. Bartlett

INFECTIONS OF THE CENTRAL NERVOUS SYSTEM

Infections of the central nervous system produce clinical expression by 3 processes: Inflammation, increased intracranial pressure and tissue necrosis. Each may cause headaches. Meningeal inflammation causes meningismus: inability to straighten a leg when the hips are flexed (Kernig's sign) and leg flexion occurs when the head is flexed (Brudzinski's sign). Primarily with chronic meningeal inflammation, cranial nerve palsies is possible. Inflammation within the brain parenchyma (encephalitis) or necrosis (cerebral abscess) may alter consciousness, and cause focal neurologic deficits or seizures. Any of the 3 may result in increased intracranial pressure with altered consciousness and fever.

Diagnostic Studies. *Cerebrospinal fluid;* Guidelines for interpretation for CSF analysis are provided in Table 26–1 for normal findings, abnormal CSF with non-infectious causes and the differential diagnosis for major infectious conditions. *CT and MRI:* Patients with focal neurologic defects or evidence of increased intracranial pressure (vomiting or papilledema) should have brain imaging prior to LP. Hypodense area in scans suggest encephalitis or meningo-encephalitis; ring-enhancing lesions suggest cerebral abscess.

Pyogenic Meningitis

Diagnosis: The CSF generally shows a total WBC exceeding 100/mm3 with a predominance of neutrophils, increased protein and decreased glucose. Blood cultures are often positive. Most cases show typical bacteria on gram stain, positive antigen assays *(S. pneumoniae, H. influenzae* type B and *N. meningitidis)* and positive cultures. Major pathogens in community-acquired and nosocomial infections are listed in Table 26–2.

Treatment: Therapeutic decisions are dictated by etiologic agent. The guidelines below are provided for initial empiric treatment assuming no specific clues with the initial evaluation pending culture results according to host status (Table 26–3). After the putative agent is identified, antibiotic treatment is simplified according to the agent recovered and, in some cases, in vitro susceptibility tests and pharmacologic properties for penetration across the blood-brain barrier (Tables 26–4a and 26–4b).

Tuberculous Meningitis (Table 26–5)

This represents hematogenous spread during miliary disease or reactivation and rupture of a latent tubercle.

Table 26–1
Cerebrospinal Fluid Analysis

	CELL COUNT/dl AND PREDOMINANT TYPE	PROTEIN (mg/dl)	GLUCOSE (mg/dl)	MICROSCOPIC EXAM	CULTURE
Normal	0–5, mononuclear cells	15–45	40–80 (>.6 × serum level)	Neg	Neg
Meningitis					
Viral	10–2,000, early-PMNs; late-mononuclear cells	Normal–100	Normal	Neg	Usually neg
Bacterial					
Untreated	100–100,000 PMNs	Normal–600	Low in 50–80%	Pos: 60–80%*	Pos: 90%
Partially treated	100–10,000 PMNs	Usually ↑	Normal or low	Variable*	Variable
Tuberculosis	10–1,000 mononuclear cells	100–500	Normal or low	Rarely pos	Usually pos
Fungal	5–1,000 mononuclear cells	50–500	Low	Antibody and antigen detection*	Usually pos
Syphilitic	5–100 mononuclear cells	50–100	Normal or low	VDRL pos in 75%*	Neg
Encephalitis	0–2,000, early-PMNs, late-monos	50–120	Normal	Neg	Neg

(continued)

Table 26–1. *(continued)*

	CELL COUNT/dl AND PREDOMINANT TYPE	PROTEIN (mg/dl)	GLUCOSE (mg/dl)	MICROSCOPIC EXAM	CULTURE
Brain abscess	5–500, variable	50–500	Normal	Neg	Neg
Non-infectious diseases**					

* Serum serology for syphilis, HIV, fungal (Coccidioidomycosis, histoplasmosis), CSF serology (Coccidioidomycosis, syphilis non-treponemal tests) and antigen detection (Cryptococcosis, *N. meninigitidis, S. pneumoniae, H. influenzae* type B)

** *Abnormal CSF with non-infectious causes*

1. Traumatic tap: ↑ protein; RBCs; WBC count and differential proportionate to RBCs in peripheral blood; clear and colorless supernatant of centrifuged CSF. Usually 1 WBC/700 RBC.
2. Chemical meningitis (injection of anesthetics, chemotherapeutic agents, air, radiographic dyes): ↑ protein, lymphocytes (occasionally PMNs).
3. Cerebral contusion, subarachnoid hemorrhage, intracerebral bleed: RBCs, ↑ protein (1 mg/1000 RBCs), disproportionately increased PMNs (peak at 72–96 hours); ↓ glucose in 15–20%).
4. Vasculitis (SLE, etc.): ↑ protein (50–100 mg/dl), ↑ WBCs (usually mononuclear cells, occasionally PMNs); normal glucose.
5. Postictal (repeated generalized seizures): RBCs (0–500/mm^3), WBCs (10–100/mm^3 with variable % PMNs with peak at 1 day), protein normal or slight ↑.
6. Tumors (esp. glioblastomas, leukemia, lymphoma, breast cancer, pancreatic cancer): Low glucose, ↑ protein, moderate PMNs.
7. Neurosurgery: Blood; ↑ protein; WBCs (disproportionate to RBCs with predominance of mononuclear cells) up to 2 weeks post-op.
8. Sarcoidosis: ↑ protein; WBCs (up to 100/mm^3 predominantly mononuclear cells); low glucose in 10%.

Table 26–2
Pathogens Causing Pyogenic Meningitis*

	COMMONLY ACQUIRED (253 CASES)	NOSOCOMIAL ACQUIRED (151 CASES)
S. pneumoniae	97 (38%)	8 (5%)
Gram neg bacilli	9 (4%)	57 (38%)
M. meningitidis	35 (14%)	1 (1%)
Streptococci	17 (7%)	13 (9%)
Enterococcus	0	4 (3%)
Staph. aureus	13 (5%)	13 (9%)
Listeria monocytogenes	29 (11%)	5 (3%)
H. influenzae	9 (4%)	6 (4%)
Mixed	6 (2%)	10 (7%)
Staphylococcus (coag-neg)	0	13 (9%)
Other	4 (2%)	5 (3%)
Neg culture	34 (13%)	16 (11%)

* Experience at Mass. General Hospital 1962–88 (Durand ML et al: New Engl J Med 328:21, 1993)

Table 26–3
Empiric Treatment of Pyogenic Meningitis

SETTING	LIKELY AGENTS	TREATMENT
Adult, community acquired, immunocompetent	*S. pneumoniae* *N. meningitidis*	Cefotaxime, 2 g IV q 4 h Ceftriaxone, 2–3 g IV q 12 h Ceftizoxime, 3 g IV q 8 h Penicillin allergy: Chloramphenicol, 1 g IV q 6 h
Immunosuppressed		
Defective humoral antibody, asplenia, complement defect	*S. pneumoniae* *N. meningitidis*	As above
Defective cell mediated immunity	Listeria Cryptococcosis	Ampicillin, 3 g IV q 6 h ± gentamicin, 1.7–2.0 mg/kg IV q 8 h Penicillin allergy: Trimethoprim sulfamethoxazole, 3–4 mg/kg (trimethoprim) IV q 6 h
Post neurosurgical procedure or cranial trauma	Enterobacteriaceae Pseudomonas sp. *Staph. aureus*	Tobramycin, 1.7–2.0 mg/kg IV q 8 h + piperacillin, mezlocillin or ticarcillin, 40 mg/kg IV q 4 h + vancomycin, 1 g IV q 12 h Alternative to penicillins is ceftazidime 2–3 g IV q 8 h
Ventricular shunt	*S. epidermidis*	Vancomycin, 1 g IV q 12 h + rifampin, 300 mg po or IV q 12 h

* Assumes negative CSF gram stain and negative tests for bacterial antigens

Table 26–4A
Treatment of Pyogenic Meningitis by Organism

ORGANISM	PREFERRED DRUG	ALTERNATIVE	COMMENT
Strep. pneumoniae	Penicillin G or ampicillin Cefotaxime Ceftriaxone	Chloramphenicol Cefuroxime Ceftizoxime	Test susceptibility to penicillin Resistant strains: chloramphenicol or vancomycin + rifampin Treat ≥10 days
Neisseria meningitidis	Penicillin G or ampicillin	(As above)	Intimate contacts should receive rifampin. Treat ≥7 days
H. influenzae	Ampicillin (Ampicillin-sensitive strains)	Chloramphenicol Cefotaxime Ceftizoxime Ceftriaxone Ceftazidime	If children <4 yrs in household, contacts should receive rifampin prophylaxis (type B only) Treat ≥10 days)
L. monocytogenes	Ampicillin ± gentamicin	Trimethoprim sulfamethoxazole	Cephalosporins are not effective Treat 14–21 days
E. coli and other coliforms	Cefotaxime Ceftizoxime Ceftriaxone Ceftazidime	Aminoglycoside ± anti-pseudomonad—penicillin or ampicillin Sulfa-trimethoprim	In vitro sensitivity tests required; MBC data preferred Chloramphenicol lacks bactericidal activity vs GNB—not recommended Aminoglycoside is given systemically ± intrathecally Treat ≥21 days Ceftazidime should be reserved for suspected or established *P. aeruginosa*
Pseudomonas aeruginosa	Aminoglycoside + ceftazidime	Aminoglycoside + antipseudomonad penicillin (ticarcillin, mezlocillin, piperacillin)	Sulfa-trimethoprim-Acinetobacter, *Ps. cepacia* and Flavobacterium Aminoglycoside is given systemically ± intrathecally
Staph. aureus	Antistaphylococcal penicillin ± rifampin	Vancomycin + rifampin Trimethoprim-sulfa + rifampin or ciprofloxacin	Vancomycin + rifampin for methicillin resistant *S. aureus*
Staph. epidermidis	Vancomycin + rifampin	Teicoplanin	

Diagnosis: With miliary disease there is often false negative PPD. With reactivated CSF disease there may be no other organ involved, but the skin test is usually positive. CSF may be similar to viral meningitis in early stages; in late stage disease there may be cranial nerve palsies and obstructive hydrocephalus, with CSF glucose often low. Positive AFB stains and positive cultures establish the diagnosis, but long delays in culture results and the organism may prove difficult to recover making empiric treatment necessary.

Table 26–4B
Doses of Drugs for CNS Infections*

1. *Aminoglycosides and vancomycin*

AGENT	SYSTEMIC	INTRATHECAL/ INTRAVENTRICULAR
Gentamicin	1.7–2.0 mg/kg q8h	4–8 mg q24h
Tobramycin	1.7–2.0 mg/kg q8h	4–8 mg q24h
Amikacin	5.0–7.5 mg/kg q8h	10–20 mg q24h
Vancomycin	1 g q12h	5–20 mg q24h

2. *Cephalosporins*
   - Cefuroxime: 9 g/day in 3 doses
   - Cefotaxime: 12 g/day in 6 doses**
   - Ceftizoxime: 9 g/day in 3 doses**
   - Ceftriaxone: 4–6 g/day in 2 doses**
   - Ceftazidime: 6–12 g/day in 3 doses**
3. *Chloramphenicol:* 4–6 g/day in 4 doses**
4. *Penicillins*
   - Ampicillin: 12 g/day in 6 doses**
   - Antipseudomonad penicillins
     - Ticarcillin: 18–24 g/day in 6 doses (40–60 mg/kg q 4 h)
     - Mezlocillin: 18–24 g/day in 6 doses (40–60 mg/kg q 4 h)
     - Azlocillin: 18–24 g/day in 6 doses (40–60 mg/kg q 4 h)
     - Pipericillin: 18–24 g/day in 6 doses (40–60 mg/kg q 4 h)
   - Antistaphylococcal penicillins
     - Nafcillin: 9–12 g/day in 6 doses
     - Oxacillin: 9–12 g/day in 6 doses
   - Penicillin G: 20–24 million units/day in 6 doses**
5. *Trimethoprim-sulfamethoxazole:* 15–20 mg/kg/day (trimethoprim) in 4 doses
   - Metronidazole: 2 g/day in 2–4 doses
   - Vancomycin: 2 g/day in 2 doses**

* Assume adult patient with normal renal function.
** Recommendations of Tunkel AR et al, Ann Intern Med 112:610, 1990.

Treatment: (Initial)
Isoniazid, 5 mg/kg/day (usually 300 mg) po or IM plus
Rifampin, 10-20 mg/kg/day (usually 600 mg) po or IV plus
Pyrazinamide, 15-30 mg/kg/day (usually 2 g) plus
Ethambutol, 15-25 mg/kg/day (usually 2.5 g) *or*
Streptomycin, 15 mg/kg/day IM (usually 1 g)

Cryptococcal Meningitis

The major fungal pathogen is *Cryptococcus neoformans,* which is the most common pathogen in patients with meningitis plus defective cell-mediated immunity including organ transplantation, AIDS, lymphoma, corticosteroid therapy and cancer chemotherapy.

Diagnosis: The *serum* cryptococcal antigen is positive in over 95% of patients with AIDS and cryptococcal meningitis. Cryptococcal antigen is virtually always positive and false negative antigen assays are extremely rare when properly done. An India ink stain will usually show

Table 26–5
Some Causes of Chronic Meningitis: The Differential Diagnosis Includes the Following Causes of Chronic Meningitis*

INFECTIOUS		NEOPLASTIC	MISCELLANEOUS
Bacteria	Fungi	Leukemia	SLE*
M. tuberculosis	Cryptococcosis	Lymphoma	Wegener's granulomatosis
Atypical mycobacteria	*Coccidioides***	Metastatic	CNS vasculitis
*T. pallidum***	*Histoplasma***	Breast	Granulomatous vasculitis
*B. burgdorferi***	*Blastomyces*	Lung	Sarcoidosis
Leptospira	*Sporotrichum*	Thyroid	Behçet's disease
Brucella	*Pseudoallescheria*	Renal	Vogt-Koyanagi and Harada's syndromes
Listeria	*Alternaria*	Melanoma	Benign lymphocytic meningitis
Actinomyces/ Arachnia	*Fusaria*	Primary CNS	
Nocardia	*Aspergillus*	Astrocytoma	
Parasites	Zygomycetes	Ependymoma	
T. gondii	*Cladosporium*	Pinealoma	
Cysticercus	Viruses	Medulloblastoma	
Angiostrongylus	HIV**		
Spinigerum	Echovirus		
Schistosoma			

* Defined as illness present for ≥4 weeks with or without therapy: CSF analysis usually shows lymphocytic pleocytosis. Analysis of 83 previously healthy persons in New Zealand showed 40% had tuberculosis, 7% had cryptococcosis, 8% had malignancy and 34% were enigmatic (Q J Med 63:283, 1987).

** Evaluation: Culture, serum serology, CT scan or MRI (brain abscess, cysticercosis, toxoplasmosis), cytology CSF (lymphoma, metastatic ca), eosinophilic (parasitic, coccidioidomycosis), CSF serology or antigen (cryptococcosis, coccidioidomycosis, syphilis, histoplasmosis), blind meningeal biopsy (rarely positive), empiric treatment (TB, then penicillin, then amphotericin B, then ? corticosteroids).

the agent and may be used as a substitute for the antigen assay when the laboratory is down (see Chapter 18).

Treatment for Patients with AIDS: Amphotericin B (0.5-0.7 mg/kg/day) IV ± flucytosine (75-100 mg/kg/day) po until total dose of Amphotericin B is 15 mg/kg *and* negative CSF culture, then Fluconazole (200 mg/day) indefinitely. Alternative for patients with favorable prognosis (normal mental status, high CSF leukocyte count and relatively low number of organisms): Amphotericin B (0.5-0.7 mg/kg/day) IV ± flucytosine (75-100 mg/kg/day) po x 10-14 days, then fluconazole (400 mg/day) po x 8 weeks, then fluconazole (200 mg/day) po indefinitely.

Treatment for Patients without AIDS: Amphotericin B (0.3 mg/kg/day) IV + flucytosine (150 mg/kg/day) po × 6 weeks. Alternative for immunocompetent host without neurologic complications: Above regimen x 4 weeks.

Syphilis

Diagnosis: Serum shows evidence of syphilis with a positive VDRL or RPR confirmed with a FTA-absorbed. Patients with syphilis should have CSF analysis in the following settings: neurologic signs or symptoms, other evidence of active syphilis (aortitis, gumma, iritis), treatment failure, HIV infection, syphilis <1 year plus a serum nontreponomal titer ≥ 1:32 or treatment with an agent other than penicillin. The CSF in neurosyphilis shows mononuclear pleocytosis (>5/ml) and increased protein; the VDRL is positive in CSF in 2/3 of cases and is considered diagnostic.

Treatment: Intravenous aqueous penicillin G, 12-24 million units/day given as 2-4 million units q 4 h x 10–14 days.

Alternative (outpatient regimen): Procaine penicillin, 2.4 million units daily plus probenecid, 500 mg po 4 times daily 10–14 days.

Follow-up: CSF analysis every six months until negative.

Viral Encephalitis

Diagnosis: The clinical picture provides minimal help with etiology, although travel and contact histories may be important. Findings include confusion, delirium, ataxia, seizures, and cranial nerve palsies. The most important to recognize because of its devastating consequences and susceptibility to effective therapy is *Herpes simplex* encephalitis which often shows evidence of a temporal lobe lesion by MRI, CT scan or EEG. A definite diagnosis is made with brain biopsy with histopathology, culture or fluorescent antibody staining. There is generally no evidence of *H. simplex* lesions on mucocutaneous surfaces.

Treatment: Acyclovir, 10 mg/kg IV q 8 h for 10-14 days.

Cerebral Pyogenic Abscess (Table 26–6)

Diagnosis: Cerebral abscess should be suspected in patients with focal neurologic signs accompanied by systemic evidence of infection (fever or leukocytosis) and/or associated conditions most often found with this complication. Fever is found in only about one half of cases so that the absence of fever fails to help in excluding this diagnosis. Common associated conditions include sinusitis, otitis/mastoiditis, head trauma, prior neurosurgery, endocarditis and congenital cyanotic heart disease. A MRI or CT scan with contrast shows a ring-enhancing lesion adjacent to the site of entry where the pathophysiologic mechanism is direct extension as with sinusitis, otitis, head trauma or prior neurosurgery. Cerebral spinal fluid shows non-specific findings with an increased protein and modest pleocytosis with a dominance of mononuclear cells. The diagnosis is established with an aspirate of the lesion or at neurosurgery with gram stain of purulent exudate showing typical bacteria. Cultures should be obtained for both aerobic and anaerobic bacteria; cultures should also be submitted for mycobacteria and fungi. Putrid discharge indicates anaerobic bacteria; a polymicrobial flora on gram stain also suggests anaerobic bacteria.

Treatment: Antibiotic selection is based on bacteriology using care to correlate clinical symptoms, gram stains and culture results. Most pyogenic cerebral abscesses involve anaerobic bacteria or mixtures of anaerobes or coliforms and/or streptococci. Empiric therapy pending cultures and in the event that surgery is not performed is based on anticipated bacteriologic patterns according to associated conditions using the guidelines shown in Table 26–6.

SOFT TISSUE INFECTIONS

Skin and soft tissue infections are classified as superficial or deep. The classical syndromes are generally superficial soft tissue infections and include impetigo, erysipelas, lymphangitis and folliculitis. The major

Table 26–6
Some Causes of Brain Abscess

ASSOCIATED CONDITION	LIKELY PATHOGEN	
Sinusitis	Anaerobic, microaerophilic and aerobic streptococci, *Bacteroides* sp.	Metronidazole, 500 mg IV or po every 6 h *plus* Penicillin G 5–6 million units IV q 6 h Chloramphenicol, 1 g IV q 6 h plus Penicillin G, 6 million units IV q 6 h
Otitis	*Bacteroides fragilis* *Bacteroides* sp., streptococci, *Enterobacteriaceae*	As above
Trauma, post-neurosurgery	*Staph. aureus*	Oxacillin or nafcillin, 2–3 g IV q 4 h *or* Vancomycin, 1 g IV every 12 h
	Enterobacteriaceae	Cefotazime, 2 g q 4 h Ceftazidime, 2–4 g q 8 h ± Aminoglycoside
	Pseudomonas aeruginosa	Tobramycin, 2 mg/kg, then 1.7 mg/kg q 8 h plus Ceftazidime, 2–4 g q 8 h *or* Piperacillin, 4 g q 6 h
Endocarditis	*Staph. aureus* *Streptococcus* sp.	Methicillin sensitive: Oxacillin or nafcillin Methicillin resistant: Vancomycin Penicillin G, 5–6 million units IV q 6 h *or* Ampicillin, 2 g IV q 4 h ± aminoglycoside
Cyanotic heart disease	*Streptococcus* sp.	As above

pathogens are group A streptococci and *S. aureus*. Most respond to antibiotics and do not require surgical intervention. Deep soft tissue infections are substantially less common, but important to recognize early due to the need for aggressive surgical treatment as well as antibiotics. These infections tend to spread along fascial lines (fascitis) or involve muscle compartments with myonecrosis.

Superficial Soft Tissue Infections

The skin consists of an outer ectodermal layer, the epidermis that is attached to an inner mesodermal layer, the dermis. The epidermis lacks a blood vessel supply; the dermis contains lymphatic and blood vessels that provide access to humoral and cellular defenses, but also facilitate circumferential spread with lymphangitis or cellulitis. Beneath the dermis is the subcutaneous tissue containing the sweat glands, hair follicles, sebaceous glands, apocynin glands and the nails, which extend into the subcutaneous tissue. Beneath the subcutaneous tissue is the fascia which envelops muscle. Skin contains resident and transient microbial flora with concentrations of 10^2-10^6 bacteria/cm^2. The term resident flora refers to a relatively stable bacteria population that includes predominately *S. epidermidis, P. acnes* and diphtheroids. Aerobic streptococci are not part of the normal flora. Gram negative bacilli are found primarily in warm, moist areas of the skin. *S. aureus* is frequently recovered from skin cultures but is usually transient rather than resident. Pathophysiologic factors include virulence of the microbe, inoculum size, the presence of occlusive dressings (that prevent desquamation and provide a moist environment for bacterial proliferation), disruption of normal cutaneous barriers, reduced blood supply, presence of a foreign body, compromised systemic defense mechanisms and disruption of lymphatic drainage or venous status.

Microbiologic Diagnosis: Most skin and soft tissue infections are bacterial. Cultures must show appropriate appreciation of the importance of distinguishing pathogens and contaminants on the basis of the method used to obtain the culture, the organisms recovered, correlation with gram stain observations and quantitation of the bacteria. Bacterial infections of the skin usually involve heavy growth with 10^5 bacteria/ml of secretions. The major exception is group A strep: it is difficult to recover and considered significant if found at all. *S. epidermidis, P. acnes* and diphtheroids almost never cause soft tissue infections except for intravenous line sepsis. Cultures obtained from open lesions such as ulcers will virtually always yield bacteria so that interpretation must be based on the virulence of the organism, quantitation on primary isolation plates and clinical correlations. Aspirates or biopsy specimens obtained avoiding surface contamination are obviously preferred.

TYPES OF INFECTIONS (TABLE 26–7)

Impetigo: This is a superficial infection of the skin which is usually caused by group A β–hemolytic streptococci, although *S. aureus* is implicated in 5-8% of cases. The infection is highly communicable, worsens by crowding and purulent drainage dries to the characteristic golden-yellow crust. The most common sites of involvement are exposed areas—new lesions usually represent autoinoculation. The infection is restricted to the epidermis so the lesions are painless and heal without scarring. Constitutional symptoms (e.g. fever) are rare. Major concerns are appearance, secondary infections, spread to others and glomerulonephritis. Preferred drugs in adults are penicillin V (500 mg po qid) with erythromycin (500 mg po qid) for penicillin-allergic patients. For cases involving *S. aureus* the usual treatment is oral cephalexin (250-500 mg po quid), cloxacillin (250-500 mg po qid) or amoxicillin-clavulanate (250-500 mg po tid). Antibiotic treatment may not prevent nephritis, but does hasten healing and prevent spread.

Erysipelas: This is a superficial cellulitis with prominent involvement of lymphatics usually caused by group A β-hemolytic streptococci; occasional cases are caused by *S. aureus* or streptococci groups B, C or G. Predisposing conditions include streptococcal respiratory tract infection, patients with nephrosis, previous lymphatic obstruction or edema. The lesion is bright red and indurated, and has a characteristic sharply demarcated elevated border. The most common site of involvement is the butterfly area of the face with erythema of the nose and cheeks. Most

Table 26–7
Superficial Soft Tissue Infections*

DISORDER	ORGANISM	USUAL HOST/SITE	CLINICAL FEATURES	TREATMENT
Impetigo	*Strep. pyogenes* (*Staph. aureus;* streptococci, group B, C, or G)	Children May be epidemic Exposed areas	Vesicles with erythematous halos, then pustules and crusted lesions; lesions are painless	Careful and frequent cleansing; penicillin (erythromycin)
Bullous impetigo	*Staph. aureus*	Newborn and young children	Vesicles which progress to flaccid bullae	Penicillinase-resistant penicillin (erythromycin)
Erysipelas	*S. pyogenes (streptococci, group B, C, or G; S. aureus*)	Young children and older adults Areas of lymphatic obstruction or edema are predisposed	Painful erythematous, edematous, indurated, raised lesions with sharply demarcated margin; fever and leukocytosis are common	Penicillin (erythromycin)
Cellulitis	*S. pyogenes* *Staph. aureus* Others	Areas of prior trauma or ulceration	Painful, tender erythema with no elevation or sharp demarcation; systemic signs are variable	Penicillin, penicillinase-resistant penicillin or a cephalosporin
Lymphangitis	*S. pyogenes (Staph. aureus)*	Extremity	Erythematous streak with regional adenopathy	Penicillin; penicillinase-resistant penicillin; cephalothin or clindamycin

Folliculitis	*Staph. aureus (P. aeruginosa, Candida albicans)*	Any area with hair follicles; areas exposed to swimming pool or whirpool *(P. aeruginosa)*	Small erythmatous papules with central pustule; no systemic signs	Saline compresses and topical antibiotics
Furuncles	*Staph. aureus*	Areas of friction, sweat and hair follicles—neck, face, axilla, and buttocks	Firm red nodule with progression to fluctuant painful mass and spontaneous drainage; fever and leukocytosis variable	Moist heat application; antibiotics (usually penicillinase-resistant penicillin) for cases with extensive cellulitis, fever, or midface involvement; surgical drainage of large, fluctuant lesions
Carbuncle	*Staph. aureus*	Diabetics; usual areas are posterior neck, back, or thigh	Multiple abscesses that connect in subcutaneous tissue and drain along hair follicles	Incision and drainage; systemic antibiotics, usually penicillinase-resistant penicillin
Paronychia	*Staph. aureus* *S. pyogenes* *P. aeruginosa* *Candida*	Frequent hand immersion; nail fold	Periungual erythema and swelling with separation of nail fold from nail plate	

* From: Bartlett JG: Bacterial Infections of Skin, Muscle and Bone. Chapter 9.4 in: The Principles and Practice of Medicine. Harvey AM, Johns RJ, McKusick VA, Owens AH and Ross RS (Editors), 22nd Edition, Appleton and Lange, Norwalk, CT, pp. 577, 1988.

patients have fever and leukocytosis. It is difficult to recover the pathogen with culture. The usual treatment is penicillin (2-10 million units/day IV), amoxicillin (500 mg po qid), erythromycin (500 mg po qid) or clindamycin (300 mg po qid or 600 mg IV q 8 h). Seriously ill patients should be treated for both streptococci and *S. aureus* using a penicillinase-resistant penicillin (nafcillin or oxacillin, 2-3 g IV q 6 h), an antistaphylococcal cephalosporin such as cefazolin (1-2 gm IV q 8 h), or cefuroxime (0.75-1.5 gm IV q 8 h) or vancomycin (1 gm IV q 12 h). Some patients with lymphedema have recurrent infections and benefit from prophylactic penicillin V (500 mg po bid) or maintain a supply in order to expedite treatment at the first sign of infection.

Lymphangitis: Acute lymphangitis is characterized by erythematous streaks that extend from a site of infection toward enlarged and tender regional lymph nodes. Cultures at the port of entry or blood cultures will often yield the responsible organism; cultures obtained by needle aspiration of the lymphangitic streaks are usually negative. Most cases are caused by group A β-hemolytic streptococci with occasional cases caused by *S. aureus*. The usual treatment is aqueous penicillin G (2-3 million units IV/day), penicillin V (500 mg po qid), erythromycin (500 mg po qid) or clindamycin (300 mg po qid or 600 mg IV q 8 h); concern for *S. aureus* may favor the initial use of cephalexin (500 mg po qid), clindamycin (above dose) or amoxicillin-clavulanate (500 mg po tid). Additional causes of acute lymphangitis include rat bite fever caused by *Spirillum minus* which is suspected when there is a history of a rat bite; this organism is demonstrated by Giemsa stain of blood or exudate and the preferred treatment is penicillin V (500 mg po qid) or tetracycline (500 mg po qid). Acute lymphangitis following recent travel to Africa, South America or Southeast Asia should suggest filariasis due to *Wuchereria bancrofti* or *Brugia malayi*.

Chronic lymphangitis: May be caused by *Sporothrix schenckii, Mycobacterium marinum, M. kansasii*, filiarisis or *Nocardia brasiliensis*. The most common form in the United States is sporotrichosis characterized by subcutaneous nodules that occur along the course of lymphatic channels. The responsible fungus is typically introduced by trauma from a barberry bush or rose bush. The other relatively common cause of this type of nodular lesions along lymphatic channels is "swimming pool granuloma" involving *M. marinum* found in swimming pools or fish tanks.

Cellulitis: This is a relatively common spreading infection involving the dermis and subcutaneous tissue that occurs most commonly in association with local trauma or a superficial ulceration that becomes secondarily infected. Some patients have no clear portal of entry: this is most common with lower extremity involvement in alcoholic and obese patients. Typical findings are tenderness, erythema, warmth and edema. Unlike erysipelas, the advanced edge is not sharply demarcated. Systemic symptoms are variable. Multiple organisms have been implicated, but most frequent are *S. aureus* and streptococci. Detection of the etiologic agent is difficult in the absence of exudate or an ulcer representing the portal of entry. Needle aspiration of the advanced edge of inflammation is often advocated, but rarely positive. Treatment pending cultures are directed against *S. aureus* and *S. pyogenes* using cephalosporins such as cephalexin (500 mg po qid), cefazolin (1-2 gm IV q 8 h) or cefuroxime (0.75-1.5 gm IV q 8 h); alternatives are clindamycin (300 mg po qid or 600 mg IV q 8 h), vancomycin (1 gm IV q 12 h) or amoxicillin-clavulanate (500 mg po tid).

Abscesses: Subcutaneous abscesses are most common in patients with folliculitis, cellulitis, trauma or infected sebaceous cysts. *S. aureus* is implicated in 25-50% of cases and is the major pathogen with infections above the waist. When found, it is usually present and it is usually a single pathogen by gram stain and culture. Subcutaneous abscesses below the waist are more likely to involve anaerobes with or without coliforms, especially with involvement of the perineal, inguinal or buttock region. The usual finding is pain, swelling, tenderness and erythema at the infected site. The major form of therapy is drainage, but timing is important. Mature lesions as indicated by fluctuance or by needle aspiration usually require incision and drainage. Antibiotics are generally not necessary in uncomplicated cases.

Infections of Hair Follicles: These include folliculitis, furunculosis and carbuncles. The sites of involvement are those subject to perspiration and friction: neck, face, buttock and axillae. *Folliculitis* is restricted to hair follicles and presents as multiple red papules. *Furunculosis* has more extensive involvement with firm, painful, tender red nodules that become fluctuant and drain. A *carbuncle* is a confluent infection with penetration to the subcutaneous tissue and large abscess that presents as a tender mass, sometimes with multiple draining sinuses. Large lesions are usually detected with CT scan. Contributing factors to the frequency and severity of these infections are obesity, neutropenia, poor hygiene, seborrhea, corticosteroid therapy, occlusive dressings, trauma such as hair plucking and diabetes mellitus. Antibiotic treatment for severe lesions should be directed at *S. aureus* using oxacillin or nafcillin (2-3 g IV q 6 h), cephalexin (500 mg po qid), vancomycin (1 g IV q 12 h) or clindamycin (300 mg po qid or 600 mg IV q 8 h). Incision and drainage are required for lesions with fluctuant masses and large confluent lesions.

Folliculitis acquired from swimming pools or whirlpools often involve *P. aeruginosa*. *C. albicans* occasionally causes folliculitis, especially in intertriginous areas. The usual treatment is warm compresses and good hygiene with frequent use of antiseptic soaps. Some patients have recurrent furunculosis over a period of years. If hygiene alone fails, low dose prophylactic clindamycin (150 mg po qid) may help.

Bite Wound Infections: Similar to other soft tissue infections, but the infecting pathogen may reflect the oral flora of the "donor" as well as the mucocutaneous flora of the recipient. Major pathogens with human bite wounds are anaerobic bacteria, *Eikonella carrodens* and streptococci from the donor's mouth and *S. aureus* from the recipient's skin. An effective oral treatment against most pathogens is amoxicillin plus clavulanate (500 mg po tid) or clindamycin (300 mg po qid). the major pathogen is infections following animal bites is *Pasteurella multocida* which may cause cellulitis, lymphangitis, lymphadenopathy, an abscess and /or osteomyelitis. Appropriate management includes wound cleansing, débridement, avoidance of primary closure if feasible, prophylaxis for rabies and prophylaxis for tetanus. Infections involving *P. multocida* may be treated or prevented with aqueous penicillin (1-3 million units IV q 6 h), penicillin V (500 mg po qid), tetracycline (500 mg po qid), amoxicillin clavulanate (500 mg po tid) or ciprofloxacin (750 mg po bid).

Infected ulcers: Infections of decubitus ulcers, diabetic foot ulcers and ischemic ulcers represent secondary invasion of sites that are rendered susceptible due to loss of the cutaneous barrier. Cultures of purulent drainage or serous fluid expressed from the edge of the lesion or biopsies from the ulcer bed usually show a polymicrobial flora containing both aerobic and anaerobic bacteria. The same organisms can be recovered from cutaneous ulcers in patients with no overt infection: careful interpretation to virulent organisms, present in large concentrations or recovered from uncontaminated specimens is essential. There is often a question regarding underlying osteomyelitis, but the diagnosis is problematic because x-rays, bone scans, gallium scans or indium-labeled white cell scans may be difficult to interpret. The scans tend to be sensitive, but not specific. The best way to resolve this diagnostic dilemma is with bone biopsy. The most important facet of treatment is local care with débridement, avoidance of pressure, and avoidance of occlusive dressings. Vascular surgery may be critical to healing and is best evaluated by assessment of peripheral circulation including Doppler measurements. The common use of topical antiseptics and local antibiotics has no established benefit. Systemic antibiotics are commonly used, but have the best justification when there is extensive cellulitis, regional adenopathy, extensive involvement of underlying soft tissue, osteomyelitis or systemic expression with fever or bacteremia. Empiric antibiotics should be directed against coliforms and anaerobes using the same regimens commonly advocated for abdominal sepsis. *Traditional regimens*: Gentamicin or tobramycin (1.7 mg/kg IV q 8) *plus* clindamycin (600 mg IV q 8 h), metronidazole (1 g IV 12 h) or cefoxitin (2-3 g IV q 6 h). *Monotherapy regimens*: Imipenem (0.5-1 g IV q 6-8 h) or ticarcillin clavulanic acid (3-4 g IV 6 h). *Oral regimens*: Amoxicillin-clavulanic acid (500 mg po tid) or ciprofloxacin (500-750 mg po tid) plus metronidazole (500 mg po qid).

Deep Soft-Tissue Infections Involving Fascia and Muscle

Deep infections are classified according to the putative agent, the tissue plain involved or selected clinical characteristics (Table 26–8). This often gives an erroneous impression that these are distinct and easily distinguished entities, but there may be significant overlap so that classification and precise categorization may prove difficult. The most important facet in management concerns the decisions regarding antibiotic selection and the recognition of the critical role of surgery. Perhaps most important are the clinical features of these infections that distinguish them from the superficial infections thus call attention to the need for early surgical intervention:

CLUES TO DEEP SOFT TISSUE INFECTION

- *Severe pain* is spontaneous (patient has severe pain even when the area not palpated). This may be absent in some of these infections, especially those associated with neuropathies such as diabetic neuropathy.
- *Bullous lesions* which result from occlusion of deep vessels that traverse the fascia. Bullous lesions may be found with erysipelas and some forms of cellulitis caused by *P. aeruginosa*, *S. aureus* and streptococci, ischemic necrosis with fulminant infections such as meningococcemia, purpura fulminans, ecthyma gangrenosum, toxic shock syndrome, disseminated intravascular coagulation(DIC), toxins such as from brown recluse spider bites or certain primary dermatologic diseases such as bullous pemphigus.
- *Gas* in the soft tissue may be detected by palpation, by x-ray or by scans; gas in soft tissue usually reflects the production of volatile fatty acids produced by anaerobic bacteria.

- *Systemic toxicity* with high fever, high leukocyte counts and/or delirium.
- *Rapid spread* which often indicates spread through fascial pains.

Diagnosis: Recommended diagnostic studies to define the anatomic location include scans, needle aspiration, biopsy for frozen section and surgical exploration. X-rays often show soft issue swelling but this is not specific or it may show gas which is more worrisome. The preferred diagnostic technique is CT with contrast that provides excellent description of the tissue plain involved. Needle aspiration either blindly with CT or ultrasound guidance may yield the putrid, thin, gray "dishwater pus" characteristic of necrotizing synergistic cellulitis. An Alternative is a full-thickness biopsy of frozen section that will provide a histologic description. Despite all of these recommendations, the preferred diagnostic test is surgical exploration for direct visualization with the patient anesthetized.

TYPES OF INFECTIONS

Clostridial Infections: clostridium species are commonly found in crepitant cellulitis, mixed anaerobic infections of various sorts and, most importantly, gas gangrene. The latter is characterized by severe pain and delirium, usually following trauma or surgery (see subsequent discussion).

Fasciitis: Necrotizing facades refers to a deep infection that spreads along the fascial plains that envelop muscle compartments. There is usually a break in the skin that provides the portal of entry such as drug injection, a decubitus ulcer, an enterostomy, perirectal abscess or wound incision. Most cases occur in patients with diabetes mellitus. Two bacteriologic patterns are commonly noted. One involves streptococci and penicillin (aqueous penicillin G, 2-24 million units/day IV) is regarded as the preferred drug with clindamycin (600 mg IV q 8 h) as the best alternative agent. The second bacteriologic pattern is a mixture of aerobic and anaerobic bacteria similar to those found in intra-abdominal sepsis, and these are treated with antibiotic regimens used for intra-abdominal sepsis. In either case, the major treatment modality is surgery with incisions to the fascial plane to fillet the lesion. Most patients require repeated incisions.

Compartment Infections: Compartments are formed by the fascia that envelop muscle groups, usually of the extremities, the psoas muscle or the abdominal wall. Involvement of the muscle results in myonecrosis. There are three bacteriologic patterns: 1) streptococcal myonecrosis, 2) necrotizing synergistic cellulitis involving aerobic + anaerobic bacteria, 3) gas gangrene due to clostridia.

Gas Gangrene: A devastating infection with profound systemic toxicity, usually as a complication of surgery or trauma with several typical clinical settings: 1) traumatic injury or penetrating wounds, 2) surgery, especially intestinal or biliary tract operations, 3) uterine gas gangrene, 4) soft tissue lesions complicating vascular insufficiency, 5) intestinal gas gangrene found with colon cancer or neutropenia and 6) spontaneous gas gangrene occurring without predisposing cause. The usual pathophysiologic mechanisms includes contamination with histotoxic clostridia and toxin production promoted by reduced oxidation reduction potential at the site of injury. The usual incubation period from wound to onset of symptoms is 2-4 days and the 1st symptom is sudden and severe pain at the site of involvement. The skin initially shows tense

Table 26–8
Deep Soft Tissue Infections*

	CLOSTRIDIAL CELLULITIS	SYNERGISTIC NECROTIZING CELLULITS	GAS GANGRENE	STREPTOCOCCAL MYONECROSIS	NECROTIZING FASCIITIS	INFECTED VASCULAR GANGRENE	STREPTOCOCCAL GANGRENE
Predisposing conditions	Trauma Surgical wound	Diabetes, prior local lesions, perirectal lesion	Trauma surgery	Trauma surgery	Diabetes, trauma surgery, perineal infection	Arterial insufficiency	Trauma, surgery
Incubation period	3 days	3–14 days	1–2 days	3–4 days	1–4 days	5 days	6 hr–2 days
Etiologic organism(s)	Clostridia	Mixed aerobic-anaerobic flora	Clostridia, esp. *C. perfringens*	Anaerobic streptococci	Mixed aerobic-anaerobic flora, esp. coliforms, *Bacteroides* and streptococci	Mixed aerobic-anaerobic flora	*S. pyogenes*
Systemic toxicity	Minimal	Moderate to severe	Severe	Minimal until late in course	Moderate to severe	Minimal	Severe
Course	Gradual	Acute	Acute	Subacute	Acute or subacute	Gradual	Acute
Wound findings							

Local pain	Minimal	Moderate to severe	Severe	Late only	Minimal to moderate	Minimal to moderate	Severe
Skin appearance	Swollen, minimal discoloration	Erythematous or gangrenous	Tense and blanched, yellow-bronze, necrosis with hemorrhagic bullae	Erythema or yellow bronze	Blanched, erythema necrosis with hemorrhagic bullae	Erythema or necrosis	Erythema, necrosis
Gas	Abundant	Variable	Usually present	Variable	Variable	Variable	No
Muscle involvement	No	Variable	Myonecrosis	Myonecrosis	No	Myonecrosis—limited to area of vascular insufficiency	No
Discharge							
Appearance	Thin dark	Dark pus or "dishwater"	Serosanguinous	Seropurulent	Seropurulent or dishwater	None	None or serosanguinous
Odor	Sweetish or foul	Putrid	Sweet or foul	Often putrid	Putrid	Putrid	No odor
Gram statin	PMNs and gram-pos. bacilli	PMNs, mixed flora	Sparse PMNs; gram-pos. bacilli	PMNs, gram-pos. cocci	PMNs, mixed flora	PMNs, mixed flora	PMNs, gram-pos. cocci in chains
Surgical therapy	Debridement	Wide filleting incisions	Extensive excision, amputation	Excision of necrotic muscle	Wide filleting incisions	Amputation	Debridement on necrotic tissue

* From: Bartlett JG: Clostridial Myonecrosis and other Clostridial Diseases. Chapter 307 in: Cecil Textbook of Medicine. Wyngaarden JB, Smith LH and Bennett JC (Editors), W. B. Saunders Co., Philadelphia, PA pp. 1670, 1992.

edema and tenderness, sometimes with gas. With progression, the skin becomes pale and progresses to a bronze discoloration with hemorrhagic bullae. Systemic findings include diaphoresis, fever and tachycardia. This progresses with hemolytic anemia, shock and renal failure. *C. perfringens* is found in about 80% of cases with positive cultures; other clostridial species implicated include *C. septicum, C. histolyticum, C. novyi, C. bifermentans* and *C. fallax*. These clostridia produce over 20 different types of endotoxins that are implicated in both local and systemic findings. The diagnosis is based on the clinical observations noted above and supporting microbiologic studies that include a gram stain of wound exudate or aspirates of bulla to show large, gram positive bacilli; about 15% of patients have clostridia bacteremia. The most important component of treatment is radical surgery with amputation and/or extensive debridement. Aqueous penicillin G (2-4 million units IV q 4-6 h) is usually regarded as the preferred drug with clindamycin (600 mg IV q 8 h) or chloramphenicol (1 g IV 6 h) as alternate agents. The role of hyperbaric oxygen is ill-defined, but many authorities recommend it if it does not cause delay of surgery.

Necrotizing synergistic cellulitis: This is the most common compartment infection involving mixtures of aerobic and anaerobic bacteria. Similar to necrotizing facades, but the infection extends beneath the fascia to involve the compartment as well. Most patients are diabetic, often obese and many have renal failure as well. The usual sites of involvement are the perirectal area or lower extremities. Common findings are bullous lesions, spontaneous pain and gas in the soft tissue. Surgical exploration or needle aspiration typically shows "dishwater pus." Gram stain and culture of the exudate shows a polymicrobial flora composed of coliforms, streptococci and anaerobes. Blood cultures are positive in 20-30% of cases, usually yielding coliforms or anaerobes. The recommended antibiotics are those commonly used for intra-abdominal sepsis. The most important therapeutic modality however, is surgical incision of involved muscle plus supportive measures including fluid and electrolyte replacement, control of acidosis and management of renal failure.

Streptococcal myonecrosis: This infection resembles gas gangrene and necrotizing synergistic cellulitis, but the tempo of the disease is usually less fulminant. Gas in the soft tissue is uncommon and gram stains of exudate typically show gram positive cocci in chains. The preferred antibiotic is aqueous penicillin G (2-4 million units IV q 4-6 h); clindamycin (600 mg IV q 8 h) or vancomycin (1 g IV q 12 h) are alternatives. Again, surgical débridement with excision of necrotic muscle is crucial.

Pyomyositis: This is a staphylococcal infection of the skeletal muscle that is substantially less severe compared to the lesions described above that cause myonecrosis. Most cases present with focal abscesses of the muscle, commonly in the tropics where it is commonly referred to as "tropical pyomositis." The usual presentation is the insidious onset of pain, swelling and tenderness at the site of involvement, usually a lower extremity or psoas. The infection is easily demonstrated by CT scans and needle aspirates typically yield purulent exudate with *S. aureus*. Some patients respond to antibiotics alone directed against *S. aureus* such as a penicillinase-resistant penicillin such a nafcillin or oxacillin (1.5-3 g IV q 6 h), an anti-staphylococcal cephalosporin such as cefazolin (1.5-2 g IV q 8 h) or vancomycin (1 g IV q 12 h). Some patients require surgical drainage, but the surgery is not the extensive, mutilating type required for the muscle infections reviewed earlier.

Tetanus

Tetanus is a neuroparalytic syndrome caused by the neurotoxin, tetanospasmin, produced by *Clostridium tetani*. Requirements for disease are a source of the organism, local conditions that promote toxin production and inadequate humoral antibody.

There are four recognized forms of tetanus:

- Generalized tetanus accounts for at least 80% of all cases. The usual incubation period between wounding and the onset of symptoms is 7–21 days. Typical initial symptoms are trismus and tonic-clonic contractures of the face, neck, jaw and abdomen. Tetanic seizures are characterized by a sudden tonic contracture of the back with flexion and adduction of the arms, clenched fists and extension of the legs. The mortality rate of this form of tetanus in the United States is 25–30%.
- *Local tetanus* is characterized by localized involvement of the extremity with the contaminated wound. More severe cases of localized tetanus are characterized by painful spasms and usually progress to generalized tetanus. This is an unusual form of tetanus and prognosis for survival is excellent.
- *Cephalic tetanus* usually follows head injury or occurs with *C. tetani* infection in the middle ear. Symptoms include dysfunction of the cranial nerves, most frequently the 7th. This may remain localized or progress to generalized tetanus and the prognosis for survival is extremely poor.
- *Tetanus neonatorium* refers to generalized tetanus in neonates, a relatively common complication in underdeveloped countries where contaminated materials are used to sever or dress the umbilical cord in unimmunized mothers. The usual incubation period is 3-7 days after birth. The child typically shows irritability, facial grimacing and severe spasms if touched. The mortality rates exceeds 70%.

Diagnosis: *C. tetani* is infrequently recovered in cultures of the wound. A confirmed history of immunization or serum antibody level exceeding 0.01 units/dl makes tetanus extremely unlikely. The differential diagnosis includes oculogyric crisis due to phenothiazine toxicity, dental abscess, meningitis, subarachnoid, seizure disorder, tetany due to alkalosis or hypocalcemia, strychnine poisoning or alcoholic withdrawal.

Treatment:

Surgery: Associated wounds should be débrided.

Antibiotics: Penicillin G (1-10 million units/day IV) for ten days; alternatives are tetracycline (500 mg po qid), erythromycin (500 mg po qid) or chloramphenical (0.5-1 g po or IV q 6 h).

Antitoxin: Human tetanus immunoglobulin (TIG) should be given as soon as possible in doses ranging from 500–6,000 units.

Active Immunization: Full course should be given, and this does not interfere with detectable levels of TIG.

Muscle Spasms: Chlorpromazine (50–150 mg every 4-8 hours), meprobamate (400 mg every 3–4 hours) or diazepam (2–20 mg intravenously every 2-8 hours).

Supportive Care: Maintenance of an airway is important, and this may require intubation followed by tracheostomy. There also needs to be careful attention to fluid balance, autonomic instability, gastrointestinal bleeding and pulmonary embili.

Prevention: Current recommendations are for DPT vaccination of children at two months, six months, fifteen months and 4-6 years. Tetanus toxoid is highly effective and provides protective levels of antitoxin for

Table 26–9
***Tetanus Prophylaxis* (MMWR 40:RR10, 1991)**

HISTORY OF TETANUS TOXOID	CLEAN, MINOR WOUNDS		OTHER WOUNDS**	
	Td*	TIG*	Td*	TIG*
Unknown or <3 doses	Yes	No	Yes	Yes
≥3 doses***	No, unless >10 yrs since last dose	No	No, unless >5 yrs since last dose	No

* Td = Tetanus toxoid; TIG = Tetanus immune globulin
** Wounds contaminated with dirt, stool, soil, saliva, etc.; puncture wounds; avulsions; wounds from missiles, crushing, burns and frostbite.
*** If only three doses or toxoid, a fourth should be given.

at least ten years. Td (tetanus and diphtheria toxoids for adult use) is recommended every ten years at the mid-decade ages. Prevention of tetanus after injury requires appropriate wound management, assurance of adequate immunity and consideration of prophylactic antibiotics. Guidelines for immunoprophylaxis are based on immunization status and characteristics of the wound as summarized in Table 26–9.

UPPER RESPIRATORY INFECTIONS

Pharyngitis

Diagnosis: The major causes are Group A β-hemolytic streptococci or viruses. The classic presentation of Group A streptococcal pharyngitis includes sore throat with dysphagia, fever and an exam showing exudative pharyngitis with cervical adenopathy; cough laryngitis and coryza are uncommon. Throat cultures is the gold standard for diagnosis, but false negative cultures are noted in up to 10% of cases, results are not available for 24–72 hours and carrier rates (false positive cultures) are found in 5–10% of healthy adults. Antigen detection provides results in 5–10 minutes, but is relatively expensive and clearly less sensitive than culture. Current recommendations of the American Academy of Pediatrics are that negative rapid test should be confirmed by culture. Serology for antistreptolysin O or anti-DNAase B requires weeks for diagnostic titers indicating tissue invasion and are primarily useful for the diagnosis of nonsuppurative sequelae (rheumatic fever and glomerulo-nephritis). Other diagnostic considerations of clinically important causes of a sore throat include:

- Diphtheria: The characteristic finding is a grayish yellow pseudomembrane over the pharynx and tonsils which spreads over the soft palate, uvula and anterior pillars; the diagnosis is confirmed by culture for Corynebacterium dipththeriae.
- Vincent angina: A grayish membrane combined with putrid discharge; stain of exudate shows typical fusiform gram-negative bacilli and culture for aerobic pathogens is negative.
- Thrush: White exudative plaques that stud the oral mucosa in immunosuppressed patient, especially those with advanced HIV infection; the diagnosis is usually recognized clinically, but may be supported by stains of exudate showing yeast and pseudomycelia.

- *Mycoplasma pneumoniae:* Nonspecific findings, but may be accompanied by bronchitis/pneumonitis, fever, typical exposure history with an incubation period of 2-3 weeks and occasional cases with extrapulmonary findings; the diagnosis is usually established with acute and convalescent serology.
- Gonococcal pharyngitis: Most are asymptomatic, but some patients show erythema or occasionally exudate; the diagnosis is established with culture accompanied by a specific request for *N. gonorrhoeae* in the patient with an exposure history.
- Herpes simplex: Vesicular lesions on an erythematous base on the mucous membranes, especially the soft palate; the diagnosis may be established by showing typical intranuclear inclusions on a Zanck prep or culture.
- Epstein Barr virus: Erythema or exudative pharyngitis with cervical adenopathy and fever, often accompanied by generalized lymphadenopathy, splenomegaly and profound fatigue; the diagnosis is supported with a CBC showing atypical lymphocytes and a positive "mono-spot test," which may be falsely negative in early stages.
- HIV-1: Pharyngitis accompanied by generalized lymphadenopathy, hepatosplenomegaly, a morbilliform rash, dysphagia, and leukopenia in a patient with sexual or needle sharing exposure 2–6 weeks previously; the diagnosis is established by showing high titers of p24 antigen of HIV with negative serology and subsequent seroconversion within 6–12 weeks.
- *Chlamydia pneumoniae:* Erythema with laryngitis, and sometimes bronchitis and pneumonitis; no diagnostic test is commonly available in clinical laboratories.
- Viruses other than EBV, HIV-1 and HSV including rhinovirus (common cold), adenovirus (nonspecific pharyngitis) and Coxsackie–A (herpangina with vesicles on the faucial pillars).

TREATMENT

Streptococcal pharyngitis: Reasons to treat are to 1) reduce symptoms (but therapeutic trials show symptoms are reduced by only one day before improvement without treatment); 2) prevention of suppurative complications, primarily peritonsillar abscess; 3) prevention of epidemiologic spread; 4) prevention of non-suppurative complications, primarily rheumatic fever (treatment with penicillin within five days of the onset of sore throat will completely prevent subsequent rheumatic fever and treatment as late as ten days has demonstrated benefit.

- Preferred treatment: Benzathine penicillin, 1.2 million units x 1 *or* penicillin VK, 250 po four times daily x 10 days.
- Alternative treatment: Erythromycin, 250 mg po four times daily x 10 days.

Diphtheria: Penicillin or erythromycin plus antitoxin.

N. gonorrhoeae: Ceftriaxone, 125 mg IM x 1 *or* ciprofloxacin, 500 mg po x 1.

Vincent angina: Penicillin VK, 250 mg po four times daily x 10 days, clindamycin, 300 mg po qid or metronidazole, 250 mg po tid.

EBV (infectious mononucleosis): Usually no therapy, but some suggest prednisone (80 mg/day x 2–3 days, then taper over two weeks) for impending airway closure, prolonged course with high fever or persistent morbidity (JAMA 256:1051, 1986).

Sinusitis

Diagnosis: Characteristic symptoms are nasal discharge and face pain often accompanied by fever. Major other diagnostic considerations are allergic rhinitis and uncomplicated viral upper respiratory tract infections. The diagnosis of sinusitis is made by demonstrating abnormal transillumination, and tenderness over the maxillary or frontal sinuses. X-rays (Waters view) shows mucosal thickening, an air-fluid level or opaque sinuses; CT or MRI provide excellent anatomical definition, but are expensive and usually not necessary for diagnosis. Cultures of the nasal discharge are generally useless; preferred specimens are obtained by aspiration of sinuses which is usually not necessary because likely pathogens are easily predicted: *S. pneumoniae, H. influenzae* and *Moraxella catarrhalis.*

Treatment: Amoxicillin, 500 mg po three times daily x 7–14 days. This is usually recommended despite lack of activity against common betalactamase-producing organisms because the results are as good as with more expensive drugs (Arch Fam Med 2:497,1993).

- Alternatives: Trimethoprim-sulfamethoxazole, 1 DS po bid x 7–14 days; erythromycin, 250-500 mg po qid x 7–14 days; cefaclor, 500 mg po bid x 7–14 days; doxycycline, 100 mg po bid x 7–14 days. Probably equally effective are cefuroxime axetil, cefpodoxime, loracarbef, cefprozil and amoxicillin plus clavulanate.
- Refractory or recurrent cases: Prolonged courses of antibiotics, 4–6 weeks, are sometimes required. Nasal decongestants are important to include in the therapeutic regimen. Some patients with refractory cases benefit from sinus lavage.
- Chronic sinusitis: The usual pathogens are anaerobic bacteria and occasionally *S. aureus*; antibiotic treatment is usually reserved for acute flares. Surgery is often required.
- Nosocomial sinusitis: This is a common complication associated with nasal intubation in seriously ill patients, usually involves *P. aeruginosa* or coliform bacteria, and is generally treated aggressively for these organisms using a 3rd generation cephalosporin or antipseudomonad penicillin combined with an aminoglycoside.

Acute Otitis Media

Diagnosis: Cardinal symptoms are earache, discharge and conductive deafness; the diagnosis is established on physical exam which shows a bulging tympanic membrane that may drain pus if perforation has occurred. Cultures may be obtained from purulent drainage that occurs spontaneously or with myringotomy.

Antibiotic treatment: Empiric selections are identical to those recommended for acute sinusitis; optimal therapy is based on results of culture when available. Myringotomy should be considered in patients with severe pain if the tympanic membrane is intact.

INTRA-ABDOMINAL SEPSIS

Intra-abdominal sepsis refers to infections within the abdominal cavity external to the lumen of the gastrointestinal tract. Included are a diverse array of processes involving peritoneal surface and parenchymal organs such as liver, spleen and pancreas.

PATHOPHYSIOLOGY

Microbiology: The usual bacteria are those that colonize the gastrointestinal tract. The usual mechanism for infections involving serosal surfaces is a break in the mucosal barrier secondary to another process such as a perforated peptic ulcer, appendicitis, inflammatory bowel disease, intestinal surgery, colonic carcinoma or diverticular disease. The types of bacteria found depends on the level of gastrointestinal tract involved. The stomach harbors a relatively sparse flora of predominantly penicillin-sensitive gram positive bacteria that originate from the oropharynx. The small bowel also has small numbers of bacteria due to constant peristalsis; in the presence of obstruction, this defense mechanism is lost and there is overgrowth with a flora comparable to the colon's. The largest microbial populations and the segment of the gastrointestinal tract responsible for most intra-abdominal sepsis is the colon. Here the bacteria reached the geometric limits for space occupation with 10^{12}/g of the intestinal contents. About 99% are anaerobic bacteria. Coliforms (especially *E. coli*) and Bacteroides species are virtually always present.

Chemical Irritants: Chemical irritants or adjuvants often contribute to the pathologic process by their chemotactic properties or by preventing phagocytosis. Adjuvants include hemoglobulin, the fiber content of stool, fibrin, necrotic tissue and barium sulfate. Chemical irritants may elicit an inflammatory response independent of bacteria and include pancreatic enzymes, bile and gastric acid.

Biphasic Disease: The sequence of events with many or most cases of intra-abdominal sepsis is sometimes referred to as the biphasic disease. The initial insult may be free perforation of the intestine with generalized peritonitis and the usual signs of an acute abdomen. Alternatively, the infection may be successfully localized to the portal of entry to form a phlegmon or localized peritonitis. The latter is a much more subtle process and often escapes detection. With either localized or generalized peritonitis, a common sequelae is the 2nd stage of the infection characterized by intra-abdominal abscesses.

DIAGNOSTIC TESTS

Nonspecific Tests: Most patients have leukocytosis, and many will have abnormal liver function tests, an abnormal chest x-ray (pleural infusion, elevated diaphragm or atelectasis) or a positive blood culture. Bacteroides bacteremia specifically suggests intra-abdominal sepsis.

Scans: Scanning (particularly CT) has revolutionized the ability to detect intra-abdominal sepsis. CT scanning generally shows sensitivity and specificity approaching 95% for detection of intra-abdominal abscesses. Results with ultrasound are somewhat less impressive, but this technique offers the advantage that it can be used for seriously ill patients because it can be done at the bedside and avoids radiation exposure. Gallium scans require 48–72 hours and fail to distinguish tumors from inflammatory masses; the gallium is also excreted into the bowel lumen with frequent confusion in interpretation. Some of the disadvantages are avoided with indium-labelled neutrophil scans, but their main advantage is ability to detect inflammatory lesions outside the abdomen.

Peritonitis

Primary Peritonitis: Primary or spontaneous peritonitis is an infection of the peritoneal cavity found in patients with ascites, usually children with nephrosis or adults with cirrhosis. The presumed mechanism is bacteremic seeding of ascites fluid which is an excellent culture medium. The major pathogens are coliform-bacteria (primarily *E. coli*) or streptococci including *S. pneumoniae*.

Diagnosis: Suspect this infection in any febrile patient with ascites. The abdomen is usually tender and blood cultures are often positive. The major diagnostic test is analysis of peritoneal fluid showing over 300 leukocytes/ml with a predominance of polymorphonuclear cells; culture of peritoneal fluid and/or blood are usually positive.

Treatment (pending culture results): Gentamicin or tobramycin, 2 mg/kg IV, then 1.7 mg/kg q 8 h *plus* a betalactam: Cefoxitin, 2 g IV q 6 h; cefotaxime, 1.5–2 g IV q 6 h; ampicillin, 2 g IV q 6 h; or piperacillin, 4–5 g IV q 6 h or cefotaxime, 1.5–2 g IV q 6 h ± ampicillin, 2 g IV q 6 h.

Peritonitis Complicating Peritoneal Dialysis: The indwelling catheter, such as a Tenckhoff device, provides a direct route for invasion either on the external surface of the catheter, or more frequently, through the catheter lumen. Major pathogens are the resident skin flora with *S. epidermidis* accounting for most cases; *S. aureus*, streptococci, coliforms, *P. aeruginosa* and *C. albicans* account for the remainder.

Diagnosis: Most patients have abdominal pain and tenderness; fever is uncommon. The major finding is a cloudy dialysate showing a leukocyte count >than 100/ml with a predominance of neutrophils. Gram stain is usually not positive, but cultures yield the responsible organism in 90–95%.

Treatment: This is a localized infection so that antimicrobial activity is required only in the peritoneal fluid. This can be achieved by giving antibiotics either systemically or intraperitoneally: Parenteral antibiotics pending cultures: Vancomycin, 1 g plus gentamicin or tobramycin, 1.7 mg/kg. Antibiotic Doses in Dialysate: Gentamicin or tobramycin: 7–140 mg/2L (initial), 8–16 mg/2L (maintenance); vancomycin: 1000–2000 mg/2L (initial), 30–50 mg/2L (maintenance); cefotaxime: 2000 mg/2L (initial), 100–250 mg/2L (maintenance); ticarcillin: 1000–2000/2L (initial), 250 mg/2L (maintenance); amphotericin b: 2–8 mg/2L.

Removal of Catheter: This is required in 10–20% of cases. Indications are the following: Tunnel infection; fungal infection (most commonly *C. albicans*); *P. aeruginosa* infection; fecal peritonitis; recurrent peritonitis involving the same organism; persistent infection, catheter malfunction with poor flow, or intra-abdominal abscess.

Secondary Peritonitis: This is the most common form of peritonitis representing bacterial contamination from direct extension of bacteria in the gastrointestinal lumen. The peritoneal surface area approximates the total cutaneous surface and usually contains less than 50 ml of clear fluid with <250 cells/ml (approximately 50% macrophages and 40% lymphocytes). Generalized peritonitis may result in a net flow of 300–500 ml of fluid/hour giving rapid hemodynamic instability requiring extensive fluid support. There is a generalized tenderness, rebound tenderness, fever, leukocytosis, nausea, vomiting, ileus and distension with diminished or scant bowel sounds. Much more frequent is localized peritonitis in which the inflammatory reaction is restricted to the site of visceral inflammation as with appendicitis or diverticulitis. These processes tend to be much more indolent with localized pain only if the parietal peritoneum is involved. Physical findings in the abdomen may be particularly deceptive with subphrenic or pelvic infections. Nearly all patients have fever and leukocytosis.

Bacteriology: Most infections are polymicrobial with multiple aerobic and anaerobic bacteria that reflect the colonic flora. *E. coli* is found in 50–80% of cases and *Bacteroides* species in 60–80%. Numerous other coliforms and anaerobes are common as well. Enterococcus is found in 10–20%.

The role of the Enterococcus in intra-abdominal sepsis is unclear and so the need to include an antibiotic against it in the empirically selected regimens is controversial. Some authorities routinely add ampicillin; others delay this decision without a more compelling indication such as Enterococcal bacteremia, predominance of this organism in culture or by gram stain, or failure to respond with antibiotics directed against other components of the infecting flora.

Antibiotic Treatment: Most cases of intra-abdominal sepsis are treated empirically using drugs effective against coliforms and anaerobes.

*Combination treatment** An aminoglycoside vs. coliforms**: Gentamicin, 2.0 mg/kg, then 1.7 mg/kg IV q 8 h (usually preferred) or Tobramycin, 2.0 mg/kg, then 1.7 mg/kg IV q 8 h *or* Amikacin, 7.5 mg/kg, then 5.0 mg/kg IV q 8 h. Plus an antianerobic: Clindamycin, 600 mg IV q 8 h *or* Cefoxitin, 2 g IV q 6 h *or* Metronidazole, 500 mg IV q 8 h

Single drug treatment: Cefoxitin, 2 g IV q 6 h (not advocated as single agent if infection acquired during hospitalization or if there has been antibiotic administration during prior two weeks). Alternatives to cefoxitin are: cefotetan, 1 g IV q 12 h or cefmetazole, 2 g q 6–12 h. Imipenem, 500 mg IV q 6–8 h (See Solomkin J et al: Ann Surg 21:581,1990). Ticarcillin, 3-4 g + clavulanic acid (Timentin IV q 4–6 h. Ampicillin, 2 g + sulbactam, 1 g (Unasyn) IV q 6 h

Drainage: Drainage is the most important component of treatment except for amebic abscesses of the liver that generally respond to medical treatment. The technique for drainage may be percutaneous or with the traditional laparotomy incision. Percutaneous drainage is usually done under ultrasonic or CT guidance. Criteria for percutaneous drainage are the following: a well-defined abscess cavity; safe percutaneous route; immediate operative ability.

Liver Abscess

Diagnosis: Liver abscesses are classified by etiologic agent as pyogenic or amebic. Pyogenic abscesses may be extremely elusive with little more than fever, chills, leukocytosis, and modest changes in liver function tests, especially the alkaline phosphatase. Some patients have positive blood cultures. The diagnosis is usually established with CT scans. The microbiology may be established with percutaneous aspiration. De-

* Some authorities add an agent for the enterococcus: Ampicillin, 1–2 g IV q 6 h

** Aztreonam (1–1.5 gm IV q 6–8 h), ceftazidime (1.5–2 g q 8 h), cefoperazane (1.5–2 g q 8–12 h), ceftriaxone (1-2 g q 24 h) or other 3rd generation cephalosporin may be used instead of aminoglycoside in combination with metronidazole or clindamycin

tection of *E. histolytica* is generally based on serology (complement fixation, indirect hemagglutination or gel-diffusion-precipitin test); stool examination for ova and parasite is occasionally positive. Many patients will have a history of presence in countries where amebiasis is prevalent. Thus, the diagnosis of liver abscess is suspected in the patient with high fever (often FUO), hepatomegaly and/or right upper quadrant tenderness, and abnormal liver function tests (especially alkaline phosphatase elevation and hypoalbuminemia). The diagnosis is generally confirmed with CT scans or ultrasound of the abdomen showing typical ring enhancing lesions of the liver. The microbiologic diagnosis is established by blood cultures for pyogenic bacteria and serology for *E. histolytica*; needle aspiration of an abscess may be required. The distinction between pyogenic and amebic abscess is important because the role of surgery, the selection of antibiotics and the prognosis are very different.

Treatment of amebic abscesses: Metronidazole (750 mg tid or 500 mg IV q 6 h) for 5–10 days. Oral absorption is nearly 100% so po preferred. The alternative is emetine (1 mg/kg/day to a maximum of 65 mg) for ten days or chloroquine (250 mg qid for seven days followed by 250 mg bid for 3–4 weeks). A luminal amebicide such as diiodohydroxyquin should be given concurrently to eliminate cysts. Needle aspiration is not indicated except to establish the diagnosis, for some large abscesses (greater than 10 cm in diameter) for impending rupture or for failure to respond after five days of antibiotic treatment. Most patients respond rapidly and completely; surgery is rarely required.

Treatment of Pyogenic Abscesses: Drainage is often required although the frequency is debated. Some patients have multiple small abscesses which cannot be drained. The prognosis is variable, but most patients with a single abscess do well and those with multiple small abscesses do poorly. Various authorities recommend three fundamentally different approaches:

- Antibiotics alone: Often advocated for patients who have multiple small abscesses which cannot be drained surgically or for patients who show an impressive clinical response to antibiotic treatment during diagnostic evaluation.
- Antibiotics combined with needle aspiration. This affords the opportunity to define bacterial pathogens and to decompress large abscesses.
- Antibiotics combined with surgical drainage or drainage with a tube placed by CT, ultrasound or fluoroscopic guidance. This is traditional management.

Antibiotic selection: The dominant bacteria are coliforms (especially *E. coli* and Klebsiella), streptococci (especially *S. milleri* and anaerobic streptococci), Enterococcus and anaerobes (especially Fusobacteria and Bacteroides sp.). Empiric antibiotics are directed against these organisms. Regimens that include metronidazole have the advantage of including treatment against *E. histolytica* if suspended: Metronidazole (500 mg po or IV q 6–8 hr) or clindamycin (600 mg IV q 8 hr) *plus* gentamicin/tobramycin (2.0 mg/kg IV; the 1.7 mg/kg q 8 hr) or 3rd generation cephalosporins such as ceftazidime (1.5–2 g q 8-12 hr) or cetriaxone (1–2 g q 24 hr) *plus* ampicillin (2 g IV q 6 hr) or aminoglycosides such as gentamicin or tobramycin (2.0 mg/kg IV then 1.7 mg/kg q 8 h) *plus* antipseudomonad penicillin such as piperacillin (4–5 gm IV q 6 hr).

Cholecystitis

Diagnosis: Typical symptoms are acute right upper quadrant pain, anorexia, nausea, vomiting and fever (about 38°C). Exam shows RUQ tenderness, guarding and Murphy's sign (increased tenderness with palpation in subhepatic area during deep inspiration). Over 95% have stones that are most easily and reliably detected with ultrasonography. Radionucleoside scan of the gallbladder with ^{99}Tc DISIDA or related compounds is the preferred method to confirm the diagnosis; filling of the gallbladder makes the diagnosis unlikely.

Treatment: Supportive measures: Nasogastric suction and intravenous hydration: Antibiotics: Early in cholecystitis the gallbladder is sterile; within a week the gallbladder is infected in 30–50% of cases. The primary pathogens in rank order are *E. coli*, other coliforms (Klebsiella, Enterobacter, etc.), Streptococcus, Enterococcus and *Clostridium* sp. Anaerobic bacteria are infrequent except with ascending cholangitis. Although bile is sterile in about 50% of gallbladders resected for acute cholecystitis, infection is responsible for some of the major complications—empyema, gangrene and perforation. Suggested antibiotics are: Ampicillin (2 g IV q 6–8 h) *plus* gentamicin or tobramycin (2.0 mg/kg IV, then 1.7 mg/kg q 8 h) *or* cefoperazone (1–2 g IV q 12 h) alone or in combination with gentamicin or tobramycin. Other 2nd or 3rd generation cephalosporins are probably equally effective.

Surgery: Surgeons continue to debate the relative merits of early or late surgical intervention. *Advantages of early intervention* (within 1–2 days of onset of symptoms) are: The procedure is as safe as with delayed procedures; resection is easier without fibrosis, the duration of hospitalization and recovery is reduced, delay may overlook serious complications such as empyema or perforation and the disease may recur during the waiting period. *Advantages of delayed intervention* are: The patient will be in optimal condition, there is time to clearly establish the diagnosis, resection may be easier if acute inflammation has resolved and the frequency of postoperative complications is reduced.

Pancreatic Abscess

Diagnosis: Abscesses complicate about 2–4% of cases of acute pancreatitis, and are most common with severe, acute first attacks of pancreatitis complicated by hypovolemic shock. The major clue is survival of the acute attack, but continued fever and leukocytosis at 10–14 days when there is deterioration with sepsis. Some patients improve and then deteriorate with fever, nausea and vomiting accompanied by abdominal pain tenderness and a mass. Serum amylase levels are often not helpful. Abdominal x-rays may show displacement of the gastric bubble. Obliteration of the psoas shadow or gas within the abscess (soap bubble sign) is considered diagnostic of a retroperitoneal abscess. The most sensitive and specific diagnostic test is scanning with ultrasound or CT.

Treatment: Most pancreatic abscesses are fatal if not drained. The usual procedure is surgical débridement with external drainage using soft-sump or closed suctioned drains. The initial experience with percutaneous drainage was poor, but this tactic is now gaining greater acceptance.

Antibiotic selection: The usual bacteria are coliforms (*E. coli*, Klebsiella, Enterobacter, Protens, etc.) and Streptococcus or Enterococcus; anaerobes are relatively infrequent. Suggestions for empiric selection based on prior observations are: Aminoglycoside such as gentamicin or tobramycin (2.0 mg/kg IV, then 1.7 mg/kg q 8 h) *or* 3rd generation cephalosporins such as ceftazidime (1.5–2 g q 8-12 h) or ceftriaxone (1–2 g q 24 h) *plus* Ampicillin (2 g IV q 6–8 h) or Aminoglycosides such as gentamicin or tobramycin (2.0 mg/kg IV, then 1.7 mg/kg q 8 h) *plus* an anti-pseudomonad penicillin such as piperacillin (4–5 g IV q 6 h). Ticarcillin + clavulanate (4-5 g IV q 6 h) ± aminoglycoside.

Single drug treatment versus combination treatment: Traditional treatment of intra-abdominal sepsis has included an agent directed against coliforms and a 2nd agent directed against anaerobic bacteria. The expanded spectrum of some drugs now permits the use of a single agent directed against both types of organisms such as imipenem or ticarcillin plus clavulanic acid. Initial studies indicate single drug therapy is equally effective although some feel these drugs should be preserved for infections involving resistant bacteria.

Diverticulitis

Diagnosis: Typical clinical features are abdominal pain (most commonly LLQ), fever (usually 38–39°C), leukocytosis and lower quadrant tenderness, sometimes with a palpable mass. Abdominal x-rays may show thickened bowel wall, displacement of the small bowel or abnormal collection of gas. Barium or hypaque enema exams will show typical diverticula, especially in postevacuation films, but caution is necessary because increased intraluminal pressure may cause perforation. Endoscopy will exclude other diagnoses, especially carcinoma. CT scans, especially with hypaque, are effective in showing inflammation of pericolic fat, diverticula, bowel thickening, fistulas and abscesses.

Treatment: Most patients can be managed without surgery. Supportive care: NPO and IV hydration; nasogastric tube suction if there are signs of obstruction or peritonitis; Antibiotics: regimens summarized above for secondary peritonitis; surgical consult: surgery is indicated for repeated attacks, and complications—perforation, bleeding, fistula formation, obstruction and suspected or established carcinoma.

Appendicitis

Diagnosis: Typical symptoms are fever, nausea, anorexia and abdominal pain that is usually epigastric or periumbilical in early disease and later localizes to the right lower quadrant. Tenderness is nearly always present and often is localized to McBurney's point. About 75% have localized rebound tenderness and 35% rectal tenderness. Flat and upright films may show free air indicating perforation and rarely show calculi in the RLQ. Compression sonography typically shows a noncompressible appendix >6 mm in diameter. CT scans are used increasingly in difficult cases to assist in detecting alternative diagnoses and complications.

Treatment: Surgical removal of the appendix is the traditional method of management. Antibiotics are directed against coliforms and anaerobes using: Combination treatment: Gentamicin *or* tobramycin, 2.0 mg/kg IV, then 1.7 mg/kg q 8 h *plus* clindamycin, 600 mg IV q 8 h, cefoxitin, 2 g IV q 6 h *or* metronidazole, 500 mg IV q 6 h. Single agent: Cefoxitin, 2 g IV q 6 h.

Intra-Abdominal Abscesses

Abscess may be on the peritoneal surface at the portal of entry, in the retroperitoneal space or in viscera such as liver, spleen or pancreas. Abscesses adjacent to the portal of entry reflect successful localization such as a diverticular abscess or periappendiceal abscess. With free perforations, eventual location of the abscesses reflect intra-abdominal flow patterns with gravity favoring caudad spread and negative intra-peritoneal pressure from diaphragmatic movement favoring cephalad spread. Consequently, there is a tendency for abscesses to localize to the subphrenic spaces, pericolic gutter and pelvis.

Microbiology: Most intra-abdominal abscesses involve the same bacteria noted previously in peritonitis, e.g. coliforms (especially *E. coli*) and anaerobes (especially *Bacteroides fragilis*). An exception is hepatic abscesses involving *E. histolytica*.

Diagnosis: Nearly all patients have fever and leukocytosis; most have abdominal pain and/or tenderness, but this varies with site. As noted, subphrenic and pelvic abscesses are often difficult to detect with abdominal exams. CT has revolutionized the ability to detect intra-abdominal abscesses so these are now rare causes of fever of unknown origin.

Antibiotic Treatment: Most cases of intra-abdominal abscess are treated empirically using drugs effective against coliforms and anaerobes.

- *Combination treatment**: An aminoglycoside vs. coliforms**: Gentamicin, 2.0 mg/kg, then 1.7 mg/kg IV q 8 h (usually preferred) *or* Tobramycin, 2.0 mg/kg, then 1.7 mg/kg IV q 8 h *or* Amikacin, 7.5 mg/kg, then 5.0 mg/kg IV q 8 h. *plus* an agent vs. anaerobes: Clindamycin, 600 mg IV q 8 h *or* Cefoxitin, 2 g IV q 6 h *or* Metronidazole, 500 mg IV q 8 h.
- *Single drug treatment*: Cefoxitin, 2 g IV q 6 h (not advocated as single agent if infection was acquired during hospitalization or if antibiotic administration during prior 2 weeks). Alternatives to cefoxitin are: cefotetan, 1 g IV q 12 h or cefmethazole, 2 g q 6–12 h. Imipenem, 500 mg IV q 6–8 h (See Solomkin J et al: Ann Surg 212:581,1990). Ticarcillin, 3–4 g + clavulanate acid (Timentin) IV q 4–6 h. Ampicillin, 2 g + sulbactam, 1 g (Unasyn) IV q 6 h.

INFECTIOUS DIARRHEA

Diarrhea reflects increased water in stools due to impaired absorption, increased secretion or both. Diarrhea is defined on the basis of stool volume (>200 g/day for adults), increased fluid content of stool (>80% for semi-solid stool and >98% for liquid stool) or the frequency and character of stool (usually defined as 2–3 liquid or semi-solid stools/day for an arbitrary period, usually at least 2–3 consecutive days). Diarrhea is also classified as acute (sudden onset with symptoms of <1 week) or chronic (usually insidious onset and long duration, usually 2-4 weeks). Infections are only one of many causes of acute and chronic diarrhea, but infectious diarrhea is 2nd only to cardiovascular disease as a cause of death in the world and the leading cause of childhood death in Asia, Africa and Latin America. Rates of gastrointestinal infections range from 1.5–2/adult/year in the U.S. and 15–20/child/year in some tropical countries. Most cases of infectious diarrhea in both adults and children are mild, self-limited and untreatable. Decisions about diagnostic evalu-

* Some authorities add an agent for the enterococcus: Ampicillin, 1–2 g IV q 6 h.
** Aztreonam (1–1.5 g IV q 6–8 h), ceftazidime (1.5–2 g q 8 h), ceftriaxone (1–2 g q 24 h), or other 3rd generation cephalosporin may be used in place of aminoglycoside in combination with metronidazole or clindamycin.

ations and antimicrobial treatment of infectious diarrhea is an important component of both the art and science of medical care.

Types of Enteric Infections

The traditional classification of infectious diarrhea is by three pathogenic mechanisms that play a central role in the differential diagnosis and management.

- Non-inflammatory diarrhea: This is the major cause of diarrheal illness that usually results from infection of the small bowel due to the action of enterotoxin (such as *V. cholera* or enterotoxigenic *E. coli* toxins) or other conditions that interfere with the absorptive function of the villus (such as infection with Cryptosporidium, Giardia, Microsporidia, Rotavirus, Norwalk virus and other small round viruses). These patients typically present with watery diarrhea without fecal leukocytes, blood or mucus. The volume of diarrhea is large, and in severe cases of cholera may actually exceed 10 L/day.
- Inflammatory diarrhea or dysentery: This usually results from colonic infection with microbial invasion of the colonic mucosa or local toxin that elicits an inflammatory response. The prototypical example is Shigellosis, although the most common cause in the United States is *Campylobacter jejuni*; other prominent causes of inflammatory diarrhea include Salmonella, Yersinia, *C. difficile*, Aeromonas, Plesiomonas, amebiasis and enterohemorrhagic *E. coli*. Patients in this category often have fecal leukocytes, and/or blood in stool. In classic dysentery there are frequent, small volume stools with gross blood or mucus accompanied by abdominal cramps, fever and tenesmus.
- Enteric fever: A 3rd type of infection is found primarily with typhoid fever, some other forms of salmonellosis and possibly Yersinia. The course of infection is initially characterized by constipation with high fever and positive blood cultures due to systemic infection following invasion of Peyer's patches; the organisms then return to the gut through the biliary tract to cause diarrhea with positive stool cultures in a later phase of the infection.

Differential Diagnosis

Diarrhea may be caused by a variety of conditions including many that are not infectious. Remember this in diagnosis (Table 26–10). The pathophysiology of diarrhea is based on 4 different mechanisms:

- Osmotic diarrhea that responds to fasting and shows a large solute gap: fecal solute gap = serum osmolality minus $2 \times (Na^+$ plus $K^+)$ in stool.
- Secretory diarrhea which results in large volume watery diarrhea that persists with fasting and the stool osmolality $[2 \times (Na^+$ plus $K^+)]$ is close to the osmolality of plasma.
- Abnormal morphology of the colon which causes diarrhea by a number of mechanisms.
- Abnormal motility which may cause diarrhea due to bacterial overgrowth, "intestinal hurry" or premature emptying of the colon.

The proper management of infectious diarrhea requires recognition of specific microbial patterns with appropriate use of laboratory diagnostic techniques and clinical correlations. Likely agents and use of diagnostic resources is largely dependent on patient age, the distinction between

Table 26–10
Diarrhea: Differential Diagnosis

- Osmotic diarrhea (responds to fasting)
  - Ingestion of poorly absorbed solutes
    - $MgSO_4$, laxatives, some antacids such as $MgOH_2$, mannitol, sorbitol
  - Maldigestion
    - Disaccharide deficiency, short bowel syndrome, postgastrectomy syndrome, intestinal ischemia, lactulose deficiency
  - Mucosal transport defects
- Secretary diarrhea (large volume, watery diarrhea)
  - Caffeine/laxatives/laxative abuse
  - Enterotoxins (ETEC, *V. cholera*)
  - Pancreatic cholera syndrome
  - Carcinoid syndrome
  - Zollinger-Ellison syndrome
- Morphologic changes in intestine
  - Viral gastroenteritis
  - Bacterial/parasitic invasion (Shigella, *E. histolytica*) or toxin mediated (*C. difficile, E. coli* 0157:H7)
  - Sprue
  - Idiopathic inflammatory bowel disease
  - Lymphoma
  - Ischemia
  - Whipple disease
  - Radiation enteritis
  - Collagen-vascular disease
  - Eosinophilic colitis/enteritis
  - AIDS enteropathy
- Abnormal motility
  - Irritable bowel syndrome (?)
  - Neuropathy–diabetic
  - Post vagotomy/postgastrectomy dumping syndrome
  - Small bowel overgrowth

secretory and inflammatory diarrhea, severity of the symptoms, and epidemiologic setting.

Diagnosis of Microbial Agents

Fecal leukocyte exam: Fresh stool (preferably mucus obtained with an applicator stick) mixed with methylene blue and examined microscopically—many PMNs is a positive; a few PMNs or none is negative.

PMNs often present	***Variable***	***Not present***
Campylobacter jejuni	*Salmonella*	*Vibrio cholerae*
Shigella	*Yersinia*	Enteroadherent *E. coli*
Enteroinvasive *E. coli*	Vibrio para$_t$	Enterotoxigenic *E. coli*
Exacerbations of inflammatory bowel disease	*C. difficile*	Food poisoning
	Aeromonas	*S. aureus*
	Plesiomonas	*B. cereus*
	Enterohemorrhagic *E. coli*	*C. perfringens*
		Viral Gastroenteritis
		Adenovirus
		Rotavirus

PMNs often present	*Variable*	*Not present*
		Norwalk agent
		Calicivirus
		Parasitic infection
		Giardia
		*E. histolytica**
		Cryptosporidia
		Isospora
		Small bowel overgrowth
		"AIDS enteropathy"

Microbial Agents

- **Stool culture:** Routine stool cultures for most labs include Salmonella, Shigella and *C. jejunii*; the routine studies or a specific request may be required for Yersinia, Aeromonas, Pleisomonas, Enterohemorrhagic *E. coli* (serotype 0157:H7), *Vibrio cholera* and *Vibrio parahaemolyticus* (or other non-cholera vibrios).
- *C. difficile*: The usual test is the tissue culture assay to detect toxin B or an EIA to detect toxin A and/or toxin B.
- *Ova and parasite*: Major pathogens detected are *E. histolytica*, Cryptosporidia, *Dientamoeba fragilis*, Isospora and *G. lamblia*; non-pathogenic commensals are common and include *Blastocystis hominis, E. nana, E. hartmanni* and *Entamoeba coli*. Repeated stool studies may be required to detect some of the pathogenic protozoan parasites, especially giardia where the yield with three stools is about 80%; alternative methods are duodenal fluid analysis, jejunal biopsy and immunodiagnostic studies of stool or DNA probes. The same concern applies to *E. histolytica* where endoscopy collected specimens may be preferred and serology (IHA titers > 1.128) is positive in > 85% with invasive disease. Modified acid fast staining is preferred for detecting Cryptosporidia and Isospora.

Host Categories

TRAVELERS' DIARRHEA

Most studies show 30–50% of persons from industrialized countries visiting underdeveloped countries will develop "travelers' diarrhea." The most common cause is enterotoxigenic *E. coli* (ETEC); this is usually a trivial, self-limited form of diarrhea that, despite a benign course, may be quite disruptive to a vacation or business trip. Clinical laboratories are not able to detect ETEC so that diagnostic studies of stool for fecal leukocytes and/or stool culture are generally positive. Other likely agents of travelers' diarrhea include Shigella, Salmonella, Aeromonas (especially in Thailand), non-Cholera vibrios (coastal areas of Asia), Cryptosporidium (Russia, especially St. Petersburg), Giardia (North America and Russia), Rotavirus and Norwalk virus (especially Mexico). Factors that influence the likelihood of travelers' diarrhea include residence of the traveler in a highly industrialized area, lack of travel to a tropical area in six months or longer, lack of adherence to careful food and drink selection, reduced gastric acidity, and immunodeficiency.

Prevention: Travelers should be advised to consume only freshly prepared food that is steaming hot, fruit that can be peeled, vegetables that

* Frequently associated with blood

have been washed with previously boiled or bottled water, syrups, jellies, bread, hot tea or coffee, and bottled beverages including alcoholic and carbonated beverages. The advisability of prophylaxis depends on the host status and travel circumstances

- **Bismuth subsalicylate:** This form of prophylaxis is not as effective as antimicrobial drugs, but is probably adequate for most high risk areas and has the fewest side effects and a relatively low cost. It is advocated for the traveler who requests prophylaxis, is unwilling to follow dietary restrictions and/or has a trip in which a modest or brief illness might cause important consequences. The dose is two 262 mg tablets qid.
- **Antibiotic prophylaxis:** Efficacy is established and most predictable with fluoroquinolones which are also most expensive; trimethoprim-sulfamethoxazole is effective in inland Mexico during the summer, but resistance is a major problem in most underdeveloped areas. The dose is 160–800 mg (1 DS/day). Doxycycline has established merit from studies done in the late 1970s, but most areas now show major resistance. Doses of these drugs recommended for prophylaxis during travel are the following which is adapted from DuPont HL and Ericsson CD: Prevention and treatment of travelers' diarrhea. New Engl J Med 328:1821, 1993:

Agent	*Dose*	*Comment*
Bismuth subsalicylate	two-262 mg tabs/day	Less effective than antibiotics; low cost; fewer side effects
Trimethoprim-sulfamethoxazole	160/800 mg (1 DS)/day	Resistance is problematic except for inland Mexico. Low price
Fluoroquinolones		
Norfloxacin	400 mg/day	Fluoroquinolones are most predictably effective
Ciprofloxacin	500 mg/day	
Ofloxacin	300 mg/day	

Treatment

- **Rehydration:** Dehydrating diarrhea is unusual so that most travelers can take virtually any beverage coupled with a source of salt such as saltine crackers. Small children may require electrolyte-containing solutions such as Pedialyte or Lytren. Glucose-electrolyte solutions are now commonly available in pharmacies and grocery stores in many countries, and these are preferred for adults and children with severe, dehydrating diarrhea.
- **Symptomatic relief:** Preferred drugs are Bismuth subsalicylate (one oz every 30 minutes for a total of 8 oz/day) and/or loperamide (4 mg initially, then 2 mg after each loose stool, not to exceed 16 mg/day). Loperamide and other antiperistaltic agents are to be avoided in patients with symptoms of dysentery with bloody stools or fever.
- **Antibiotic treatment:** Recommended for patients with moderate diarrhea defined as at least three stools per day with tolerable symptoms that do not interfere with activities. The recommendation is a loading dose of the antimicrobial followed by standard dose for three days. Loperamide may be taken with antibiotics for moderate diarrhea, but should be avoided in patients with dysentery. These recommendations are summarized below (adapted from Ericsson CD and DuPont HL: Travelers' diarrhea: Approaches to Prevention and Treatment. Clin Infect Dis 16:616,1993):

Severity of diarrhea	*Preferred treatment*
Mild: 1-2 loose stools/ 24 h	None
Moderate: ≥3 loose stools/24 h and tolerable symptoms	Loperamide: 4 mg, then 2 mg after each loose stool up to 16 mg/day. Symptoms persist >2 days: Antibiotic treatment
Moderately severe: ≥3 loose stools/24 h with distressing symptoms (interferes with activities)	Loperamide (above dose) plus Single dose antibiotic TMP- SMX: 2 DS tabs × 1 Norfloxacin: 800 mg × 1 Ciprofloxacin: 1000 mg × 1 Ofloxacin: 600 mg × 1
Severe diarrhea: ≥3 loose stools/24 h incapacitating symptoms, fever or bloody stools	Avoid loperamide Antibiotic-loading dose followed by 3-day course TMP-SMX: 2 DS, then 1 DS bid × 3 days Norfloxacin: 800 mg, then 400 mg bid × 3 days Ciproflaxacin: 1000 mg, then 500 mg bid × 3 days Ofloxacin: 600 mg, then 300 mg bid × 3 days

FOODBORNE AND WATERBORNE OUTBREAKS

There are about 400–600 outbreaks annually in the U.S., although most are not reported; current estimate is about 6 million cases of waterborne and foodborne illness/year. Most foodborne outbreaks involve bacteria. The major pathogen is Salmonella; less common, but important to consider, are food poisoning due to enteric toxin-producing bacteria (*C. perfringens* type A, *S. aureus*, *B. cereus*), enterotoxigenic *E. coli*, Enterohemorrhagic *E. coli*, *V. cholera*, Yersinia, Aeromonas and *V. parahaemolyticus*. In recent years there has been a 10 × increase in the number of infections involving *S. enteritidis* in the northeast U.S., primarily for infected eggs now subject to stricter regulations. Parasites are less frequent and may include *G. lamblia*, *E. histolytica*, *Diphyllobothrium latum* and cryptosporidia. Waterborne outbreaks most often involve *G. lamblia* or cryptosporidium, and both have been implicated with ingestion of chlorinated but inadequately filtered water. Neurologic symptoms that occur rapidly after a meal with or without gastrointestinal dinoflagellate symptoms suggests histamine-like serombrotoxin, neurotoxins, mushrooms, solanine, pesticides or monosodium glutamate.

Differential diagnosis: The differential diagnosis of food poisoning syndromes based on symptoms and incubation period from the time of exposure is listed in Table 26–11.

Diagnostic evaluation: Diagnostic studies depend largely on the suspected pathogen based on the epidemiologic setting and incubation period in Table 26–12. In many cases, the diagnostic studies are done primarily in the interest of public health since most of the conditions listed are brief, self-limited, cause minimal morbidity and are not treatable. With regard to antimicrobial therapy, the agents listed that would require specific forms of antimicrobial treatment include all cases of Shigella, giardiasis, amebiasis; some cases of enterotoxigenic *E. coli* and *C. jejunii* are rare cases of salmonellosis.

Table 26–11
Differential Diagnosis of Diarrhea Associated with Food or Water Contamination

INCUBATION PERIOD	VOMITING	FEVER	CAUSES	DIAGNOSIS
1–6 hrs.	+ +	0	Preformed toxins: *S. aureus* or *B. cereus* Anisakis, heavy metals *D. latam*	Detection of toxin in food; usually clinical diagnosis
8–16 hrs.	±	0	Toxin produced in vivo: *C. perfringens* type A and *B. cereus*	Isolation of organism from food or stool
6–72 hrs.	±	±	Salmonella, Shigella, *C. jejunii, V. parahemolyticus,* Enterotoxigenic *E. coli* *Enterohemorrhagic E. coli* *V. cholera,* Yersinia, Aeromonas, Giardia, Cryptosporidia	Stool culture and O&P exam
12–72 hrs.	+ +	±	Norwalk agent	Research lab only

ANTIBIOTIC EXPOSURE

Diarrhea is a common complication of antibiotic treatment and the only etiologic agent identified in the majority of cases is *C. difficile*. Any antimicrobial may cause this complication, but clindamycin has the highest frequency. As with most enteric pathogens, there is a spectrum of disease in which many patients have rather trivial, self-limited diarrhea; at the other end of the spectrum are patients with severe, life threatening pseudomembranous colitis (PMC). The frequency of *C. difficile* among all patients with antibiotic-associated diarrhea is 10–25%, for antibiotic-associated diarrhea with colitis 50–70% and for antibiotic-associated PMC 90–100%. This diagnosis should be suspected in any patient with diarrhea complicating antibiotic exposure, but the frequency of positive *C. difficile* toxin assays and the need to make this diagnosis is magnified when there is severe diarrhea despite discontinuation of the implicated agent, chronic diarrhea, enigmatic diarrhea, diarrhea complicated by systemic findings (fever and leukocytosis), hypoalbuminemia, toxic megacolon or suspected intra-abdominal sepsis.

Diagnosis: Approximately 1/2 patients have fecal leukocytes. Endoscopy may show PMC which is considered nearly diagnostic of *C. difficile*-induced disease, although there are occasional other causes such as intestinal ischemia, Crohn disease, shigellosis, heavy metal poisoning, etc. A CT scan of the abdomen often shows a characteristic thickened colonic mucosa with ascites, lack of small bowel involvement and contrast material giving the characteristic "accordion sign." The preferred test for a specific diagnosis is an assay for *C. difficile* toxin, preferably with the standard tissue culture assay or the more recently introduced enzyme immunoassay (EIA).

Treatment: Many patients with mild symptoms do not require therapy except to discontinue the implicated agent. Patients with severe diarrhea should be treated with the less expensive metronidazole (500 mg po bid) or vancomycin (125 mg po qid). Vancomycin is more expensive, and highly effective with response rates of 95–99%. Most patients have resolution of fever within 24–48 hours and gradual resolution of

Table 26–12
Treatment of Infectious Diarrhea

MICROBIAL AGENT	PREFERRED	ALTERNATIVE	COMMENT
Bacteria			
Aeromonas hydrophilia	Sulfa-trimethoprim 1 DS bid × 5 days Ciprofloxacin, 500 mg po bid × 5 days	Tetracycline, 500 mg po qid × 5 days Gentamicin, 1.7 mg/kg IV q8h × 5 days	Efficacy of treatment not established and should be reserved for patients with severe disease, immunosuppression, extraintestinal infection or prolonged diarrhea.
Campylobacter jejuni	Erythromycin, 250–500 mg po qid × 7 days Ciprofloxacin, 500 mg po bid × 7 days	Doxycycline, 100 mg po bid × 7 days Furazolidone, 100 mg po qid × 7 days	May not alter course unless given early or for severe Sx. Indications include: acutely ill, persistent fever, bloody diarrhea >8 stools/day, dehydration symptoms <4 days or to prevent transmission. Resistance to erythromycin has been described. Clinical course not altered when started >4 days after onset of symptoms.
Clostridium difficile	Vancomycin, 125 mg po q6h × 10–14 days Metronidazole, 250 mg po qid × 10–14 days	Bacitracin, 25,000 units po qid × 10–14 days Cholestyramine, 4 gm packet tid	Vancomycin is preferred for severe disease. Discontinuation of implicated antibiotic is often adequate. Some strains are highly resistant to bacitracin. Relapses: Vancomycin or metronidazole × 10–14 days, *then* cholestyramine (4 gm po tid), vancomycin (125 mg qid) or lactobacilli (1 gm qid) × 21 days *or* vancomycin + rifampin (600 mg/day). When oral treatment is not possible: metronidazole, 500 mg q8h IV.
E. coli			Laboratory confirmation for *E. coli*—associated diarrhea is usually not available except for EHEC.
Enterotoxigenic *E. coli* (ETEC)	Sulfa-trimethoprim 1 DS po bid × 3 days Ciprofloxacin, 500 mg po bid × 3 days	Trimethoprim, 200 mg po bid × 3 days Doxycycline, 100 mg po bid × 3 days	
Enteroadherent			Efficacy not established except for enterotoxin

E. coli (EAEC)	Ofloxacin 300 mg po bid × 3 days	Bismuth subsalicylate 60 ml qid × 5 days	producing strains, e.g., ETEC (traveler's diarrhea). Many ETEC strains are now resistant to doxycycline and TMP-SMX
Enterohemorrhagic *E. coli* (EHEC)	Ciprofloxacin, 500–750 mg po bid × 5–7 days		Efficacy not established. Sulfa-trimethoprim may increase toxin production.
Enteroinvasive *E. coli* (EIEC)	Ampicillin, 500 mg po or 1 gm IV qid × 5 days Sulfa-trimethoprim 1 DS po bid × 5 days	Ciprofloxacin, 500 mg po bid × 5 days	Associated with hemolytic-uremic syndrome and TTP. Laboratory detection: stool culture for *E. coli* serotype 0157:H7 or analysis for Shiga toxin
Enteropathogenic *E. coli* (EPEC)	Sulfa-trimethoprim 1 DS po bid × 3–5 days	Neomycin, 100 mg/kg/day po × 3–5 days Furazolidone, 100 mg po qid × 3–5 days	Presentation is dysentery as with Shigella
Food poisoning *Clostridium perfringens, Staph. aureus, Bacillus cereus, Listeria*	None		Self-limited and toxin mediated: antimicrobial treatment is not indicated
Plesiomonas shigelloides	Sulfa-trimethoprim, 1 DS po bid × 5 days Ciprofloxacin, 500 mg po bid × 5 days	Tetracycline, 500 mg po qid × 5 days	Efficacy or treatment is not established and should be reserved for patients with extraintestinal infection, prolonged diarrhea or immunosuppression.
Salmonella Thyphoid fever *(S. typhi)* Non-typhoid *(Salmonella)* Enteric fever (non-typhoid Salmonella) Metastatic infection Chronic bacteremia	Sulfa-trimethoprim 1–2 DS po bid × 14 days Ampicillin, 2–6 gm po or IV/day × 14 days Amoxicillin, 2–4 gm po/day × 14 days Chloramphenicol, 3–4 gm/day IV or po × 14 days Cefotaxime, 4–8 gm/day IV × 14 days	Ciprofloxacin, 500 mg po qid × 14 days	Antibiotic treatment is contraindicated in patients with uncomplicated enterocolitis; indications are typhoid fever, chronic bacteremia, metastatic infection or enterocolitis in compromised host (AIDS, sickle cell hemoglobinopathy, lymphoma, etc.) AIDS patients may require long term suppressive treatment with ampicillin or ciprofloxacin.

(continued)

Table 26–12. *(continued)*

MICROBIAL AGENT	PREFERRED	ALTERNATIVE	COMMENT
Enterocolitis in compromised host	Cefoperazone, 1 gm bid IV × 14 days Ceftriaxone, 1 gm IV bid × 14 days		Patients with typhoid fever or enteric fever should receive antibiotics in high doses initially; with severe toxicity give dexamethasone (3 mg/kg × 1, then 1 mg/kg q6h × 48 hr) or prednisone (60 mg/day 20 mg/day over 3 days).
Carrier	Ampicillin, 4–6 gm/day or amoxicillin, 6 gm/day + probenecid, 2 gm/day × 6 weeks	Ciprofloxacin, 500–750 mg po bid × 6 wks Rifampin, 300 mg bid + sulfa-trimethoprim, 1 DS bid × 6 wks	Cholecystectomy for cholelithiasis and carriers who relapse.
Shigella	Ciprofloxacin, 500 mg po bid or norfloxacin, 400 mg po bid × 3–5 days Sulfa-trimethoprim 1 DS po bid × 3–5 days	Ampicillin, 500 mg po or 1 gm IV qid × 3–5 days Nalidixic acid, 1 gm po qid × 5–7 days Cefoperazone, 1–2 gm IV q12h × 5–7 days	Preferred agents for empiric treatment are sulfa-trimethoprim or ciprofloxacin/norfloxacin. Ampicillin-resistant strains are common; for ampicillin-susceptible strains, amoxicillin should not be used. Sulfa-trimethoprim resistance is increasing and is common in strains from underdeveloped areas.
Vibrio cholerae	Tetracycline, 500 mg po qid × 3–5 days Doxycycline, 300 mg po × 1	Sulfa-trimethoprim, 1 DS po bid × 3 days Furazolidine, 100 mg po qid × 3 days Erythromycin, 250 mg po qid × 3 days	
Vibrio sp. (*V. parahaemolyticus, V. fluvialis, V. mimicus, V. hollisae, V. furnissii, V. vulnificus)*	Tetracycline (as above—see comments)	Ciprofloxacin, 500 mg po bid × 5 days	Efficacy of treatment is not established and should be reserved for severe disease.

Yersinia enterocolitica	Sulfa-trimethoprim 1 DS po bid × 7 days Gentamicin, 1.7 mg/kg IV q8h × 7 days	Ciprofloxacin, 500–750 po bid × 7 days Doxycycline, 100 mg po bid × 7 days Chloramphenicol, 3–4 gm/day po or IV × 7 days	Efficacy of treatment for enterocolitis or mesenteric adenitis is not established, especially when instituted late; major indications are prolonged diarrhea or generalized infection
Parasites			
Cryptosporidia	Symptomatic treatment: Loparamide, lomotil etc. plus nutritional support Compromised host: Consider octretide (5–80 μg tid SC) paromomycin (500 mg po qid) or azithromycin (1500 mg/day, then 600 mg/day × 27 days, than 100 mg/day)		Consider treatment only for chronic diarrhea in compromised host. No antimicrobial agent has established efficacy
Balantidium coli	Tetracycline, 500 mg po qid × 10 days	Iodoquinol, 650 mg tid × 21 days Metronidazole, 500 mg po tid × 10 days	No antimicrobial agent has established efficacy
Blastocystis hominis (see comments)	Metronidazole, 1.5–2.0 gm/day × 7 days		Role as enteric pathogen is not clear
Entamoeba histolytica			
Acute dysentery	Metronidazole, 750 mg po tid × 5–10 days *then* diloxanide furoate, 500 mg po tid × 10 days or Iodoquinol 650 mg po tid × 21 days	Dehydroemetine, 1–1.5 mg/kg/day IM × 5 days, then diloxanide furoate	Alternatives to diloxanide furoate as oral luminal-acting drug are: iodoquinol, 650 mg po tid × 21 days, and paromomycin, 500 mg po tid × 7 days. Metronidazole may be given IV for severely ill patients (7.5 mg/kg q6h). Diloxanide furoate is available from the CDC.

(continued)

Table 26–12. *(continued)*

MICROBIAL AGENT	PREFERRED	ALTERNATIVE	COMMENT
Mild disease	Metronidazole, 500 mg po tid × 5–10 days, then diloxanide furoate (as above)	Paromomycin, 500 mg po tid × 7 days Metronidazole, 2.4 gm/day × 2–3 days, then diloxanide furoate Metronidazole, 50 mg/kg × 1, then diloxanide furoate	
Cyst passer	Iodoquinol, 650 mg po tid × 21 days Diloxanide furoate, 500 mg po tid × 10 days Paromomycin, 500 mg po tid × 7 days	Metronidazole, 500–750 mg po tid × 10 days	Need to treat is arbitrary, but luminal amebicides (diloxanide furoate, paromomycin or iodoquinol) are preferred. Diloxanide furoate is available from CDC 404-639-3670
Giardia lamblia	Quinacrine, 100 mg po tid × 5–7 days)	Metronidazole, 250 mg po tid × 7 days Furazolidone, 8 mg/kg/day po × 10 days Tinidazole, 2 gm single dose	Metronidazole is less effective than quinacrine, but better tolerated. Pregnancy: Consider paromomycin, 25–30 mg/kg/day × 5–10 days.
Isospora belli	Sulfa-trimethoprim 2 DS po bid × 2–4 wks	Pyrimethamine, 25 mg + folonic acid, 5–10 mg/day × 1 month	Patients with AIDS and other immunosuppressive disorders usually require prolonged maintenance treatment

From Bartlett JG: Pocket Book of Infectious Disease Therapy, Williams and Wilkins, Baltimore, MD 1993—pages 222–226.

diarrhea with a normal bowel pattern at an average of 4 days after starting treatment. Metronidazole or vancomycin therapy allows relapse in 15–40% of patients when treatment is discontinued and the occasional case complicated by ileus or toxic megacolon if oral drugs cannot reach the site of infection.

COMPROMISED HOSTS

Diarrhea in the immunocompromised host is caused by multiple enteric pathogens with a frequency dictated by the specific defect:

- Humoral immunity deficit (hypogammoglobulinemia, IgA and IgM deficiency, modular lymphoid hyperplasia): Giardiasis and cryptosporidiosis.
- Neutropenia: Typhlitis due to *Clostridium septicum* and *C. tertium*.
- Cytotoxic chemotherapy and antibiotic treatment: *C. difficile* associated with diarrhea/colitis (Previous discussion).
- Defective cell mediated immunity (cancer chemotherapy, organ transplant recipients, chronic corticosteroid administration, lymphoma and AIDS). Table 26–13 applies to other populations with defective cell mediated immunity.

URINARY TRACT INFECTIONS (UTIs)

UTIs include clinical conditions which vary in clinical presentation, the susceptible host and the pathogen involved. Nevertheless, most can be easily diagnosed with simple urine culture and can be successfully treated with an array of antibiotics selected based on cost and patient convenience.

Classification: Complicated vs. Uncomplicated UTIs

UTIs are classified based on anatomic site (urethritis, cystitis, pyelonephritis); they are also classified as complicated or uncomplicated depending on persistence of infection, recurrent infections, infections involving resistant organisms and renal destruction. Most young adult women with cystitis and pyelonephritis have no urologic abnormalities and the symptoms, although sometimes annoying, do not lead to the complications noted. Patients with anatomic abnormalities of the genitourinary system, diabetics and patients with indwelling catheters are more problematic. Uncomplicated infections usually involve *E. coli* sensitive to nearly all antimicrobial agents, other antibiotic-sensitive coliforms, *S. saprophyticus* and occasionally the enterococcus. Complicated infections associated with a urologic abnormality, calculus, catheterization or nosocomial acquisition are far more likely to involve antibiotic-resistant strains of coliforms, *P. aeruginosa* and the Enterococcus. The goals of therapy are also somewhat different. With uncomplicated UTIs, appropriate therapy can eliminate the putative agents with relative ease. By contrast, patients with indwelling catheters or obstruction are likely to have persistent or recurrent bacteriuria when antibiotics are discontinued. In many instances, the objective of therapy with complicated UTI is to simply eliminate symptoms.

Table 26–13
Microbial Agents Associated with Diarrhea In Patients with HIV Infection and AIDS

AGENT	FREQUENCY	DETECTION	TREATMENT	COMMENT
Acute diarrhea				
Salmonella	5–15%	Stool culture	TMP-SMX Fluoroquinolones Cephalosporin-3d generation	Acute diarrhea ± enteric fever
Shigella	1–3%	Stool culture	Fluoroquinone TMP-SMX	Acute diarrhea dysentery
C. difficile	10–15%	Stool toxin assay	Oral vancomycin Oral metronidazole	Acute diarrhea Usually associated with clindamycin, ampicillin or cephalosporin CT scan shows thickened colonic mucosa
Campylobacter	4–8%	Stool culture	Erythromycin Fluoroquinolone	Acute diarrhea
Enteric viruses	15–30%	Research labs only	None	Acute diarrhea, no fecal WBCs
Chronic diarrhea				
Cytomegalovirus	15–40%	Gut biopsy	Ganciclovir 5 mg/kg IV bid × 3 wks	Chronic diarrhea May involve any level of GI tract. CT scan shows bowel wall thickening Cramps and fever common Complications include hemorrhage and perforation Enteritis or colitis

Cryptosporidia	10–30%	AFB stain of stool	Paromomycin (efficacy is?)	Chronic diarrhea with fluctuating severity, no fever or fecal WBCs. Enteritis
Microsporidia	20–40%	Small bowel biopsy-EM or Giemsa stain Recently developed stool exam	No antimicrobial with extablished merit	Chronic diarrhea No fever or fecal WBCs Enteritis
M. avium	10–20%	Blood cultures AFB stain of stool	Clarithromycin plus ethambutol and/or clofazimine	Chronic diarrhea, cramps, fever and pos blood cultures, Enteritis
Isospora	1–3%	AFB stain of stool	TMP-SMX	Chronic diarrhea Similar to cryptosporidia but treatable and less common
Small bowel overgrowth	10–20% (?)	Breath test Quantitative culture of small bowel aspirate	Amoxicillin + clavulanate Doxycycline	Achlorhydria and SBO is common, but role in causing diarrhea is often obscure

* Based on: Goodman GS et al: New Engl J Med 329:14, 1993 (viral agents), Nelson MR et al: AIDS 6:1495, 1992, Bartlett JG et al: Clin Infect Dis 15:726, 1992, Kotler DP et al: Am Intern Med 113:444, 1990.

DIAGNOSIS

Symptoms: Clinical expression is variable ranging from asymptomatic bacteriuria to the readily recognized symptoms of cystitis (frequency, urgency and dysuria) and pyelonephritis (flank pain, fever, frequency and dysuria). The diagnosis is established with urine culture and urine analysis.

Urine Culture: Urine is usually collected by catheter or voiding. The latter is subject to contamination so that quantitative cultures are required to separate pathogens and contaminants. The traditional criterion for a positive culture is 10^5 bacteria/ml. However, about 1/3 of women with acute cystitis have colony counts in mid-stream urine samples of only 10^2–10^4/ml. Thus, the use of 10^2 may be a more appropriate criterion in some cases when accompanied by topical symptoms and a typical organism, primarily *E. coli*. Many microbiology laboratories still use techniques that detect only 10^3/ml and some identify and report pathogens only when present in concentrations of 10^5/ml, unless advised otherwise. Some laboratories have adopted alternatives to culture using photometry or bioluminescence that may give results within two hours. These show good sensitivity and specificity when compared to concentrations by culture of 10^5/ml, but these tests are substantially less sensitive with counts of 10^2–10^4/ml.

Setting	*Significant bacteriuria*
Acute cystitis	$\geq 10^3$/ml
Acute pyelonephritis	$\geq 10^4$/ml
UTI in men	$\geq 10^4$/ml
Asymptomatic bacteriuria	$\geq 10^5$/ml $\times$ 2

Urine Analysis: Pyuria is found in nearly all cases of urinary tract infections. The optimal method is voided sample using a hemocytometer with uncentrifuged urine. A concentration of $\geq$10 WBC/mm^3 indicates pyuria.

ASYMPTOMATIC BACTERIURIA

Diagnosis: Positive urine culture done routinely in the absence of symptoms suggesting a UTI. The diagnosis is secure only if the concentration is 10^5 bacteria/ml and is confirmed with a repeat culture yielding the same bacteria.

Treatment: No treatment is recommended in the great majority with limited exceptions as follows: Young children, pregnant women, renal transplant patients, some diabetics, some immunocompromised patients undergoing instrumentation and patients undergoing surgery such as prosthetic hip replacement, and prosthetic resection. The typical elderly patient with asymptomatic bacteriuria with 10^5 bacteria/ml in a urine culture obtained for whatever reason should not be treated. At the same time, urine culture and treatment is clearly indicated when elderly patients have otherwise unexplained fever, increased urinary frequency, new incontinence or low abdominal pain.

Antimicrobial agents are indicated according to guidelines noted above. The agent is selected on the basis of in vitro sensitivity tests, cost and tolerance usually using one of the 3–7 day regimens suggested for cystitis.

Acute Cystitis

Diagnosis: The most common host is a young, sexually active woman, although this may be seen in nearly any patient population. Typical symptoms are dysuria, frequency, urgency and suprapubic pain. The major differential diagnosis is vaginitis or urethritis. The diagnosis is established by urine culture showing typical urinary tract pathogens, primarily *E. coli* or *S. sasprophyticus*:; urine analysis will show ≥10 leukocytes/ml un-spun urine. For the healthy woman with classical symptoms without fever, flank pain or systemic toxicity, many authorities treat empirically or test only for pyuria; this avoids the expense of urine cultures.

Treatment: The relative merits of antimicrobial treatment with 1 dose versus 3 days are debated. Response rates are somewhat better with the 3 day course, but the complications and cost of antibiotics are also higher. Single dose therapy should be reserved for patients who are not pregnant, have no evidence of pyelonephritis, have symptoms <7 days and will comply with necessary follow-up evaluations.

Cystitis: Single dose (only for uncomplicated cases)

Trimethoprim, 400 mg*	Ampicillin, 3 g
Sulfa-trimethoprim, 320/1600 mg (2 DS)*	Cephalexin, 2 g
Nitrofurantoin, 200 mg*	Sulfisoxazole, 2 g
Amoxicillin, 3 g	Ciprofloxacin, 250 mg
Amoxicillin + clavulanate, 500 mg	Norfloxacin, 400 mg

Cystitis: Multidose regimens (3–7 days)

Trimethoprim, 100 mg q 12 h*
Sulfa-trimethoprim, 160/800 mg q 12 h*
Nitrofurantoin, 100 mg q 6 h*
Amoxicillin, 500 mg q 8 h
Amoxicillin + clavulanate, 500 mg q 8 h

Relapse: "Test-of-cure" urine culture at 1 week after single dose or 3 day therapy is controversial. Patients who fail to respond or relapse within 96 hours are usually considered to have a silent renal infection and should be treated for 2–6 weeks with an antibiotic selected based on in vitro sensitivity tests. A classic distinction is made between relapses and reinfection. Relapse means a recurrent infection, usually within 2 weeks, caused by involvement of the same organism according to species and sensitivity tests. The recommendation for relapse is to rule out a structural abnormality or chronic prostatitis; antibiotic treatment should be for 6 weeks based on vitro sensitivity of the urinary pathogen. Reinfection means a recurrent infection with a different organism; this mechanism accounts for over 80% of recurrent infections in women.

Treatment of Multiple Reinfections: If the episodes/year exceeds three, the following are recommended for long-term prophylaxis: Trimethoprim-sulfamethoxazole, 1/2 tab daily or 3 days/week or Nitrofurantoin macrocrystals, 50 mg daily or Trimethoprim, 50 mg daily or Trimethoprim-sulfamethoxazole, 1 single strength or double strength tab after intercourse.

* Preferred

Acute Urethritis

Diagnosis: The symptoms are the same as those noted with acute cystitis with dysuria, frequency and urgency, but urine cultures fail to reveal even low concentrations of any urinary pathogen. The usual cause in women is cervicitis involving *C. trichomatis* or *N. gonorrhoeae*; Herpes simplex virus is less common. In most instances, the symptoms are mild, onset gradual and pelvic exam reveals cervical mucopus.

Treatment: In the absence of a positive urine culture and negative culture for *N. gonorrhoeae:* doxycycline, 100 mg bid for 10 days.

Pyelonephritis

Diagnosis: The usual symptoms are flank pain, systemic symptoms (fever, nausea, vomiting, malaise) and lower urinary tract symptoms. Occasional complications include bacteremia or, less frequently, perinephric abscesses or intra-renal abscesses. Severe infections and complicated infections are commonest in patients with obstruction in the urinary tract, diabetes or immunosuppression. The diagnosis of the UTI is established by urine culture and demonstration of pyuria; evidence of upper tract involvement is based on the constellation of symptoms noted above including systemic findings, relapsing infection as defined above, urine analysis showing white cell casts, and ultrasonography or computed tomography showing nephric enlargement or a suppurative complication.

Treatment: Most patients with pyelonephritis can be treated with oral antibiotics. Indications for parenteral treatment are severe systemic toxicity, failure to respond to oral agents or a urinary tract pathogen insensitive to drugs that can be given po. The selection of an antibiotic is based on in vitro sensitivity tests, although empiric treatment based on anticipated pathogens is necessary for the first 24–48 hours. Recommended options for oral or parenteral administration are the following:

Pyelonephritis, oral therapy for mild pyelonephritis (treat ≥14 days)

Trimethoprim, 100 mg q 12 h*	Amoxicillin, + clavulanate 500 mg q 8 h
Sulfa-trimethoprim, 160/800 q 12 h*	Ciprofloxacin, 250 mg q 12 h
Cephalexin, 500 mg q 6 h	Norfloxacin, 400 mg q 12 h
Amoxicillin 500 mg q 8 h	

Pyelonephritis, parenteral therapy (Intravenous administration until afebrile and improved, then oral therapy to complete total of 14 days)

Gentamicin, 1.5 mg/kg q 8 h*	Ampicillin + gentamicin (above doses) q 8 h
Ceftriaxone, 1 g q 12	Cefazolin, 1 g (or higher) q 8 h
Sulfa-trimethoprim, 160/800 mg q 12 h*	Mezlocillin, 1 g (or higher) q 6 h*
Ampicillin, 1 g (or higher) q 8 h	

Refractory infections: Persistence of fever >48 hours after appropriate antibiotic therapy suggests a complicated infection with obstruction, stone or abscess. Patients with this complication should be evaluated with ultrasound, CT or intravenous pyelography.

* Preferred regimens

Prostatitis

The major forms of prostatitis are acute bacterial prostatitis, chronic bacterial prostatitis and nonbacterial prostatitis (sometimes referred to as prostosis). These have distinct presentation and management guidelines.

ACUTE BACTERIAL PROSTATITIS

Diagnosis: This is an abrupt, febrile illness associated with topical constitutional and urinary tract symptoms. The prostate gland is typically tender, indurated and enlarged. Urine culture and sometimes blood cultures yield the responsible pathogen which is usually a coliform or *P. aeruginosa.*

Treatment: Antibiotic selection is based on in vitro sensitivity tests; there may also be a need to relieve obstruction. Antibiotics should be continued at least 4 weeks to prevent chronic bacterial prostatitis.

CHRONIC BACTERIAL PROSTATITIS

Diagnosis: The typical presentation is a relapsing UTI without the systemic response noted with acute bacterial prostatitis. The usual symptoms are frequency, urgency, dysuria and perineal pain. Prostatitic exam is normal. The diagnosis is established with the "three glass test" consisting of a first voided specimen (urethral specimen), a midstream urine sample (bladder specimen) and a post-prostatic massage specimen (expressed prostatic secretions) followed by the next 10 ml of urine (post-prostatic culture). Quantitative cultures are all 4 specimens show disproportionately in the EPS and the post-prostatic culture. Low counts or negative cultures are noted in the urethral and midstream urine cultures unless there is a concurrent cystitis. Examination of the four specimens shows significant pyuria with at least 15 white blood cells per high powered field in EPS specimen.

Treatment: Antimicrobial agents should penetrate the prostate gland and have in vitro activity against the bacteria involved. Agents with the best track record in this condition are: Trimethoprim-sulfamethoxazole, one double strength tablet bid for 4–16 weeks. The cure rate with this treatment is a poor 30–40%, but better with than most other antimicrobial regimens.

Fluoroquinolones such as ciprofloxacin, 500–750 mg bid for 4-8 weeks. Cure rates appear to be higher than with TMP-SMX and this treatment is definitely preferred for selected pathogens such as *Ps. aeruginosa.* Patients who cannot be cured may benefit from long-term suppressive treatment using trimethoprim-sulfamethoxazole, one single strength tablet daily or nitrofurantoin, 100 mg once or bid.

Nonbacterial Prostatitis: Patients with this condition have the same symptom noted with chronic bacterial prostatitis, but urine cultures and EPS samples in the "three glass test" are negative. Nevertheless, the EPS sample shows leukocytes. Numerous fastidious pathogens have been suggested causes of this syndrome, but none of this work has shown conclusive results. Antibiotic treatment is usually not successful, although some authorities favor a course of doxycycline (100 mg bid for 14 days) to eliminate a possible role of chlamydia or ureaplasmas.

SEXUALLY TRANSMITTED DISEASES (STDs)

There has been a major change in STDs during the past decade which now includes over 25 known pathogenic organisms. The consequences of these infections may be substantial and include the following: HIV infection/AIDS; pelvic inflammatory disease with complications of infertility, ectopic pregnancy and chronic pain; neonatal or prenatal complications and malignancies including cervical cancer, lymphoma, hepatocellar carcinoma and Kaposi sarcoma. The approach here will be by syndrome for diagnosis and management, but a few general principles apply to all patients being evaluated for STDs:

- Risk-reduction counseling should include emphasis on abstinence, careful selection of sexual partners, use of condoms and spermicides.
- Most patients with STDs should be treated without waiting for diagnostic tests.
- Partner notification is voluntary although legal precedents have established that the right of exposed persons to be informed supersedes the desires of patient for nearly all STDs.
- Patients with 1 STD are often silent carriers of other STD pathogens so screening is often desired; this silent carriage applies to HIV, gonorrhea, *C. trachomatis* and syphilis.
- Patients exposed to STDs should usually be evaluated and treated empirically.
- All required STDs should be reported to health authorities according to local regulations.
- Recommendations for treatment of nearly all STDs is available from Centers for Disease Control. The recommendations given below are based on these guidelines.

Urethritis

Diagnosis: The two likely pathogens are *N. gonorrhoeae* and *C. trachomatis*. The distinction is made by gram stain of urethal discharge. In the absence of discharge, an intraurethal swab may be used instead. Patients with gonococcal urethritis will show typical gram-negative diplococci within PMNs. Nongonococcal urethritis (NGU) is characterized by mucoid or purulent urethral discharge with over 5 PMNs/oil immersion field without intracellular gram-negative diplococci. *C. trachomatis* is the usual cause, but occasional cases are due to *Ureaplasma urealyticum, Trichomonas vaginalis, Herpes simplex* virus and occasional cases are due to unknown agents. Many labs now offer cultures and/or rapid diagnostic tests for detection of *C. trachomatis*. The need to culture urethral discharge is arbitrary; advantages are the ability to detect gonorrhea in patients with false-negative smear (>5%) and the opportunity for in vitro sensitivity testing of isolates.

Treatment: Nongonococcal urethritis: Doxycycline, 100 mg po bid x 7 days. Alternative regimens are erythromycin base, 500 mg Po qid x 7 days or erythromycinethylsuccinate, 800 mg po qid x 7 days.

Follow-up: Patients should return for evaluation if symptoms recur. Recurrent or persistent discharge generally represents noncompliance, new exposure or failure to respond. The original treatment should be repeated if there is noncompliance or a new exposure; if this appears to be a failure to respond, a urethral specimen should be obtained for culture and wet mount for *T. vaginalis*; if negative, the patient should be treated with the alternative regimen for 14 days. Referral to a urologist is rarely helpful.

Sex partners: Evaluate and treat contacts during the 30 days prior to the onset of symptoms in symptomatic patients and 60 days if asymptomatic. Patients should avoid sex until the patient and partner therapy is completed and both are asymptomatic. Reporting: Most states require reporting of infections involving *C. trachomatis*.

Gonococcal Urethritis: Treatment includes an agent directed against *N. gonorrhoeae* and a second agent for possible co-infection with *C. trachomatis*: Ceftriaxone, 125 mg IM x 1 *or* Ciprofloxacin, 500 mg po x 1 *or* Cefixime, 400 mg po x 1 *or* Ofloxacin, 400 mg po x 1 *PLUS* Doxycycline, 100 mg po bid x 7 days.

Note: Regimens recommended for *N. gonorrhoeae* have been shown to cure over 95% of anal and genital infections; ceftriaxone and ciprofloxacin are preferred for pharyngeal infections. Disadvantages of the ceftriaxone regimen are the expense, lack of availability in vials of <250 mg and the requirement for an injection. No ceftriaxone-resistant stains of *N. gonorrhoeae* have been reported. Quinolones are contraindicated for pregnant or nursing women and for children <18 years of age; these drugs are not active against *T. pallidum*. Alternative regimens with established merit for uncomplicated anal and genital infections are the following: Ceftriaxone, 500 mg IM x 1; Cefotaxime, 500 mg IM x 1; Cefotetan, 1 g IM x 1, Cefoxitin, 1 g IM x 1; Cefuroxime axetil, 1 g po x 1; Cefpodoxime proxetil, 200 mg po x 1; Enoxacin, 400 mg po x 1; Lomefloxacin, 400 mg po x 1; Norfloxacin, 800 mg po x 1; Spectinomycin, 2 g IM x 1.

Syphilis: Patients treated for gonorrhea should be screened for syphilis with serology when first seen. Treatment with Ceftriaxone or the 7 day course of doxycycline or erythromycin may cure incubating syphilis, but supporting data are not available.

Follow-up: Patients with uncomplicated gonorrhea do not need the test-of-cure as once thought. Patients with persistent symptoms should be evaluated by culture for *N. gonorrhoeae* and isolates tested for antimicrobial sensitivity. Recurrence of symptoms is usually due to a new infection and emphasizes the need for patient education and improved sex-partner referral or infection caused by *C. trachomatis*.

Sex partners: Evaluate and treat contacts during the 30 days prior to symptoms in symptomatic patients and 60 days if asymptomatic.

Reporting: All states require reporting of gonorrhea.

Mucopurulent Cervicitis (MPC)

Diagnosis: MPC is comparable to urethritis in the male and is characterized by a yellow endocervical exudate visible in the endocervical canal on an endocervical swab specimen or by demonstrating PMNs on cervical gram stain. Most patients are asymptomatic, but some will note vaginal discharge or bleeding. Major pathogens are *C. trachomatis* and *N. gonorrhoeae*. Cervical specimens should be cultured for *N. gonorrhoeae* and tested for *C. trachomatis* (culture or rapid diagnostic tests using Gen-Probe or EIA) if the technology is available.

Treatment: This is based on results of tests for *C. trachomatis* and *N. gonorrhoeae*. In the event that the likelihood of infection with either organism is high or the patient is unlikely to return for treatment, the following recommendations are made

- Populations with high prevalence of both infections: Treat empirically for *N. gonorrhoeae* and *C. trachomatis.*
- If the prevalence of *N. gonorrhoeae* is low, but the likelihood of chlamydia is significant, treat for *C. trachomatis.*
- If prevalence of both infections is low and patient is likely to return: Await results of diagnostic test.

Gonococcal MPC: Treat for *N. gonorrhoeae* and *C. trachomatis* using one of the following regimens: Cetriaxone, 125 mg IM x 1 *or* Ciprofloxacin, 500 mg po x 1 *or* Cefixime, 400 mg po x 1 *or* Ofloxacin, 400 mg po x 1 *PLUS* Doxycycline, 100 mg po bid x 7 days *Note:* See comments above for treatment of gonococcal urethritis

Chlamydia trachomatis MPC: Doxycycline, 100 mg po bid x 7 days *or* Azithromycin, 1 g x 1. Alternative regimens include: Ofloxacin, 300 mg po bid x 7 days *or* Erythromycin base, 500 mg po qid x 7 days *or* Erythromycin ethylsuccinate, 800 mg po qid daily x 7 *or* Sulfisoxazole, 500 mg po qid x 10 days.

Note: Azithromycin and quinolones are substantially more expensive than doxycycline. For pregnant patients, doxycycline is contraindicated, fluoroquinolones are contraindicated during pregnancy and in persons under 18 years of age, safety of azithromycin has not been established for pregnancy, and Sulfisoxazole is contraindicated in pregnancy near term. The recommendation for pregnant women is erythromycin base, 500 mg po qid x 7 days; alternatives if this cannot be tolerated are erythromycin, 250 mg po qid x 14 days *or* erythromycin ethylsuccinate, 400 mg po qid x 7 days *or* 400 mg po qid x 14 days *or* (if erythromycin cannot be tolerated) amoxicillin, 500 mg po tid x 7 days.

Follow-up: Patients do not need retesting unless symptoms persist or there is recurrence. *Sex partners*: Sex partners should be referred including all with sexual contact within 30 days of the onset of symptoms in symptomatic patients and within 60 days if asymptomatic. Patients with established exposure to *N. gonorrhoeae* should be treated with the regimen noted for uncomplicated gonococcal infection (which includes treatment directed against *C. trachomatis*). Patients with exposure to *C. trachomatis* should be evaluated and treated for infection involving that organism, preferably using doxycycline or azithromycin.

Genital Ulcers

Diagnosis: The usual causes are Herpes simplex, syphilis or chancroid, although relative frequency varies by geographic area, patient population, history and physical examination. Evaluation should include a serologic test for syphilis and the following:

- Dark field exam or direct immunofluorescence test for *T. pallidum.*
- Culture or Tzanck test for HSV.
- Culture for *Haemophilus ducreyi.*

Treatment: Treatment should be initiated against the most likely diagnosis while therapeutic tests are pending. About 1/4 of patients with genital ulcers have no laboratory confirmation or any diagnosis. For empiric therapy and cases with no diagnosis, treatment should be directed against the most likely cause.

Chancroid: The diagnosis is established if *H. ducreyi* is recovered, but the special media required is not commercially available and even when it is the sensitivity is under 80%. Probable diagnosis is based on epidemiology, the finding of a painful genital ulcer, and ulcer with tender inguinal adenopathy (especially if there is suppurative adenopathy) or a painful ulcer combined with negative studies for *T. pallidum* plus a clinical presentation that is atypical for HSV.

Preferred treatment: Azithormycin, 1 g po x 1 *or* Cetriaxone, 250 mg IM x 1 *or* Erythromycin base, 500 mg po qid x 7 days. *Alternative regimens*: Amoxicillin, 500 mg + clavulanate (Augmentin) po tid x 7 days *or Ciprofloxacin*, 500 mg po bid x 3 days.

Follow-up and sex partners: Patients should be examined 3–7 days after treatment. There should be symptomatic improvement within three days. The time for healing depends on the ulcer, large ulcers require over 2 weeks. Sex partners within 10 days before the onset of symptoms should be examined and treated whether symptomatic or not.

Genital Herpes Simplex: Approximately 20% of all adults in the U.S. have serologic evidence of HSV-2 infection. At least 75% have no history suggestive of genital herpes. Most of the remaining 25% will have a single episode with no recurrences, and a minority will have recurrent episodes of genital herpes. The diagnosis is generally established on the basis of exposure (which is often lacking due to the large reservoir of asymptomatic patients who shed virus intermittently despite absence of symptoms), typical ulcers showing vesicular lesions on an erythematous base that break down to form the typical genital ulcer and/or laboratory confirmation with culture or Tzanck test.

Treatment: First episode: Acyclovir, 200 mg po 5 x daily x 7–10 days. Herpes proctitis: Acyclovir, 400 mg po 5 x daily x 10 days.

Recurrent genital herpes: Most patients do not benefit from treatment, but it is sometimes recommended if instituted during the prodrome or within 2 days of the onset of lesions. If given, the recommendation is acyclovir, 200 mg po 5 x daily x 5 days *or* acyclovir, 400 mg po tid x 5 days.

Suppressive therapy; Patients with 6 or more episodes per year may be treated with acyclovir, 400 mg bid; safety and effectiveness has been documented for up to 5 years of continuous therapy, although it is recommended that this be discontinued after one year to evaluate the recurrence rate.

Pregnancy: Safety of acyclovir during pregnancy is not established. The Burroughs Wellcome Company and CDC maintain a registry to access safety in pregnancy which shows no risk to the infant in reports to date; the registry may be contacted at (800) 722-9292, x 8465. The risk of transmission of HSV to the neonate from an infected mother appears to be highest in women with first episode genital herpes near the time of delivery and it is low (less than 3%) in women with recurrent disease. The current recommendations is caesarean section in women who have active lesions at the time of labor, preferably before rupture of membranes. Women with a history of genital herpes or sex partner(s) with genital herpes should have cultures of the birth canal at the time of delivery to assist in decisions concerning the neonate.

Syphilis

Stages of syphilis are primary (genital ulcer of chancre), secondary (rash, mucocutaneous lesions, adenopathy), tertiary (neurologic, ophthalmic, cardiac, auditory or gummatous) or latent (early — <1 year or late — >1 year). The following guidelines deal with all stages.

Diagnosis: Genital ulcer indicates early syphilis in which preferred diagnostic studies are dark-field exam or direct fluorescent antibody tests are done on lesion exudate or tissue. Serologic tests for syphilis include the nontreponemal tests (VDRL and the RPR) and treponemal test (FTA-ABS). The nontreponemal titers correlate with disease activity, are reported as reactive or non-reactive and generally remain positive for life regardless of treatment or disease activity.

	Stage Nontreponemal VDRL or RPR	***Test Treponemal FTA-abs***
Primary	70-80%	80-90%
Secondary	99%	100%
Latent	*	
Treated	1%	98%
Untreated	99%	98%

The diagnosis of neurosyphilis is based on positive serum serologic test results and abnormal cerebrospinal fluid with over 5 WBC/mm^3 plus elevated protein; the CSF VDRL is positive in about 60–70% of patients with neurosyphilis and, when present, is considered diagnostic of neurosyphilis.

Treatment: *Primary and secondary syphilis:* Benzathine penicillin G, 2.4 million units IM x 1. Penicillin allergy in non-pregnant patient: Doxycycline, 100 mg po bid daily x 2 weeks *or* Tetracycline, 500 mg po qid daily x 2 weeks. Considerations for non-pregnant patients in whom compliance and follow-up is assured include erythromycin, 500 mg po qid x 2 weeks and ceftriaxone.

Follow-up: Persistence or recurrence of signs or symptoms, and failure of nontreponemal titers to decrease by 4 fold at 3 months following treatments for primary syphilis or 6 months after treatment for secondary syphilis indicates probable treatment failure. These patients should have HIV serology (if not already done) and should have retreatment with benzathine penicillin, 2.4 million units IM x 3 at weekly intervals.

- *Latent syphilis*: The definition is individuals with serologic evidence of syphilis but without other clinical evidence of disease. Early latent syphilis implies a duration of less than one year; syphilis of unknown duration or more than one is considered latent syphilis.
- *Early latent syphilis*: Benzathine penicillin G, 2.4 million units IM x 1. Patients with penicillin allergy should be treated with doxycycline, 100 mg po bid x 2 weeks or tetracycline, 500 mg po qid x 2 weeks.
- *Late latent syphilis or latent syphilis of unknown duration:* Benzathine penicillin G, 2.4 million units IM x 3 given weekly. Alternatives for non-pregnant, penicillin-allergic patients are doxycycline, 100 mg po bid x 4 weeks or tetracycline, 500 mg po qid x 4 weeks.
- *Neurosyphilis*: Penicillin G, 12-24 million units daily x 10-14 days. Alternative regimen for outpatients is procaine penicillin IM, 2.4 million units IM daily plus probenecid, 500 mg po qid, both for 10–14 days. Patients with neurosyphilis and penicillin allergy should be desensitized and treated with penicillin.

Sex partners: Persons exposure to primary, secondary or early latent syphilis should be evaluated including serologic tests and treated accordingly. Persons exposed within 90 days should be treated even if seronegative.

* "Chronic persisters" are patients with positive results (especially with titer >1:4) at 1 year after treatment of primary syphilis, 2 years after treatment of secondary syphilis and 5 years after treatment of late syphilis.

Pregnancy: Penicillin is the only drug with documented efficacy for preventing transmission to the fetus and treating established fetal infection. The usual dose regimens based on stage are appropriate. Tetracyclines are contraindicated in pregnancy and erythromycin should not be used since it does not reliably treat infection in the fetus. The recommendation is for penicillin desensitization with penicillin treatment.

Vaginitis

Diagnosis: The 3 major causes of vaginal discharge are trichonomiasis, *Candida albicans* and bacterial vaginosis which are diagnosed and treated as follows

- *Trichonomiasis*: The yellow-green discharge is malodorous and with vulvar irritation; the diagnosis is established with wet mount of vaginal discharge showing typical motile organisms. *Treatment*: Metronidazole, 2 g po x 1; Alternative regimens: Metronidazole, 500 mg bid x 7 days. Sex partners: Should be treated with either of the 2 regimens noted above.
- *Vulvovaginal candidiasis*: The discharge is typically white and associated with vulvar pruritus; wet preparation or gram stain of discharge shows yeast or pseudohyphae. *Treatment*: Single dose treatment is reserved for uncomplicated and moderately severe cases; multi-dose regimens (3–7 days) are preferred for severe or complicated cases. There are numerous intravaginal formulations including: Chlortrimazole, 1% cream, 5 g x 7–14 days; Chlortrimazole, 100 mg vaginal tab x 7 days or two tab x 3 days; Chlortrimazole 500 mg vaginal tab x 1; Miconazole, 2% cream, 5 g x 7 days; Miconazole, 200 mg vaginal suppository, bid x 3 days or a 100 mg vaginal suppository daily x 7 days; Teiocomazole, 6.5% ointment, 5 g x 1; Terconazole, 0.4% cream, 5 g x 7 days; Terconazole, 80 mg suppository, 1 daily x 3 days. Both miconazole and chlortrimazole are now available OTC. *Sex partners:* Notification or treatment is not indicated because Candida vaginitis is not considered a STD.

Bacterial vaginosis: The discharge is thin and malodorous; diagnostic studies on discharge show: 1) high pH (over 4.5), 2) typical "clue cells" with a gram stain or wet mount, 3) sparse lactobacilli and large numbers of other forms, especially gram-negative or gram-variable rods (Gardnerella or Bacteroides species) and curved gram-variable rods (Mobiluneus sp.) on gram stain, 4) fishy odor with 10% KOH, and 5) abnormal succinate/lactate ratio with gas liquid chromatography.

Treatment: Metronidazole, 2 g po x 1. Alternatives are: Metronidazole, 500 mg bid x 7 days; intravaginal metronidazole, 100 mg/day x 7 days; clindamycin, 300 mg po bid x 7 days or intravaginal clindamycin 2% cream bid x 7 days. The preferred regimen for pregnant women is topical clindamycin.

Pelvic Inflammatory Disease

Diagnosis: Minimum criteria are lower abdominal, adnexal and cervical tendernesses. Additional criteria that increase specificity include fever (oral temperature over 38.3°C), cervical or vaginal discharge, elevated ESR, positive C-reactive protein, culture or other evidence of cervical infection with *N. gonorrhoeae* or *C. trichomatis*, laparoscopy evidence of ID, ultrasound evidence of tubo-ovarian abscess or histopathologic evidence by endometrial biopsy.

Treatment: Hospitalized patients: Two regimens are considered equally effective

- Cefoxitin, 2 g IV q 6 h or cefotetan IV, 2 g IV q 12 h for at least 48 hours after clinical improvement *plus* doxycycline, 100 mg po or IV q 12 h x 14 days.
- Clindamycin, 900 mg IV q 8 h + gentamicin, 2 g kg IV and then 1.5 mg/kg q 8 h; this regimen is given at least 48 hours after clinical improvement. After hospital discharge, doxycycline, 100 mg po bid for 10–14 days or clindamycin, 450 mg po qid x 14 days.

Outpatient treatment: Two regimens are considered equally effective. Ofloxacin, 400 mg bid *plus* clindamycin, 450 mg qid or metronidazole, 500 mg bid for 14 days. Cefoxitin, 2 g IM plus probenecid, 1 g po concurrently or ceftriaxone, 250 mg IM (or ceftrizoxime or cefotaxime) *plus* doxycycline, 100 mg po bid x 14 days.

Sex partners: Sex partners should be treated empirically with regimens effective for *C. trachomatis* and *N. gonorrhoeae.*

HIV Infection

See Chapter 18 for information on pneumocystis and other infections in patients with AIDS. Chapter 25 gives information on hepatobiliary complications of HIV infection.

Appendix 26–1
Preferred Antimicrobial Agents for Specific Pathogens
(Adapted in part from The Medical Letter on Drugs and Therapeutics 34:49, 1992)

ORGANISM	USUAL DISEASE	PREFERRED AGENT	ALTERNATIVES
Achromobacter xylosoxidans	Meningitis, septicemia	Antipseudomonad penicillin (2) Imipenem	Cephalosporins - 3rd gen (5) Sulfa-trimethoprim Imipenem Ticarcillin + clavulanic acid
Acinetobacter calcoaceticus var antitratum (Herellea vaginicola); var Iwoffi (Mima polymorpha)	Sepsis (esp line sepsis) Pneumonia	Imipenem Aminoglycoside (tobramycin or amikacin) + ceftazidime *or* antipseudomonad penicillin (2)	Fluoroquinolone (6) Cephalosporin - 3rd gen (5) Tetracycline (4) Antipseudomonad penicillin (2)
Actinobacillus actinomycetemcomitans	Actinomycosis	Penicillin	Clindamycin Tetracycline (4) Erythromycin Cephalosporins (5)
	Endocarditis	Penicillin + aminoglycoside (1)	Cephalosporin (5) + aminoglycoside (1)
Actinomyces israelii (also A. naeslundii, A. viscosus, A. odontolyticus and Arachnia proprionica)	Actinomycosis	Penicillin G	Clindamycin Tetracycline (4) Erythromycin
Aeromonas hydrophila	Diarrhea	Fluoroquinolone (6) Sulfa-trimethoprim	Tetracycline (4)
	Bacteremia	Cephalosporin (3rd gen)	Sulfa-trimethoprim Aminoglycoside (1)
	Cellulitis/myositis/ osteomyelitis	Fluoroquinolone (6) Sulfa-trimethoprim	Aminoglycoside (1) Imipenem

Appendix 26–1 *(continued)*
(Adapted in part from The Medical Letter on Drugs and Therapeutics 34:49, 1992)

ORGANISM	USUAL DISEASE	PREFERRED AGENT	ALTERNATIVES
Afipia felix	Cat scratch disease	Fluoroquinolone (6) (usually not treated)	Sulfa-trimethoprim Gentamicin Amoxicillin-clavulanate
Bacillus anthracis	Anthrax	Penicillin G Penicillin + streptomycin (meningitis or inhalation anthrax)	Erythromycin Tetracycline (4) Chloramphenicol
Bacillus cereus	Food poisoning Invasive disease	Not treated Clindamycin, erythromycin, vancomycin	
Bacillus species	Septicemia (comp host)	Vancomycin	Imipenem Aminoglycosides (1) Fluoroquinolones (6)
Bacteroides bivius	Female genital tract infections	Metronidazole Clindamycin Cefoxitin Cefotetan	Chloramphenicol Antipseudomonad penicillin (2) Imipenem Betalactam-betalactamase inhibitor (7)
"*B. fragilis* group"	Abscesses Bacteremia Intra-abdominal sepsis	Metronidazole Clindamycin Cefoxitin	Chloramphenicol Antipseudomonad penicillin (2) Imipenem Betalactam-betalactamase inhibitor (7) Cefmetazole

"*B. melaninogenicus* group"	Oral-dental & pulmonary infections Female genital tract infections	Metronidazole Clindamycin Cefoxitin	Chloramphenicol Betalactam-betalactamase inhibitor (7) Imipenem Cefotetan Cefmetazole
Bartonella bacilliformis	Bartonellosis	Chloramphenicol Penicillin	Tetracycline + streptomycin
Bordetella pertussis	Pertussis	Erythromycin	Sulfa-trimethoprim Ampicillin
Borrelia burgdorferi	Lyme disease	Tetracycline (4) (early disease) Ceftriaxone (late complications)	Penicillin G po or IV Amoxicillin Cefuroxime axetil Erythromycin/Azithromycin (?) Cefotaxime Penicillin G
Borrelia recurrentis	Relapsing fever	Tetracycline (4)	Erythromycin Chloramphenicol
Brucella	Brucellosis	Doxycycline + rifampin Doxycycline + gentamicin or streptomycin	Chloramphenicol ± streptomycin Sulfa-trimethoprim Rifampin + cephalosporin (3rd gen) (5) (CNS involvement)
Calymmatobacterium granulomatis	Granuloma inguinale	Tetracycline (4)	Sulfa-trimethoprim Erythromycin (pregnancy)
Campylobacter fetus	Septicemia, vascular infections, meningitis	Gentamicin Imipenem	Chloramphenicol Erythromycin Clindamycin Tetracycline (4)

Appendix 26–1 *(continued)*
(Adapted in part from The Medical Letter on Drugs and Therapeutics 34:49, 1992)

ORGANISM	USUAL DISEASE	PREFERRED AGENT	ALTERNATIVES
Campylobacter jejuni	Diarrhea	Erythromycin Fluoroquinolone (6)	Tetracycline (4) Furazolidine Gentamicin
Capnocytophaga ochracea	Periodontal disease Bacteremia in neutropenic host Tonsillitis (?)	Clindamycin Erythromycin	Amoxicillin-clavulanic acid Imipenem Cefoxitin Cephalosporins (3rd gen) (5) Fluoroquinolone (6) Tetracycline
Capnocytophaga canimorus (DF_2)	Dog and cat bites Bacteremia meningitis (asplenia)	Penicillin Clindamycin	Cephalosporins (3rd gen) (5) Imipenem Vancomycin Fluoroquinolones (6)
Cardiobacterium	Bacteremia Endocarditis	Penicillin + aminoglycoside	Cephalosporin (5) ± aminoglycoside
Cat scratch disease, agent of	Cat scratch disease with lymphadenitis	Fluoroquinolone (6)	Gentamicin Amoxicillin-clavulanate Trimethoprim-sulfamethoxazole
Chlamydia pneumoniae (TWAR agent)	Pneumonia	Tetracycline (4) Erythromycin	Clarithromycin Azithromycin
Chlamydia psittaci	Psittacosis	Tetracycline (4)	Chloramphenicol
Chlamydia trachomatis	Urethritis Endocervicitis PID	Tetracycline (4) Azithromycin	Erythromycin Ofloxacin Sulfisoxazole

	Epididymitis		
	Urethral syndrome		
	Trachoma	Tetracycline (4) (topical + oral)	Sulfonamide (topical + oral)
	Lymphogranuloma venereum	Tetracycline (4)	Erythromycin
	Inclusion conjunctivitis	Erythromycin (topical or oral)	Sulfonamide
Citrobacter diversus	Urinary tract infections, pneumonia	Aminoglycoside (1) Cephalosporin (2nd & 3rd gen) (5) Sulfa-trimethoprim	Tetracycline (4) Fluoroquinolone (6) Imipenem Piperacillin
Citrobacter freundii	Urinary tract infection, wound infection, septicemia, pneumonia	Imipenem Fluoroquinolone (6) Sulfa-trimethoprim Aminoglycoside (1)	Tetracycline (4) Cephalosporin (3rd gen) (5)
Clostridium difficile	Antibiotic-associated colitis	Vancomycin (oral) Metronidazole (oral)	Bacitracin (oral) Cholestyramine Lactobacilli Vancomycin + rifampin
Clostridium sp.	Gas gangrene Sepsis	Penicillin G	Chloramphenicol Metronidazole
	Tetanus	Tetanus immune globulin or IGIV	Antipseudomonad penicillin
	Botulism	Trivalent equine antitoxin (CDC)*	Clindamycin
	Crepitant cellulitis		Imipenem
Corynebacterium diphtheriae	Diphtheria	Penicillin *or* erythromycin + antitoxin (CDC)*	
Corynebacterium JK strain	Septicemia	Vancomycin	Penicillin G + gentamicin Fluoroquinolone (6)

Appendix 26–1 *(continued)*
(Adapted in part from The Medical Letter on Drugs and Therapeutics 34:49, 1992)

ORGANISM	USUAL DISEASE	PREFERRED AGENT	ALTERNATIVES
Corynebacterium minutissimum	Erythrasma	Erythromycin	
Corynebacterium ulcerans	Pharyngitis	Erythromycin	
Coxiella burnetii	Q fever	Tetracycline (4)	Chloramphenicol Ciprofloxacin (6) Rifampin (?)
Dysgonic fermenter type 2 (DF_2)	See *Capnocytophaga canimoris*		
Edwardsiella tarda	Gastroenteritis (usually not treated) Wound infection Bacteremia, liver abscesses	Ampicillin	Cephalosporin (5) Aminoglycoside (1) Chloramphenicol Tetracycline (4)
Ehrlichia canis	Ehrlichiosis	Tetracycline (4)	Chloramphenicol (?)
Eikenella corrodens	Oral infections, bite wounds	Ampicillin/amoxicillin Penicillin G	Tetracycline (4) Amoxicillin-clavulanic acid Cephalosporin (5) Imipenem
Enterobacter aerogenes, E. cloacae	Sepsis, pneumonia, wound infections	Aminoglycoside (1) Sulfa-trimethoprim Fluoroquinolone (6)	Aztreonam Imipenem Antipseudomonad penicillin (2) Cephalosporin-3rd gen (5)
	Urinary tract infection	Sulfa-trimethoprim Cephalosporin-3rd gen (5)	Antipseudomonad penicillin (2) Aminoglycoside Fluoroquinolone (6) Imipenem

Enterococcus (E. faecalis and *E. faecium)*	Urinary tract infections	Ampicillin/amoxicillin	Penicillin + aminoglycoside (1) Vancomycin Nitrofurantoin Fluoroquinolone (6)
	Wound infections, intra-abdominal sepsis	Ampicillin	Vancomycin Penicillin + aminoglycoside (1) Imipenem (*E. faecalis*)
	Endocarditis	Penicillin G/ampicillin + gentamicin, streptomycin or amikacin	Vancomycin + gentamicin or streptomycin
Enterococcus (Vancomycin-resistant)		Moderate resistance: high dose penicillin + vancomycin ± aminoglycoside (MIC ≤ 32 μg/ml) High resistance + deep infection: ciprofloxacin ± rifampin and gentamicin	Teicoplanin (many strains resistant)
Erwinia agglomerans	Urinary tract infections Bacteremia Pneumonia	Aminogycosides (1)	Fluoroquinolone (6) Chloramphenicol Cephalosporins (5)
Erysipelothrix rhusiopathiae	Localized cutaneous	Penicillin	Erythromycin
	Endocarditis/ disseminated	Penicillin	Cephalosporins (5)

Appendix 26–1 *(continued)*
(Adapted in part from The Medical Letter on Drugs and Therapeutics 34:49, 1992)

ORGANISM	USUAL DISEASE	PREFERRED AGENT	ALTERNATIVES
E. coli	Septicemia Intra-abdominal sepsis Wound infection	Cephalosporin (3rd gen) (5) Ampicillin (if sensitive)	Aminoglycoside (1) Sulfa-trimethoprim Imipenem Fluoroquinolone (6) Cephalosporin (1st or 2nd gen) (5) Aztreonam Antipseudomonad penicillin (2)
	Urinary tract infection	Ampicillin (if sensitive) Tetracycline (4) Sulfa-trimethoprim Aminoglycoside (1) Cephalosporin (5) Antipseudomonad penicillin (2)	Imipenem Aztreonam Fluoroquinolone (6) Sulfonamide
Flavobacterium meningosepticum	Sepsis	Vancomycin	Sulfa-trimethoprim Erythromycin Clindamycin Imipenem Fluoroquinolone (6)
Francisella tularensis	Tularemia	Streptomycin or gentamicin	Tetracycline (4) Chloramphenicol (?)
Fusobacterium	Oral/dental/pulmonary infection; liver abscess	Penicillin G Metronidazole	Cefoxitin/cefotetan Chloramphenicol Imipenem Clindamycin

Gardnerella vaginalis	Vaginitis	Metronidazole	Clindamycin (po or topical)
Haemophilus aphrophilus	Sepsis, endocarditis	Penicillin G + aminoglycoside (1)	Cephalosporin-3rd gen (5) + aminoglycoside (1)
H. ducreyi	Chancroid	Ceftriaxone	Sulfa-trimethoprim
		Erythromycin	Amoxicillin + clavulanic acid
			Fluoroquinolone (6)
H. influenzae	Meningitis	Cefotaxime, ceftriaxone	
		Chloramphenicol	
	Epiglottis	Cephalosporin - 3rd gen (5)	Chloramphenicol ± ampicillin
	Pneumonia	Sulfa-trimethoprim	Betalactam-betalactamase inhibitor (7)
	Arthritis	Cefamandole/cefuroxime	
	Cellulitis	Ampicillin (if sensitive)	
	Otitis	Sulfa-trimethoprim	Erythromycin - sulfonamide
	Sinusitis	Ampicillin/amoxicillin (if sensitive)	Cephalosporin - 2nd or 3rd gen (5)
	Bronchitis		Tetracycline (4)
			Betalactam-betalactamase inhibitor (7)
			Fluoroquinolone (6)
Hafnia alvei	Pneumonia, wound infection, urinary tract infection	Aminoglycosides (1)	Ciprofloxacin (6)
			Chloramphenicol
			Antipseudomonad penicillin (2)
Helicobacter pylori (Campylobacter pylori)	Gastritis	Bismuth subcitrate *plus* metronidazole *plus* tetracycline	Bismuth *plus* metronidazole *plus* amoxicillin
	Recurrent duodenal ulcer disease		Omeprazole *plus* amoxicillin
Kingella sp.	Endocarditis	Penicillin + aminoglycoside	Cephalosporin (5) + aminoglycoside
	Septic arthritis		

Appendix 26–1 *(continued)*
(Adapted in part from The Medical Letter on Drugs and Therapeutics 34:49, 1992)

ORGANISM	USUAL DISEASE	PREFERRED AGENT	ALTERNATIVES
Klebsiella pneumoniae, K. oxytoca	Septicemia Pneumonia Intra-abdominal sepsis	Cephalosporin (3rd gen) (5)	Aminoglycoside (1) Sulfa-trimethoprim Piperacillin/mezlocillin Imipenem Betalactam-betalactamase inhibitor (7) Aztreonam Fluoroquinolone (6)
Klebsiella sp.	Urinary tract infection	Sulfa-trimethoprim Cephalosporin (5) Tetracycline (4)	Aminoglycoside (1) Betalactam-betalactamase inhibitor (7) Fluoroquinolone (6) Piperacillin/mezlocillin Imipenem
Legionella sp.	Legionnaires' disease	Erythromycin ± rifampin	Sulfa-trimethoprim + rifampin Fluoroquinolone (6) + rifampin Clarithromycin (?) Azithromycin (?)
Leptospira	Leptospirosis	Penicillin G or ampicillin	Tetracycline (4)
Leptotrichia buccalis	Orodental infections "Vincent's infection"	Penicillin G	Tetracycline (4) Clindamycin Erythromycin Metronidazole

Listeria monocytogenes	Meningitis Septicemia	Ampicillin or penicillin ± gentamicin	Sulfa-trimethoprim
Moraxella	Ocular infections Bacteremia	Aminoglycoside (1) Penicillins	Cephalosporin - 3rd gen (5) Imipenem Fluoroquinolone (6) Antipseudomonad penicillin (2)
Moraxella catarrhalis (Branhamella catarrhalis)	Otitis, sinusitis, pneumonitis	Sulfa-trimethoprim	Amoxicillin-clavulanic acid Erythromycin Clarithromycin/azithromycin Tetracycline (4) Cephalosporin (5) Fluoroquinolone (6)
Morganella morganii	Bacteremia Urinary tract infection Pneumonia Wound infection	Aminoglycoside Fluoroquinolone (6) Imipenem Cephalosporin (3rd gen) (5)	Sulfa-trimethoprim Aztreonam Antipseudomonad penicillin (2) Betalactam-betalactamase inhibitor (7) Tetracycline (4)
Mycobacterium tuberculosis (See page 126)	Tuberculosis	INH + rifampin pyrazinamide, ± ethambutol	Streptomycin, Capreomycin or Kanamycin Ciprofloxacin or Ofloxacin Ethionamide PAS Cycloserine
M. kansasii (See page 133)	Pulmonary infection	INH + rifampin + ethambutol ± streptomycin	Ethionamide Cycloserine

Appendix 26–1 *(continued)*
(Adapted in part from The Medical Letter on Drugs and Therapeutics 34:49, 1992)

ORGANISM	USUAL DISEASE	PREFERRED AGENT	ALTERNATIVES
M. avium-intracellulare (See page 133)	Pulmonary infection	INH + rifampin + ethambutol + streptomycin	Clofazimine (extrapul dis) Clarithromycin Ethionamide Amikacin Cycloserine Ciprofloxacin/Ofloxacin
	Disseminated infection (AIDS)	Clarithromycin + ethambutol or clofazimine ± ciprofloxacin (6) 3-5 of the following: rifampin, ethambutol, amikacin, kanamycin, clofazimine, clarithromycin, ciprofloxacin	Rifampin or rifabutin Eithionamide Cycloserine Pyrazinamide Imipenem Amikacin
M. chelonae (See page 134)	Skin and soft tissue	Amikacin and/or cefoxitin, clofazimine or clarithromycin, then sulfonamide, rifampin, doxycycline or erythromycin	
M. fortuitum (See page 133)	Soft tissue and wound infections	Amikacin, ciprofloxacin + sulfonamide	Clofaximine Clarithromycin Cefoxitin Doxycycline Imipenem
M. marinum (See page 133)	Soft tissue infections	Rifampin + ethambutol *or* Sulfa-trimethoprim or Minocycline (doxycycline)	Ciprofloxacin (6)

M. ulcerans	Pulmonary	INH, rifampin + ethambutal	
M. leprae	Leprosy	Sulfone sensitive strains: Dapsone + rifampin Sulfone resistant strains: Clofazimine ± rifampin	Ethionamide (Protionamide) Minocycline Ofloxacin
Mycoplasma fermentans	Genital tract infections	Doxycycline	
Mycoplasma pneumoniae	Pneumonia	Erythromycin Tetracycline (4)	Clarithromycin (?) Azithromycin (?) Fluoroquinolone (?)
Neisseria gonorrhoeae	Urethritis Salpingitis Cervicitis Arthritis-dermatitis	Ceftriaxone Cefixime Fluoroquinolone (6)	Spectinomycin Sulfa-trimethoprim Cefotaxime, Cefoxitin Ceftizoxime Cefuroxime axetil
N. meningitidis	Meningitis Bacteremia Pericarditis Pneumonia	Penicillin G	Ampicillin Chloramphenicol Sulfa-trimethoprim Cephalosporin-cefotaxime, ceftizoxime, ceftriaxone
	Prophylaxis	Rifampin Fluoroquinolone (6)	
Nocardia asteroides	Nocardiosis: pulmonary infection, abscesses - skin, lung, brain	Sulfonamide (usually sulfadiazine) Sulfa-trimethoprim (sulfa level maintained at 10–20 mg/dl)	Sulfasoxazole Imipenem ± amikacin Minocycline ± sulfa Amikacin ± sulfa Cycloserine

Appendix 26–1 *(continued)*
(Adapted in part from The Medical Letter on Drugs and Therapeutics 34:49, 1992)

ORGANISM	USUAL DISEASE	PREFERRED AGENT	ALTERNATIVES
Pasteurella multocida	Animal bite wound	Penicillin G	Tetracycline (4) Ciprofloxacin (6) Amoxicillin-clavulanic acid
	Septicemia Septic arthritis/ osteomyelitis	Penicillin G	Cephalosporins (5) Betalactam-betalactamase inhibitor (7) Chloramphenicol
Peptostreptococcus	Oral/dental/pulmonary infection; intra-abdominal sepsis; gynecologic infection	Penicillin G Ampicillin/amoxicillin	Clindamycin Metronidazole Cephalosporin (5) Chloramphenicol Erythromycin Vancomycin Imipenem
Plesiomonas shigelloides	Diarrhea (usually not treated)	Sulfa-trimethoprim Tetracycline (4) Fluoroquinolone (6)	Chloramphenicol Aminoglycosides (1)
	Extra-intestinal infection	Cephalosporin-3rd gen (3) Aminoglycoside (1)	Aztreonam Sulfa-trimethoprim Imipenem Fluoroquinolone (6)
Propionibacterium acnes	Acne	Tetracycline (4)	Clindamycin (topical)
	Systemic infection	Penicillin	Clindamycin

Proteus mirabilis	Septicemia Urinary tract infection Intra-abdominal sepsis Wound infection	Ampicillin	Aminoglycosides (1) Cephalosporins (5) Sulfa-trimethoprim Antipseudomonad penicillin Aztreonam Imipenem Fluoroquinolone (6)
Proteus indole positive	Septicemia Urinary tract infection	Cephalosporin-3rd gen (5)	Aminoglycoside (1) Sulfa-trimethoprim Antipseudomonad penicillin (2) Aztreonam Imipenem Betalactam-betalactamase inhibitor (7) Fluoroquinolone (6)
Providencia rettgeri	Septicemia Urinary tract infection	Cephalosporin-3rd gen (5)	Aminoglycoside (1) Antipseudomonad penicillin (2) Imipenem Aztreonam Sulfa-trimethoprim Fluoroquinolone (6)
Providencia stuartii	Septicemia Urinary tract infection	Cephalosporin-3rd gen (5)	Aminoglycoside (1) Antipseudomonad penicillin (2) Sulfa-trimethoprim Imipenem Aztreonam Fluoroquinolone (6) Betalactam-betalactamase inhibitor (7)

Pseudomonas aeruginosa	Septicemia, pneumonia Intra-abdominal sepsis	Aminoglycoside (tobramycin) ± antipseudomonad penicillin (2)	Aminoglycoside (1) ± cefoperazone, imipenem or ceftazidime Aztreonam Ciprofloxacin (6)
	Urinary tract infections	Aminoglycoside (1) Antipseudomonad penicillin (2) Fluoroquinolone (6)	Imipenem Ceftazidime Cefoperazone Aztreonam
Ps. cepacia	Septicemia Pneumonia	Sulfa-trimethoprim	Betalactam-betalactamase inhibitor (7) Ceftazidime Fluoroquinolone (6)
Ps. mallei	Glanders	Streptomycin + tetracycline	Chloramphenicol + streptomycin
Ps. maltophilia (*Xanthomonas maltophilia*)	Septicemia	Sulfa-trimethoprim	Ticarcillin-clavulanic acid
Ps. pseudomallei	Melioidosis	Ceftazidime ± sulfa-trimethoprim	Sulfa-trimethoprim Tetracycline (4) + chloramphenicol Imipenem Cefotaxime Amoxicillin + clavulanate

Ps. putida	Septicemia, pneumonia, urinary tract infections	Aminoglycosides (1) Fluoroquinolone (6)	
Rhodococcus equi	Pneumonia, pulmonary abscess, bacteremia	Vancomycin ± ciprofloxacin, imipenem or amikacin	Imipenem Erythromycin Ciprofloxacin (6) Amikacin
Rickettsia	Rocky Mountain spotted fever, Q fever, tick bite fever, murine typhus, scrub typhus, typhus, trench fever	Tetracycline (4)	Chloramphenicol Fluoroquinolone (6)
Rochalimaea henselae *Rochalimaea quintana*	(See Afipia felix) Bacillary angiomatosis	Erythromycin	Aminoglucosides Aztreonam Sulfa-trimethoprim Tetracycline (4)
Salmonella typhi	Typhoid fever	Ceftriaxone	Chloramphenicol Sulfa-trimethoprim Ampicillin/amoxicillin Fluoroquinolones (6) Cefotaxime/cefoperazone/ceftriaxone
Salmonella sp. (other)	Enteric fever Mycotic aneurysm	Cefotaxime/cefoperazone/ceftriaxone	Ampicillin/amoxicillin Sulfa-trimethoprim Chloramphenicol Fluoroquinolone (6)

Appendix 26–1 *(continued)*
(Adapted in part from The Medical Letter on Drugs and Therapeutics 34:49, 1992)

ORGANISM	USUAL DISEASE	PREFERRED AGENT	ALTERNATIVES
Serratia marcescens	Septicemia Urinary tract infection Pneumonia	Cephalosporin-3rd gen (5)	Gentamicin or amikacin ± antipseudomonad penicillin or cephalosporin-3rd gen (5) Cephalosporins-3rd gen (5) Sulfa-trimethoprim Antipseudomonad penicillin (2) Imipenem Fluoroquinolone (6) Aztreonam
Shigella	Colitis	Sulfa-trimethoprim	Ampicillin Tetracycline (4) Ciprofloxacin/nalidixic acid (6)
Spirillum minus	Rat bite fever	Penicillin G	Tetracycline (4) Streptomycin
Staphylococcus aureus			
Methicillin-sensitive	Septicemia Pneumonia Wound infection	Penicillinase resistant penicillin (3) ± rifampin or gentamicin Cephalosporins-1st gen (5) Cefuroxime/cefamandole	Erythromycin/clindamycin Vancomycin Betalactam-betalactamase inhibitor (7) Imipenem Fluoroquinolone (6) Clindamycin
Methicillin-resistant		Vancomycin ± rifampin or gentamicin	Sulfa-trimethoprim Fluoroquinolones (6) Minocycline Teicoplanin (investigational)

Staph. saprophyticus	Urinary tract infections	Sulfa-trimethoprim Ampicillin/amoxicillin Fluoroquinolone (6)	Cephalosporins (5) Tetracycline (4)
Staph. epidermidis	Septicemia Infected prosthetic devices	Vancomycin	Sulfa-trimethoprim Penicillinase resistant penicillin (3) Cephalosporin (5) Fluoroquinolone (6) Imipenem
Streptococcus, Group A, B, C, G; *bovis, milleri, pneumoniae, viridans*, anaerobic	Pharyngitis Soft tissue infection Pneumonia Abscesses	Penicillin G or V	Cephalosporin (5) Clindamycin Vancomycin Erythromycin Clarithromycin
	Endocarditis	Penicillin G ± streptomycin or gentamicin	Cephalosporin (5) Vancomycin
	Meningitis	Penicillin G	Chloramphenicol Cephalosporin-3rd gen (5)
S. pneumoniae (resistant strains)		Vancomycin ± rifampin (for meningitis) Erythromycin	Chloramphenicol Sulfa-trimethoprim Tetracycline
Streptobacillus moniliformis	Rat bite fever Haverhill fever	Penicillin G	Tetracycline (4) Streptomycin
Treponema carateum	Pinta	Penicillin G	Tetracycline
Treponema pallidum	Syphilis	Penicillin G	Tetracycline (4) Erythromycin Ceftriaxone
Treponema pallidum ss endemicum	Bejel	Penicillin G	
Treponema pallidum ss *pertenue*	Yaws	Penicillin G	Tetracycline (4)

Appendix 26–1 *(continued)*
(Adapted in part from The Medical Letter on Drugs and Therapeutics 34:49, 1992)

ORGANISM	USUAL DISEASE	PREFERRED AGENT	ALTERNATIVES
Ureaplasma urealyticum	Urethritis Endocervicitis PID (?)	Erythromycin	Tetracycline (4)
Vibrio cholerae	Cholera	Tetracycline (4)	Erythromycin Sulfa-trimethoprim Furazolidone Fluoroquinolone (6)
Vibrio vulnificus	Septicemia Wound infection	Tetracycline (4)	Cefotaxime
Xanthomonas maltophilia	Septicemia UTI Pneumonia	Sulfa-trimethoprim	Ceftazidine Fluoroquinolone (6)
Yersinia enterocolitica	Enterocolitis (usually not treated) Mesenteric adenitis (usually not treated)	Sulfa-trimethoprim	Cephalosporin-3rd gen (5) Ciprofloxacin (6) Tetracycline (4)
	Septicemia	Aminoglycoside (gentamicin)	Chloramphenicol Cephalosporins-3rd gen (5)

Yersinia pestis	Plague	Streptomycin	Chloramphenicol Tetracycline (4) Gentamicin
Yersinia pseudotuberculosis	Mesenteric adenitis (usually not treated) Septicemia	Aminoglycoside (1) Ampicillin	Sulfa-trimethoprim Tetracycline (4)

* Available from CDC 404-639-3670

1. Aminoglycosides = Gentamicin, tobramycin, amikacin, netilmicin
2. Antipseudomonad penicillin = Ticarcillin, piperacillin, mezlocillin; carbenicillin and azocillin are no longer available
3. Penicillinase resistant penicillins: Nafcillin, oxacillin, methicillin, cloxacillin, dicloxacillin
4. Tetracycline = Tetracycline, doxycycline, minocycline
5. Cephalosporins
   1st generation: Cefadroxil, cefprozil, cefazolin, cephalexin, cephalothin, cephapirin, cephradine
   2nd generation: Cefaclor, cefamandole, cefonicid, ceforanide, cefotetan, cefoxitin, cefuroxime, cefmetazole
   3rd generation: Cefotaxime, ceftizoxime, ceftazidime, cefoperazone, ceftriaxone, moxalactam, cefixime, cefpodoxime, ceftibutin, Carbaceferms: Loracarbef, cefprozil
6. Fluoroquinolones: Norfloxacin, ciprofloxacin, ofloxacin and lomefloxacin. Systemic infections are usually treated with ciprofloxacin, exoxacin, lomefloxacin or ofloxacin; all may be used for urinary tract infections With regard to spectrum: Ps. aeruginosa—ciprofloxacin; S. pneumoniae—ofloxacin; Mycobacteria—ciprofloxacin or ofloxacin; C. trachomatis—ofloxacin
7. Betalactam-betalactamase inhibitor: Amoxicillin + clavulanate, ticarcillin + clavulanate and ampicillin + sulbactam

Appendix 26–2
Preparations and Recommended Dosing Regimens for Antimicrobial Agents (Adapted from Drug Information 92, American Hospital Formulary Service, 1992 pp 33–481)

AGENT	TRADE NAMES	DOSAGE FORM	USUAL ADULT REGIMEN: DAILY DOSE, ROUTE & DOSE INTERVAL
Acyclovir	Zovirax	5% ointment 3 & 15 gm tubes	Topical q3h
		200 mg caps	200 mg po; ×3–5/day
		800 mg tabs	800 mg po; ×5/day
		200 mg/5 ml susp	200–800 mg po; ×3–5/day
		500; 1000 mg vials (IV)	15–36 mg/kg/day IV over 1hr q8h
Amantadine	Symmetrel	100 mg cap & tabs 50 mg/5 ml syrup	100–200 mg/day po q12–24h
Amdinocillin	Coactin	0.5; 1 gm vial	40–60 mg/kg/day IM or IV q4–6h
Amikacin	Amikin	0.1; 0.5; 1 gm vials	15 mg/kg/day IV q8–12h
Aminosalicylic acid	PAS	0.5 gm tabs	150 mg/kg/day po q6–12h
Amoxicillin	Amoxil, Polymox, Trimox, Utimox, Wymox, Larotid	250; 500 mg caps 125; 250 mg/5 ml syrup	.75–2 gm/day po q6–8h
Amoxicillin + K clavulanate	Augmentin	125/31 mg/5 ml susp 250/62 mg/5 ml susp 125/31 mg tabs 250/125 mg tabs 500/125 mg tabs	.75–1.5 gm/day (amoxicillin) po q8h
Amphotericin B	Fungizone	50 mg vial	0.3–1 mg/kg/day IV over 4–8 hr q 1–2 days

Ampicillin	Omnipen, Amcill, Penamp, Polycillin, Principen, Totacillin	250; 500 mg caps 125; 250; 500 mg/5 ml susp 3.5 gm + probenecid, 1 gm (for GC)	1–2 gm/day po q6h
Ampicillin sodium	Omnipen-N, Polycillin-N, Totacillin-N	0.125; 0.25; 0.5; 1; 2; 10 gm vials	2–8 gm/day IV q4–6h
Ampicillin + sulbactam	Unasyn	1:0.5 gm + 2:1.0 gm vials (Amp:sulbactam)	4–8 gm ampicillin/day IV or IM q6h
Atovaquone	Mepron	250 mg tabs	750 mg po 3×/day w/food
Azithromycin	Zithromax	250 mg tabs	500 mg po first day, then 250 mg q24h × 5
Azlocillin	Azlin	2; 3; 4 gm vials	8–24 gm/day IV q6–8h
AZT	(see zidovudine)		
Aztreonam	Azactam	0.5; 1; 2 gm vials	1.5–6 gm/day IV or IM q6–8h
Bacampicillin	Spectrobid	400 mg tabs (equivalent to 280 mg ampicillin) 125 mg/5 ml syrup (equiv to 87 mg amp)	.8–1.6 gm/day po q12h
Bacitracin	Baci-IM	50,000 unit vials	10,000–25,000 units IM q6h; 25,000 units po q6h
Capreomycin	Capastat	1 gm vial	1 gm/day IM
Carbenicillin indanyl sodium	Geocillin	382 mg tabs	382–764 mg po q6h
Cefaclor	Ceclor	250; 500 mg caps 125; 187; 250 & 375 mg/5 ml susp	1–2 gm/day po q8h

Appendix 26–2
(continued)

AGENT	TRADE NAMES	DOSAGE FORM	USUAL ADULT REGIMEN: DAILY DOSE, ROUTE & DOSE INTERVAL
Cefadroxil	Duricef, Ultracef	500 mg caps; 1 gm tab; 125; 250; 500 mg/5 ml susp	1–2 gm/day po 1–2 x/day
Cefamandole nafate	Mandol	0.5; 1; 2; 10 gm vials	2–18 gm/day IM or IV q4–6h
Cefazolin	Ancef, Kefzol, Zolicef	0.25; 0.5; 1; 5; 10; 20 gm vials	2–6 gm/day IV or IM q8h
Cefixime	Suprax	200; 400 mg tabs; 100 mg/5 ml susp	400 mg/day po, 1–2 ×/day
Cefmetazole	Zefazone	1; 2 gm vials	4–8 gm/day IV q6–12h
Cefonicid	Monocid	0.5; 1; 10 gm vials	1–2 gm/day IV or IM in 1 dose/day
Cefoperazone	Cefobid	1; 2; 10 gm vials	2–8 gm/day IM or IV q8–12h
Ceforanide lysine	Precef	0.5; 1 gm vials	1–3 gm/day IV or IM q12h
Cefotaxime sodium	Claforan	0.5; 1; 2; 10 gm vials	2–12 gm/day IV or IM q6h
Cefotetan	Cefotan	1; 2; 10 gm vials	2–4 gm/day IV or IM q12h
Cefoxitin sodium	Mefoxin	1; 2; 10 gm vials	2–18 gm/day IV or IM q4–6h
Cefpodoxime proxetil	Vantin	100; 200 mg tabs 50 mg/5 ml; 100 mg/5 ml susp	200–800 mg/day po, q12h
Cefprozil	Cefzil	250; 500 mg tabs 125; 250 mg/5 ml susp	0.5–2 gm/day po, q12–24h usually 500 mg qd or bid
Ceftazidime	Fortaz, Tazidime, Tazicef, Ceptaz	0.5; 1; 2; 6 gm vials	3–6 gm/day IV or IM q8–12h
Ceftizoxime sodium	Cefizox	1; 2; 10 gm vials	2–12 gm/day IV or IM q6–8h
Ceftriaxone	Rocephin	0.25; 0.5; 1; 2; 10 gm vial	1–2 gm IV or IM q12–24h
Cefuroxime	Zinacef	0.75; 1.5 gm vial	2.25–4.5 gm/day IV or IM q6–8h

Cefuroxime axetil	Ceftin	0.125; 0.25; 0.5 gm tabs	0.5–1.0 gm/day po q12h
Cephalexin monohydrate	Keflex, Keftab, Cefanex, Keflet	0.25; 0.5 gm caps	1–2 gm/day po q6h
		0.25; 0.5 gm tabs	
		125; 250 mg/5 ml susp	
Cephalothin sodium	Keflin	1; 2; 20 gm vials	2–12 gm/day IV q4–6h
Cephapirin sodium	Cefadyl	0.5; 1; 2; 4 gm vials	2–4 gm/day IV q6h
Cephradine	Anspor	250; 500 mg caps	1–2 gm/day po q6h
		125; 250 mg/5 ml susp	
	Velosef	0.25; 0.5; 1; 2 gm vials	2–8 gm/day IV or IM q6h
Chloramphenicol	Chloromycetin	250 mg caps	1–2 gm/day po q6h
Chloramphenicol palmitate	Chloromycetin	150 mg/5 ml syrup	1–2 gm/day po q6h
Chloramphenicol Na succinate	Chloromycetin sodium succinate	1 gm vial	2–4 gm/day IV q6h
Chloroquine HCl	Aralen HCl	250 mg amp (150 mg base)	200–250 mg base q6h IM or IV
Chloroquine PO_4	Aralen PO_4	500 mg tabs (300 mg base)	300–600 mg (base) qd–q week
		250 mg tabs (150 mg base)	
Chloroquine hydroxy	Plaquenil	200 mg tabs (155 mg base)	10 mg/kg/day po q24h
Cinoxacin	Cinobac	250; 500 mg cap	1 gm/day po q6–12h
Ciprofloxacin	Cipro	250; 500; 750 mg tabs	0.5–1.5 gm/day po q12h
	Cipro IV	200; 400 mg vials	800 mg/day IV q12h
Clarithromycin	Biaxin	250; 500 mg tabs	500 mg/day po q12h
Clindamycin HCl	Cleocin HCl	75; 150; 300 mg cap	0.6–1.8 gm/day po q6–8h
Clindamycin PO_4	Cleocin PO_4	150 mg/ml in vials (2, 4, 6 ml)	1.8–2.7 gm/day IV q6–8h
Clindamycin palmitate HCl	Cleocin pediatric	75 mg/5 ml solution	0.6–1.8 gm/day po q6–8h
Clindamycin vaginal cream	Cleocin VC	2% 40 gm tube	Topical: 1/day × 7 days

Appendix 26–2
(continued)

AGENT	TRADE NAMES	DOSAGE FORM	USUAL ADULT REGIMEN: DAILY DOSE, ROUTE & DOSE INTERVAL
Clofazimine	Lamprene	50; 100 mg caps	50–300 mg/day po q8–24h
Cloxacillin	Tegopen	250; 500 mg caps	1–2 gm/day po q6h
	Cloxapen	125 mg/5 ml solution	
Colistin	Coly-Mycin S	25 mg/5 ml susp	2.5–5.0 mg/kg/day IV q6–12h
	Coly-Mycin M	150 mg vial (IV)	
Cyclacillin	Cyclapen-W	250; 500 mg cap	1–2 gm/day po q6h
		125; 250 mg/5 ml susp	
Cycloserine	Seromycin	250 mg caps	0.5–1 gm/day po in 2 doses
Dapsone		25; 100 mg tabs	25–100 mg/day po q24h
Demeclocycline	Declomycin	150; 300 mg caps	600 mg/day po q6–12h
Dicloxacillin	Dycill, Dynapen	125; 250; 500 mg cap	1–2 gm/day po q6h
	Pathocil	62.5 mg/5 ml susp	
Didanosine (Dideoxyinosine) (ddI)	Videx	25; 50; 100; 150 mg tabs and 100; 167; 250; 375 mg packets	>60 kg:200 mg (tabs) bid <60 kg:125 mg (tabs) bid
Dideoxycytidine (ddC)	HIVID	0.375; 0.75 mg tabs	0.75 mg po tid
Diethylcarbamazine	Hetrazan	50 mg tabs	6–13 mg/kg/day, 1–3 doses
Diloxanide	Furamide		500 mg po q8h

Doxycycline	Vibramycin	50 mg/5 ml susp	100–200 mg/day po q12–24h
	Doxy caps, Doxy tabs	100 mg tabs	
	Vibra-tabs	50; 100 mg caps	200 mg/day IV q12h
	Doxy-100, 200	100; 200 mg vial	
Eflornithine	Ornidyl		400 mg/kg/day IV; 100 mg/kg po q8h
Emetine HCl		65 mg/ml (1 ml vial)	1–1.5 mg/kg/day up to 90 mg/day; IM or
Enoxacin	Penetrex	200; 400 mg tabs	400–800 mg/day po q12h
Erythromycin	E-mycin; ERYC; Ery-Tab; E-Base Erythromycin Base Iotycin, PCE, RP-Mycin, Robimycin	250 mg caps 250; 333; 500 mg tabs 2% topical	1–2 gm/day po q6h (topical for acne)
Erythromycin estolate	Ilosone	250 mg caps, 500 mg tabs 125; 250 mg/5 ml susp	1–2 gm/day po q6h
Erythromycin ethylsuccinate	E.E.S.	200; 400 mg tabs	1.6–3.2 gm/day po q6h
	EryPed	200; 400 mg/5 ml susp	
Erythromycin gluceptate	Ilotycin gluceptate	1 gm vial	2–4 gm/day IV q6h
Erythromycin lactobionate	Erythrocin lactobionate	0.5; 1 gm vial	1–4 gm/day IV q6h
Erythromycin stearate	Eramycin Erypar; Erythrocin stearate; Ethril; Wyamycin S SK-erythromycin	250; 500 mg tabs	1–2 gm/day po q6h
Ethambutol	Myambutol	100; 400 mg tabs	15 mg/kg/day po q24h
Ethionamide	Trecator-SC	250 mg tabs	0.5–1 gm/day po in 1–3 daily doses

Appendix 26–2
(continued)

AGENT	TRADE NAMES	DOSAGE FORM	USUAL ADULT REGIMEN: DAILY DOSE, ROUTE & DOSE INTERVAL
Fluconazole	Diflucan	50; 100; 200 mg tabs 100; 200 mg vials	100–200 mg/day po or IV q24h
Flucytosine	Ancobon	250; 500 mg cap	50–150 mg/kg/day po q6h
Foscarnet	Foscavir	24 mg/ml, 500 ml	90–180 mg/kg/day IV qd or tid
Furazolidone	Furoxone	100 mg tabs 50 mg/15 ml susp	100 mg po q6h
Ganciclovir	Cytovene	0.5 gm vial	5 mg/kg IV bid (induction) or qd (maintenance)
Gentamicin	Garamycin Gentamicin SO_4 Injection Isotonic (NaCl) Gentamicin SO_4 ADD-Vantage Gentamicin SO_4 in 5% dextrose piggyback	40; 60; 70; 80; 90; 100; 120 mg vials 2 mg/ml for intrathecal use	3–5 mg/kg/day IV or IM q8h
Griseofulvin	Grisactin Fulvicin Grifulvin V Gris-PEG Grisactin Ultra Fulvicin P/G	microsize: 250 caps, 250; 500 mg tabs 125 mg/5 ml susp ultramicrosize: 125; 165; 250; 330 mg tabs	500 mg–1 gm po/day 330–750 mg po/day

Imipenem/Cilastatin	Primaxin	0.25; 0.5; 0.75 gm vials (Imipenem: cilastatin is 1:1)	1–4 gm/day IV q6h
Interferon Alfa 2a	Roferon-A	3, 18, 36 mil unit vials	3 mil units 3×/wk (HCV)
			30–35 mil units/wk (HBV)
			30 mil units/m2 3×/wk (Kaposi Sarcoma)
			1 mil units intralesion (condylomata)
Alfa 2b	Intron A	3, 5, 10, 25, 50 mil unit vials	As above
Iodoquinol	Yodoxin	210 mg tabs	650 mg/day po q8h
	Diquinol	650 mg tabs	
	Yodoquinol		
Isoniazid	Laniazid	50; 100; 300 mg tabs	300 mg/day po q24h
	Tubizid	50 mg/5 ml (oral solu)	
	Nydrazid	1 gm vial (IM)	300 mg/day IM q12–24h
Itraconazole	Sporanox	100 mg caps	200–400 mg/day po q12–24h
Kanamycin	Kantrex	.075; 0.5; 1 gm vial	15 mg/kg/day IV q8h
	Klebcil	500 mg caps	
Ketoconazole	Nizoral	200 mg tabs	200–400 mg/day po q12–24h up to 1.6 gm/day
Lincomycin	Lincocin	250; 500 mg caps	1.5–2.0 gm/d po q6–8h
		300 mg/ml (2, 10 ml)	1.8–8 gm/d IV q8–12h
Loracarbef	Lorabid	200 mg parvule	400–800 mg/day po q12h
Lomefloxacin	Maxaquin	400 mg caps	400 mg/day po q24h

Appendix 26–2
(continued)

AGENT	TRADE NAMES	DOSAGE FORM	USUAL ADULT REGIMEN: DAILY DOSE, ROUTE & DOSE INTERVAL
Mefloquine	Lariam	250 mg tabs	1250 mg po × 1 (treatment); 250 mg po q wk (prophylaxis)
Mebendazole	Vermox	100 mg tabs	100 mg po × 1–2 up to 2 gm/day
Methacycline	Rondomycin	150; 300 mg caps	600 mg/d po
Methenamine hippurate	Hiprex	1 gm tabs	1–2 gm/day po q12h
Methenamine mandelate	Mandelamine	0.35; 0.5; 1 gm tabs 250; 500 mg/5 ml syrup 0.5; 1 gm granules	1–4 gm/day po q6h
Methicillin	Staphcillin	1; 4; 6; 10 gm vial	4–12 gm/day IV or IM q6h
Metronidazole	Flagyl, Metryl Metizol, Protostat Metric 21, Satric	250; 500 mg tabs 500 mg vial	0.75–2 gm/day po q12h 0.75–2 gm/day IV q6–12h
Mezlocillin Na	Mezlin	1; 2; 3; 4 gm vial	6–24 gm/day IV q 4–6h
Miconazole	Monistat	200 mg amp 200 mg vaginal supp	0.6–3.6 gm/day IV q8h qd × 3
Minocycline	Minocin	50; 100 mg caps & tabs 50 mg/5 ml syrup 100 mg vial	200 mg/day po q6–12h 200 mg/day IV q6–12h
Moxalactam	Moxam	1 gm vial	2–8 gm/day IV q6–8h

Nafcillin	Unipen	250 mg caps; 500 mg tabs	1–2 gm/day po q6h
	Nafcil, Nallpen, Unipen	0.5; 1; 2; 10 gm vial	2–12 gm/day IV or IM q4–6h
Nalidixic acid	NegGram	0.25; 0.5; 1 gm tabs	4 gm/day po q6h
		250 mg/5 ml susp	
Neomycin	Mycifradin	500 mg tabs	3–12 gm po/day
		125 mg/5 ml solu	
Netilmicin	Netromycin	100 mg/ml vials	4–6.5 mg/kg/day IV or IM q8h
Niclosamide	Niclocide	500 mg tabs	2 gm (single dose)
Nitrofurantoin	Macrodantin	macrocrystals:	50–100 mg po q6h
	Furadantin	25; 50; 100 mg caps	Suppressive treatment: 50–100 mg qd
	Furaton	microcrystals:	
	Furalan	50; 100 caps/tabs	
	Faran	25 mg/5 ml susp	
Norfloxacin	Noroxin	400 mg tabs	400 mg po bid
Novobiocin	Albamycin	250 mg caps	1–2 gm/day po q6–12h
Nystatin	Mycostatin	100,000 units/ml	5 ml swish, swallow or 5–10 ml po 3–5 × daily
	Nystex	500,000 unit tab	
	Nilstat	0.05; 0.15; 0.25; 0.5; 1; 2; 5; 10 billion units powder	
Ofloxacin	Floxin	200; 300; 400 mg tabs	200–400 mg po q12h
Oxacillin	Bactocill, Prostaphlin	250; 500 mg caps	2–4 gm/day po q12h
		250 mg/5 ml solu	
		0.25; 0.5; 1; 2; 4; 10 gm vials	2–12 gm/day IV or IM q4–6h

Appendix 26–2
(continued)

AGENT	TRADE NAMES	DOSAGE FORM	USUAL ADULT REGIMEN: DAILY DOSE, ROUTE & DOSE INTERVAL
Oxamniquine	Vansil	250 mg caps	12–15 mg/kg × 1 15 mg/kg q12h × 4
Paromomycin	Humatin	250 mg caps	2–4 gm/day po q6–12h
Penicillin G and V		(1 unit = 0.6 mcg)	
Crystalline G potassium	Pentids	0.2; 0.25; 0.4; 0.8 million unit tabs 0.4 million units/5 ml	1–2 gm po/day q6h
	Penicillin G for injection	1; 2; 3; 5; 10; 20 million unit vials	2–20 million units/day IV q4–6h
	Pfizerpen		
Crystalline G sodium	Penicillin G sodium for injection	5 million unit vial	2–20 million units IV/day q4–6h
Benzathine	Bicillin	200,000 unit tabs	Not recommended po
	Bicillin L-A	3 million unit vial;	1.2–2.4 mil units IM
	Permapen	600,000 units/ml vial (1, 2, 4, 10 ml vials)	
Benzathine + procaine	Bicillin C-R	Benzathine: procaine/ml 150,000:150,000 units (10 ml) 300,000:150,000 (1, 2, 4 ml) 450,000:150,000 units (2 ml)	1.2–2.4 mil units IM

Procaine	Crysticillin	300,000 units (10 ml)	0.6–4.8 mil units/day IM q6–12h
	Pfizerpen	500,000 units (12 ml)	
	Wycillin	600,000 units (1, 2, 4 ml syringe)	
Phenoxyethyl penicillin (V)	Beepen VK, Betapen VK, Pen-Vee K, V-C llin K, Veetids, Ledercillin VK, Rcbicillin VK	125; 250; 500 mg tabs	1–2 gm/day po q6h
		125; 250 ml/5 ml susp	
Pentamidine	Pentam 300	300 mg vial	4 mg/kg/day IV qd
	NebuPent	300 mg aerosol	300 mg/day/mo (prophylaxis)
Piperacillin	Pipracil	2; 3; 4; 40 gm vials	6–24 gm/day IV q4–6h
Piperazine		250 mg tabs	3.5–5 gm/day
		500 mg/5 ml	
Polymyxin B	Aerosporin	500,000 unit vials	1.5–2.5 mg/kg/day IM or IV q4–6h
		1 mg = 1,000 units	
		200,000 units + 40 mg neomycin	
Praziquantel	Biltricide	600 mg tabs	20–75 mg/kg/day po in 3 doses
Primaquine		15 mg (base) tabs	15 mg po qd
Pyrantel	Antiminth	50 mg/ml susp	11 mg/kg × 1
Pyrazinamide		500 mg tabs	15–30 mg/kg/day po in 6–8 doses
Pyrimethamine	Daraprim	25 mg tabs	25 mg po q wk or daily up to 200 mg/day
Pyrimethamine + sulfadoxine	Fansidar	Sulfa-500 mg plus pyrimeth-25 mg	1 tab/wk
			3 tabs (1 dose)
Quinacrine	Atabrine	100 mg	300–800 mg po/day
Quinine	Legatrin	130; 200; 300; 325 mg caps	325 mg bid
	Quine 200, 300		650 mg q8h po
	Quin-260 etc	260; 325 mg tabs	
Quinine dihydrochloride		IV available from CDC	600 mg IV q8h

Appendix 26–2
(continued)

AGENT	TRADE NAMES	DOSAGE FORM	USUAL ADULT REGIMEN: DAILY DOSE, ROUTE & DOSE INTERVAL
Rifabutin	Mycobutin	150 mg caps	600 mg/day po
Rifampin	Rifadin	150; 300 mg caps	600 mg/day po (TB)
	Rifamate	300 mg cap with 150 mg INH	600–1200 mg/day po (other indications)
		600 mg vials	600 mg/day IV
Spectinomycin	Trobicin	2; 4 gm vials	2 gm IM × 1
Streptomycin		1 & 5 gm vial	1–2 gm IM/day
Sulfonamides			
Trisulfapyrimidines	Triple sulfa Neotrizine Terfonyl	Sulfadiazine, Sulfamerazine & Sulfamethazine, 167 mg (each) tabs and 167 mg (each) 5 ml susp	2–4 gm/day po q4–8h
Sulfadiazine	Microsulfon	0.5 gm tabs	2–4 gm/day po q4–8h
Sulfamethoxazole	Gantanol	0.5; 1 gm tabs	2–4 gm/day po q8–12h
Sulfapyridine		0.5 gm tabs	1–4 gm/day po q6h
Sulfasalazine	Azulfidine	0.5 gm tabs 0.25 mg/5 ml susp	3–4 gm/day po q6h
Sulfisoxazole	Gantrisin	0.5 gm tabs	4–8 gm/day po q4–6h

Teicoplanin	Targocid	400 mg vials	6–12 mg/kg/day IV q24h
Tetracyclines			
Demeclocycline	Declomycin	150 mg cap 150; 300 mg tab	600 mg/day po q6–12h
Doxycycline	Vibramycin	50; 100 mg tabs 50; 100 mg caps 50 mg/5 ml susp 100 mg vials	100–200 mg/day po q12–24h 200 mg/day IV q12–24h
Minocycline	Minocin	50; 100 mg caps 50; 100 mg tabs 100 mg vials	200 mg/day po or IV q12h
Oxytetracycline	Terramycin Uri-Tet	250 mg cap 50; 125 mg/ml with lidocaine (IM)	1–2 gm/day po q6h 0.5–1 gm/day IM q12h
Tetracycline	Achromycin; Tetralan Brodspec; Panmycin Robitet; Sumycin, etc.	100; 250; 500 mg caps 250; 500 mg tabs 125 mg/5 ml susp	1–2 gm/day po q6h
Thiabendazole	Mintezol	500 mg tabs 500 mg/5 ml susp	1–3 gm po/day
Ticarcillin	Ticar	1; 3; 6; 20; 30 gm vials	4–24 gm/day IV q4–6h
Ticarcillin + clavulanic acid	Timentin	3 gm ticarcillin + 100 mg CA vials	4–24 gm/day (ticarcillin) IV q4–6h
Tobramycin	Nebcin	20; 60; 80 & 1200 mg vials	3–5 mg/kg/day IV or IM q8h
Trimethoprim	Proloprim; Trimpex	100; 200 mg tabs	200 mg/day po q12–24h

Appendix 26–2
(continued)

AGENT	TRADE NAMES	DOSAGE FORM	USUAL ADULT REGIMEN: DAILY DOSE, ROUTE & DOSE INTERVAL
Trimethoprim-sulfamethoxazole	Bactrim, Septra Cotrim	Trimethoprim:sulfa 40 mg:200 mg/5 ml susp 80 mg:400 mg tabs 160 mg:800 mg DS tabs 16 mg:80 mg/ml (IV) (5, 10, 20 ml vials)	2–20 mg/kg/day (trimethoprim) po or IV q6–8h
Vancomycin	Vancocin pulvules Vancocin HCl (oral solu)	125; 250 mg caps	0.5–2 gm/day po q6h
	Vancocin HCl IV	1; 10 gm vials	
	Lyphocin	0.5; 1 gm vials (IV)	1–2 gm/day IV q6–12h
Vidarabine	Vira-A, Ara-A	200 mg/ml	15 mg/kg/day IV
Zidovudine	Retrovir, AZT	100 mg caps; 50 mg/5 ml syrup 240 ml	500–600 mg/day po q4–8h
		Infusion—10 mg/ml (20 ml)	1–2 mg/kg IV q4h

Neurologic Disorders

27

Richard Lechtenberg

COMA

Altered consciousness or loss of consciousness is one of the most worrisome of neurologic problems. Therapy is dictated by the etiology, and rapidity of diagnosis is essential for a good prognosis. In many cases, the pattern of progression or resolution of the problem is highly informative.

To help monitor the severity of altered consciousness, several rating scales have been developed. The one most widely used is the **Glasgow Coma Scale** (Table 27–1). On this scale a low score (0–7) correlates with profoundly impaired consciousness or severe psychiatric disturbance. The unimpaired individual scores 15

- If a history can be obtained, items of special interest include a history of substance abuse; prescription drug use; chronic diseases, such as diabetes mellitus and epilepsy; and head trauma
- The examination must include a rigorous search for evidence of head trauma, substance abuse, and metabolic problems. The possibility of a psychiatric disturbance, such as catatonia, must be kept in mind, but no case of altered consciousness should be dismissed as a purely psychiatric problem even if the patient has a history of schizophrenia or severe depressive reactions. Pay special attention to eye signs (Table 27–2)

Blood from the ears must be considered probable evidence of a basilar skull fracture until proven otherwise. Fluid from the nose should be checked for glucose to determine whether or not it is CSF leaking through a meningeal tear.

Unless there is reason not to expect alcohol abuse, the patient should be given thiamine 100 mg IV prior to dextrose (see Wernicke's encephalopathy below). Hypoglycemia should be assessed as part of the examination with a bedside test

- In addition to routine blood chemistries, ABGs, and hematologic studies, in case of unexplained coma, the patient's urine should be screened for amphetamines, barbiturates, cocaine, opiates, opioids, and any substances that are abuse problems in the region. A blood alcohol level may be informative if the patient's breath smells of ethanol. An ECG should be obtained routinely to look for arrhythmias. The stomach contents should be pumped out and examined
- With coma or even transient loss of consciousness associated with head trauma, a CT or MRI scan should be obtained. This is cost effective because substantial head trauma or intracranial abnormalities are less likely to be missed. Benign intracranial findings will support the decision to allow the patient to leave the hospital. Traditionally, x rays and observation are used to screen patients with head trauma or other causes of transient loss of consciousness. During observation, other tests may be obtained, but the presumption is that significant

Table 27–1
Glasglow Coma Scale

TESTING	RESPONSE	SCORE
Verbal response	Oriented	5
	Disoriented, but in context	4
	Inappropriate words	3
	Incomprehensible sounds	2
	Mute	1
Motor response	Obeys verbal instruction	6
	Localizes to stimulus	5
	Withdraws from noxious stimulus	4
	Postures with arm flexion	3
	Postures with arm extension	2
	No response to noxious stimulus	1
Eye opening	Spontaneous	4
	With verbal inducement	3
	With pain	2
	No voluntary eye opening	1

With permission from Lechtenberg R. Synopsis of Neurology. Philadelphia, Lea and Febiger, 1991.

intracranial problems, such as subdural hematomas, cerebral contusions, and meningeal tears, will be obvious after 24–48 h of observations. With MRI and CT techniques, the likelihood of significant intracranial lesions can be much more directly assessed. The patient who has a brief (<15 min) loss of consciousness after head trauma but a normal CT or MRI scan may more confidently be sent home to be watched by a friend or relative than the individual assessed with little more than a skull x ray and careful physical examination. Because a basilar skull fracture may be inapparent on a CT scan, many physicians recommend getting a skull x ray with basilar views to further assess the victim of head trauma if the CT is negative

Table 27–2
Eye Signs in Comatose Patients

CLINICAL FINDING	POSSIBLE CAUSES
1. Pupils midposition (4–6 mm) and fixed	Midbrain damage
2. Pupils dilated and fixed unilaterally	Third nerve damage Uncal herniation
3. Pupils dilated and fixed bilaterally	Protracted anoxia Methyl alcohol Scopolamine
4. Pupils small and reactive	Metabolic encephalopathy Opiates or opioids Pontine damage Diencephalic damage
5. Dysconjugate gaze	Cranial nerve damage Brainstem damage
6. Absence of all eye movements	Pontine damage Metabolic encephalopathy Drug overdose

- Further studies and therapy should be performed as dictated by the probable cause of the coma. However, the physician must maintain adequate ventilation, circulation, and body temperature, regardless of the cause.

EPILEPSY

Seizures are episodes of disorganized electrical activity in the brain. This disorganized electrical activity may produce loss of consciousness, alteration of consciousness, focal sensory disturbances, focal motor activity, inappropriate affective displays, or other neurologic or psychologic phenomena. These signs of disorganized electrical activity may occur individually or in combination.

Diagnosis. Seizures are considered generalized or partial according to whether or not the electrical disturbance in the cortex appears to arise diffusely or focally. Generalized seizures described as tonic-clonic involve loss of consciousness and transient tonic muscle contractions followed by transient clonic muscle contractions. With some generalized seizures, such as generalized absence seizures, the loss of consciousness may be so brief and so isolated that it goes unrecognized. Some types of partial seizures need not involve loss of consciousness, but those described as complex partial seizures invariably involve alteration or loss of consciousness.

Pathophysiology. Seizures are assumed to arise because of disorganized electrical activity in the cerebral cortex. The many forms that seizures assume suggests that >1 defect underlies this problem. This idea is supported by the vast differences in treatability exhibited by different types of seizures.

Therapy. Recurrent seizures often prompt visits to emergency rooms but are not usually true emergencies. The patient who has a seizure because of poor compliance with medication instructions often needs little more than a change in drug regimen to ensure better compliance (Table 27–3). Drug levels should be checked at the time of the seizure recurrence, and a routine reevaluation of the patient's overall health status is appropriate, but IV or IM administration of antiepileptic medications is usually unnecessary and inappropriate.

Table 27–3
Antiepileptic Dosage for Adults

DRUG NAME	BRAND NAME	USUAL DOSE (mg/kg/day)	THERAPEUTIC LEVEL (μg/ml)	DAYS TO STEADY STATE	SERUM HALF-LIFE (hrs)
Carbamazepine	Tegretol	10–25	6–12	3–6	8–19
Valporate	Depakote	10–70	50–100	2–4	7–17
Valproic acid	Depakene	10–70	50–100	2–4	7–17
Phenytoin	Dilantin	4–10	10–20	5–10	22–40
Ethosuximide	Zarontin	20–40	40–100	6–12	50–60
Primidone	Mysoline	10–25	6–12	1–5	8–16
Phenobarbital	—	1–5	15–35	16–21	50–96
Clonazepam	Klonopin	.03–.10	.013–.072	6	16–60

With permission from Lechtenberg R. Synopsis of Neurology. Philadelphia, Lea and Febiger, 1991.

Drug-Related Seizures

Seizures may develop because of withdrawal from or intoxication with drugs, the most common of which is ethanol.

Diagnosis. Many patients exhibit signs of drug use when they present with drug-related seizures, but toxicologic screens may be needed to establish which drug was taken closest to the time of seizure. Signs of alcohol use do not ↓ the probability of concurrent cocaine or opiate use. If a consistent history of ethanol or cocaine use can be established, the seizure should be assumed to be related to use of the substance most implicated and treated accordingly. Other causes or consequences of seizures, such as subarachnoid hemorrhage, meningitis, or post-traumatic epilepsy, should not be dismissed simply because circumstantial evidence points convincingly at substance abuse.

Pathophysiology. Seizures are presumed to occur with neuroexcitatory agents, such as amphetamines and cocaine, because of a direct effect of the substances on neurotransmitters in the brain. Inhibitory circuits responsible for coordinating neural activity may be disturbed by the stimulant drugs. A similar mechanism is also presumed for seizures that develop because of withdrawal from depressant drugs.

With barbiturate or benzodiazepine withdrawal, excess membrane channels created by neurons to deal with the burden of drug-related ion channel blockade may seriously impair maintenance of ion balances across the cell membranes. With ethanol abuse, changes in membrane channel populations are established, and seizures with ethanol withdrawal are assumed to develop because ion dysequilibriums develop as channels blocked by ethanol become active.

Therapy (for adults only)

- Ethanol withdrawal. Administer 100 mg thiamin IV prior to dextrose infusion and for ≥2 days thereafter. Detoxify with chlordiazepoxide 25–100 mg po 4–6 times daily
- Barbiturate withdrawal. Administer phenobarbital 200 mg IV acutely. Give phenobarbital 100 mg IV or po once daily for 2 days after the seizure. Taper by 35 mg qd over the subsequent 3 days
- Cocaine, amphetamines, and methaqualone. Stabilize autonomic functions. Monitor cardiac function closely and intervene if arrhythmias develop. Hold antiepileptic medication unless >1 seizure occurs. Phenobarbital 100 mg IV for 2 days if recurrent seizures develop. Taper phenobarbital with IV or po doses over the course of 3 days

Febrile Seizures

A seizure associated with high fever may be a sign of meningitis or encephalitis in adults but is more likely benign when it occurs in children. These childhood febrile seizures are considered simple if they are not likely to manifest debilitating CNS disease or epilepsy.

Diagnosis. For the child <5 years old, simple febrile seizures are

- Generalized, tonic-clonic movements may be observed in all limbs, and focal weakness is not evident during the postictal period
- Seen between 1 and 5 years of age. Seizures with fever before 6 months of age must be assumed to be a consequence of meningitis or encephalitis

- No more than 15 min long. The postictal period may extend for several mins or hrs after the obvious seizure ictus, but the ictus itself should persist for <15 mins
- Associated with a normal neurologic examination
- Unassociated with a family history of epilepsy

Complex febrile seizures are

- Complex partial or simple (usually focal motor) seizures
- Apparent before 1 year of age. Seizures in feverish children who are >5 years old must be viewed with as much suspicion as fever-associated seizures in adults
- Longer than 15 min in duration
- Associated with a persistent neurologic deficit
- Associated with a family history of epilepsy

Complex febrile seizures must be investigated aggressively with metabolic, electroencephalographic, bacteriologic, and neuroimaging studies. Simple febrile seizures are usually not investigated beyond metabolic and electroencephalographic studies.

Pathophysiology. The cause of simple febrile seizures is unknown. The susceptibility of the young child's brain to pyrexia is presumed to be related to its immaturity.

Therapy

- Simple febrile seizures: Antipyretics, such as acetaminophen orally or by suppository, alcohol rubs, cooling baths
- Complex febrile seizures: Antiepileptic medication (phenobarbital, valproate sodium) (Table 27–4); treat cause if established

Status Epilepticus

Diagnosis. Status epilepticus is seizure activity that is unremitting. The patient does not recover from the postictal state before the next seizure occurs. The most common, obvious, and lethal form of status epilepticus is tonic-clonic status. The most common settings for status epilepticus are after withdrawal of antiepileptic medications (patient compliance problems), with substance abuse (alcohol or barbiturate use

Table 27–4
Antiepileptic Dosage for Children

DRUG NAME	BRAND NAME	USUAL DOSE (mg/kg/day)	SERUM HALF-LIFE (hrs)
Phenobarbital	—	3–5	30–50
Phenytoin	Dilantin	4–7	3–11
Primidone	Mysoline	10–25	6–8
Carbamazepine	Tegretol	20–30	6–16
Valproate	Depakote	15–60	4–14
Clonazepam	Klonopin	0.01–0.20	16–60
Ethosuximide	Zarontin	20–40	24–30

With permission from Lechtenberg R. Synopsis of Neurology. Philadelphia, Lea and Febiger, 1991.

especially), and with new onset seizure activity (previously undiagnosed epilepsy). Individuals with no prior history of seizures who develop status epilepticus should be investigated for intracranial lesions, such as neoplasms and A-V malformations; metabolic disturbances, such as hyperglycemia and hyponatremia; acute infections, such as meningitis and encephalitis; and substance abuse.

Pathophysiology. The physiologic basis for status epilepticus is unknown. Presumably, inhibitory controls over some neural circuits are completely disabled, and disorganized neuronal activity continues unabated after the initial episode occurs.

Therapy. Status epilepticus is a potentially lethal condition, so the management of this problem must be aggressive and comprehensive (Table 27–5). Autonomic problems associated with status epilepticus include hyperthermia, BP instability, and impaired respiratory control

- Breathing disturbances are usually quite obvious, but not usually life threatening. Many clinicians intubate patients as soon as status epilepticus is diagnosed, but most patients do not require ventilatory support. Intubation may provide some protection against aspiration, but the principal advantage of the maneuver is to simplify mechanical ventilation if respiratory depression develops during drug treatment
- Hyperthermia should be managed with a cooling blanket and antipyretics
- Hypotension may develop with the seizure activity, but it is more commonly seen as a consequence of antiepileptic therapy. In any case, BP must be monitored and managed
- Renal problems may develop secondary to myoglobinuria. This is especially likely with violent seizure activity that produces considerable muscle injury. Dehydration and hypovolemia must be avoided to minimize the risk of myoglobin accumulation in the kidneys
- If hypoglycemia is probable, a 50 ml bolus of $D_{50}W$ should be given IV
- If alcohol abuse is probable, thiamine 100 mg IV prior to dextrose should be given as soon as possible and repeated po qd for 3 days

Drug therapy should be administered IV. The doses of antiepileptic medications used for status epilepticus are higher than those conventionally applicable in seizure management (Table 27–6). The physician should wait ≥10 min, but no >20 min, between successive treatments to determine whether or not seizures are persisting.

Table 27–5
Treating Patients with Status Epilepticus

Stabilize autonomic function
Check blood gases, glucose, electrolytes, magnesium, calcium
Administer thiamine 100 mg IV if alcohol abuse is probable
Administer glucose as $D_{50}W$ in a 50-ml bolus IV if hypoglycemia is probable
Start intravenous antiepileptic medications
Intubate if respiratory effort is depressed
Monitor vital signs and cardiac rhythm
MRI or CT if cause not apparent
EEG if diagnosis is in doubt

Table 26–6
Antiepileptic Medication for Status Epilepticus in Adults

Phenytoin (Dilantin) 500 mg at no more than 50 mg/min IV
Repeat phenytoin 500 mg every 30 minutes until seizures stop
  up to maximum of 20 mg/kg/day
Lorazepam 5 mg at no more than 2 mg/min IV
Repeat lorazepam 5 mg IV every 10 minutes until seizures stop
  up to maximum of 0.1 mg/kg/day
Phenobarbital 260 mg at no more than 100 mg/min IV
Repeat phenobarbital 260 mg IV every 20 minutes until seizures
  stop
  up to maximum of 20 mg/kg/day
Diazepam (Valium) 10 mg at no more than 5 mg/min IV
Repeat diazepam 10 mg IV every 10 minutes until seizures stop
  up to maximum of 0.25 mg/kg/day
Consider general anesthesia if all else fails

Phenytoin. Most clinicians use phenytoin as their first-choice drug in the management of status epilepticus. It is given IV up to a total daily dose of 20 mg/kg. Individual doses are usually about 500 mg (5–12 mg/kg) and are infused at a rate not >50 mg/min. This drug should be pushed directly into the IV line (albeit very slowly) to avoid its precipitation into holding chambers or IV bottles and to avoid accidental delivery of a bolus more rapidly than is appropriate. (Dilute in 0.9% NaCl; avoid mixing with dextrose to prevent precipitation; flush the vein immediately with saline to avoid thrombosis.) After the first dose of phenytoin (500 mg), lorazepam or diazepam may be given. If seizures have not stopped after 2 or 3 boluses of benzodiazepine, the second dose (500 mg) of phenytoin may be administered. Contraindications: complete heart block, CHF. Do not administer concomitantly with dopamine or lidocaine.

Lorazepam and diazepam are favored as second-choice drugs because of their rapid onset of action. They are cleared from the body much more quickly than phenytoin, and so phenytoin should be given first to provide continuing antiepileptic drug levels. Diazepam is given IV (never IM) at a max daily dose of 0.25 mg/kg at an infusion rate of no >5 mg/min. Lorazepam is given IV at a max daily dose of 0.10 mg/kg at an infusion rate of not >2 mg/min. Diazepam is usually given in individual boluses of 10 mg with doses repeated q 10–20 min until seizure activity stops, autonomic problems (i.e., hypotension) develop, or a max dose (usually not more than a total of 40 mg in 1 day) has been administered. Lorazepam is usually administered in boluses of 5–7 mg.

Phenobarbital. If phenytoin and a short-acting benzodiazepine have not stopped seizure activity, phenobarbital may be tried. This barbiturate is usually given in 260- to 300-mg boluses administered at a rate of 100 mg/min. The max tolerated dose is usually <1200 mg or a total daily dose of <20 mg/kg. Successive doses of phenobarbital should be ≥20 min apart. Hypotension or respiratory depression are likely if >1000 mg of phenobarbital is delivered over the course of 1 h.

If all these measures fail, the patient may need general anesthesia. Most anesthetic agents have little or no antiepileptic activity, but the anesthetic agent will at least alter brain activity and simplify immobilization of the patient.

WERNICKE'S ENCEPHALOPATHY

Diagnosis. Features of Wernicke's encephalopathy include

- Abnormal eye movements, such as ophthalmoplegia, ophthalmoparesis, or nystagmus
- Altered mentation, such as obtundation, disorientation, apathy, or confabulation
- Gait disorders, such as ataxia or disturbed tandem gait

More worrisome, but less constant features include dysautonomia with hypothermia and hypotension. Individuals with autonomic abnormalities are at more immediate risk of dying.

The severity of the syndrome is quite variable, and individuals with relatively mild cases may appear to recover substantially with little or no treatment. The individual at risk is usually one with a nutritional disturbance, either as a result of dietary habits or concurrent illness.

Pathophysiology. The underlying disorder is thiamine deficiency. Symptomatic individuals are most often alcoholic. An acute deterioration often occurs when the individual at risk is given IV glucose or dextrose. CNS lesions evident in patients dying from Wernicke's encephalopathy include hemorrhagic necrosis in periventricular thalamic and hypothalamic gray matter (especially in the mamillary bodies), periaqueductal gray matter, and brain stem and cerebellar midline structures. Acute changes are evident in these structures on MRI scanning, but are not usually apparent on CT scanning until hemorrhage into necrotic tissue is substantial.

Therapy. Any reason to suspect this potentially lethal condition justifies parenteral thiamine administration. Thiamine 100 mg IV should be given as soon as the condition is suspected. It is preferable to give the thiamin prior to the patient's receiving dextrose because a glucose challenge will often precipitate an acute attack of Wernicke's encephalopathy. Supplements of 50–100 mg of thiamine should be given po or IV for 3 days.

Ocular and gait changes are sensitive to even low doses of thiamine. Improvement of an ophthalmoplegia to slight nystagmus and of severe ataxia to a disturbance of tandem gait should not be taken as an indication of adequate treatment. If treatment is delayed or inadequate, cognitive changes may be permanently disabling, with amnestic syndromes the most apparent.

NEUROLEPTIC MALIGNANT SYNDROME

Diagnosis. Core features of NMS include

- Encephalopathy (disorientation, agitation, catatonia, altered consciousness)
- Hyperthermia (fever)
- Dysautonomia (labile BP, tachycardia, diaphoresis, cutaneous vasoconstriction)
- Muscular rigidity (lead-pipe rigidity, bradykinesia)

Occasional features include tremor, dyskinetic movements, sustained postures (waxy rigidity), gaze abnormalities, dysphagia, elevated CPK myoglobinuria, and acute renal failure

- The evolution of signs and symptoms may be limited to hours or develop over days. Most cases occur within the first 2 weeks after the start of neuroleptics
- NMS may develop with first exposure to neuroleptics at relatively low doses. Alternatively, it may evolve when the neuroleptic dose is ↑ or the type of neuroleptic changed
- Men are more commonly affected than women. The incidence for patients on neuroleptics is <1%. Patients with psychotic disorders are more at risk for the syndrome. Lethal catatonia is often indistinguishable from NMS. Malignant hyperthermia may also seem similar to NMS, but it invariably develops after exposure to an anesthetic agent and is not associated with the early appearance of encephalopathy and dysautonomia
- Syndromes difficult to distinguish from NMS may develop with exposure to amphetamines; tricyclic antidepressants in combination with monoamine oxidase inhibitors, tryptophan, or lithium; cocaine; reserpine; or tetrabenazine, and with withdrawal from antiparkinsonian medications

Pathophysiology. Neuroleptic agents probably act primarily on the D_2 dopamine receptor because they produce postsynaptic blockade and interfere with the dopaminergic system

- Responsible neuroleptic agents include phenothiazines (especially fluphenazine), butyrophenones (especially haloperidol), and substituted benzamides (such as metoclopramide and droperidol)
- NMS is an idiosyncratic reaction: It is not dose related

Therapy. Without treatment, mortality >20%. Death usually results from cardiopulmonary failure, aspiration pneumonia, or renal failure. Complications of NMS include disseminated intravascular coagulation, renal tubular acidosis, inappropriate antidiuretic hormone, hyperglycemia, and pancreatic necrosis. Most important in treatment is the withdrawal of the neuroleptic agent. The patient must be observed in a CCU to manage the dysautonomia. Cooling blankets, rehydration, antipyretics, and other supportive measures should be instituted as problems appear. Pharmacotherapy of NMS includes using dantrolene or dopaminergic drugs (bromocriptine, L-DOPA, lisuride, pergolide, amantadine). The dose of drug necessary to ↓ the NMS symptoms is usually arrived at empirically. The useful range of bromocriptine doses is from <10 mg qd to >100 mg qd. One dopaminergic agent may be effective when others are not. If dantrolene is used it may be given as 0.25 mg/kg IV bid.

MIGRAINE

Diagnosis

- Pain over 1 side of the head usually develops after premonitory signs. These signs may be transient visual obscurations or more dramatic focal neurologic deficits (hemiplegia, ophthalmoplegia)
- Women are more likely to be affected than men, and there often is a

family history of similar attacks. Attacks usually begin during adolescence and abate in the sixth or seventh decade of life

- The most common premonitory sign is an evolving scotoma, often surrounded by a scintillating border. The scotoma may enlarge over the course of 10–60 min. The pulsatile pain characteristic of the migraine usually develops as the premonitory signs resolve. Nausea and vomiting in association with the attacks is common
- Symptoms during migraine attacks include photophobia, phonophobia, and irritability as well as headache
- Other types of hemicranial pain include the cluster headache. This typically occurs in men, develops late at night, awakens the sufferer from sleep, and is associated with personality changes during the attack. The episodes usually start with pain behind one eye that extends to much of the rest of the hemicranium

Pathophysiology

- Migraines are called vascular headaches and are assumed to arise with disturbances in the autoregulation of intracranial (and to a lesser extent extracranial) vasculature. A variety of neurotransmitters have been implicated as participants in the evolution of the headaches, but none has been convincingly established as the cause
- Inflammation around sensory nerves and dilation of large intracranial blood vessels may produce much of the pain that is experienced

Therapy

- Ergotamine in various forms is the traditional therapy for acute attacks of migraine. It is available in oral, sublingual, intranasal, IM, and rectal preparations. It is often used in fixed combination with caffeine (Cafergot). Dihydroergotamine (DHE 45) is used for IM injection. The tolerable dose of ergotamine varies with the type of preparation, route of administration, and individual sensitivity. It is usually taken in multiple small doses, starting at the first indication of a migraine attack. The dose is titrated up to a max daily and max weekly allowance. For example, oral ergotamine tartrate 1 mg tablets should be taken no >4 times qd and no >2 days consecutively in any week. Individual doses of 1 or 2 mg may be repeated at 1- or 2-hour intervals during a migraine attack
- More conventional analgesics, such as acetaminophen, naproxen, propoxyphene, and aspirin, and NSAIDs are sometimes useful for mild attacks. Several popular preparations include a barbiturate (butalbital) along with analgesic or anti-inflammatory medications
- For many individuals, prophylaxis is simpler and more effective than treatment of an acute attack. Beta adrenergic blocking agents, such as propranolol (Inderal), have been especially useful, but they are contraindicated in individuals with COPD. Low doses (propranolol 40–120 mg qd) are usually effective in susceptible individuals. The ergot alkaloid methysergide (Sansert) is useful in prophylaxis, but has been associated with some reports of retroperitoneal fibrosis. Some physicians use NSAIDs, amitriptyline (Elavil), or Ca channel blocking agents, such as verapamil (Calan), for prophylaxis, but the effectiveness of these agents is quite variable from individual to individual
- Sumatriptan is a serotonin-receptor agonist, the drug seems to abort migraine episodes by acting selectively at 5-SHT_1 (A and D subtypes) receptors in the carotid circulation. The presumption is that sumatriptan inhibits the development of perivascular inflammation that evolves with inappropriate stimulation of pain fibers.

<u>Dosage</u> SQ (6–12 mg). Repeat in 1 hr. if needed; orally: 100 mg tablet, max 300 mg/d. It appears effective in many individuals with either migraine or cluster headaches. Contraindications: Angina or CHD

DIZZINESS/VERTIGO

Diagnosis

- Acute or chronic positional instability develops with damage to or irritation of the inner ear, the VIIIth cranial nerve, the brain stem, or the brain. Feelings of instability are usually considered dizziness. The perception of environmental movement in association with the feeling of instability is usually considered vertigo. Nausea and vomiting routinely occur with severe vertigo
- If the vertigo that develops is short-lived and evident only when the head assumes certain positions, it is often classified as benign paroxysmal positional vertigo. With this type of vertigo, nystagmus can be consistently elicited when the head is positioned appropriately
- Ménière syndrome is the association of recurrent episodes of vertigo with episodes of tinnitus and progressive hearing loss
- Persistent vertigo should be investigated with CT and MRI studies of the posterior fossa. If structural lesions are not evident, the vertigo is probably attributable to labyrinthine damage or dysfunction. In patients at risk for ischemia, digital subtraction angiography or MRI angiography of the vertebrobasilar circulation may point to a vascular basis for the complaint

Pathophysiology

- Most cases of dizziness or vertigo remain unexplained after routine evaluations. If the symptom remains independent of other more localizing signs and symptoms, the patient should be periodically reassessed to be sure that a slowly evolving but treatable lesion, such as an acoustic schwannoma, is not responsible for the symptom
- In any case of labyrinthine dysfunction, exposure to ototoxic drugs or other substances must be considered
- An acute inflammatory lesion of the labyrinth (acute labyrinthitis) may produce a vertigo that is substantially exacerbated by abrupt changes in head position
- Ménière's is often ascribed to an endolymphatic hydrops, but the underlying problem may be a disturbance of ion balance in the endolymph
- Brainstem and cerebellar lesions routinely produce vertigo or dysequilibrium. With structural damage to these structures, instability may persist for years. Transient episodes may occur with ischemia

Therapy

- Because the cause of dizziness or vertigo is often unknown, much of the treatment must be symptomatic. Antiemetic agents are helpful with vertigo severe enough to elicit vomiting. These medications include droperidol (Inapsine) 2.5–5.0 mg IM, prochlorperazine (Compazine) 10 mg IM, and promethazine (Phenergan) 25 mg po or pr. Problems associated with these antiemetic agents include sedation, dystonia, and extrapyramidal reactions. Consequently, they should be used at the lowest feasible doses. Sublingual and rectal preparations are available for some of them
- Drugs believed to act more directly on the labyrinth to suppress vertigo include diazepam (Valium) 5–10 mg po, IM, or IV; meclizine

(Antivert) 25 mg po, and dimenhydrinate (Dramamine) 50 mg po. Scopolamine is also believed to suppress vertigo and is available as a patch (Transdermscop)

- Ménière's syndrome may respond to diuretic (HCTZ) treatment, but many physicians will attempt an endolymphic shunt to ↓ symptoms in long-suffering patients
- Destruction of part of the vestibular nerve is sometimes attempted with intractable vertigo, but the risk of damaging the cochlear division of the auditory nerve is high, and the likelihood of permanently eliminating the vertigo is low. The vertigo may have started at the end organ and evolved as central (brain stem) mechanisms became disabled by the persistence of misleading sensory input

TRANSIENT ISCHEMIC ATTACKS

Diagnosis. A TIA is an episode of focal neurologic deficit that lasts <24 h and is caused by vascular insufficiency. Identifying a TIA early is important because individuals suffering them are at high risk of developing stroke. The intracranial problem may be secondary to acute MI, valvular heart disease, or arrhythmia

Diagnostic measures appropriate on an emergency basis include

- Neuroimaging studies to establish that infarction has not occurred. A good MRI scan may detect ischemic damage as small as 5 mm across. This should be done as an emergency procedure the first time the patient presents with what appears to be a TIA, because cerebral, cerebellar, or brain stem infarction will require a different approach from that appropriate for a TIA
- Screening blood and urine tests to establish that the focal deficits are not a result of a metabolic or hematologic disorder. Elderly individuals with severe anemia may develop focal neurologic deficits. Hyperglycemia, hyponatremia, and hypercalcemia may all produce neurologic changes easily confused with a TIA. Coagulopathies, vasculitides (systemic lupus), and hemoglobinopathies (sickle cell disease) must also be investigated
- ECG to exclude MI or a cardiac arrhythmia; echocardiography and Holter monitoring are selectively requested

Pathophysiology. The prevailing assumption is that TIA produces no structural damage; but improvements in neuroimaging have weakened this assumption. What can be said of structural CNS damage is that it is relatively occult and may only be evident in a redundant system if the brain or spinal cord deteriorate.

Therapy. Attempts to arrive at a consensus on the management of TIAs have only emphasized the diversity of opinions in this area. Many physicians believe that TIAs suggestive of the carotid system should be managed with carotid endarterectomy. Most advocate some type of anticoagulation in the management. Typical approaches include

- Reducing postural stress by keeping the patient recumbent. With focal ischemia, local autoregulation of blood flow is disturbed, and postural changes may stress the ischemic tissue to the point that infarction occurs
- Limiting serum glucose levels. Many investigators believe that abnormally high glucose levels may worsen the stress imposed upon neurons by ischemia. This means that glucose infusions are ill advised

- Hospitalizing the patient and monitoring the course of the TIA. In many cases the patient presents after the episode has completely resolved, but observation is still warranted. How long the patient should be watched is controversial. After the first episode of TIA, recommendations range from days to >1 week. If the patient has had several prior episodes of TIA, protracted observation is less warranted (and less likely to be acceptable to the patient), especially if the TIA is much the same each time it occurs. A change in the pattern of the TIA or a shortening of the interval between TIAs is more worrisome and should prompt closer observation of the patient
- IV heparin for 3 days to 2 weeks if there is no evidence of hemorrhage associated with the neurologic problem and if the patient has no apparent coagulation problem. If valvular heart disease or an arrhythmia appear to be at least partially responsible for thromboembolic lesions precipitating the TIAs, anticoagulation may be continued for a longer interval
- After a few days with heparin, most physicians will gradually switch to aspirin or warfarin to simplify drug administration and monitoring. A prothrombin time of 1.5 times the control value (INR 2–3) is usually taken as an indication of adequate anticoagulation with warfarin (see Chap. 11). Anticoagulation with warfarin is usually continued for ≤3 months. If AF is present, anticoagulation is continued indefinitely. Throughout the period of anticoagulation, extreme vigilance must be maintained to detect the first sign of bleeding. Interactions between warfarin and concomitant medications must be considered (see Chap. 11)
- Carotid endarterectomy has been in and out of favor for several decades, but it is currently favored in cases of TIA or even nondisabling stroke in which a high-grade carotid stenosis is found on the same side as the neurologic deficits
- Whether or not endarterectomy is being contemplated, the patient with TIAs should have an evaluation of the aortic arch and the vasculature supplying the head. Improvements in transcranial Doppler studies and MRI angiography have made this an increasingly atraumatic investigation. Problems with resolution of the blood vessels may ultimately require angiography, but vascular anomalies and large lesions should indicate considerably less invasive studies
- Patients at risk for stroke and not on warfarin or heparin are usually given aspirin daily, in doses ranging from 80 qd to 325 mg tid. The addition of dipyridamole appears to have no clinical value in individuals with occlusive vascular disease. Ticlopidine 250 mg bid is advisable for patients who cannot tolerate aspirin; rare neutropenia is a problem with ticlopidine, and fatalities have been reported
- After endarterectomy, many physicians prescribe aspirin and dipyridamole. They are ineffective in reducing the frequency or extent of restenosis. Restenosis of carotid vessels managed with endarterectomy occurs in as many as 1 out of 4 patients within 1 year of the surgery

STROKE

Diagnosis. The individual who acutely develops focal neurologic deficits, such as hemiparesis, aphasia, ataxia, dysarthria, hemisensory deficits, or cranial nerve disturbances, may have suffered a stroke: an acute vascular injury to the CNS.

Alternative explanations for the neurologic findings include

- Transient ischemia. If the deficits clear within 24 h, there may prove to be no structural damage to the CNS
- Seizure. The deficits rarely persist for >1 h, but some individuals may exhibit a Todd's paralysis that persists for >1 day
- Acute decompensation from a chronic lesion, such as a tumor
- Profound metabolic disturbances, such as hypoglycemia

Seizures may be the first sign of a stroke and may delay diagnosis. Focal deficits are difficult to assess during the ictal and postictal periods associated with seizure activity. Individuals with hemorrhagic stroke, especially if the hemorrhage extends into the subarachnoid space, may give severe headache as the first complaint.

Risk factors for stroke include hypertension, diabetes mellitus, hypercholesterolemia, cigarette smoking, AF, valvular heart disease, and LV hypertrophy. Hemorrhagic strokes must be considered likely in any individuals on anticoagulant therapy who acutely develop focal neurologic deficits.

In many cases, stroke is suggested by the combination of signs and symptoms reported or exhibited by the patient. Concurrent face and ipsilateral hand numbness or weakness suggests damage to the cerebral cortex about the central sulcus in the distribution of the middle cerebral artery. Hemiparesis, affecting the dominant hand, associated with aphasia suggests damage to the dominant frontal lobe. A hemisensory deficit that extends onto the face from the affected side of the body suggests a thalamic injury, such as that seen with hypertension and lacunar infarction.

Pathophysiology. Stroke is irreversible brain damage secondary to occlusive or hemorrhagic vascular disease. Occlusive lesions may develop with arterial thrombosis, spasm, dissection, atherosclerosis, or inflammation. Even an adjacent neoplasm may produce stroke by compressing the arterial lumen. With hemorrhage into the parenchyma of the brain or spinal cord, damage to CNS tissue may be very direct and immediate. Hemorrhage into the subarachnoid space may produce focal or nonfocal disturbances which are often complicated by ischemic damage as vascular spasm develops in association with the subarachnoid blood.

Intracranial hemorrhage is most commonly seen with chronic hypertension or with rupture of an intracranial aneurysm. The latter is more likely to produce subarachnoid accumulation of blood (subarachnoid hemorrhage) than an intraparenchymal blood clot. Rupture of a vessel damaged by chronic hypertension is more likely to produce an intraparenchymal clot than a subarachnoid hemorrhage.

Ischemic injuries to the brain are especially likely with: systemic hypoperfusion, such as that associated with cardiac arrest; intracranial vasculitis, such as that developing with SLE; emboli, arising in the heart, emissary vessels to the head, or intracranially as reflux from occluded vessels; or thrombosis, such as that commonly occurring in association with atherosclerosis

- Focal neurologic deficits developing after trauma suggest a subdural, epidural, or subarachnoid hemorrhage. Deficits noted on awakening in the morning are likely to be ischemic injuries associated with intracranial thrombosis. A pre-existing infection, such as a pneumonia or otitis media, which evolved shortly before the appearance of the neurologic deficits, may point to a meningoencephalitis or vasculitis as the cause of the stroke syndrome

Investigations. These are similar to those required for TIAs

- Patients believed to have suffered a stroke should have emergency neuroimaging studies. CT scanning is especially useful in revealing hemorrhagic lesions. MRI scanning reveals ischemic injuries early in their evolution. With evidence of intracranial hemorrhage, an angiogram should be performed to determine the site of bleeding and to assess the likelihood of subsequent hemorrhage. The patient with multiple aneurysms should have surgical intervention to ↓ the risk of recurrent bleeding. CBC, urinalysis, and ECG are routine; echocardiography is required if embolic stroke is suspected

- There are some situations in which an LP is clearly appropriate or inappropriate, but in many cases the clinician must decide whether or not to do an LP on the basis of how comfortable he or she is with the diagnosis. Ischemic stroke developing in the setting of an acute infection should be investigated with an LP so that CSF can be collected for culture. A hemorrhagic stroke with substantial distortion of the brain, especially if posterior fossa structures are involved, should make the clinician forgo an LP

Therapy

- Much of acute stroke therapy is supportive. IV hydration must be started as soon as possible so that the patient can be made NPO and intravascular volume readily adjusted. Because of concern over the deleterious effects of IV dextrose, as already discussed for TIA, many clinicians start with a saline infusion at 30 ml/h
- If a seizure occurs at the time of the stroke, antiepileptic medications are usually administered, unless there is an associated metabolic disturbance to which the seizure activity may be attributed. The antiepileptic of choice is phenytoin; the preferred route is IV. A loading dose of 10–15 mg/kg infused at a rate of no >50 mg/min is usually sufficient to control seizures during the first day after the stroke appears. If seizures recur, phenytoin 300 mg qd should be administered as a single dose (see earlier discussion)
- A respiratory arrest may occur, especially if aspiration has complicated the stroke

The high risk of aspiration makes oral intake of nutrition or drugs inadvisable. The patient should be kept NPO for at least the first day or 2 if there is any evidence of speech, swallowing, or alertness problems

- Autonomic disturbances may cause substantial damage. Falling BP associated with changes in position may exacerbate the ischemia that caused the dysautonomia. Patients with even minor strokes should be kept recumbent or nearly so until their deficits have stabilized for at least a few days. Hypertension may develop acutely with the stroke, but must be managed cautiously (see Chap. 1). An expanding intracranial hematoma may produce the Cushing effect (rising BP and slowing pulse), but aggressive lowering of the systemic BP may impair cerebral perfusion and ↑ the area of ischemic injury surrounding the area of initial infarction or hemorrhage
- Antihypertensives given to the stroke patient with hypertensive emergency should be titrated to produce a slow and only moderate ↓ in BP: not >20% ↓ in the baseline systolic and never to <140 mm Hg. Many clinicians use sodium nitroprusside (see Chap. 1). If volume status is normal, gentle diuresis will suffice
- Thrombolytic agents are not yet approved for use outside research protocols, and experience with those currently available suggests that they may be of value only in highly selected patients, under well-controlled conditions, and if treatment can be initiated within the first 2 h after deficits appear

- Surgery is not considered a viable option for acute stroke, but opinions are changing as surgical and anesthetic techniques produce less morbidity and mortality in these extremely unstable patients, and as neuroimaging techniques help to select patients most likely to profit from invasive strategies. The carotid system, rather than the vertebrobasilar system, is the most amenable to surgical intervention. The patients most likely to profit from acute surgical intervention are those with acute occlusive disease of the internal carotid artery who do not have profound neurologic deficits—such as impaired consciousness, aphasia, or hemiplegia—or intracerebral hemorrhage, and who do evidence contrast medium reflux in the petrous portion of the internal carotid artery
- Successful surgical procedures on appropriate patients include internal carotid thromboendarterectomies, proximal remnant angioplasties (stumpectomies) with concurrent external carotid endarterectomies, and superficial temporal-to-middle cerebral artery bypass procedures

Managing catastrophic deterioration. Strokes occasionally produce a catastrophic deterioration, such as brain herniation, status epilepticus, massive intracranial hemorrhage after infarction, or vasospasm after intracranial hemorrhage (see previous discussion)

- Herniation may be transfalcial (across the falx cerebri), transtentorial (across the tentorium cerebelli), or transforaminal (through the foramen magnum). It should be suspected in any stroke victim, whether that stroke is ischemic or hemorrhagic, who exhibits rapid deterioration, especially if that deterioration involves clouding of consciousness and autonomic dysfunction

A variety of measures ↓ the risk of herniation. These include minimizing agitation, restricting fluids, and inducing hyperventilation

- Acutely, the patient may be given a rapid (5- to 20-min) infusion of 20% mannitol solution at a dose of 0.5 g/kg. With this infusion, the patient must be watched closely for hypervolemia
- May clinicians use megadoses (10–100 mg) of dexamethasone or other corticosteroids as a single injection at the first sign of herniation
- Centers with aggressive neurosurgical teams may opt for surgical decompression if an extensive area of necrotic tissue is evident. The surgical evacuation of intracerebral hemorrhages has generally produced poor results. Removal of intracerebellar hemorrhages and infarction has had much better outcomes

Ischemia associated with vasospasm. The patient with subarachnoid bleeding or extension of intracerebral or intracerebellar hemorrhage into the subarachnoid space is at high risk for vasospasm. Consequently, the individual with few symptoms of subarachnoid blood may acutely develop evidence of extensive cerebral ischemia. Ca channel blockers, such as nimodipine, seem to ↓ the risk of vasospasm associated with subarachnoid hemorrhage and improve the outcome in patients with signs of cerebral vasospasm. _Dosage:_ Nimodipine 60 mg po q 4 h for 3 weeks, commenced within 4 days of symptoms.

PARKINSON'S DISEASE

Diagnosis

- There are 4 characteristic features of Parkinson's disease: rigidity, tremor, bradykinesia, and dementia. If any or all of these signs occur with conditions that are not Parkinson's disease but imitate it, the situation is referred to as parkinsonism

- The tremor associated with Parkinson disease and parkinsonism is a resting tremor. It is less evident or remits completely when a movement is initiated in the affected limb
- The rigidity is usually lead pipe or cogwheel in character. Lead-pipe rigidity is a fairly constant resistance to movement while the affected limb is passively moved. With cogwheel rigidity, the examiner can feel abrupt, but very brief, changes in the degree of resistance to movement. The cogwheel character of the tremor is especially likely to be evident if the affected limb is moved passively while the patient tries to perform mental calculations
- Causes of parkinsonism include drugs (phenothiazines and butyrophenones), hereditary basal ganglia disease (Wilson's hepatolenticular degeneration, progressive supranuclear palsy), and metabolic encephalopathy (carbon monoxide poisoning, MPTP poisoning)

Pathophysiology

- Parkinson's disease develops with disease of the brain stem and diencephalon; the substantia nigra is severely damaged early in the course of the disease. Dopamine-dependent pathways in the basal ganglia are disturbed and eventually degenerate. Neuronal loss is obvious and extensive

Therapy

- Within the past few years, therapy has focused on neuroprotective drugs. Whether or not any of the currently available drugs are truly neuroprotective remains unresolved
- Most physicians feel obliged to start deprenyl (Eldepryl, selegiline) 5 mg bid early in the course of disease. This MAO B inhibitor may scavenge free radicals thought to produce much of the neuronal damage in dopaminergic cells that eventually degenerate
- Early in the course of Parkinson disease, anticholinergic drugs such as trihexyphenidyl (Artane) 2 mg bid or tid and benztropine mesylate (Cogentin) 0.5 mg bid or tid, may keep the patient virtually symptom free for months or years. As the disease progresses, these same drugs may be useful in reducing symptoms and tolerated at somewhat higher doses
- The anti-influenzal drug amantadine (Symmetrel) 100 mg bid may also ameliorate symptoms during the course of the deterioration, but is rarely effective for >6 months and is routinely used as supplemental therapy in combination with more typically dopaminergic drugs, such as L-DOPA or bromocriptine (Parlodel)
- Dopamine does not cross the blood-brain barrier, and so L-DOPA, which is converted to dopamine in the CNS, is used to ↑ the overall level of dopamine in the CNS. Dopamine produces GI disturbances when it reaches appreciable levels in the systemic circulation, and so a DOPA decarboxylase inhibitor (e.g., carbidopa) is usually combined with L-DOPA (as in Sinemet) to ↓ the total dose of L-DOPA needed to achieve therapeutic levels in the CNS. DOPA decarboxylase inhibitors like carbidopa cross the blood-brain barrier poorly. Most physicians delay the introduction of L-DOPA/carbidopa treatment until other treatments fail to control the patient's symptoms. When treatment is started, a tablet with 25 mg carbidopa and 100 mg L-DOPA (Sinemet 25/100) is given bid or tid. The dose is ↑ to maximize the benefit

unless akathisia, GI distress, hallucinations, or other serious adverse effects develop

- Alternative dopaminergic drugs include bromocriptine, lisuride, and pergolide mesylate. These drugs are usually introduced when L-DOPA preparations fail to produce substantial improvement. Bromocriptine (Parlodel) is usually started at a dose of 1.25 mg qd and gradually ↑ to as much as 7.5 mg per day. Pergolide mesylate (Permax) is given 0.05 mg each day initially and gradually ↑ to ≤1 mg tid. Hallucinations and agitation are common problems with these dopaminergic drugs and are often dose limiting
- Attempts to restore dopaminergic function in the brain have included the transplantation of adrenal or fetal tissues into the basal ganglia. The experience with this approach has been very inconsistent, but some groups have demonstrated convincing improvement in patients receiving transplants of fetal tissue

MYASTHENIA GRAVIS

Diagnosis

- Myasthenia gravis is a disease of the neuromuscular junction that produces muscle weakness. It is characterized by antibodies to and consequent degeneration of the postsynaptic elements of the junction. The muscles most often symptomatic early in the disease are the ocular motor muscles and the levator palpebrae. Women are more commonly affected than men. Changes in the thymus, ranging from hyperplasia to malignancies, often appear in association with the disease. Hyperthyroidism may occur with myasthenia or as an independent cause of muscle weakness
- The affected individual typically weakens as an activity is continued or the day passes. Strength usually peaks shortly after awakening
- An IV injection of ≤1 mg edrophonium chloride (Tensilon), a short-acting, cholinesterase inhibitor, will produce a transient improvement in strength in affected individuals. An alternative, but much more hazardous, screening test involves the injection of a minuscule (1/70th of a curarizing dose) amount of curare. The individual with myasthenia is excessively sensitive to this neuromuscular blocking agent
- The diagnosis is usually confirmed with EMG and nerve conduction studies. The affected individual will exhibit decreasing amplitudes of muscle action potentials with repeated (several times per second) stimulation of the nerve innervating the muscle. Muscles not obviously symptomatic will exhibit this decrementing pattern of action potentials, as will those which are symptomatic
- Antiacetylcholine receptor antibodies are usually detectable in the serum. CT studies of the mediastinum may reveal thymic enlargement
- Several conditions produce myasthenic syndromes, that is, disorders symptomatically similar to myasthenia gravis but arising from distinctly different causes. These include the Eaton-Lambert syndrome, in which disease of the presynaptic elements of the neuromuscular junction develops in the setting of a malignancy. The most common malignancy to produce the Eaton-Lambert syndrome is bronchogenic carcinoma

Pathophysiology

- Myasthenia is presumed to arise because of damage to the acetylcholine receptor on the postsynaptic membrane of skeletal and ocular motor muscles. Cardiac muscle is not affected, but the diaphragm is often involved. Prior to the development of successful therapies, death usually occurred because of respiratory insufficiency. The affected individual would have a respiratory arrest or develop pneumonia because of inadvertent aspiration or recurrent hypoventilation

Therapy

- Anticholinesterase inhibitors have been used successfully for several decades. By interfering with the breakdown of the neurotransmitter acetylcholine at the synapse, these drugs ↑ the exposure of the defective postsynaptic receptor to acetylcholine and potentiate the effect of acetylcholine. Pyridostigmine bromide (Mestinon) 60 mg po q 4 h during the day is a common regimen. The major disadvantage of these drugs is their cholinergic activity independent of the skeletal muscles. GI motility is ↑ and may be especially disabling. Attempts to modulate this nonmuscular effect of cholinesterase inhibitors with atropine and similar anticholinergic drugs have been problematic because of the risks of overdose
- Mediastinal exploration and resection of thymic tissue has been associated with substantially improved longterm prognoses in individuals with myasthenia gravis. Complete thymectomy is now generally recommended for all young (<40 years old) individuals who become symptomatic. Some physicians recommend the procedure at any age, once the diagnosis has been firmly established
- Because this is presumed to be an autoimmune disorder, a variety of immunosuppressant approaches have been tried. The most successful has been treatment with corticosteroids. After initiating treatment with relatively high doses (prednisone 60–100 mg each morning for days or a few weeks), maintenance therapy may require little more than a few mgs every other day. Strength may deteriorate when the steroids are started; some physicians start at low doses of prednisone and gradually ↑ the daily dose to avoid this deterioration
- Many physicians use Azathioprine (Imuran) as adjunctive immunosuppressant therapy for a few months at the start of treatment. The dose is 2.5–4 mg/kg/day, tapered over the course of weeks, unless the patient exhibits leukopenia or other serious reactions to the drug

ACUTE POLYNEUROPATHY

Diagnosis

- Guillain Barré syndrome is one of the most common and most lethal forms of acute polyneuropathy. It is an inflammatory, pure-motor neuropathy, or nearly so. The affected individual usually develops progressive weakness, starting in the legs and progressing cephalad over the course of 2 weeks. The deficits usually appear within weeks of a URI. Bladder and bowel control are retained, but diaphragmatic paralysis may develop. Sensation is usually preserved throughout the

limbs, but many patients note paresthesias about the feet or ankles and occasionally in the hands. Areflexia or hyporeflexia are invariably present at some time during the course of the illness
- Transient autonomic disturbances, such as hypertension, tachycardia, mydriasis, and disturbances of sweating, commonly develop during the course of the illness and usually do not require treatment
- Ocular motor control is usually unaffected. In the rare Miller-Fisher variant, strength may be relatively little affected, but ataxia, areflexia, and ophthalmoplegia prominent
- At the time the weakness (or ophthalmoplegia) evolves, the patient is afebrile. The CSF exhibits a high protein content (usually >100 mg/dl), with little or no associated ↑ in the white cell content. This is usually referred to as cytoalbuminemic dissociation and was originally used to differentiate acute polyneuropathy from poliomyelitis
- EMG and nerve conduction studies will establish that a neuropathy is present, but this test may give deceptively normal results early in the evolution of symptoms. Within days or weeks of the first signs of weakness, the patient will have a conduction block

Pathophysiology

- Guillain Barré is idiopathic, but there are forms of acute polyneuropathy that are attributable to specific infectious agents, such as diphtheritic polyneuropathy. The underlying defect in acute inflammatory polyneuropathy is demyelination of peripheral nerves

Therapy

- The most important measure is supportive treatment. At the first sign of respiratory embarrassment the patient must be intubated. Individuals with respiratory insufficiency must be maintained on ventilators, and care must be taken to manage any pulmonary problems, such as atelectasis or pneumonia, that develop
- Repeated trials with corticosteroids have demonstrated no efficacy for this traditional therapy
- Plasmapheresis has been attempted in several trials. There is a growing consensus that this is efficacious in acute inflammatory polyneuropathy. Routinely, 5 exchanges are completed over the course of 7–14 days
- IV gamma globulin infusions appear to be as effective, if not more effective, than plasmapheresis. Immunosuppressive therapy does not improve the outcome
- None of the treatments currently available influence the severity of the deficits that evolve, but plasmapheresis and gamma globulin do ↓ the duration of hospitalization. Only 15% of patients will recover with no residua. Three to 8% die from complications, such as infection

ACUTE SPINAL CORD COMPRESSION

Diagnosis

- Cord compression usually produces sensory and motor deficits at or below the level of the compression. The sensory level is 3–4 dermato-

mal levels lower than the motor level and is most apparent contralateral to the motor deficits. Both of these features of the sensory level are related to the crossing of the spinothalamic tracts after ascending in Lissauer's tract (substantia gelatinosa). With massive compression, deficits will be evident bilaterally, and quadriplegia or hemiplegia associated with hypesthesia or anesthesia below the level of the motor deficit will develop
- Bladder and bowel control may be lost relatively early in the course of spinal cord compression. With involvement of the cauda equina alone, bladder and bowel dysfunction are likely to be prominent elements of the symptomatology

Pathophysiology

- Common causes of spinal cord compression include malignancies, benign neoplasms, trauma, and infection. Malignancies impinging upon or arising in the spinal cord are usually metastatic lesions. The most common benign neoplasms impinging upon the cord are meningiomas and neurofibromas. Trauma sufficient to cause cord compression is usually in the cervical region. Trauma to the lumbar region may produce spinal root compression, but is unlikely to involve the cord because the conus medullaris in the adult rarely extends much below the L1 vertebral body. Infections involving the vertebral bodies or the intervertebral discs may impinge directly on the cord or produce cord compression as tissues around the cord are damaged and vertebrae sublux
- Subluxation of the atlas and the axis (C1 and C2) may develop in juvenile rheumatoid arthritis and produce cervical spinal cord compression that is insidiously progressive
- Cord compression develops in some instances secondary to enlargement of a cyst (syrinx) within the cord. Syringomyelia is most commonly seen in the cervical or lumbar cord regions. Pain and temperature sensory deficits may be substantial early in the course of the cyst enlargement, presumably because the anterior decussation of the spinothalamic tract is compressed by the syrinx
- Patients from regions in which the parasite Schistosoma mansoni is endemic, such as Puerto Rico, may develop a rapidly enlarging granulomatous reaction to the ova of this worm as they accumulate in the lumbar spinal cord. The affected individual will have paraparesis; sensory deficits in the legs; and bladder, bowel, and sexual dysfunction evolving over the course of days

Therapy

- What is causing the cord compression must be ascertained as soon as cord compression is suspected. This is often evident on MRI of the spinal cord. The histologic character of the lesion may be suggested by the image, but in many cases an ambiguous mass must be biopsied
- With acute deterioration, high-dose corticosteroids usually help ↓ symptoms and provide additional time for more definitive treatment. Dexamethasone 40–100 mg IV is administered as soon as the cord injury can be ascribed to compression. Subsequent treatment with 4–10 mg IV q 6 h may be useful on a shortterm basis
- If a circumscribed, extraparenchymal mass is evident, surgical resection is usually appropriate. Surgery should be performed as soon as feasible: Protracted cord compression will produce irreparable dam-

age. If functional transection of the cord persists for much >24 h, the probability of recovering much function is remote

- Patients with metastatic disease impinging on the cord should have radiation therapy on an emergency basis. Decompressive surgery along with radiation provides little if any additional benefit, but it is often performed when the diagnosis is uncertain. Radiation therapy of the tumor may produce a transient ↑ in the local mass effect of the lesion; steroids are usually continued for several days or weeks to counter this phenomenon. The dose of radiation and character of the ports are determined by the probable nature of the tumor. Surgery is curative for some infectious lesions such as epidural abscesses

Suggested Reading

Bracken MB, Shepard MJ, Collins WF, et al.: Methylprednisolone or naloxone treatment after acute spinal cord injury. Results of the Second National Acute Spinal Cord Injury Study. J Neurosurg, *76*:23–31, 1992.

Calne DB: Treatment of Parkinson's Disease. N Engl J Med *329*:1021, 1993.

Gilman S: Advances in Neurology. N Engl J Med, *326*: 1671, 1992.

Lance JW: Treatment of migraine. Lancet, *339*: 1207–1209, 1992.

Lechtenberg R: Seizure Recognition and Treatment. New York, Churchill Livingstone, 1990.

Lechtenberg R: Synopsis of Neurology. Philadelphia, Lea & Febiger, 1991.

North American Symptomatic Carotid Endarterectomy Trial Collaborators: Beneficial effect of carotid endarterectomy in symptomatic patients with high-grade carotid stenosis. N Engl J Med, *325*: 445–453, 1991.

Ropper AH: The Guillain-Barré syndrome. N Engl J Med, *326*: 1130–1136, 1992.

Sandercock P, Willems H: Medical treatment of acute ischemic stroke. Lancet, *339*: 537–39,1992.

Stein SC, O'Malley KF, Ross SE: Is routine computed tomography scanning too expensive for mild head injury? Ann Emerg Med, *20*:1286–89, 1991.

Sundaresan N, Digiacinto GV, Hughes JEO, Cafferty M, Vallejo A: Treatment of neoplastic spinal cord compression: Results of a prospective study. Neurosurgery, *29*:645–650, 1991.

Welch KMA: Drug therapy of migraine. N Engl J Med, *329*:1476–1482, 1993.

Renal Diseases

28

Shiv L. Jindal and J. Charles Jennette

Because the kidneys are required for many homeostatic functions, renal diseases can manifest in a wide variety of ways, including: fluid, electrolyte, and acid-base disorders; renal failure with accumulation of nitrogenous wastes in the blood; hypertension; and abnormal urinary excretion of blood cells, leukocytes, and protein. This chapter will focus primarily on the diagnosis and management of the causes of acute and chronic renal failure and glomerular diseases.

ACUTE RENAL FAILURE

Renal failure is categorized as acute or chronic, either of which will result in ESRD if not reversed (Table 28–1). ARF is defined as rapid or abrupt onset of renal failure in a few hours or days of this illness characterized usually but not always by oliguria (urine volume <400 ml/day) with severe ↓ in GFR, ↑ BUN and creatinine, and abnormality of other renal functions.

The major causes of ARF are classified anatomically into: prerenal, renal, and postrenal

Prerenal ARF

The causes of prerenal ARF are listed in Table 28–2. Structurally, the kidneys are normal and respond appropriately to the various prerenal causes, in particular, sudden marked ↓ in vascular volume and/or cardiac output, which leads to hemodynamic changes such as low BP and ↓ renal perfusion, and hormonal changes. The end result is:

- ↓ renal blood flow, ↓ GFR
- ↑ tubular absorption of Na^+, H_2O, and urea (not creatinine)

The final outcome is

- Oliguria
- More concentrated urine
- Low urine Na^+ concentration

Diagnosis. A relevant history and physical examination will often reveal the correct diagnosis. Urinalysis is normal (Table 28–3), Urinary indices in the diagnosis of ARF are given in Table 28–3. Renal ultrasound is normal

Management. Early recognition and treatment of the underlying cause before the more severe form of ATN (acute tubular necrosis) sets in is crucial

- Conditions with contracted intravascular volume often require CVP line to monitor volume replacement with 0.9% saline, blood, or albu-

Table 28–1
Categories of Renal Failure

1. Acute Renal Failure
   - Prerenal
     - Contraction of intravascular volume
     - Low cardiac output
     - Acute renal artery disease
   - Renal
     - Acute glomerular disease
     - Acute vascular disease
     - Acute tubular and interstitial disease
   - Postrenal
     - Acute urinary tract obstruction
2. Chronic Renal Failure
3. End Stage Renal Disease [ESRD]

min, depending on the type of loss. Typically, 1 l 0.9% saline is infused over 30–60 min then titrated to achieve adequate urine output and BP

- Third-space losses can be reversed by using colloids (albumin or blood) and fewer crystalloids (isotonic saline)
- Cardiogenic shock requires the insertion of a Swan-Ganz catheter to monitor PCWP
- Low-dose dopamine and dobutamine are titrated to maintain BP (see Chap. 4 discussion of cardiogenic shock)

The following cautions should be taken

Table 28–2
Causes of Prerenal Acute Renal Failure

- Intravascular volume depletion
  - Acutal losses
    - Hemorrhage
    - GI . . diarrhea, vomiting
    - Renal . . salt wasting, diuretics
    - Skin . . burns, exudative dermatitis
- Reduced effective circulating volume
  - Redistribution of fluid
    - Ascites
    - Peritonitis
    - Pancreatitis
    - Abdominal surgery
  - Peripheral vasodilation
    - Sepsis
    - Anaphylaxis
- Cardiac dysfunction with low cardiac output
  - Mycocardial infarction
  - Cardiac tamponade
  - Other causes of cardiogenic shock (Table 4–4)
- Acute renal artery disease
  - Acute stenosis
  - Acute thrombosis
  - Acute embolism

Table 28–3
Urinary Indices in the Diagnosis of Acute Renal Failure

	PRERENAL	RENAL ATN
Urine volume	Low	Low
Urinalysis	Normal	Active, i.e, protein, RBC, epithelial cells epithelial cell casts, pigmented granular casts
Urine (Na^+) mEq/l	<20	>40
Urine (osm) mOsm/l	>500	<300
U/P creatinine	>40	<20
RFI (UNa)/(U/P Cr)	<1%	>3%
Fractional Excretion of Na^+ (U/P Na^+)/(U/P Cr) × 100	<1%	>3%

U/P = urine:plasma ratio
RFI = renal failure index

- Avoid furosemide if the patient is volume depleted
- Avoid NSAIDs which may further aggravate ARF
- Urinary indices are of no value if the patient is already given furosemide or has underlying chronic renal failure (CRF)

Postrenal ARF

Obstruction to the flow of urine leads to oliguria or complete anuria. Oliguria or anuria interspersed with polyuria are indicators of urinary tract obstruction. Sites and common conditions causing urinary tract obstruction include the following

- Urethra and bladder neck: prostatic hypertrophy, urethral stricture or valves, meatal stenosis, phimosis
- Bladder: neurogenic, calculus, carcinoma, blood clot
- Ureter: intrinsic obstruction (calculus, sloughed necrotic renal papilla, clots, carcinoma), extrinsic obstruction (uterine prolapse, ureterocele, strictures, pelvic or retroperitoneal tumors), retroperitoneal fibrosis
- Ureteropelvic junction: intrinsic (calculus, clots, sloughed necrotic renal papilla); extrinsic (stricture, fibrous bands, aberrant arteries)
- Renal pelvis: calculus, clots, papilla, carcinoma, TB

Look for suprapubic fullness indicating distended urinary bladder usually caused by bladder neck obstruction (e.g., enlarged prostate). If trauma, consider bladder rupture. Obstruction higher up—e.g., bilateral calculi—leads to hydronephrosis. Ultrasound may show dilation of the collecting system; however, retrograde pyelogram may be necessary to rule out postrenal obstruction. Obstruction leads to

- ↑ intratubular pressure
- ↓ glomerular transcapillary pressure and GFR
- Afferent arteriolar vasoconstriction
- Further ↓ in GFR

Management comprises removal of obstruction surgically or by percutaneous nephrostomy

Renal ARF

Causes include

- Most commonly: ATN
- Glomerular nephritis (GN)—rapidly progressive GN and acute diffuse proliferative GN (e.g., poststreptococcal)
- Tubulointerstitial disorders such as acute HTIN (see p. 558) and intratubular obstruction (abnormal proteins or drugs)
- Vascular disorders, such as thrombotic microangiopathies (e.g., malignant hypertension, TTP, HUS), thromboembolic disorders (e.g., DIC, cholesterol embolization), vasculitis

ACUTE TUBULAR NECROSIS

Various terms describe this condition at different stages: e.g., ARF (clinical), ATN (pathologic), and vasomotor nephropathy (pathophysiologic).
The 2 basic pathogenic mechanisms for ATN are ischemia and nephrotoxicity (Table 28–4)

- Ischemia is caused by the mechanisms listed in Table 28–2. If the hypoperfusion that causes prerenal failure continues, a second mechanism sets in that maintains oliguria. This involves tubular epithelial injury resulting in tubular permeability causing leak and reabsorption of fluid back into the circulation (back leak theory) and tubular obstruction due to debris (cells, casts, etc.) (obstructive theory). There is also vasoconstriction of the afferent arteriole leading to ↓ GFR (tubuloglomerular feedback)
- Drug nephrotoxicity is a major cause of nosocomial nephrotoxic ARF. Aminoglycosides remain the most common cause of drug-induced ATN. Although some aminoglycosides (e.g., gentamicin) are more nephrotoxic than others (e.g., tobramycin), all have nephrotoxic potential
- Patients with pre-existing renal disease, multiple myeloma, or dehydration are at greatest risk for developing radiocontrast-induced ATN
- In patients with ATN associated with hemoglobinuria and myoglobinuria, poorly understood factors in addition to urine excretion of Hb and

Table 28–4
Causes of Ischemic and Nephrotoxic ATN

Ischemic ATN
  Same as Table 28–2
Nephrotoxic ATN
  Endogenous toxins
    Hemoglobin
    Myoglobin
  Exogenous toxins
    Drugs (e.g., aminoglycosides and other antibiotics, chemotherapeutics)
    Radiocontrast dyes
    Heavy metals (e.g., mercury, arsenic)
    Organic solvents (e.g., carbon tetrachloride, ethylene glycol)
    Anesthetics (e.g., methoxyflurance, enflurane)

Table 28–5
Causes of Hemoglobinuria and Myoglobinuria

Hemoglobinuria
Transfusion reactions
Snake and arthropod venoms
Hemolytic anemia
Amnionic fluid leak
Rhabdomyolysis
Crushing trauma
Muscular ischemia
Muscular overexertion (e.g., seizures)
Hyperthermia
Hypothermia
Infection (e.g., influenza)
Snake and arthropod venoms
Drugs and toxins (e.g., alcohol)
Inflammation (e.g., dermatomyositis)
Hereditary enzyme defects

myoglobin contribute to the nephrotoxicity. Table 28–5 lists causes for hemoglobinuria and myoglobinuria.

Diagnosis is clarified by

- The clinical identification of the causes listed in Tables 28–4 and 28–5
- Urinalysis and urinary indices (see Table 28–3)
- Urinalysis for myoglobin and Hb

Prevention involves the following

- Maintenance of intravascular volume, cardiac output, BP, and thereby adequate renal perfusion is crucial to prevention of ischemic ATN; it also reduces the toxicity of most nephrotoxins. Adequacy of intravascular volume can be achieved by giving crystalloids (0.9% saline), albumin, or blood and mannitol. These measures are particularly important in cardiac or cardiovascular surgery, in patients at high risk for hemoglobinuria or myoglobinuria, and when radiocontrast dyes are used
- Alkaline diuresis (urine pH >7.0) is recommended to prevent ARF in conditions with high uric acid load, myoglobinuria, or salicylate overdose
- Allopurinol 600 mg prior to and 300 mg qd after chemotherapy in various myeloproliferative disorders
- Avoid NSAIDs in high-risk cases, such as the elderly, in patients with volume-depleted status with high renin activity, and in those with compromised renal function. Avoid concomitant use of triamterene-containing diuretics
- Avoid using multiple nephrotoxic drugs, e.g., aminoglycoside antibiotic and methoxyflurane anesthesia

Management of ATN focuses on its 2 phases: oliguric and diuretic

Oliguric Phase

- Most ischemic ATN is oliguric. Nonoliguric ATN is more often nephrotoxic; thus, the recognition of renal failure may be delayed, resulting in hyperkalemia and fluid overload. Morbidity and mortality is reported to be less if patients are nonoliguric to start with or are converted to a nonoliguric state with high-dose furosemide (≤1000 mg).

Do not exceed 4 mg/min infusion since ototoxicity may occur with high-dose bolus

- Maintain meticulous fluid and electrolyte control: Dialysis can be delayed if the fluid and electrolyte balance is maintained tightly and intake and output are carefully monitored. Intake is calculated based on the daily losses. Good guidelines are the daily weight (usually 0.5 lb weight loss daily), presence or absence of edema, and BP status. Protein is restricted to 0.6–0.8 g/kg body weight, Na^+ to 2 g qd, K^+ to 40–60 mEq qd

Hyperkalemia can be controlled by a combination of the following measures

- Strict reduction of K^+ in the diet; eliminate oral K^+ supplements and drugs containing K^+
- Correct acidosis with $NaHCO_3$ po; 600 mg bid, up to 1.2 g tid; goal CO_2 16–20 mEq/l, with care not to cause volume overload and/or CHF
- Glucose-insulin infusion, e.g., 2 g glucose with 1 U of regular insulin (50 cc 50% D/W with 10 U of regular insulin over 15–20 min)
- Resins. Kayexalate po or as a rectal enema; or Ca resonium po
- Cardioprotection with IV CaCl or Ca gluconate (see Chap. 31)

Hemodialysis or peritoneal dialysis may be required. Indications for dialysis are

- Clinical signs of uremia (encephalopathy, nausea and vomiting, GI hemorrhage, pericarditis) and fluid overload causing intractable CHF and pulmonary congestion
- Biochemical BUN (>120 mg/dl), uncontrollable hyperkalemia, acidosis

Diuretic Phase

Carefully monitor fluid and electrolyte balance to prevent severe volume depletion that can result in significant morbidity and mortality.

Prognosis. Despite modern technology, morbidity and mortality remain high, mostly because of the underlying conditions that caused the ATN, e.g., postcardiac or vascular surgery, sepsis, cardiogenic shock. Death is usually caused by these underlying conditions, hyperkalemia, fluid overload, or GI hemorrhage.

ACUTE HYPERSENSITIVITY TUBULOINTERSTITIAL NEPHRITIS

HTIN accounts for 15–20% of ARF. Acute infectious TIN (acute pyelonephritis) rarely causes ARF but may lead to chronic pyelonephritis and CRF. The most common causes of AHTIN are drugs, e.g., penicillins, sulfonamides, NSAIDs, cephalosporins, furosemide, rifampin, and phenytoin.

Diagnosis. The classic signs and symptoms begin 1–2 weeks after initiation of drug administration: Fever, rash, and eosinophilia. However, all 3 features occur only in 1/3 of patients. Eosinophilia is most frequent (80% of patients). Typical urinalysis findings are sterile pyuria, eosinophiluria, WBC casts, proteinuria (<2 g/24 h) and slight hematuria.

Management. Identify and remove potential inciting agent (renal function should begin to improve within several days). If no response to discontinuation of drugs or no inciting agent identified, steroid therapy may facilitate recovery (prednisone 1 mg/kg/day po for 4–6 weeks). If

ARF is severe, dialysis and management of fluid and electrolytes as described previously for ATN is required

Prognosis. If an inciting agent is identified and removed, full recovery usually ensues within 1–2 weeks. However, recovery may take ≤2 months. Persistence of ARF for >2 weeks and absence of an apparent inciting agent are signs of poorer prognosis.

CHRONIC RENAL FAILURE

CRF occurs slowly over many years. It is irreversible. As the nephron population ↓, the remaining nephrons adapt (intact nephron hypothesis), ultimately leading to additional nephron loss through sclerosis. There is also extrarenal adaptation and trade-off. Therefore, these patients enjoy a symptom-free life until the GFR drops to <25% of normal. Life support with dialysis and/or renal transplant is necessary when the nephron population is <5%.

Causes in Adults. Diabetic glomerulosclerosis, Chronic glomerulonephritis, Hypertensive arterionephrosclerosis, Renovascular disease, Adult polycystic kidney disease, Chronic pyelonephritis, Analgesic abuse, Hereditary disorders

Natural history. Hemodynamic, hormonal, structural, and adaptive events occur during the progression of CRF

- Hemodynamic. Initially there is ↑ renal blood flow (hyperperfusion), leading to ↑ intraglomerular pressure and ↑ GFR per remaining nephron and therefore ↑ filtered load of nonprotein nitrogen (urea, creatinine, uric acid), electrolytes, and other solutes
- Hormonal changes predominantly regulate the tubular functions of absorption and secretion (e.g., aldosterone, atrial natriuretic hormone, ADH, and PTH, which control Na^+, K^+, H_2O, Ca^{++}, and PO_4, respectively). A steady state is maintained for a long time and the patient is asymptomatic until progressive glomerulosclerosis leads to azotemia and uremia
- Structural. Progressive glomerulosclerosis may develop as a result of glomerular hyperfiltration
- Extrarenal adaptations and tradeoffs. As the Hb concentration ↓, there is a shift to the right of the O_2-Hb dissociation curve, unloading O_2 at the tissue level (favorable). Therefore blood transfusion is usually not needed until the Hb drops to <7–8 g/dl (70–80 g/l), at which time the patient becomes symptomatic
- As the serum PO_4 level rises, serum Ca^{++} falls. This in turn stimulates PTH, causing phosphaturia and mobilization of Ca^{++} from bones. With the progression of renal failure, metabolic bone disease can appear in the form of renal rickets/osteomalacia (deficiency of vitamin D), osteitis fibrosa (↑ PTH), and metastatic calcification (increased PO_4 x Ca^{++} product)
- Chronic acidosis is associated with mobilization of $CaCO_3$ from bones (which are rich reserves of $CaCO_3$), which may ultimately contribute to metabolic bone disease

Signs and Symptoms. Almost any system can be affected during the course of CRF. The earliest symptoms are related to

- GI system: morning nausea, anorexia, intermittent vomiting, and weight loss

- CNS: leg cramps (especially at night), fatigue, asterixis, and lack of concentration

Late and usually severe and alarming features are

- CVS: uremic pericarditis, cardiac tamponade
- CNS: encephalopathy, neuropathy
- MSK: metabolic bone disease, intractable itching

Diagnosis. See Table 28–6 for features that differentiate between ARF and CRF.

Management. The goals are to slow the progression of renal failure, control the manifestations of uremia, and maintain proper nutritional status. In order to slow the progression of CRF

- Control hemodynamic factors, i.e., hyperperfusion, ↑ intraglomerular pressure, and hyperfiltration in remaining nephrons. Dietary restriction of protein is very important: Research data indicate that diets low in protein and phosphorus slow the progression of CRF, whereas diets high in lipids may accelerate it. There is increasing evidence that ACE inhibitors may retard the progression of CRF by reducing intraglomerular pressure in residual hyperfunctioning glomeruli, which is thought to cause progressive glomerulosclerosis
- Control both systolic and diastolic hypertension
- Control factors known to aggravate renal failure: prerenal factors such as volume depletion and hypotension; CHF; infection; and drug toxicity due to aminoglycosides, radiocontrast dyes, NSAIDs, and postrenal obstruction
- Control the underlying disease process that is causing CRF, e.g., diabetes mellitus

General treatment of CRF requires management of protein intake, fluid balance, K^+, Ca, phosphorus, acidosis, hypertension, and anemia

- Fluid and Na^+ balance. CRF impairs the ability to handle a Na^+ load and to conserve Na^+. Because of reduced glomerular filtration and tubular reabsorption, Na^+ intake $>$ the limited renal capacity for excretion results in Na^+ and H_2O retention, which can cause hypertension, edema, and CHF. Conversely, because of impaired renal conservation of Na^+, inadequate Na^+ intake causes Na^+ depletion and reduced extracellular fluid volume, which can cause reduced renal blood flow and worse renal failure. Na^+ intake of 2–3 g qd is appropriate in most circumstances in nondialyzed CRF patients, depending upon BP and presence of edema. Na^+ intake of 1–2 g/day is usually more appropriate for dialysis patients. Some CRF patients with salt-losing nephropathy may require more Na^+ intake to prevent volume depletion and further ↓ in GFR. If Na^+ balance is maintained, thirst will usually maintain normal H_2O balance until the GFR is $<$5 ml/min. Thereafter, careful control of fluid intake may be required
- Protein and calorie control. Experimental and clinical studies suggest that protein restriction slows the progression of CRF. Protein should be restricted to 0.6–1.0 g/kg body weight, 1/3 of which should be of high biological value (i.e., rich in essential amino acids), e.g., milk, eggs, fish, meat. To prevent malnutrition and catabolism, the diet should contain 35–40 kcal/kg/day. In patients with proteinuria, the protein intake must be increased by approximately 1 g/day for every 1 g/day proteinuria
- Potassium. Usually not a problem unless the patient is oliguric or has a sudden overload of K^+. Contributing factors that may cause hyperkalemia include: The use of nonselective β blockers, ACE inhibitors, K^+-sparing diuretics, salt substitute, NSAIDs; and severe meta-

Table 28–6
Guidelines to Differentiating Between Acute and Chronic Renal Failure

	ACUTE	CHRONIC
Etiology	Prerenal Renal Postrenal	Diabetes mellitus Chronic glomerulonephritis Hypertensive arterionephrosclerosis Adult polyscytic kidney disease Chronic prylonephritis Hereditary disorders Analgesic abuse
Urine volume	Usually oliguric	Usually polyuric until late stages
Endocrine Function	Usually normal	Abnormal
Hb	Normal	Anemia
Ca	Normal	Abnormalities of vitamin D metabolism and 2° ↑ PTH (e.g., ↓ Ca, ↑ $CaPO_4$
PO_4	Normal	↑ PO_4
Blood Pressure	Normal or Low	High with hypertensive changes: fundi and ECG/LVH pattern
Kidney size	Normal	Small in chronic glomerulonephritis, nephrosclerosis and chronic pyelonephritis Large in polycytstic kidneys, amyloidosis, hydronephrosis, and diabetes
Course	Usually reversible	Irreversible with slow deterioration

bolic acidosis and hyporeninemic hypoaldosteronism, especially in NIDDM (see Chap. 31, treatment of hyperkalemia)

- Ca and PO_4. CRF can cause vitamin D deficiency and resistance to vitamin D. Ca supplement and an active form of vitamin D are usually given to prevent metabolic bone disease. Phosphorus should be restricted to minimize hyperparathyroidism and possibly to retard progression of CRF. Besides dietary restriction of PO_4 to 300–700 mg/day, $CaCO_3$ 0.5–1 g tid, which binds PO_4 in the gut, may be administered to keep serum levels of PO_4 at a lower concentration; $CaCO_3$ avoids aluminum overload, which may occur with aluminum compounds
- Acidosis. Because of impaired excretion of acidic metabolites and renal loss of bicarbonate, metabolic acidosis is common in patients with CRF who are not on dialysis. Keep serum HCO_3 level close to 20 mEq/l and arterial pH <7.35. Mild acidosis can be controlled with $NaHCO_3$ 600 mg bid or tid or $CaCO_3$ 500–1000 mg bid or tid. More severe acidosis may require IV alkali or dialysis
- Hypertension. CRF alters the metabolism and excretion of some antihypertensive drugs. Antihypertensive drugs can beneficially influence problems in CRF patients in addition to hypertension, e.g., fluid overload (diuretics) and glomerular hyperfiltration (ACE inhibitors). ACE inhibitors may have special significance because they not only reduce systemic BP but also intraglomerular pressure. Volume overload often requires diuretics, especially furosemide, because thiazides are not effective in patients with severe CRF. The action of antihypertensive drugs, as well as other drugs, may be altered in CRF because of ↓ renal excretion, altered metabolism, altered volume of distribution, and, in patients on dialysis, removal by dialysis. This requires appropriate dose adjustment
- Anemia. Avoid transfusions unless the patient is symptomatic because of low Hb. Patients with CRF usually tolerate a Hb of 7 g/dl without symptoms except those with concomitant angina or CHF, who require judicious infusion of packed RBCs with added furosemide. Recombinant human erythropoietin (EPO) should be used in order to ↓ the need for blood transfusion. The usual dose of EPO is 40–100 IU/kg SC 3 times/week. The dose of EPO can be adjusted depending on the response (Hb should be kept $\leq$12 g/dl)
- Dialysis. A point will be reached in the course of the disease when conservative management with diet and drugs fails to control signs and symptoms of uremia and hyperkalemia. At this point dialysis and/or renal transplant is indicated. Consider dialysis at the early manifestation of uremia, which can appear when urea is approaching 30–40 mEq/l (BUN 80–100 mg/dl, 28.5–35 mmol/l) and creatinine 8–10 mg/dl (800–1000 μmol/l)
- Types of Dialysis. Hemodialysis can be done in hospital, or the patient can be trained to do the same at home or in a self-care unit. A-V vistula or a graft provide vascular access. Sometimes a subclavian catheter can be inserted for urgent or shortterm dialysis. The most common form of peritoneal dialysis is continuous ambulatory peritoneal dialysis (CAPD). This type is preferable for elderly people with difficult vascular access, individuals with cardiovascular instability, and diabetics. CAPD is easier than hemodialysis and can be done without much extra assistance. Some of the common problems with CAPD are peritonitis, protein loss, hyperglycemia, and respiratory embarrassment in patients with COPD
- Transplantation is the preferred replacement therapy for end stage renal disease. It may restore the quality of life to normal and is more economical than chronic dialysis in the long run.

GLOMERULAR DISEASE

The steps in the assessment and management of a patient with glomerular disease are

- Clinical recognition of glomerular disease
- Determination of the type of glomerular disease
- Identification of the cause or pathogenic category
- Determination of the prognosis and selection of treatment

Clinical Recognition. Glomerular injury manifests as

- Evidence of *structural* damage to the glomerulus: abnormal urinalysis demonstrating proteinuria, casts, hematuria, and other cells
- Evidence of *functional* damage to the glomerulus: azotemia, salt and H_2O retention, hypertension, oliguria

With structural and functional damage to the glomerulus, certain clinical syndromes result that indicate the presence of glomerular disease

- Nephritic syndrome: Hematuria, proteinuria ($<$3.0 g/day), cells in the urine (RBC, WBC), urine casts (all types, with RBC casts most specific), azotemia ($\uparrow$ BUN, creatinine), hypertension, edema
- Nephrotic syndrome: Proteinuria $>$3 g/day, lipiduria (free fat droplets and oval fat bodies with Maltese crosses under polarized light), hypoalbuminemia, hypercholesterolemia, and edema
- Combined nephritic and nephrotic syndrome
- Asymptomatic proteinuria or hematuria: Proteinuria or hematuria without the other features of nephritis or nephrotic syndrome
- Rapidly progressive GN: $\geq$50% loss of renal function within 3 months, often with oliguria or anuria
- Chronic glomerulonephritis: Nephritis or nephrotic with gradual progression of renal failure over many years

Determination of Type of Glomerular Disease. Once the clinical diagnosis is made, the second step is to determine the type of glomerular injury responsible for the clinical syndrome (Tables 28–7, 28–8, and 28–9). Accurate diagnosis, therapeutic decisions, and prognostication may require renal biopsy. Pathologic evaluation usually requires 3 procedures: light, immunofluorescence, and electron microscopy.

Light Microscopy. Morphologic changes involve glomeruli primarily. However, tubules, interstitium, and blood vessels often are involved secondarily. Glomerular injury can be diffuse (most or all glomeruli involved), focal (only some glomeruli involved), segmental (segments of glomeruli involved), or global (whole glomeruli involved). Blood vessels may be involved by the same inflammatory process that is in the glomeruli in some forms of systemic vasculitis, e.g., microscopic polyarteritis and Wegener's granulomatosis.

Glomerular morphologic changes can be classified into

- Proliferative disorders involving proliferation of various cells located in the glomerulus, e.g., mesangial cells (mesangial proliferative GN), endothelial cells, and epithelial cells (crescentic GN); and sometimes accompanied by influx of leukocytes
- Nonproliferative disorders in which glomeruli may have no histologic abnormalities (minimal change glomerulopathy), thickening of capillary walls (membranous GN), segmental scarring (focal segmental glomerulosclerosis), nodular sclerosis (diabetic glomerulosclerosis), or infiltration by proteinaceous material (amyloidosis)

Table 28–7
Characteristics of Some of the Common Types of Proliferative and Mixed Glomerulonephritis

	LIGHT MICROSCOPY	IMMUNOFLUORESCENCE MICROSCOPY	ELECTRON MICROSCOPY	CAUSE, THERAPY AND PROGNOSIS
1. Mesangial GN	(a) Mesangial proliferation (focal segmental)	IgA-dominant C3 granular, mesangial	Mesangial deposits	IgA nephropathy (Berger's disease) Rx: Supportive Prognosis: Variable (Features of poor prognosis: Nephrotic syndrome, hypertension) Differential diagnosis: Henoch-Schönlein purpura, liver cirrhosis
	(b) Same as 1(a)	IgG-dominant C3, C1q, IgM, IgA	Same as 1(a)	SLE (Type II) Rx: None Prognosis: Generally good
2. Diffuse Proliferative GN	(a) Hypercellularity: endothelial, mesangial ± epithelial (± crescents) proliferation and leukocyte influx	IgG C3 granular capillary wall	Subepthelial humps	Post-infectious GN Rx: Supportive Prognosis: Good, especially in children
	(b) Same as 2(a) plus wire loop lesions	IgG, IgA, IgM C3, C1q (full house)	Mesangial, subendothelial, & subepithelial deposits Microtubular arrays	SLE (Type IV) Rx: Steroids, Imuran, Cyclophosphamide Prognosis: Variable, guarded

3. Cresentic GN/ Rapidly Progressive GN (RPGN)	(a) Crescents (cellular, fibrous, mixed)	IgG C3 linear GBM	No dense deposits	Anti-GBM GN, (Goodpasture's disease) Rx: Steroids, Imuran, plasmapheresis Prognosis: Variable, guarded
	(b) Same as 3(a)	IgG C3 granular	Subendothelial Subepithelial humps	SLE. post-infectious GN, other immune complex GN Rx: Steroids, Imuran, Cyclophosphamide for SLE Prognosis: Fair
	(c) Same as 3(a)	No deposits	No dense deposits	Pauci-immune GN, Wegener's granulomatosis, microscopic polyarteritis Rx: Steroids, Cyclophosphamide Prognosis: Variable
4. MPGN Type I	Mesangial proliferation, thick capillary walls, lobular pattern, double contour of BM	C3-dominance IgG, IgM	Subendothelial and mesangial deposits	(a) Idiopathic (most common in children) Rx: No therapy Prognosis: Poor (b) Secondary to infection, neoplasm, cryoglobulinemia Rx: Treat primary cause Prognosis: Variable
5. MPGN Type II (dense deposit disease)	Lobular, pattern, ribbon-like thickening of capillary walls	C3 capillary, mesangial	Intramembranous dense deposits	(a) Idiopathic (b) Secondary to partial lipodystrophy Rx: No therapy Prognosis; Poor

Table 28–8
Characteristics of Non-Proliferative Glomerular Disorders

	LIGHT MICROSCOPY	IMMUNOFLUORESCENCE MICROSCOPY	ELECTRON MICROSCOPY	CAUSE, THERAPY AND PROGNOSIS
1. Minimal Change glomerulopathy	Normal	Negative	Non-specific fusion of foot processes. No dense deposits	(a) Idiopathic (most common in children) Rx: Usually steroids alone or with cyclophosphamides for poor responders Prognosis: Excellent; relapse is common but responds to retreatment (b) Secondary to lymphoid malignancy Rx: Treat neoplasm
2. Focal segmental glomerulosclerosis	Sclerosis of part of glomerular tuft	IgM and C3 in sclerosis	Non-specific fusion of foot processes. No dense deposits	(a) Idiopathic (most common in children) Rx: No therapy Prognosis: Slow progression to renal failure (b) Secondary to obesity, reduced renal mass Reflux nephropathy

3. Membranous glomerulopathy	Thickening of capillary walls, no proliferation of cells Spike formation	IgG-dominant C3 granular capillary	Subepithelial dense deposits (staging I–IV)	(a) Idiopathic (most common in adults) Rx: Steroids, chlorambucil, cyclophosphamide; varying reports of benefits Prognosis: Spontaneous remission in 20–25%; slow progression to renal failure (b) Secondary to malignancy, lymphoma, SLE, drugs, hepatitis
4. Diabetic glomerulosclerosis	Nodular sclerosis and thicknened GBM	IgG linear GBM	Thick GBM	Diabetes mellitus Rx: Control diabetes, ACE inhibitor Prognosis: Poor
5. Amyloidosis				
AL	Acidophilic effacement of tufts	Immunoglobulin light chains ($\lambda > \kappa$)	10 nm fibrils	May be secondary to B cell neoplasm Rx: Treat neoplasm
AA	Same as AL	Amyloid A protein	10 nm fibrils	May be secondary to chronic inflammatory disease (e.g., TB, rheumatoid arthritis) Rx: Treat inflammatory disease

Table 28–9
Characteristics of Glomerular Injury in Systemic Diseases

	LIGHT MICROSCOPY	IMMUNOFLUORESCENCE MICROSCOPY	ELECTRON MICROSCOPY	THERAPY AND PROGNOSIS
1. SLE (WHO Classification: Types I–V)				
Type I	Normal	Negative	Negative	No therapy
Type II (Mesangial)				
IIa	Normal	IgG, IgM, IgA C3, C1q granular, mesangial	Mesangial dense deposits	No therapy
IIb	Mesangial proliferation	Same as IIa	Same as IIa	No therapy
Type III (focal [<50%] glomeruli involved)	Proliferation of endothelial mesangial and ± epithelial cells, leukocyte influx, necrosis	IgG, IgM, IgA C3, C1q	Subendothelial and mesangial dense deposits	No therapy unless severe
Type IV (diffuse [>50%] glomeruli involved	Proliferation of endothelial mesangial and epithelial cells, vessel necrosis	IgG, IgM, IgA C3, C1q	Subendothelial and mesangial dense deposits	Rx: Steroids, imuran, cyclophosphamide Variable response Prognosis: Guarded

Type V (Membranous GN)	Thickening of capillary walls	IgG, IgM, IgA C3, C1q	Subepithelial dense deposits most numerous	No therapy
2. Microscopic polyarterits	Necrotizing glomerulonephritis and vasculitis, usually crescents	Negative	No dense deposits	Rx: Steroids, cyclophosphamide Prognosis: Fair
3. Wegener's granulomatosis	Necrotizing glomerulonephritis and vasculitis, usually crescents	Negative	No dense deposits	Rx: Steroids, cyclophosphamide Prognosis: Fair
4. Thrombotic microangiopathies (HUS, TTP, PSS, malignant hypertension)	Glomerular consolidation, arteriolar necrosis, arterial intimal expansion, thrombi	Negative or fibrin	Lucent subendothelial expansion	Rx: Plasmapheresis, control hypertension Prognosis: Guarded
5. Mixed cryoglobulinemia	Same as MPGN Type I	IgG, IgM C3	Subendothelial and mesangial dense deposits	Rx: Steroids, cyclophosphamide, plasmapheresis
6. Henoch-Schönlein purpura	Same as I, A nephropathy	I, A-dominant C3	Mesangial dense deposits	No therapy unless very severe Prognosis good

- Mixed disorders with both proliferative and nonproliferative changes (types I and II membranoproliferative GN)

Immunofluorescence Microscopy. This is of great value in defining specific categories of disease based on

- Patterns of immune deposits. Granular (lumpy-bumpy), signifying injury due to immune complex localization, as seen in postinfectious GN or lupus nephritis. Linear deposition of immunoglobulin signifying injury due to antiglomerular basement membrane antibodies (anti-GM Ab), as seen in Goodpasture's syndrome
- Composition of immune deposits, e.g., IgA-dominance of immunoglobulin in IgA nephropathy, Henoch-Schönlein purpura and cirrhotic liver disease; IgG and conspicuous C1q in lupus nephritis; C3-dominance in MPGN
- Absence of immune deposits, e.g., idiopathic (pauci-immune) crescentic GN, microscopic polyarteritis GN, and Wegener's granulomatosis GN

Electron Microscopy. This defines

- Epithelial foot process effacement (fusion), which is a nonspecific finding seen in any condition with significant proteinuria
- Electron-dense deposits and their locations, e.g., mesangial (IgA nephritis, lupus nephritis), subendothelial (lupus and MPGN type I), subepithelial (membranous GN, post-streptococcal GN), and intramembranous (MPGN Type II)
- Abnormal material, e.g., amyloid deposits

Identification of Cause or Pathogenic Category. The third step in defining glomerular injury is to determine the cause or pathogenesis

- Granular immune deposits by IM and dense deposits by EM indicate immune complex disease. The composition of the immune deposits, other laboratory data (serology, complement levels), and additional clinical data (associated diseases: SLE, cryoglobulinemia, endocarditis, streptococcal infection, hepatitis, malaria) may indicate specific forms of immune complex GN, such as IgA nephropathy, lupus nephritis, or poststreptococcal GN
- Linear immunoglobulin binding to GBM by IM and detection of anti-GBM antibodies by serology indicate anti-GBM GN. Concurrent pulmonary hemorrhage indicates Goodpasture's syndrome
- No immune deposition is characteristic of idiopathic (pauci-immune) crescentic GN and the GN in patients with microscopic polyarteritis and Wegener's granulomatosis. Antineutrophil cytoplasmic autoantibodies are a serologic marker for these diseases
- A concurrent systemic disease may be the cause of glomerular diseases: diabetes, amyloidosis, systemic sclerosis, SLE

Prognosis and Treatment. The final step is to determine the prognosis and to select the treatment for glomerular injury (see Tables 28–7, 28–8, and 28–9). The treatment of glomerulonephritis generally consists of

- Supportive measures in keeping with the functional changes in the glomerulus, e.g., fluid and electrolyte balance, and control of BP. If ARF or CRF ensue, treat as detailed earlier in this chapter
- Treatment of the primary cause, if possible, e.g., diabetes, infection, neoplasm, drug exposure
- Steroid and immunosuppressive treatment of inflammatory diseases and immune-mediated diseases

Suggested Reading

Brenner BM, Rector FC Jr: The Kidney. 4th Ed. Philadelphia, W. B. Saunders, 1991

Glassock RJ: Current Therapy in Nephrology and Hypertension. 3rd Ed. Philadelphia, B C Decker, 1992

Lewis EJ, Hunsicker LG, Bain RP, et al: The effect of angiotensin-converting-enzyme inhibition on diabetic nephropathy. N Engl J Med *329*:1456, 1993.

Hematologic Disorders

29

Stuart Roath and Samuel Gross

ANEMIAS

The history and physical should reveal the likely cause of anemia. A classification of anemias is given in Table 29–1.

The MCV taken in context with the peripheral blood smear should yield a presumptive diagnosis (Table 29–2). (N.B.: Reticulocytes have a large diameter and will ↑ MCV.) Corrected reticulocyte count = measured reticulocyte count x hematocrit ÷ by 40. Further tests requested and interpreted in logical steps should confirm the diagnosis. Table 29–3 gives appropriate lab tests and results that may be helpful in evaluating the cause of microcytic anemias.

Normocytic, Normochromic Anemias

MEMBRANE DISORDERS

The red cell membrane is composed of a highly mobile bilayer of intercalated phospholipids, glycolipids, and non-esterified cholesterol penetrated by a protein structure that includes antigens, receptors, and

Table 29–1
Classification of Anemias (morphological)

A. Normocytic Normochromic
   1. membrane defects
   2. metabolic disorders
   3. aplastic anemia
   4. pure red blood cell aplasia
   5. secondary anemias (simple chronic anemias)
   6. anemias with marrow disruption
   7. defects in globin chain synthesis
   8. hemolytic anemias

B. Microcytic Hypochromic
   1. iron deficiency
   2. thalassemias
   3. erythropoietic porphyrias

C. Macrocytic (Megaloblastic)
   1. folic deficiency
   2. B_{12} deficiency
   3. orotic aciduria
   4. refractory
   5. drug induced

Table 29–2
Peripheral Blood Morphology—Diagnostic Aids

MCV (FL)	RBC'S	SUGGEST
<78	Microcytic hypochromic	Iron deficiency
		Thalassemias
		Sideroblastic
		Chronic disease
78–98	Normocytic	Acute blood loss, hemolytic anemia
		Neoplasm, renal failure
		Hypothyroidism, aplasia
		Chronic disease
>100	Macrocytic	
	Oval macrocytes	B_{12} or folate deficiency
	Normal macrocytes	Liver disease
		Rarely: aplasia, myelodysplasia
	Dimorphic	Sideroblastic
		Treated iron deficiency
		Megaloblastic and iron deficiency
		Hemolytic anemia
	Reticulocytes ↑	Blood loss
		Hemolysis
		Response to therapy
	Fragmented cells	Fragmentation
	Helmet, schistocytes	Hemolysis
	Irregular contracted cells	DIC
	Basophilic stippling	Sideroblastic
		Thalassemias, lead poisoning
	Target cells	Thalassemias
		Sickle cell disease
		Liver disease
		Post-splenectomy states
	Spherocytes	Hereditary spherocytosis
		Warm immune hemolysis
		Burns
		Gas gangrene
		Rarely G6PD
	Sickle forms	Sickle cell anemia
	Spiculated (Burr cells)	Liver
		Splenectomy, uremia
		Severe malnutrition
	Blister cells	G6PD
	Rouleaux formation	Myeloma, macroglobulinemia
	Howell-Jolly bodies (Nuclear fragments)	Megaloblastic, splenectomy
		Hemolytic anemia
	Nucleated red cells	Leuko erythroblastic:
	Myelocytes metamyelocytes	Infiltration
		Severe hypoxemia
		Blood loss (severe)
		Severe hemolysis
		Neonates
	Hypersegmented neutrophils	Megaloblastic (characteristic)
		Inflammatory processes
		Renal failure
		Rarely hereditary

Table 29–3
Lab Aids to Microcytic Anemias

NORMAL	IRON DEFICIENCY	THALASSEMIA*	CHRONIC DISEASE	SIDEROBLASTIC
MCV 78–98 fl	<78	<70	N or <78	<78 to 110
Ferritin M 20–250 ng/ml (2–250 μg/L) F 12–250 ng/ml (12–250 μg/L)	<12**	N or ↑	20–1000 (usually ↑)	>250
Serum iron 65–175 μg/dL (12–32 μmol/L)	<30 μg/dL <5 μmol/L	N or ↑	<30 μg/dL <5 μmol/L	>200
TIBC 250–410 μg/dL 45–73 μmol/L	>360 μg/dL >64 μmol/L	N	<300 μg/dL <54 μmol/L	N
Transferrin saturation 25–50%	>16	N or ↑	<16	>80
Basophilic stippling	no	yes/no	no	yes/no
Marrow iron stores	absent	N or ↑	N or ↑	↑ Abnormal sideroblasts
RDW 12–15	16–24	<15	Variable, usually >15	>18

* in minor or intermediate cases
** diagnostic only if low; may be normal with infections, malignancies, severe liver disease
N = normal
RDW = red cell distribution width
M = male
F = female

transport proteins on a supporting submembrane lattice of spectrin and actin, which in turn control H_2O content in combination with an ATP energy-derived cation pump.

Hereditary Spherocytosis is the single most common membrane defect. It is inherited as an autosomal dominant by about 0.02% of the U.S. population. Classical findings often include neonatal jaundice, pallor, modest splenomegaly, abdominal pain (with gallstones), and after the neonatal period, intermittent non-obstructive jaundice. Patients may go for years with minimal symptoms or may experience waxing and waning periods of heightened hemolysis on aplasia following either viral or bacterial infections.

Hematologic findings include anemia, reticulocytosis, ↑ indirect reacting bilirubin, spherocytes, and increased osmotic fragility in hypotonic saline. The defect, which resides in the spectrin fraction of the membrane impairs membrane flexibility and results in splenic trapping. The RBC membrane in HS is also highly permeable to Na.

Treatment of choice is splenectomy, preferably after the patient reaches <3 years of age or at a time when the patient is responsive to active immunization with polyvalent pneumococcal and H. flu. Post-splenectomy penicillin is administered for ≥5 years. This approach applies to any splenectomized individual, irrespective of the underlying disorder.

Hereditary Elliptocytosis is twice as common but much less severe than HS. It is inherited as a single dominant, and codominant inheritance may be fatal. A peripheral blood film reveals prominent elliptocytosis. The defect resides in the spectrin-actin interface of the red cell membrane. It often presents in the newborn with prominent jaundice. The osmotic fragilities mimic that of HS.

Splenectomy is rarely if ever required, and HE is less pronounced in the older patient.

Cation Permeability Disorders induce minimal hemolysis, the result of either Na^+ or K^+ losses. In the former the picture is that of stomatocytosis, the result of ↑ H_2O absorption. In the K^+-loss group, the cells tend to desiccate (desiccocytosis).

Inheritance is unclear, and splenectomy is effective in the occasional serious case.

Disorders of Physical or Thermal Injury include the so-called "Waring Blender Syndrome" defects, which result from vascular damage and are known as microangiopathic hemolytic anemia. Mechanical factors, as in eddy currents initiated by prosthetic material (e.g., heart valves), may also effect similar findings which, on occasion, may be so severe as to initiate consumption of clotting factors, leading to DIC. Thermal injury produces a cell bubble effect, not unlike yeast, which has all the clinical and laboratory features of HS.

Paroxysmal Nocturnal Hemoglobinuria (PNH): See page 4.

METABOLIC DISORDERS

Hexose Monophosphate Pathway. G6PD deficiency is the classic example of the hexose monophosphate shunt disorder, with millions of people affected by a sex-linked inheritance of an abnormality that includes >100 variants. The 2 most common variants are the type that occurs predominantly in American Blacks and the type that is most common in the Mediterranean basin, or the more unstable "African" type.

The gene for G6PD is inherited as an X-linked recessive and is characterized by inability to summon electrons (e.g., hydrogen atoms) to respond to oxidant-induced membrane stress. Common inducers of oxidant stress are drugs and infections. With infections, hydrogen peroxide generated during phagocytosis is very likely the initiating agent. Drug-induced stress is produced by agents that impair the electron transfer system (the list is extensive). Fava bean-induced hemolysis occurs mainly in the Mediterranean population, is usually severe—even lethal—and may occur merely by inhalation of the pollen. Dopa quinone, a metabolite of L-DOPA, is a powerful oxidant, and is probably responsible for the severe hemolysis in a limited number of fava bean-sensitive populations. The reason for the dopa quinone effect is probably a distinctly separate, gene-related inability to metabolize L-DOPA.

Treatment consists of separation from the offending agent (when possible), aggressive hydration to minimize heme-induced renal damage, red cell transfusions for symptomatic anemia, and iron to replace hemoglobinuric losses. Counseling is a necessary prophylactic course.

Apart from the (often massive) hemoglobinuria, and the anemia and reactive reticulocytosis (which contain sufficient G6PD to limit further oxidant attack at the same dose level, e.g., tachyphylaxis), the peripheral smear reveals occasional red cells with retracted areas of hemoglobinization (blister cells) (Table 29–2).

Embden-Meyerhof Pathway. PK deficiency is the most common example of a glycolytic enzymopathy. Because the defect occurs subsequent to 2–3 DPG formation, patients with PK deficiency tend to be more symptomatic than those with G6PD deficiency. In addition, the abnormality is constant and not triggered by an external source. Although inherited as an autosomal recessive, the disease varies in severity, very likely due to subsets. Infection-induced marrow hypoplasia also adds to the severity.

Hematologic findings include chronic anemia of variable severity, reactive reticulocytosis, and nonspecific anisocytosis. All patients have degrees of splenomegaly. The hemolysis is entirely within the RE system.

Treatment may include red cell transfusion for symptomatic anemia. Splenectomy helps only in patients who develop hypersplenic events. Folate supplementation probably helps those individuals whose dietary folate is inadequate to replace red cell synthesis demands. Iron administration is contraindicated.

APLASTIC DISORDERS

Anemias characterized by normal MCHC and reticulocytopenia are hypoproliferative (anemia of marrow failure or ineffective erythropoiesis). Aplastic anemia is a classic example of such a disorder, although only rarely if ever is the marrow totally acellular. Scattered areas of trilineage activity are usually present in such individuals.

Acquired Disorders. Factors known to induce marrow aplasia include: ionizing radiation, aromatic hydrocarbons (e.g., benzene and toluene), virtually all anticancer agents, a variety of inorganic poisons (e.g., arsenicals), certain antimicrobials (e.g., chloramphenicol), anticonvulsants (e.g., phenylhydantoins), antithyroid agents (e.g., tapizol), hypoglycemics, mood elevators, insecticides (e.g., DDT), solvents (e.g., carbon tetrachloride), viruses such as those that cause hepatitis, bacterial agents (e.g., tubercle bacillus), and certain immune-mediate hemolytic anemias (e.g., PNH) that often terminate in either aplastic anemia or malignancy. In >1/2 of the affected population, the etiologic agent is unknown.

Inherited Disorders. Inherited, or constitutional aplastic anemia, also referred to as Fanconi Anemia and often accompanied by various combinations of abnormalities involving the skin, bones, and kidneys, has an associated high risk of late-occurring leukemia, usually of the monocytic type.

Aplastic anemia is usually slow in onset and characterized by petechiae, frequent infections, and signs and symptoms specifically related to low levels of circulating Hb. Hematologic findings, as noted, include reticulocytopenia with a normocytic-normochromic anemia, thrombopenia, and granulocytopenia. Marrow biopsy usually reveals skip areas of hematopoietic activity, most commonly lymphocytes and plasma cells, as well as reticulin, fat, and supporting tissue.

Severe aplastic anemia by definition is characterized by a reticulocyte count $\leq 0.1\%$, an absolute granulocyte count $\leq 500/mm^3$, and a platelet count $\leq 20{,}000/mm^3$. Iron turnover is marginal; the iron-binding protein (β_1 globulin, transferrin) is highly saturated, with much of the iron present in the reticuloendothelial system. Organomegaly is an uncommon finding and, when present, suggests an underlying malignancy, infectious disorder, or autoimmune process.

Treatment of choice for all severe aplastic anemias, including the Fanconi type, is bone marrow transplantation preferably with a matched related donor, with therapy designed to minimize GVHD. MUDs are acceptable, although they carry a high risk for severe GVHD and its associated ↑ in morbidity. The response to matched sibling donor BMT is a 75% disease-free survival leading to cure. In the absence of an appropriate donor, leukocyte-poor, carefully screened, and temporally sequenced red cell and platelet transfusions are needed in order to maintain adequate function and minimize the occurrence of alloimmunization and platelet refractoriness, respectively. Rigid infection surveillance is also warranted in order to minimize the chances of overwhelming sepsis. Red cell and platelet transfusions should be performed at levels of 6 g/L and 10,000/mm^3 or less, respectively. HLA-matched platelets are the preferred donor source.

The use of such cytokines as Epo, G-CSF, or GM-CSF has provided modest, albeit unsustained success, but only in the less severely affected patients. Combination IL-3 and Epo may prove to be somewhat more successful in effecting tri-lineage responses, but responses, when they occur, are sustained only as long as the cytokines are administered. In patients with evidence of T-cell–mediated suppression, the use of antithymocyte globulin, CSA, or even cyclophosphamide has achieved limited success. Spontaneous remissions occur in approximately 15% of cases and are essentially unpredictable. Combinations of corticosteroids and androgens offer only marginal responses.

SECONDARY ANEMIAS

Red cell hypoplasia or aplasia has been identified in patients with renal failure whose severity is roughly proportional to the degree of uremia. Both red cell mass and plasma volume are depressed in these patients, who are further compromised by a shortened red cell survival and bleeding secondary to impaired platelet function. Although platelet and white cell levels are usually normal, 10% of ESRD patients have granulopenia, apparently the result of HDL-induced suppression of granulopoiesis. Red cell deformation with helmet cells is a common feature of this disease.

Treatment. For anemic, uremic patients unresponsive to Epo (25 mg/kg twice weekly), carefully monitored red cell transfusion is the only efficacious therapy.

Deficiencies in pituitary, thyroid, adrenocortical, or gonadal hormonal function can produce a normochromic-normocytic anemia, although the anemia of thyroid deficiency may be microcytic and hypochromic, the result of inadequate foodstuff iron absorption in association with hypometabolic states; or macrocytic if the major inadequacy is folate.

ANEMIAS WITH MARROW DISRUPTION

Primary or marrow metastatic disorders, or marrow encumbered by increased numbers of metabolically inert cells (as in the lipid storage disease) may also lead to severe pancytopenia. Agnogenic myeloid metaplasia, a rare disease of unknown etiology resulting in marrow fibrosis accompanied by extramedullary myeloproliferation, ultimately results in pancytopenia with massive splenomegaly. The peripheral blood film is characterized by distorted and fragmented cells (ordinarily captured and removed from the circulation by the spleen), schiztocytes, tear drops, giant platelets, and immature forms. Proper diagnosis mandates proper evaluation of biopsy material. There is no known effective therapy. Fibrosis is relentless but usually slow (upwards of 5–7 years), and the disease terminates either in hematopoietic failure or refractory myeloid leukemia.

Splenectomy does not effect cures and may actually be counterproductive if the spleen is both reticulo-endothelial tissue and a major hematopoietic organ.

Sickle Cell Disease

Of the 200 known hemoglobinopathies, sickle cell disease is the most common and the most destructive. In most of these disorders, the physical defect is a single amino acid substitution in either the α, β, γ, or δ subunits. Virtually all the diseases are inherited as an autosomal codominant, and in the vast majority of cases detection is readily apparent by gel electrophoresis at variously adjusted pHs.

Molecular features of human Hb variants fall into 5 major groups of single or double amino acid substitution.

Examples of single substitution include Hb S, C, D, E, and G on the β chain, Hb I on the α chain, Hb F on the γ chain, and Hb A_2 on the δ chain.

Of the amino acid deletions identified to date, all are found on the β chain. None produces serious clinical findings, the classic sample being Hb Freiberg.

A third category is the fusion hemoglobins, which result in nonhomologous crossing over, e.g., Hb Lepore, a γ-β fusion with clinical findings consistent with the thalassemias.

A fourth group includes the elongated subunits, which have either a base substitution or a frame shift. An example of the former is Hb Constant Spring, and of the latter, Hb Wayne, both occurring on the α chain. There are no known β-chain frame shifts. Symptomatology is minimal.

A fifth classification includes the unstable hemoglobins: those producing the Heinz bodies and hemolysis, those with high O_2 affinity without cyanosis (e.g., familiar erythrocytosis), and those that result in cyanosis (e.g., M-hemoglobins). The unstable variants as well as the high O_2-affinity group, including the M-hemoglobins, appear only as heterozygotes. The homozygous state is felt to be lethal.

Of all African Americans, 1.5% are homozygous and 8% heterozygous for sickle cell disease. Of all homozygous sickle cell disease patients, 30% have approximately 80% of all the major symptomatology, and it is postulated, although unproven, that a haploid subtype of the disease accounts for the severity of findings. Sickle cell disease is the only hemolytic disorder marked by serious intravascular clotting. Major untoward events include strokes, relentless priapism, and infarction of any system, including the renal medulla or segments of the GI tract. Early in life, splenic sequestration presents a hazard and may result in >50% of the total blood volume being acutely trapped in the splenic circulation at a given time.

Treatment of sequestration includes cautious transfusion and monitoring for autoreinfusion of entrapped cells. Because of the propensity for repeated episodes, splenectomy following a second event is appropriate.

By 5–7 years of age, the spleen tends to shrink in size following repetitive infarctions, but it may be enlarged and become nonfunctional before it involutes.

It is likely that minor repetitive CNS infarctions account for changes in mental function. There are data to support the likelihood that CNS vascular reserve is impaired as a result of these episodes. Infarction-induced changes in the renal medulla impair concentrating ability; most SS patients consequently develop hyposthenuria by age 10, necessitating frequent trips to the drinking fountain and toilet.

The single most effective diagnostic test of hemoglobinopathy is electrophoresis of peripheral blood. Abnormal Hb can also be identified in utero via analysis of amniocentesis fluid. The solubility test, which depends on differences in the solubility of deoxyhemoglobin-S when compared to other hemoglobins, is far less reliable.

The pathophysiology of sickle disease results from β-chain substitution of valine for glutamine. It occurs in the deoxy form wherein Hb elongates into bundles of fibers which ultimately gel into "permanent" sickle forms. The extent of this phenomenon is controlled by the initiating insult and the nature of the associated β chain. A normal associated β chain (e.g., Hb A), as in sickle cell trait, ↓ the degree of gelation, whereas Hb C on the paired chain enhances this phenomenon. For example, homozygous (100%) deoxyhemoglobin-S requires 24 g Hgb S/100 ml red cells to induce gelation. Equal concentrations of deoxyhemoglobin-S and deoxyhemoglobin-C require 30 g/100 ml for gelation to occur, and equal concentrations of Hgb S and F require 36.9 g/100 ml. The obvious combination for maintenance of a symptom-free disorder is the S-F or the β-d combination. The net effect of the elongated and rigid red cells is obstruction of blood flow, initially at the capillary level and subsequently, as the clot propagates, to larger vessels. Reoxygenation may effect a reversal of sickle cells to a normal shape only prior to gelation, i.e., only prior to their assumption of the permanent sickled form. Prolonged minimal deoxygenation, abrupt severe deoxygenation, or an environment, will induce the appearance of irreversible, sickled forms, the most prominent symptom of which is pain and the worst finding of which is stroke.

Treatment. Pain crises require analgesia and hydration. The patient with a serious vascular event should receive exchange transfusion in order to maintain Hgb S <30% in the presence of a hematocrit ≤33% in order to minimize the risk of viscosity-induced stroke.

With impaired splenic function, there is an associated immunologic deficit, including diminution ion IGM production and opponization, the latter resulting in ↓ ability to recognize encapsulated organisms.

As a consequence, patients with Hb S disease or sickle cell Hb in combination with another abnormal Hb should receive pneumococcus, H. flu., and meningococcus vaccines. Because of the uncertainty of the efficacy of vaccination <2 years of age, all patients should also receive 5 years of penicillin, commencing in the first 4 months of life.

Sickle cell Hb electrophoretic patterns in older patients are the inverse of those of the newborn: i.e., 5% F and 95% S. By the time the patient presents to the doctor with local or diffuse pain, it is usually hard to distinguish between infarction and infection. Radionuclide scanning is helpful at times, but infections may include an infarction component, and many infarctions result in secondary infections. It is best to treat any suspected infarction as both infarction and infection, irrespective of the presence or absence of fever. Another area of major concern is the abdominal pain crisis. The distinction between sickle cell-induced abdominal pain crises and so-called "surgical" abdomens is the absence of bowel sounds, or the hypodynamic bowel, in sickle pain crisis. Bowel sounds in inflammatory bowel disease are hyperactive, save for the onset of typhlitis or septic shock.

Genetic counseling is a major therapeutic endeavor and is designed to enable parents to make decisions about risks and consequences. Male sickle cell disease patients produce variably viable sperm, and sickle cell disease females are generally able to conceive and bear children but only with careful Hb control and prolonged obstetrical monitoring.

For severe sickle cell disease, i.e., those with stroke or repeated infections/infarction, bone marrow transplantation is the treatment of choice.

Sickle cell disease can occur, as noted, with other hemoglobinopathies, including thalassemia and Hb C. Heterozygous Hgb S-Hgb C disease is less symptomatic than the former and occurs about 25% as commonly as Hb S disease, but it is almost as common among adults because of the diminished life expectancy of Hgb SS disease. Hgb CC anemia is mild to moderate, and includes target cells and occasional precipitated Hb clumps. Splenomegaly is common.

Red cell transfusion for sickle cell disease is rarely indicted. Its value is essentially limited to patients with prolonged symptomatic aplastic crises or who acquire "adult" Hb prior to surgery (reduction of S Hb to ≤30%) or who develop massive pneumonias with ineffective oxygenation. The advantage of supplemental folate (1 mg/day) as a means of addressing ↑ utilization needs remains controversial

- There are around 55 unstable hemoglobins, all of which cause varying degrees of hemolysis in the heterozygous state. The homozygous disorder is apparently lethal. The amino acid substitution occurs in the heme pocket of the β chain, which enhances oxidization to methemoglobin, following which the heme forms precipitate out (Heinz bodies). Symptomatology is minimal and does not require therapy

IMMUNOHEMOLYTIC ANEMIAS

Immunohemolytic diseases are characterized by a group of disorders in which hemolysis is mediated by autoantibodies of the IgG or IgM type and ≥1 components of complement—usually activated C3 and occasionally C4—coating the red cell. Antibody identification is carried out by the direct Coombs', aka antiglobulin, test. Antibodies of the IgG type coat, but do not agglutinate, red cells in vitro in the absence of antiglobulin, and are accordingly termed "incomplete antibodies." A direct positive test is the *sine qua non* of the immunohemolytic process. The indirect test detects serum antibodies. Any serum with suspected antibody is incubated for 30 min at 37° C with red cells, following which the serum is washed away and the red cells are treated with reagent to determine both presence and antibody specificity. Classification of immunohemolytic anemias includes chemical and structural relationships: (1) warm activation (primarily at body temperature), (2) cold activation (room temperature or lower), (3) whether it is an IgG (m.w. 160,000) or an IgM (m.w. 1,000,000), and (4) ability to activate complement. Warm antibodies do not injure the red cell membrane per se, although they bring about spheroid changes in shape and corresponding ↑ in osmotic fragility. In summary, the IgG antibodies have a m.w. in the 160,000 range, an optimal temperature of 37° C, little or no activation of complement, a positive direct Coombs' test, a frequently positive indirect Coombs' test, and only rare specificity but strong avidity for red cell antigens. Most of the cases of IgG autohemolytic anemia are of unknown etiology; approximately 20% are the result of drug-induced phenomena, and 10–15% the result of malignancies. Because of the "incomplete" nature of these antibodies and the fact that they rarely activate complement, phagocytosis occurs within the reticuloendothelial system, the net effect of the anemia being ↑ bilirubin production.

Antibodies that activate complement usually cause abrupt and extensive hemolysis, usually in the intravascular space, resulting in rapid utilization of haptoglobin and resultant levels of ≤5 mg. Unlike 7S warm (IgG) antibodies, the 19S cold (IgM) antibodies are optimally reactive at 2–4° C. Above 10° C, affinity ↓, and at about 30° C antibodies dissociate from the cell itself. In effect, IgM antibodies remain bound to red cell antigens only at low temperatures. Agglutination is therefore often limited to the peripheral circulation of the extremities. Warming an extremity may cause the disappearance of the cold antibody effect. In any suspected cases of cold antibody disease, studies ideally should be carried out at bedside using serially diluted anticoagulated blood drawn from a cold extremity in order to determine the lowest concentration at which hemagglutination is observed. Factors determining the potency of hemolysis include

- Mechanical destruction when cold exposure is accompanied by muscular exertion
- Complement activation inducing profound intravascular hemolysis
- Temperature controlling the distribution and reactivity of the antigen on the red cell membrane
- Antigen

Complement-mediated hemolysis is an orderly sequence of interactions that usually creates perforations in the red cell membrane. Activation begins with the C1q subunit. Conversion of C4 and C2 into activated components leads to an unstable complex activating C3, which, in turn, causes segments of C5–C9 to alter lipids and bind proteins, thereby creating membrane depressions. The properdin system is an alternate activation pathway that bypasses the first 3 components. Why one or the other of the pathways occurs is unclear, but either should be looked for in any patient with massive intravascular hemolysis leading to hemoglobinuria.

IgG disorders are usually self-limited but on occasion progress to a chronic and unremitting state. Icterus, as opposed to hemoglobinuria, is its common pathologic expression. Splenomegaly is a rare occurrence. Reticulocytosis and leukocytosis usually accompany hemolysis. In some patients there is an associated thrombocytopenia, aka Evan's syndrome. Drugs known to induce warm autoimmune hemolytic disease—such as quinine, quinidine, and sulfonamides—form an antigenic protein complex. Penicillin may also induce an autoimmune process that differs from other drug complexes in that the cell-drug complex is antigenic, which elicits IgG antibodies directed against penicillinized red cells.

Therapy for warm autoantibody disease depends on the underlying situation. Most patients respond to the administration of glucocorticosteroids, which poison monocyte function and impair lymphocyte (antibody) production. Patients refractory to corticosteroids usually respond to a high-dose gammoglobulin or splenectomy.

10% of patients are refractory to all forms of therapy. For any identifiable etiologic mechanism, effective treatment must eliminate the autoimmune process. Immunohemolytic anemia secondary to cold antibodies may occur in patients with mycoplasma pneumonia and similar infectious disorders or be associated with certain myeloproliferative diseases. Symptoms are due to a vasocclusion in portions of the circulation exposed to cooling. Hemolysis may range from mild to severe, with impressive amounts of intravascular lysis leading to free Hb, followed by conversion to methemoglobin and, following consumption of haptoglobin, to methemalbumin, which is then released in the kidneys as methemoglobinuria. Splenomegaly is uncommon.

Because the IgM is largely confined to the circulation, corticosteroids and/or hyperimmune globulin are not effective, and the single most effective approach is the intense use of plasmapheresis, usually every 3–4 weeks, until the process subsides. When transfusions are needed to raise the Hb levels in the severe cases, we must recognize the likelihood of an impaired cross-match, followed by an attempt to identify a basis for intravascular lysis and hemoglobinuria. In these situations, a large volume of IV fluids is required to "wash out" excess free Hb and avoid renal damage.

Microcytic, Hypochromic Anemias

IRON DEFICIENCY

The classic example of a microcytic, hypochromic anemia is iron deficiency. In the newborn infant, iron deficiency may be a consequence of premature delivery, or from nutrition inadequate to the task of supplying the growing hematopoietic mass.

Total body iron in a term infant is about 220 mg and in a 70 kg adult 3.5 g (range 2–5 g). In the newborn, 85% of the iron is in the red cell; in the adult, it is 65%. Smaller amounts are present in the tissues as storage iron, with significantly lesser amounts as enzyme and transport iron. With the exception of the actively menstruating female, iron requirements for a normal adult are very small—usually no more than 0.5 mg/kg per day. Iron-rich foods contain more than adequate amounts of iron and, save for the premature infant and/or the childbearing or menstruating female, iron supplementation is unnecessary.

Iron absorption is governed by demand and occurs in the duodenum and jejunum following a complex uncoupling process of apoferritin to ferritin. It is then transported in the plasma on a β_1-globulin (transferrin) to nursing cells in the marrow, where it is injected by pinocytosis into developing red cell precursors, at which point it is stored in the mitochondria for subsequent attachment to protoporphyrin to form heme.

Iron deficiency is not expressed clinically until iron stores are used up and demands for further utilization of iron go unmet. The net effect is a ↑ in the free transferrin and the appearance of hypochromic, microcytic anemia.

In the older patient, lassitude, stomatitis, esophageal webbing, koilonychia, and achlorhydria are progressive entities. In the term infant, the most common cause is inadequate dietary iron. In the adult, the most likely causes are GI bleeding and excessive menstrual losses. In the tropics, hookworm infestation plays a role.

Adult treatment consists of $FeSO_4$ or equivalent (1–3 x 325 mg) po qd between meals. Orange juice (citric acid) enhances iron absorption by hastening its valence change. Milk or milk products and cereals, impair iron absorption because of the high phosphate load characteristic of these and similar foodstuffs and which render the iron insoluble. Therapy is usually continued for about 3 months, by which time the anemia is corrected and the stores are replaced. Of all the iron preparations, ferrous sulfate tablets are the most effective and least expensive. Red cell transfusions are rarely, if ever, indicated. Parenteral iron is often prescribed when oral iron is intolerable. Intramuscular iron is never indicated.

Normal bound iron: 60–90 μg/dl; total iron bonding capacity: 180–270 μg/dl. Normal ferritin: 30–120 mg/dl (20–250 μg/ml). (See Table 29–3).

THALASSEMIAS

Unlike sickle cell disease and related disorders where defective globin production results in a shortened red cell life span, the thalassemias are characterized by impaired production of otherwise normally structured globin chains. The net result is ineffective erythropoiesis

- α-chain development begins early in fetal life; β-chain development begins shortly before parturition, with a typical distribution at birth as follows: 100% α chains, 75% γ chains, 25% β chains. By 6 months there is a 50% decline in γ-chain, and a corresponding ↑ in β-chain production. The significance of the embryonic chains, epsilon, zeta, etc., the production of which ceases at around the 12th week of gestation, is unknown

- Whereas β-thalassemia is characterized by ↓ synthesis, β°-thalassemia has essentially *no* β-chain synthesis. Save for β°-thalassemia, incorporation of radioactive material in β-thalassemia is ≤30% of that incorporated into the α chains
- Both α- and β-thalassemia are inherited as autosomal dominants: 50% chance for heterozygous offspring (25% chance for homozygous disease and 25% chance for normal offspring) from 2 heterozygous parents. β-thalassemia is common to the Mediterranean sub-basin of southern Italy and Greece. In the Orient, α-thalassemia is the common form. In Africa, both α- and β-thalassemia occur with almost equal frequency

In the heterozygous form, the anemia varies from nil to mild. In the homozygous form, anemia is severe and characterized by marked microcytosis, targeting, fragmentation, tear drops, and stippling. In heterozygotes, there is a corresponding elevation in δ-chain synthesis (Hb A_2) to 4–6% (normal, <3%) and in γ-chain synthesis (Hb F) to as much as 20%. Neither Hb A_2 nor Hb F is ↑ in heterozygous α-thalassemia. Although the reason for the differences in Hb F synthesis among the various β-thalassemia patients is unknown, those with ↑ Hb F synthesis tend to have milder symptoms than those who do not

- δ-β–thalassemia, an uncommon type, occurs as the result of deficient δ-β–chain synthesis and is accompanied by a corresponding ↑ in fetal δ-chain production to ≥5%. Hb Lepore is another uncommon disorder that consists of 2 α chains and the fusion products of 1 β and 1 δ chain. Both δ-β and Lepore disorders are essentially asymptomatic. However, the combination of Hb Lepore and β-thalassemia minor will produce a double heterozygote of Hb Lepore-β thalassemia minor, which is clinically indistinguishable from homozygous β-thalassemia. Although the thalassemias morphologically appear to be iron deficient, these patients have ↑ iron stores. Treatment would add further oxidant stress and ↑ the risks of already existing iron overload, progressing to irreversible hemosiderosis
- Clinically, homozygous thalassemia is classified as thalassemia major, a classification particularly germane to the β-thalassemias and which is expressed as severe (major) or moderate (intermedia). With the ↓ in β chains, there are ↑ numbers of residual, or unattached, α chains which, in the free form, are unstable and tend to precipitate out as inclusion bodies. These bodies damage the cell membrane and effect a corresponding ↑ in permeability, with concomitant loss of ATP and premature uptake by the reticuloendothelial system, leading to ↓ survival.

Untreated, β-thalassemia major results in severe debilitation. Blood transfusions and folate supplementation (the latter designed to address ↑ demands), in association with aggressive chelation therapy, will enhance life span and quality of life. However, transfusion carries a high risk of alloimmunization and hemosiderosis (even with aggressive chelation).

Overall, growth and development are poor. The typical habitus is one characterized by hepatosplenomegaly, massive medullary and extramedullary hematopoiesis, multiple exocrine disorders, and, as noted, transfusion-induced hemosiderosis

- Patients with Hb H disease have 20–30% β chains in tetrads (B^4). Typical findings include hypochromia, poikilocytosis, and mild anemia.

Treatment: With the exception of the occasional aplastic crisis, patients with Hb H disease uncommonly require blood transfusions. In the rare extreme case, splenectomy is moderately effective in combating the severity of the anemia.

Patients with a-thalassemia major have only tetrads of δ chains—e.g., Hb Bart—which, as the sole Hb, is ineffective in providing O_2 delivery. a-thalassemia homozygotes are virtually hypoxic and, if not still born, die within minutes of birth with classic hydropic features, including macerated placentae

Genetic counseling of heterozygotes is an important part of overall medical care. Prenatal diagnosis can be made by amniocentesis during the first trimester using either 2-dimensional chromatography or by polymerase chain expansion of DNA molecules.

Treatment of choice for thalassemia major is bone marrow transplantation. In the absence of an appropriately matched related or unrelated donor, blood transfusion, folate supplementation, and, in many cases, splenectomy (with immunization) represent the only life-sustaining alternatives

PORPHYRIAS

The porphyrias are a unique group of multisystem disorders with microcytic hypochromic anemia, characterized by ↑ production of uroporphyrins and their precursors—viz., aminulovulenic acid and porphrobilingen—as a result of blocks along various steps in the heme biosynthetic pathway.

Glycine and succinyl CoA combine to form ALA in the presence of ALA synthetase and pyridoxal phosphate. Condensation of 2 ALAs catalyzed by ALA dehydrase forms PBG, a red, H_2O-soluble compound which is a diagnostic end-product of acute intermittent porphyria.

Increased production of porphyrin or porphyrin precursors results in erythopoietic porphyria or hepatic porphyria. Erythropoietic porphyria is characterized by dermatitis with bullous lesions, stained teeth, ineffective production as well as ↑ destruction of red cells, and splenomegaly. As in hepatic porphyria, a less severe disorder of little hematologic significance, large amounts of uro- and coproporphyrin-1 are present in bone marrow cells as well as in urine, stool, and tissues. The light sensitivity of the fluorescent porphyrins causes the skin and teeth changes. PBG imparts a red color to the urine, which also fluoresces in the presence of UV light as the result of the concomitant presence of porphyrins. Tests that identify PBG also identify UBG, which is distinguished from the former compound by solubility; e.g., the addition of a fat solvent such as chloroform to a red solution suspected of being either PBG or UBG will entrap the UBG if it is present.

Treatment. Erythopoietic porphyria and erythropoietic protoporphyria require red cell transfusion support for maintenance of life. The only curative therapy is marrow transplantation, without which patients rarely live beyond 20–25 years of life.

Macrocytic (Megaloblastic) Anemias

The classic example of megaloblastic anemia is that secondary to vitamin B_{12} or folic acid deficiency. Megaloblastic anemia is a disorder resulting from impairment of DNA synthesis and involving changes in any or all hematopoietic cell lines. As a consequence, megaloblastic erythroid cells are larger (macro-ovalocytes), have a higher cytoplasmic-to-nuclear ratio, and possess more granular chromatin than do normal erythroid forms. The white cell series are also larger than their normal components and have strangely shaped nuclei with ragged chromatin which, in the mature form, become hypersegmented. Granulation tends to be deficient. Megakaryocytes are sometimes bizarrely shaped but may be normal in appearance.

MCVs usually exceed 100 μ^3 (Table 29–2); the reticulocyte count is low and sometimes absent. With progressive disease, erythroid precursors with obvious megaloblastic features may be found in the circulation. Neutrophil nuclei usually exhibit 5–6 segments, sometimes as many as 18 (Table 29–2). The marrow is usually cellular and characterized by megaloblastic transformation and frequent mitotic figures. Pancytopenia may ensue.

Clinically, the anemia is slow in onset and characterized by fatigue, shortness of breath. Patients appear both pale and lemony yellow.

Serum bilirubin, serum iron, LDH, and muramidase levels are invariably ↑.

FOLIC ACID DEFICIENCY

The role of the pterins in human nutrition assumed major importance following the discovery of pteroylmonoglutamic acid (folic acid), which consists of 3 components: a pteridine, an amino-benzoic acid, and a glutamic acid. Its nomenclature is N-(2-amino-4-hydroxpteridin-6-ethyl)-p-amino-benzoic acid, an acyl radical with the generic term "pteroylglutamate." The catalytic reduction of folic acid by dihydrofolate reductase to 5, 6, 7, 8-tetrahydrofolic acid ensures its role in enzyme reactions. Dihydrofolate reductase is sensitive to folic acid analogs, which contain the 4-amino group, which is the fundamental reason for its anticancer activity.

In humans, the major form of folate is N^5 methyltetrahydrofolic acid. The N^5 methyl group is a Leuconostoc Citrovorum growth factor, which accounts for one of its earlier names: Citrovorum factor. It is also commonly referred to as folinic acid. Functionally, this family of folate compounds, or 1-carbon constituents, serves as the source for DNA synthesis.

Although widely distributed in nature, the richest sources are vegetables such as asparagus, spinach, and lettuce. The minimum daily requirements for adults is 40–60 μg, and approximately twice that amount for the premature newborn.

Folates are absorbed primarily in the proximal jejunum. Most of what is ingested is absorbed, following which it is protein bound for transportation.

With both bioassay (Lactobacillus casei systems) and chemical assay, the normal range of bound serum folate is 4–20 ng/ml.

Folate deficiency leads to a megaloblastic anemia associated with glossitis, ↑ levels of LDH, and weight loss. Neurologic changes do not occur as a consequence of folic acid deficiency.

Typical laboratory findings include ↓ serum and red cell folate and ↑ excretion of folic acid intermediates (e.g., formaminoglutaic acid following a loading dose of histidine).

Infants fed solely goat's milk, which is essentially folate free, develop folic acid deficiency. Ascorbic acid participates in the reduction of folic acid to tetrahydrofolic acid. As a consequence, dietary deficiency of vitamin C may induce folic deficiency in an individual whose folate intake is marginal.

The commonest cause of folate deficiency is inadequate intake or aggressive cooking of foodstuffs. With poor intake, folate deficiency may become manifest in <3 months.

Malabsorptive disorders, so-called celiac diseases, and parasitic infestations induce folate deficiency because of changes in the GI mucosa. Oral administration of folic acid, even in the presence of celiac syndrome, will result in improvement in serum folate levels.

Certain pharmacologic agents (dilantin) may also impair folate absorption.

Additionally, oral contraceptives have been shown to block absorption.

Increased requirements are imposed by pregnancy or in patients with various chronic hemolytic anemias. Patients with severe anorexia secondary to neoplastic diseases profit from the additional administration of folic acid.

Folic acid antagonists used in the treatment of leukemia and related diseases interfere with the conversion of folic acid to tetrahydrofolate by blocking dihydrofolate reductase. This is corrected only via tetrahydrofolate (Citrovorum factor) administration.

Treatment of folic acid deficiency with as little as 1 mg/day for 7–10 days is sufficient to correct the disorder, but 5 mg is usually given to adults. Folinic acid is rarely needed in deficiency states.

VITAMIN B_{12} DEFICIENCY

Both ineffective production and ↑ hemolysis contribute to vitamin B_{12} deficiency anemia. Normal red cells transfused into B_{12}-deficient patients have ↓ survival.

The source of vitamin B_{12} in human nutrition is essentially tissues of animal origin as well as fish, eggs, and milk. The total daily dietary requirement is 2–5 μg.

Because vitamin B_{12} is stored and re-used deficiency states take 2–3 years to develop after cessation of B_{12} ingestion. Functionally, vitamin B_{12} is a cyanocobalamin molecule.

Systems impaired by vitamin B_{12} deficiency include those involved with methionine-methyl synthesis (which relates ultimately to tetrahydrofolic regeneration) and methylmelanyl coA isomerization (which relates to metabolism of proprionic acid). The impairment in DNA synthesis accounts for the megaloblastic transformation and all related features. More specifically, defective methylmelanyl coA metabolism impairs the neurologic processes, a feature prominent in such patients. Absorption occurs in the ileum following its conjugation with parietal cell secreted intrinsic factor, which is enhanced by histamine, methacholine, and gastrin production and eliminated by gastrectomy.

Plasma B_{12} levels are 150–500 pg/ml, all of which is transcobalamine bound.

Transcobalamines prevent loss of body secretions and provide transport through cell membranes. Transcobalamine-2 is the initial transport mechanism. Transcobalamine-1 carries most of the vitamin B_{12} in plasma, and the role of transcobalamine-3 is uncertain, although much of it appears to rise from granulocytes. Neurologic abnormalities consist of combined system disease of the spinal cord. Vitamin B_{12} levels are determined by bioassay or isotope dilutions. In the absence of a coexisting folate deficiency, folate levels are ↑ in the presence of vitamin B_{12} deficiency.

Vitamin B_{12} deficiency is rarely the result of inadequate diet except in Vegans. It is most often due to

- Diminished intestinal absorption, secondary to either intrinsic factor deficiency (defective synthesis or antibody blocked)
- Gastric resection
- Overgrowth of intestinal bacteria, as in the blind loop syndrome
- Intestinal statis
- Infestation by the vitamin B_{12}-utilizing fish tapeworm
- Organic disease of the bowel wall itself, or
- Increased requirements during pregnancy and in premature infants

Occasionally, low folate levels may give a falsely low B_{12} result.

The term "pernicious anemia" is reserved for deficiencies of intrinsic factor irrespective of the basic underlying pathology.

The Schilling test measures absorption of vitamin B_{12} and is an effective means of identifying the various etiologic factors. Variations of this test with and without intrinsic factors are available.

Treatment. Response to therapy is dramatic. As little as 100 μg of cyanocobalamine will induce a marked reticulocyte rise, and maintenance with 100-1,000 μg every 4-6 weeks will maintain adequate levels. Most patients are given 4 x 1,000 μg over 2-3 weeks as a loading dose and then maintained on 1,000 μg IM monthly for the rest of their lives.

It is inappropriate to treat vitamin B_{12}-deficient patients with folic acid unless there is an associated folic acid deficiency, in which case both folate and B_{12} are used simultaneously. In the solely B_{12}-deficient patient, folate administration will produce a modest hematologic response and a marked impairment in the neurologic abnormalities.

DISORDERS OF HEMOSTASIS

Patient may bleed inappropriately, clot excessively and undesirably, or have disorders where combinations of these occur. The individual patient's problem must be accurately diagnosed, often in a stepwise fashion, as appropriate management must be precisely directed. A brief understanding of the systems involved in hemostasis and of the tests that may be applied to localize defects within the system is essential before proceeding to list clinical problems and their management.

Hemostasis is complex and by no means fully understood. Its major components are

- The vessel wall: Musculature, endothelial lining, products
- Blood platelets: Contractile mechanisms, products, surface characteristics
- Blood leukocytes: Relationships with platelets and vessel walls; production or surface siting of coagulation proteins
- Hemostatic factors: Classical coagulation factor pathways, natural coagulation inhibitors, fibrinolytic factors, inflammatory cascade factors influencing coagulation

Table 29–4 illustrates the characteristics of blood coagulation factors. Figures 29–1 to 29–4 demonstrate some of the characters of these systems; tests that are relevant to various components of these systems are listed in Table 29–5.

Diagnosis

Unexpected bleeding in the newborn (e.g., from the umbilical cord or from needle stick punctures) and major bleeding events (such as intracranial hemorrhage or scalp hematomas) arising within the first few days of life should raise the possibility of a quantitative or qualitative deficiency of a clotting factor. In those societies where circumcision is performed at this time, undue bleeding following this procedure is also especially significant.

Assuming that vitamin K has been given, assessment should take place as follows

- If not already available, a thorough family history for bleeding disor-

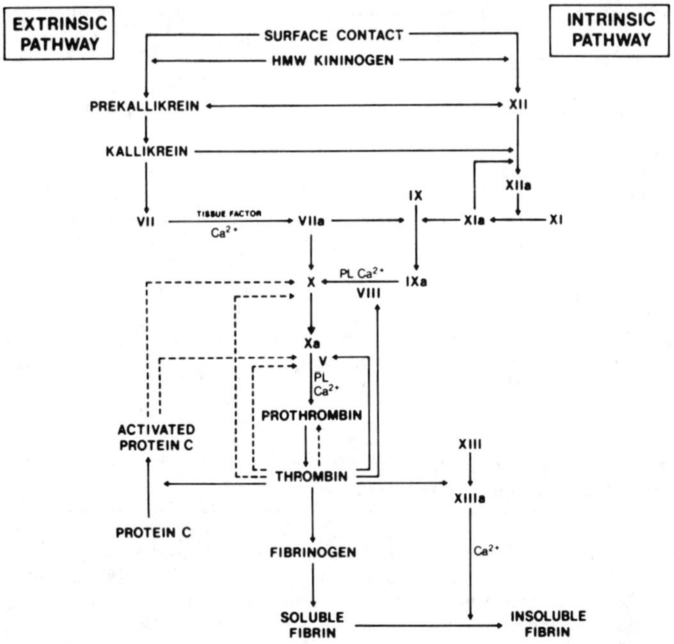
EXTRINSIC PATHWAY
INTRINSIC PATHWAY
SURFACE CONTACT
HMW KININOGEN
PREKALLIKREIN
XII
KALLIKREIN
XIIa
IX
VII
TISSUE FACTOR
Ca2+
VIIa
XIa
XI
PL Ca2+
X
IXa
VIII
Xa
V
PL
Ca2+
PROTHROMBIN
ACTIVATED PROTEIN C
XIII
THROMBIN
XIIIa
PROTEIN C
FIBRINOGEN
Ca2+
SOLUBLE FIBRIN
INSOLUBLE FIBRIN

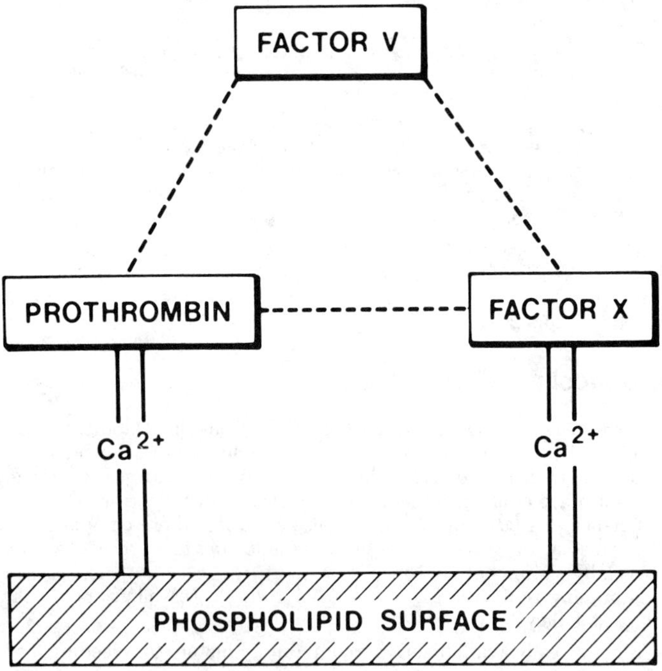
FACTOR V
PROTHROMBIN
FACTOR X
Ca2+
Ca2+
PHOSPHOLIPID SURFACE

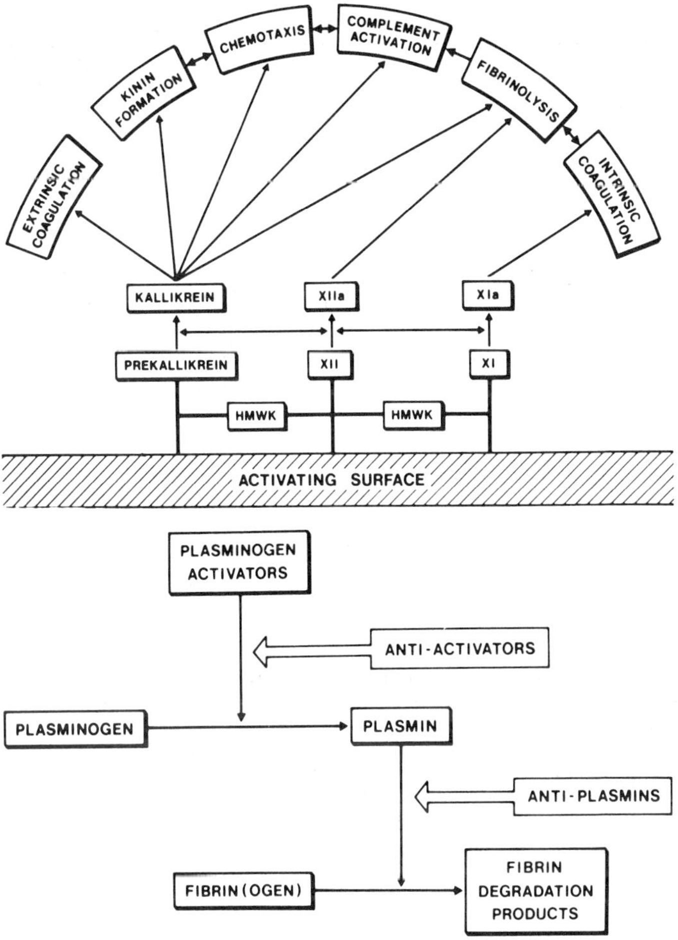

Figures 29–1–4. Characteristics of blood coagulation systems.

ders must be undertaken. Even if this is negative, if there is a strong suspicion that a factor deficiency is involved, the neonatal period is often an excellent occasion in which to take blood samples from relatives. With a definitive family history, it should be possible to institute therapy as soon as screening or assessment blood tests have been done, without waiting for results

- In the absence of a positive family history, a drug history must be taken. Anti-convulsants may have an effect on K vitamin-dependent coagulation-factor production and, rarely, other maternal medications may be significant
- If no "leading" information is available, then the routine screening tests for the commoner coagulation defects should be carried out (prothrombin time [INR], PTT, and fibrinogen level). A plasma sample should be retained frozen for a more precise factor assay. *Bleeding time*

Table 29–4
Characteristics of Blood Coagulation Factors

FACTOR NUMBER	COMMON SYNONYM	APPROX. MOLECULAR WEIGHT	APPROX. PLASMA HALF-LIFE (HRS)
I	*Fibrinogen*	340,000	120
II	*Prothrombin*	68,000	85
III	*Tissue factor*	. . .	. . .
IV	*Calcium ions*	. . .	. . .
V	Labile factor	350,000	15
VII	Stable factor	60,000	5
VIII	Antihemophiliac factor	1,200,000	14
IX	Christmas factor	55,000	20
X	Stuart-Prower factor	63,000	60
XI	Plasma thromboplastin antecedent (PTA)	160,000	60
XII	Hageman factor	82,000	60
XIII	Fibrin stabilizing factor	350,000	100
. . .	*High-molecular weight kininogen (HMWK)*	110,000	. . .
. . .	*Prekallikrein*	80,000	. . .

Note: Italicized synonyms indicate that the synonym is used more commonly than the factor number.

determinations: The bleeding time is of little value in the newborn as a screening test, but the observation of protracted or recurrent bleeding (e.g., from heel prick) is important

- The most common factor deficiencies are the hemophilias and related disorders. Factor VIII, IX, and vWD and, less likely, Factor XIII, V, VII, and dysfibrinogenaemias (fibrinogen is Factor I, but name rather than Factor number tends to be used clinically).
- *Hemophilia:* in hemophilia A, Factor VIII deficiency–the role of mole-

Table 29–5
Clotting Problems and Relevant Tests

Platelet defects	Bleeding time (template) Aggregation (aggregometer) Adhesion (glass beads)
Platelet numbers (thrombocytopenia or thrombocythemia)	Platelet count
K-dependent factor defects (qualitative and quantitative) (V, VII, X)	Prothrombin time (I.N.R.)
VIII, IX, V, XI, XII deficits	Partial thromboplastin time (APTT or ≡)
Anticoagulants (natural or added)	PT ± APTT
Fibrinogen defects	Thrombin time (TT) Direct fibrinogen assay
Fibrinolysis	Fibrin degradation products (FDPs, XDPs, D-Dimer)

cule in Factor X activation and thereby thrombin formation is well recognized. The carrier mother may be unaware of her status, new mutations occur in hemophilia (at a rate of as high as 25%), and bleeding due to Factor VIII (C) deficiency may occur in females. The Lyonisation hypothesis for activation of the X chromosome would account for a small percentage of carrier females who have very low Factor VIII C levels, and, of course, individuals with a single X chromosome (Turner's syndrome) might also be unfortunate enough to have the hemophilia gene on this chromosome. The diagnosis is usually made in newborn males who are severely affected. 10% of hemophiliac infants may be expected to show bleeding in the newborn period. Circumcision bleeding, intracranial hemorrhage and cephalohematomas, and bleeding from the umbilical cord stump are probably the most common sites of bleeding in these newborn. *Diagnosis*: A PTT >50 seconds in the presence of a normal prothrombin time (no >2 seconds prolonged over the top of the normal range for your laboratory) would make one suspect hemophilia A. The test is repeated adding a normal pooled plasma sample that will correct it if due to a factor deficiency (but in the presence of an anticoagulant mimicking Factor VIII deficiency, normalization of the APTT will not take place). A specific coagulation factor assay should then be carried out using correction tests and antigenic determination against a precipitable antibody. The approach for Hemophilia B is very much the same as that for A, and vWD rarely presents and is quite difficult to diagnose in the newborn. Although the Type 3 might show itself by bleeding from the umbilical stump or following heel prick, only in this form the bleeding time is markedly prolonged.

Most individuals with congenital acquired defects of coagulation (both bleeding and clotting tendencies) develop symptoms in childhood or adult life. Some will come to light as a result of family studies, some will bleed on provocation (dental extraction, minor surgery, trauma), and others will be investigated for, e.g., epistaxis or unexpected menstrual spotting. Another group will come to light because of apparently unprovoked thrombosis. Some will have mixed thrombotic and hemostatic problems, and sometimes the state of the vessel wall itself will contribute toward bleeding. Conditions include

- Thrombocytopenias and thrombopathies
- Factor deficiencies
- Thrombotic states
- Mixed thrombotic/bleeding states (DIC and TTP)
- Acquired inhibitors of clotting factors

FUNCTIONAL PLATELET DISORDERS

Most are discovered during the investigation of the patient with a bleeding problem. They are characterized by a bleeding time (>10 min). Aspirin, NSAIDs, penicillins, and cephalosporins can cause platelet dysfunction. A few rare hereditary thrombopathics are difficult to distinguish from each other: Glanzmann's thrombopathy, Bernard Soulier Syndrome, vWD variants, Glycoprotein 1a deficiency, the grey platelet syndrome, and Storage pool deficiency. In these disorders membrane defects and platelets associated with poor adhesion or aggregation can be found. There is usually a positive family history. Management, if indicated, is by platelet transfusion or bone marrow transplantation.

Inherited Coagulation Defects

HEMOPHILIA A

Hemophiliacs are graded for severity according to the percentage of Factor VIII coagulant present (VIIIC). The most severe have <2%, moderate 2–10%, and mild >10% normal levels. Severe hemophiliacs will have persistent abnormal bleeding at any site, although characteristically into the joints, muscles, and soft tissues. This is an enormous problem, especially during early childhood, and if untreated will result in considerable morbidity and crippling deformations. Bleeding from cuts is often unimpressive, and epistaxis, e.g., tends only to follow injury. Occasionally intrarenal or GI hemorrhage, or hematuria occur. Individuals tend to follow the same disease bleeding pattern throughout their childhood. Those with moderate or mild hemophilia tend to bleed only after significant trauma, dental extraction, surgery, etc. These divisions are guidelines only and shouldn't influence management in an individual patient.

The individual should regularly attend a hemophilia clinic and wear an identity bracelet or hemophilia card. The parents should be aware of the problem.

Treatment of the Acute Bleeding Episode. The principle of treatment is to raise the Factor VIII C level to 2–4 times its basal level and hopefully bring it into the lower end of the hemostatic functional range. Many mildly affected hemophiliacs benefit from Desmopressin (DDAVP) 0.3 μg/kg in saline by IV infusion, but this can only be used for a few days as patients may be refractory to a second dose. When a major bleeding episode has occurred, most hemophiliacs, and certainly severely affected ones as well as many mildly affected ones, will need Factor VIII concentrates. Enough needs to be given to raise the Factor level to about 50% of the normal value and to keep it there for 3–4 days. Many older hemophiliacs will present early on during the bleeding episode, as they are aware that this is taking place and that rapid induction of treatment can often prevent a more severe episode. As little as 15 U/kg of Factor VIII may abort a major hemarthrosis. Brief periods of bed rest only are usually recommended, and rapid mobilization in the case of muscle and joint problems is currently recommended with physiotherapy under cover with Factor VIII concentrate. Adequate analgesia is necessary during the acute event; drugs such as acetaminophen (paracetamol) and codeine are recommended. Aspirin is contraindicated.

Patients with head injuries should receive a CT or equivalent scan. All hemophiliacs with head injuries should be hospitalized and given prophylactic Factor VIII treatment. If there is documented evidence of intracranial hemorrhage, therapy should normalize their factor levels initially and they should be so treated for 10–14 days thereafter. Neurosurgery is not contraindicated in these patients.

Dental treatment is a problem in hemophiliacs. First dentition gives surprisingly little trouble, and fillings under local anesthetic could be covered without factor replacement treatment (use DDAVP). Extractions certainly need to be covered as well as being given tranexamic acid 25 mg/kg tid for 5 days. Surgery such as sinovectomy should be covered in much the same way as intracranial hemorrhage; levels should be maximized initially to approaching 100% and kept around 50% for the next 10 days.

Prophylactic Treatment. Depending on the programs available, severely affected boys with frequent hemorrhages may need prophylactic treatment with Factor VIII concentrate. 20 U/kg twice a week IV is effective, and parents can be trained to give such treatment, as indeed can older hemophiliacs themselves. DDAVP before scheduled minor surgery reduces the need for blood products.

Treatment of the Hemophiliac with an Inhibitor. 5–10% of patients with hemophilia will develop antibodies to Factor VIII. This makes their bleeding much more difficult to control because of their inability to have their Factor VIII levels ↑ by concentrates. The factors influencing both the development and the aggressiveness of antibody production are poorly understood and may be genetic. They present a considerable management problem and, if low levels of inhibitors are present (<10 plasma U), they may respond to increasing the dose of Factor VIII concentrate. The clinical response is clearly critical rather than the measurement of the rise in plasma units. The use of recombinant Factor VIII, prothrombin complexes, and activated Factor VIII may be of value, and porcine Factor VIII has been lifesaving in covering severe serious bleeds. However, this is highly antigenic, and its use in any one individual is bound to be very limited. Exchange plasmapheresis to reduce the inhibitor has been used. DDAVP appears to retain its effectiveness, presumably because native Factor VIII may be less affected by antibody. Certainly any hemophiliac who has received numerous Factor VIII concentrates should have his antibody status checked, especially before planned surgery. Differing administrative schedules for Factor VIII use and even immunosuppressive treatment have been promoted to minimize this problem. Success seems to be variable at best.

VON WILLEBRAND'S DISEASE

The vWF, genetically controlled form chromosome 12, is non-Vitamin K dependent and produced by the endothelium. It acts as a cofactor with VIIIC and, because of its action in facilitating platelet adhesion to the endothelium, its manifestations are largely those of a bleeding tendency rather than a hemostatic defect. However, because it "carries" VIIIC, there is often a functional ↓ in this factor that may be enough to give a coagulation defect as well.

Diagnosis. If there is a bleeding diathesis associated with a prolonged bleeding time, in the presence of a normal platelet count and in the absence of drugs such as aspirin, some form of vWD may be present (excluding acutely ill patients who may have acquired severe disorders of hemostasis). The APTT, *always* prolonged in hemophilia A, is not diagnostic of vWD although it is *often* prolonged. Similarly, the Factor VIIIC level is *often* but not *always* below the normal range. The vWF antigen may be quantitated immunologically. Most patients with vWF deficiency will have absent or reduced ristocetin-induced platelet aggregation. However, one type (2B) behaves aberrantly in this fashion. A direct assay for the ristocetin cofactor is probably the best assay for the diagnosis.

Table 29–6 shows the main subtypes of vWD; this is an incomplete description and new subtypes continue to be described. The types are based on the quantity and quality of polymer (multimer) circulating or found on platelets. The largest multimers appear to be most effective in attaching to platelets. In type 1 vWD, these forms are still detectable; type 2 shows loss of these large multimers and generally speaking the disease is worse than type 1. Type 3 shows minimal levels of all components of the VIII vWF complex and tends to resemble hemophilia with the addition of vWD, and often presents in infancy.

Table 29–6
Classification and Characteristics of von Willebrand's Disease

TYPE	B.T.	VWF PLASMA	VIIIC LEVEL	MULTIMER	PL. AGG (RISTO)	RISTO COFACTOR
I	Inc	reduced	reduced	normal	normal or ↓	reduced
IIa	"	normal or ↓	normal or ↓	large absent	reduced	reduced
IIb	"	"	"	"	enhanced	normal or ↓
IIc	"	"	"	small and abnormal	reduced	reduced
III	"	"	"	variable and abnormal	very reduced	reduced

Management. This depends largely on the type and severity of the vWD. DDAVP (Desmopressin) seems to be the treatment of choice for type 1 and certainly transiently corrects the bleeding time. It is less effective in type 2, but subtype 2a may respond relatively well. Tranexamic acid is sometimes recommended with DDAVP for its effect on inhibiting plasminogen activation. Factor VIII concentrates need to be used in the remainder of vWFs but do have a variability of vWD multimer content. Cryoprecipitate, however, contains everything needed to correct the defects in vWD but, of course, like any biological product, carries the risk of disease transmission, however well the donor is screened. Single-donor rather than pooled units should always be used if possible.

Individuals with vWD bruise easily and bleed from cuts and from the gums and nose. Menorrhagia is also common, and some of the most severe type-3 vWDs have tissue and joint hemorrhages characteristic of classic hemophilia. Most cases, however, are very mild and are diagnosed in family studies or because of bleeding, e.g., following dental extraction. It is thought that the incidence may be as high as 1% of the population at large.

FACTOR IX DEFICIENCY (HEMOPHILIA B; CHRISTMAS DISEASE)

Most of what has been said about classic hemophilia (Hemophilia A) is true for Hemophilia B. It is about 5 times less common than Hemophilia A, the frequency being 1 per 10,000 of the population. Factor IX is produced by the liver and is Vitamin K dependent. The APTT is still the best screening test to indicate that this form of hemophilia is present, and direct estimation of the Factor IX level would confirm the diagnosis. Unlike classic hemophilia, where a dysfunctional form of the clotting factor appears to be present, Factor IX-deficient individuals may also have failure to synthesize the molecule in any form. Carriers are often highly symptomatic in this disorder as well. Other variations from classic hemophilia include a lesser tendency to form antibodies, and the relatively long half-life of Factor IX means that less frequent doses need to be given.

Management is as for Hemophilia A, but IX concentrate rather than VIII is used.

Acquired Coagulation Factor Deficiencies

HEPATIC FAILURE

Most patients with established hepatocellular failure will have some abnormality in their coagulation tests (see prothrombin time and APTT) but are often asymptomatic insofar as their coagulation is concerned. It has to be remembered that some of both procoagulant- and anticoagulant-produced factors depend on hepatocytes and Vitamin K for their synthesis. If there is a coagulopathy associated with liver disease, it is always worth giving Vitamin K in adequate amounts (1 mg I.M. as a test dose) initially. If, however, factor replacement is necessary (e.g., for an investigative or surgical procedure), then covering with FFP to bring the prothrombin time to within about 3 sec of normal and the APTT to within about 5 sec of normal should be adequate. Fibrinogen levels tend not to be markedly diminished in stable liver disease, and fibrinogen itself or cryoprecipitate rarely needs to be given.

CHRONIC MALABSORPTION SYNDROMES

These present with a functional Vitamin K deficiency and a hemostatic defect that is correctable by I.M. Vitamin K.

DISSEMINATED INTRAVASCULAR COAGULATION

This condition invariably presents with bleeding. However, thrombosis in small vessels can be the main feature (e.g., in hemolytic uremic syndrome or TTP). DIC has been reported in several clinical situations: Infections, malignancies, obstetric emergencies, following major surgery, and a host of other conditions. Patients with clinically significant DIC show a consumptive coagulopathy associated with heightened fibrinolysis: Low levels of those factors which are consumed in the coagulation process, particularly Factors V, VIII, and X, and fibrinogen and prothrombin themselves. Thus, both the prothrombin time and APTT or equivalent will be prolonged. In addition, platelets will be consumed; sometimes markedly so, especially in states where bone marrow function is impaired (e.g., leukemias, severe infections). The procoagulant side of DIC that results in thrombin formation also triggers protein C activity and plasmin formation. This degrades the increased amount of fibrin produced, resulting in an excessive level of fibrin split products: Fragments X, Y, D, and E. Most laboratories are capable of measuring ≥1 of these.

5–10% of patients who develop acute myeloid leukemias have a partially differentiated promyelocytic form and its characteristic cytogenetic karyotype (15 17 T). Many patients have died of hemorrhage either prior to or during induction treatment. The role of the leukemic cells in activating DIC is still not completely certain, but the syndrome, if unrecognized, carries a considerable mortality.

The principal treatment of DIC is the removal of the underlying insult. However, while this is being managed, the patient will need to be supported through the period of risk from DIC. Replacement of clotting factors, usually with fresh frozen plasma and, if necessary, cryoprecipitate or even Factor VIII concentrates, should be undertaken. Assuming that thrombocytopenia is present, platelet concentrates should also be given. The use of these products should be monitored by INR, APTT, and platelet counts. There is no merit in giving fresh blood that cannot be obtained by specific correction of factors as described above. Hb levels, however, should be maintained, as should adequate BP; shock itself may contribute to DIC. Prednisolone and heparin have been recommended for the treatment of DIC, but their firm role has never been established. Generally, defibrinolytic treatment is said to be contraindicated, but newer antiproteases such as Aprotinin may well be strikingly valuable in this situation, especially for shortterm use.

HEMOLYTIC UREMIC SYNDROME AND THROMBOTIC THROMBOCYTOPENIC PURPURA

These syndromes represent microangiopathies with clotting and are predominantly those of intravascular coagulation. The former is associated in childhood with a febrile illness and is characterized by renal failure. TTP affects adults where many of the manifestations are neurologic, variable, and difficult to assemble diagnostically. It has been suggested that abnormally high levels of vWF may be related to the onset of both these diseases. HUS tends to be self-limiting and, with supportive care and, if necessary, renal dialysis, recovery can be expected.

Treatment of TTP is uncertain, but plasmapheresis is of proven value.

ACQUIRED INHIBITORS OF COAGULATION

Apart from inhibitors acquired in hemophilia itself, by far the commonest is the lupus anticoagulant. This is so called because of its association with SLE or other autoimmune disorders, but can certainly be diagnosed in the absence of these underlying problems. The anticoagulant itself is an immunoglobulin that reacts with platelet membranes, particularly activating prothrombin production. Patients with the lupus anticoagulant therefore are at risk from clotting as well as bleeding, and principally show thromboses, pulmonary embolism, and, in pregnant women, a high incidence of abortion. Patients with the lupus anticoagulant will not often need treatment as they will not have a bleeding problem. Corticosteroids diminish or abolish the clotting abnormalities, as will immunosuppressive drugs.

OTHER CONDITIONS ASSOCIATED WITH COAGULATION FAILURE

Patients receiving massive blood transfusions may develop dilution of clotting factors and platelet deficiencies. Patients receiving plasmapheresis or on extracorporeal circulation may also show the same phenomena and citrate intoxication may complicate this. Such patients may need replacement clotting factors and platelets.

Thrombotic Disorders

The natural hemostatic balance is maintained by inhibitors of the procoagulation system, and fibrinolytic mechanisms. The level of natural coagulation inhibitors is normally genetically regulated, and they include protein C, S, and ATIII

- Protein C deficiency can present at any age from the neonatal period onward; presentation neonatally is usually of DIC-like syndrome characterized by a widespread thrombosis and purpura; most such patients often die during this period. Most, however, present later, and the heterozygotes of the autosomal variety will have characteristically recurrent venous thromboses. Protein C is Vitamin K dependent and is produced by the liver, as are many other coagulation factors. Its level is also affected by Warfarin treatment, so its assay, which is usually immunologic, cannot be carried out in patients who are on this anticoagulant. Family studies in individuals with protein C deficiency are essential, especially in the recessive type, and antenatal diagnosis is now possible. Management is generally with Warfarin, but human Protein C concentrates may become available. Factor IX concentrates are also rich in Protein C. Although Warfarin is the treatment of choice in adults, in children, of course, with indefinite administration of the drug there may be longterm problems with bone growth and development

- Protein S acts as a cofactor for Protein C. Two types of patients have been described: One with Protein S complexed to C4B binding protein and less available functionally, and another where manufacture of the protein seems to be severely affected. Few cases have been reported, but the management would appear to be similar to that for Protein C deficiency
- ATIII deficiency is probably incompatible with life in the homozygous form, and heterozygotes are variably affected, but rarely in the neonatal period (1 or 2 cases have been reported, but they have been homozygous cases). Children and adults have a tendency to both venous and arterial thromboses, and as ATIII provides most of the plasma antithrombin activity, the chance of being affected by recurrent venous thrombus or embolism is almost 100%. Treatment with heparin is effective in the short term, and longterm anticoagulation with Warfarin is usually recommended
- Problems of the vessel wall: Vasculidities include mainly the so-called allergic purpuras (Henoch Schönlein type), some drug-induced purpuras that are non-thrombocytopenic, and those associated with a variety of infections. Rarely such purpuras may also be seen because of defects in connective tissue or paraproteinemias
- Allergic purpuras occur most often in children or adolescents but can be seen at any age, usually as an acute illness with systemic symptoms such as headache, fever, or abdominal or joint pain. The purpura, which is often over the joints, fingers, or ear tips, may be accompanied by urticaria or erythema. Frank hemorrhage may often occur, and renal involvement resembling acute nephritis may be found. There are no characteristic blood findings, but the vascular injury has been demonstrated to be a result of IgA based immune complexes, and IgA levels may be ↑ in some cases of the disease. Drug-induced vascular purpuras may have a similar skin lesion, but patients are usually less ill. Treatment is supportive.

Platelet Disorders: Thrombocytopenias and Thrombopathies

In the adult the normal platelet count is 150–400 x 10°/l. Platelet counts of 450–1,000 may be seen in patients with chronic hemolytic disease, severe iron deficiency and malignancy, and following splenectomy.

Thrombocytopenia is due to either failure of platelet production or increased platelet loss. Some causes of impaired platelet production include

- Aplastic and hypoplastic anemias

- Vitamin B_{12} or folate deficiency
- Occupation of the marrow by, e.g., tumor, leukemia, or fibrosis
- Anti-tumor chemotherapy

Disorders causing increased platelet loss include

- Immune (iso- and auto-) thrombocytopenic purpuras (iso-, e.g., associated with previous platelet transfusions or pregnancy; autoimmune, e.g., ITP; other immune purpuras associated, e.g., with SLE or hemolytic anemia—Evans' Syndrome)
- Hypersplenism with platelet sequestration
- Consumptive coagulopathies (DIC, TTP, and some vascular purpuras)
- Drugs can cause both immune and occasionally non-immune thrombocytopenias

IMMUNE THROMBOCYTOPENIC PURPURAS

ITP occurs in about 4 per 100,000 children per year and a lesser incidence in adults. Most cases present acutely, often after viral illnesses, and a number may be associated with infectious mononucleosis. A few present in the chronic phase. The acute disease manifests with the sudden onset of spectacular bruising with widespread petechiae and purpuric lesions. There is often epistaxis and occasionally conjunctival or retinal hemorrhages. Hematuria, intra-joint bleeding, or widespread ecchymoses often point to coagulation defects rather than ITP. Physical examination is otherwise unremarkable, and it is said that splenomegaly does not occur in this condition. Frequent splenic palpation may cause subcapsular hemorrhages or rupture, so they should be limited and gentle. The pathologic findings include platelet counts of levels such as 10 x 10°/l, and recent studies have shown the presence of platelet-associated immunoglobulins, including IgM and IgG antibodies and to Glycoproteins 1V, 2V or 3A. It is assumed that these are virally induced but also recognize a platelet-based antigen. The rest of the blood count should be normal, but if there is any doubt, bone marrow aspirate should be undertaken, especially if steroids are to be given, as the steroids might mask, e.g., an underlying leukemia. The marrow shows plentiful megakaryocytes and is otherwise normal.

Management of Acute ITP. The disease is often self-limiting, but the impressive clinical findings and the occasional risk of cerebral hemorrhage indicate positive management. Although there are no good data regarding survival of patients given different treatment, conventionally, Prednisolone in doses of 1 mg/kg/day until the platelet count rises to normal levels and then reduced over the next 6 weeks would be orthodox treatment. IVIG may be equally effective, but individuals given Prednisolone can often be quickly discharged from hospital and monitored easily on an outpatient basis. Most individuals will remit and spontaneously be cured on this regimen, but a few, often identifiable by suboptimal responses, will become cases of chronic ITP.

Chronic ITP may well have a somewhat different etiology from the acute form, and the platelet-associated immunoglobulin is often IgG rather than M and should be found in most cases. Some cases of chronic ITP will be subclinical, with platelet counts of ≥25–50 x 10°/l. They need no management but should be observed, and a careful search for associated autoimmune states should be made. Those that need treatment can be offered a course of IVIG. This is often again of temporary benefit, as is pulsed steroid therapy. Vinca alkaloids and cytotoxic immunosuppression probably have little place in the treatment of chronic ITP. Newer treatments include α Interferon and, more successfully, danazol. In some reports half of patients with chronic ITP make an excellent and sustained response, but this drug would need to be given for ≥6 months. The initial dose should be 800 mg/day, but it may be tapered to 200 mg/day after about 2 months.

Splenectomy is the established treatment for chronic ITP, and in children the success rate is about 2/3; many adults will at least have higher platelet counts following a splenectomy, which makes their management easier. The operation, however, is not without morbidity, and in children especially there is always a risk of sepsis, especially from encapsulated organisms. Vaccination against pneumococcal and hemophilus should be undertaken preferably prior to splenectomy. Children should be given penicillin V po bid for many years following splenectomy, and adults for ≥1 year.

OTHER IMMUNE PURPURAS

- That associated with infectious mononucleosis may be indistinguishable from ITP but is usually of ≤6 weeks duration and may not be as severe. Splenic rupture is a possible complication in this combination of disorders
- HIV-associated immune thrombocytopenia is a complication of AIDS and can be an early finding. The disease mimics chronic ITP and can be managed in much the same way
- Drug-induced immune thrombocytopenia behaves like chronic ITP, but the offending antibody seems to be addressed against a drug, so the mechanism of platelet involvement is not well understood. The platelet count normalizes when the drug is removed. Drugs implicated include: Cimetidine, heparin, phenytoin, sodium valporate, rifampicin, sulfa compounds, and NSAIDs.

PROBLEMS WITH LEUKOCYTES AND THEIR MANAGEMENT

Clinical problems due to, or associated with, leukocytes fall into natural categories: Too few, too many, or poorly functioning leukocytes

Leucopenias

Most problems associated with leucopenias are due to inadequate numbers of neutrophils/neutropenias. In children <12, neutrophil counts as low as 1.5 x 10^9/L probably represent the lower limits of the normal range, except in the first few months of life after the immediate neonatal period when they may drop as low as 1 x 10°/l. In adults, anything <1.8 should be regarded as significantly low.

It is essential to establish that neutropenia actually exists. A cause or association should be detected for the neutropenia. Assuming morbidity to be associated with a neutropenia, steps need to be taken to eliminate the cause of the neutropenia or ameliorate its effects

- Serial full blood counts need to be carried out to make sure this is not one of the cyclic phenomena occasionally described and associated with cyclic changes in other blood cells, platelets, and oral ulcers
- Assuming the neutropenia is persistent, if longstanding and relatively

asymptomatic, it is worth carrying out a neutrophil mobilization test, preferably using both hydrocortisone and adrenaline as stressor agents (5 ml/kg of hydrocortisone hemisuccinate IV and 0.03 ml/kg of 1–10,000 adrenaline SC. Monitor neutrophil counts at 15-min intervals for 1 h and hourly thereafter, up to 6 h. Functionally neutropenic patients fail to show a normal neutrophil count during either part of this procedure, whereas those who have adequate reserves but slightly low circulating numbers of neutrophils show responses well within the normal range

True persistent neutropenia can be due to

- Congenital (extremely rare) conditions e.g., Kostmann's syndrome
- Immune neutropenias: The isoimmune neutropenia of the neonatal period and autoimmune neutropenias, occasionally detected later (disorders analogous to idiopathic autoimmune thrombocytopenic purpura)
- Generalized disorders of bone marrow: bone marrow failure e.g., aplastic anemia
- Drug-induced neutropenias
- Miscellaneous causes such as Felty's syndrome
- Some infections

ANTIBIOTIC POLICY IN SEVERE NEUTROPENIA

"Neutropenic fever" should be assessed through cultures of blood or other materials, but therapy should be initiated as soon as these are taken, not awaiting the results. There is no fixed protocol for such treatment, but combinations of, e.g., aminoglycosides such as gentamicin or amikacin with a synthetic penicillin such as Azlocillin, are often used. Many such protocols for children, however, use cephalosporins such as cephtrioxasole, which appear to be equally effective and avoid the renal and ototoxicity and the necessary monitoring of aminoglycoside blood levels. Frequently no organism will be found, and hopefully the symptoms will resolve within 48 h. Antibiotics should be administered for ≥5 days and for 24 h following the dehiscence of fever. If pyrexia persists, further microbial culture should be attempted, including fungal and viral studies. A switch to "second-line" antimicrobial therapy, including a potent antifungal agent, should be considered. (For discussion of therapy for viral and fungal infections, see Chapters 18 and 26.)

PREVENTION OF NEUTROPENIC FEVER

Prophylaxis of infection in neutropenic and other immunocompromised patients should be considered, especially when the host defensive mechanisms are temporarily defective. The use of "barrier" procedures or protective isolation accompanied by careful personal hygiene on the part of the patient and all visitors and attendants is more important than prophylactic antibiotics or other measures. Laminar air flow and aggressive decontamination of patient cubicles is also effective, but expensive. Oral antibiotics should not be necessary under ideal isolated conditions. All blood products should be carefully screened, as described earlier, and there may be a case for a simple oral antifungal agent such as Fluconazole. Acyclovir 215 mg/m^2 tid is effective in reducing the incidence of recrudescent herpetic infection and may have some value against CMV. TMP SMX, as described, is also known to prevent pneumocystis infection—certainly in some groups of patients. It may also be effective against toxoplasmosis. Longterm prophylactic antibiotics are rarely used except in splenectomized patients or those with recurrent single-site infection.

Leukocytosis

All blood counts reporting *leukocytosis* are not necessarily due to leukemia. It is also true that many patients with leukemia do not have leukocytosis or may indeed be leucopenic as far as the peripheral blood is concerned. Generally, *leukocytosis* shows an increase in mature or near-mature forms of white cells, with essentially normal bone marrow processes and, unless there are separate causes for them, no involvement of the nonleucocytic elements of the bone marrow (red cells, platelets).

Leukocyte counts of ≤100 x 10^9/l have been observed in severe infections. Reactive leukocytosis can present a diagnostic problem, especially in children and with some of the less common infections. Lymphocytes or monocytes may be raised (e.g., in mycoplasma pneumonia or pertussis), and modest raises may be seen in, e.g., pregnancy or Hodgkin's disease and some patients with progressive cancer. In the latter, especially the myelophthisic, appearance in the blood of immature forms may initially give rise to diagnostic difficulties, especially in relation to some of the more indolent myeloproliferative disorders.

Leukemia

Leukemias can be conveniently divided into the acute and chronic myeloid and lymphatic types. The diagnosis can only be safely made through examination of bone marrow material when the number of immature cells can be assessed, cytochemistry, cell markers and cytogenetics carried out, and gene rearrangement noted, where appropriate.

ACUTE MYELOID LEUKEMIA (AML)

Patients may present with: Anemia, bleeding, and/or fever; skin lesions (infiltrates and/or bleeding); gum infiltrates (especially in M4 and M5 varieties); and, less often, testicular, ophthalmic, or CNS manifestations. The bone marrow should contain >30% blasts, most of which should type antigenically as myeloid cells and, in the more differentiated forms, should show at least the cytochemical characteristics of development with, e.g., myeloperoxidase or nonspecific esterase. TDT is occasionally positive (10–15%). Seven subtypes of AML are known (Table 29–7).

M1, 2, and 3 Leukemias represent different degrees of myeloid differentiation, but the M3 variety has special features that include very prominent granules and bundles of Auer rods. This seems to be a rather precisely defined group of patients with a specific karyotypic abnormality (T15:17) and a clinical course initially accentuated by severe bleeding associated with a DIC-like syndrome. The morbidity and mortality in the presentation and early treatment induction phase of this disease is high, but if patients survive this period, their prognosis is said to be better than with other myeloid acute leukemias. The M1 and M2 leukemias have no special features and are associated with a number of different cytogenetic abnormalities. The M4 and M5 types involve monocytes and myeloblasts in different proportions, and the M6 is an erythroleukemia known earlier as the di Guglielmo type; many patients have multinucleated marrow erythroblasts that may be PAS positive. Some of these leukemias may terminate in what appear to be myeloblastic forms. The

Table 29–7
AML and ALL FAB Classifications

AML FAB Classification

M0	Undifferentiated (+ve myeloid markers)
M1	Poorly differentiated
M2	Differentiated
M3	Promyelocytic
M4	Myelomonocytic
M5	Monocytic
M6	Erythroid
M7	Megakaryocytic

ALL FAB Classification

	CELLS	CYTOPLASM	NUCLEOLI
L1	Small	Scanty	Indistinct
L2	Large (or mixed)	Abundant	Prominent
L3	Large	Abundant (often vacuolated)	Prominent

M7 variety involves megakaryocytes and may be associated with considerable marrow fibrosis.

Management of Acute Myeloid Leukemias. This is similar for all types, with the exception of M3. Treatment consists of a regimen designed to induce remission: Usually chemotherapy with an anthracycline, and cytarabine. Usually 2 courses are given, followed by consolidation treatment using similar drugs, with the addition of e.g., etoposide and μ-amsacrine. Thioguanine is often used somewhere in the scheme. There are a number of programs available, and there is little evidence that any one is superior to any other at present. The response of the different leukemic subtypes is also similar, although it is said that the M5 variety does more poorly in childhood. Overall, survivals at 5 years vary with age, being about 50% in childhood and 20% overall in adults <55. M3 leukemias deserve special attention during the induction phase, where ATRA has recently been shown to have an excellent effect in inducing differentiation and giving a form of remission with good platelet counts and hemoglobins. The white count may rise considerably, however, and such remissions are not durable, so in practice such patients should be admitted to "orthodox" induction programs as soon as is practical.

Allogenic bone marrow transplantation with a matched sibling donor gives the best survival in acute myelogenous leukemia in children and young adults. Such allogenic transplantation is carried out early in first remission. All patients should be tissue typed early in their disease, when peripheral blood leukocytes are available and their family members matched. Matched, unrelated donor transplants can also be successful, assuming there is access to a donor registry and a successful search is made. The problems associated with GVH disease are greater in this latter group of patients, and the morbidity and mortality due to this phenomenon is increased.

Autologous bone marrow transplantation is now a part of many AML treatment programs. This is usually carried out by marrow harvesting following completion of remission induction and consolidation treatment and the bone marrow either given back directly following further chemotherapy or held in reserve in case relapse should occur. Currently, purging programs for AML are not established, but such processing, e.g., with Mafosphamide, has been recommended. T-lymphocyte reducing purges may be of value in allogenic donors, especially MUDs, but there is evidence that there is an inverse relationship between the efficacy of purging and the relapse of the AML (the graft versus leukemia effect).

ACUTE LYMPHATIC LEUKEMIA (ACUTE LYMPHOBLASTIC LEUKEMIA) (ALL)

This is the commonest form of childhood cancer that, although more frequent in children, occurs in adults at all ages. The etiology is unknown although, like AML, there is a relationship between sizable doses of radiation, either accidental or related to treatment of other disorders, and the incidence of disease. A virus has been implicated in one rare form of ALL—the HTLV1—which appears to be passed on in maternal milk.

Classification of ALL is by a FAB classification into L1, 2, and 3. L1 consists mostly of smaller lymphocytes, L2 larger, and L3 more Burkitt cell-like. Phenotypically, most belong to a common "pre-β" ALL type and are CD10 (CALLA) positive. A few, especially very young children, are null cell ALLs, where immunophenotyping is not helpful; about 10% are T and about 3% B cell. Most ALLs will be TDT positive.

Prognostic features in ALL are related to the height of the WBC (poor if 50 x 10^9/L), age, and sex (males do worse than females). Cytogenetic abnormalities are common, and those with most hyperdiploidy do worse, as do those with the Philadelphia chromosome. Other cytogenetic abnormalities involve a number of chromosomes and, although related to B- or T-cell lineage, may not be related to prognosis in aggressively treated patients.

Treatment. Long, complex, and usually consists of an induction program with vincristine, prednisolone (prednisone) and L-Asparaginase. Intensification programs typically use cyclophosphamide, methotrexate, L-Asparaginase, and an anthracycline and corticosteroids, specifically directed CNS treatment with radiotherapy and/or intrathecal methotrexate followed by continuing maintenance treatment, usually with oral drugs on an outpatient basis. Typically, vincristine and methotrexate are used in such regimens. About 2 years' continuing therapy is the minimum requirement for relapse prevention. This complicated treatment regimen, with many side effects and problems with growth and mental development in children, needs a considerable amount of support. Also, in older patients, since the chances of cure ↓ with age, this prolonged treatment is often abbreviated (i.e., no maintenance). About 1/2 of all children may expect to be cured by current treatment; some may relapse with new clonal leukemias. The incidence of cure is probably about 25% in young adults, and is minimal over age 50.

Bone Marrow Transplantation. Because of the high cure rate in childhood, most centers reserve bone marrow transplantation for high-risk cases (males with high counts, Ph chromosome, or hyperdiploidy) where matched donors are available. Even if a suitable donor presents, many centers will not treat "average" ALL cases in this manner unless they relapse. Since the chances of obtaining a second remission are good, this is usually found to be an acceptable philosophy. Autologous bone marrow, usually with purging of the appropriate lymphoid population, has been used, but it is not yet clear whether this is an established treatment for either primary or relapsed ALL.

Although relapse most commonly occurs in the bone marrow, as does AML, about 10% of patients with this disease will relapse in the CNS despite the preventive treatment that is part of the induction program. This is *meningeal leukemia* and presents very much as meningitis. Blasts can usually be found in the CNS fluid, although the numbers may be quite low. Quite often such patients are not in overt hematologic relapse. The treatment is by methotrexate and craniospinal irradiation. Cytosine arabinoside is probably equally effective. Patients treated in this way have historically been neurologically or intellectually limited in follow-up. It is probably also best to treat as if there were a systemic (bone marrow) relapse as well, with the same kind of treatment as was used for initial induction and consolidation. Occasionally AML will relapse similarly and should be treated in the same way.

Testicular Relapse is a relatively common relapse in boys and may occur in ≤10% of treated individuals. (It is much less common in AML, although it certainly occurs.) Testicular irradiation is not recommended, but treatment as for a systemic relapse is effective.

Rarely, relapse occurs at other sites, such as the ovary or eye. Ocular radiotherapy is recommended for the rare cases with eye disease and, again, systemic treatment as for bone marrow relapse should be carried out.

CHRONIC MYELOGENOUS LEUKEMIA (CML)

This disease occurs at all ages, although its peak frequency is in mature adults 40–60 years of age. Many patients present without impressive clinical or laboratory findings, except for an ↑ WBC. The WBC differential invariably shows immature WBCs and frequently a mild basophilia or eosinophilia. More florid cases have the full-blown disorder with splenomegaly and very high WBCs up to 500 x 10°/l, with all types of bone marrow cells, including normoblasts and sometimes precursor megakaryocyte fragments in the peripheral blood. Presentation may be with anemia, splenic pain, sudden visual failure, gout, and rarely bleeding. Some of these symptoms are due to leucostasis.

The biology of CML is well worked out, and 90% of cases have the Philadelphia chromosome (9/21 translocation). Most that do not have this exchange of chromative material in an overt manner will still have the presence of the *bcr abl* oncogene arrangement.

Management. Drug treatment of CML is palliative. The mean survival is around 4 years, a figure that has not changed since the introduction of Busulphan about 30 years ago. This drug and Hydroxyurea are the main standbys. Allopurinol should be given (300 mg once daily) to all patients with CML when treatment is proposed. Rarely, the Philadelphia chromosome disappears or is found in a smaller percentage of cells under such treatment, but latterly α-Interferon has been introduced and in about 1/2 the cases of CML seems to be able to suppress leukocyte production after initial cytoreduction with conventional chemotherapy. About 1/3 of these patients will achieve some kind of lessening of the percentage of Philadelphia positive cells present. The only other longstanding management for this disorder is radiotherapy, which is effective in reducing the spleen size where this is a particular problem, and, when bony pain occurs, presumably due to infiltration, it is also effective. AML-type treatment has been tried and is still being evaluated in some centers. At present, its value is unproven.

Allogenic bone marrow transplantation is the only hope for cure in CML at present, and all individuals who have a matched sibling donor should be offered allogenic bone marrow transplantation. This has been carried out in patients up the age of 60 with success. About 50% of patients overall may be cured by this technique. There are, of course, the usual problems with GVH disorders and, if matched unrelated donors are used, these are enhanced.

CHRONIC LYMPHATIC LEUKEMIA (CLL)

Peak incidence is over the age of 65. Most patients run an indolent course. Presentation is often incidental: The patient is observed to have an increased lymphocyte count. Patients may present with anemia, adenopathy, and/or splenomegaly, infections, or, rarely, thrombocytopenic bleeding. The pathology of the disorder involves proliferation of mature B lymphocytes in ≥95% of cases. T-lymphocyte CLL is also described, and there are a number of CLL variants with special features. Attempts have been made to stage CLL so that prognosis and, more importantly perhaps, management can be appropriately recommended. Two systems have been used, one described by Rai and Binet. Table 29–8 describes these categories. Unfortunately, although these are of some value in a nosologic sense, their use in assessing individual patients at a single point in time is not always satisfactory.

Management. Many patients need no specific therapy. If the patient is not anemic and does not have troublesome adenopathy or splenomegaly, despite a high peripheral blood lymphocyte count and the presence of considerable bone marrow disease, there is no urgency in initiating treatment. Treatment is indicated for symptomatic anemia, falling Hb, progressive thrombocytopenia, uncomfortably enlarging lymph nodes, or rarely, spleen.

Immune dysfunction is a complication of chronic lymphatic leukemia. It may present as autoimmune disease, particularly hemolytic anemia, and less often thrombocytopenia. Deficient immunoglobulin production may be associated with recurrent infections of the upper respiratory tract, lung, and urinary tract.

Treatment. Many will respond, although will not be cured, by chlorambucil in doses of, e.g., 20 mg/week. Patients with CLL are usually elderly and frail, and if it is possible to treat in a simple manner and they are kept well, this is probably the treatment of choice. Patients who fail this regimen, or who are younger and have bulky disease, may be considered for a more aggressive combination of chemotherapy, e.g.,

Table 29–8
CLL Classifications

Rai	
0	Blood lymphocytes
1	Blood lymphocytes + enlarged nodes
2	Blood lymphocytes + splenomegaly
3	Blood lymphocytes + anemia
4	Blood lymphocytes + thrombocytopenia

	Hb.G/L	Pl × 10^9/L	CLINICAL INVOLVEMENT
Binet A	≥100	≥100	<3 areas
B	≥100	≥100	≥3 areas
C	<100 +/or	<100	any

monthly CHOP (Cyclophosphamide and an Anthracycline, Oncovin, and Prednisone) for 6 months. There seems to be little vogue for single-agent anthracyclines, but Fludarabine at monthly intervals for 6 months has shown considerable success in patients who have failed on other therapy; new agents such as Chlordeoxydaenosine also look promising. Prednisolone may be useful in the treatment of complications such as acquired hemolytic anemia or immune thrombocytopenia, but is not recommended in the usual management of CLL, although it certainly is lympholytic.

Radiotherapy to bulky disease areas or enlarged spleen is effective in reducing tumor mass. In patients with immune suppression and history of recurrent infections, a program of IV immunoglobulin at monthly intervals is of value.

A very small number of "young" patients have received allogenic matched bone marrow transplantations with success rates comparable to, e.g., CML. Such younger patients are in a considerable minority and may represent a fundamentally more aggressive form of CLL, so the usual palliative approach may certainly be amended for this group of patients.

Although a disorder such as a B-cell CLL would seem a tempting target for immunotherapy, trials with interferons have been disappointing, and monoclonal antibodies, either against CLL-associated antigens or linked with cytotoxins, have not fulfilled some animal work-based promise.

CLL VARIANTS

A "splenic" form of CLL has been described where the major problem is splenomegaly accompanied by anemia and/or thrombocytopenia. Frequently these latter become accentuated when drug treatment is given, while the spleen size stays persistently large. This group of patients seems to benefit from splenectomy, which reduces the tumor bulk and may restore good quality survival and freedom from transfusion. X irradiation of the spleen is also effective but may be of less permanent benefit. The borderline between CLL and small-cell lymphocytic leukemia is poorly defined, and, when in doubt, especially in younger patients, if therapy is needed, the more aggressive protocols are probably indicated.

Prolymphocytic Leukemia. This is usually a B- but occasionally a T-cell variant. It may be a transformed chronic leukemia, although it certainly presents de novo from time to time. The morphologic features of this disease are an increased number of prolymphocytes with their characteristic large single nucleoli and an increased cytoplasmic content compared with "adult" small lymphocytes. The disorder has a high mortality.

Hairy Cell Leukemia is a proliferation of what are hybrid lymphocytes with many B-cell features, some T-cell features, and some conforming to those of histiocytes. The presence of both heavy- and light-chain gene rearrangements suggests its B-cell origin. There are probably a number of hairy cell leukemia-like disorders!

The syndrome usually presents with nonspecific symptoms, such as malaise, fever, and weight loss. Patients present with abdominal discomfort, splenomegaly, adenopathy, anemia, and associated asymptomatic thrombocytopenia. Most patients show hairy cells in the peripheral blood on close examination. The bone marrow shows a characteristic morphologic picture where the cells' oval or indented nuclei are separated widely from each other. The cells show the typical hairy features and are defined by their tartrate resistant acid phosphatase activity. Several karyotypic abnormalities have been reported: 14q plus or abnormalities of chromosome 12 are most common, but there is no specific abnormality. Treatment of hairy cell leukemia is usually splenectomy, which should not be done until the patient is symptomatic, as many will have a very indolent course. The use of corticosteroids and lymphoma-type chemotherapy has not been helpful in the past, but successful results have been obtained with α Interferon, Desoxycorfomycine, and Chlordioxyadenosine. All these agents appear to be effective in inducing remission; hopefully, some kind of intermittent/maintenance regimen can be established that will allow longterm survival, but at the moment even these regimens do not appear to be curative.

MYELOPROLIFERATIVE DISORDERS

Polycythemia is either "true" (PV) or secondary. PV is a panmyelopathy where, sooner or later, all 3 of the major bone marrow products are increased in the peripheral blood: Red cells, neutrophils, and platelets. In secondary polycythemias, sometimes called erythemias, only the red cell component is increased. There are also pseudo polycythemias. If all the classic features are present, PV is clearly distinguishable from the others, but in some cases the distinction may be blurred, at least initially.

POLYCYTHEMIA VERA (PV)

PV is a disorder affecting mature adults with a peak incidence in the mid 50s. The presentation may be with plethora, headaches, vertigo, stroke, or MI. Peripheral vascular disease with endangered digits or limbs may occur, the incidence of gout is increased, and, paradoxically, a number of patients may present with bleeding from the GI tract. On examination, if the full-blown syndrome is present, splenomegaly will undoubtedly be found or detected on abdominal ultrasound. Hepatomegaly is usually not prominent, and adenopathy is unusual.

The peripheral blood contains ↑ RBCs. This may be matched by a high Hb and hematocrit; but, if the patient has bled, these may be normal or low. The neutrophil count should be raised but with no immature cells circulating. The platelet count should be raised with variations in platelet size but not all of these features may be present.

All patients suspected of being polycythemic should have a red blood cell mass. This should be accompanied by a plasma volume. Males living at sea level or thereabouts should have ≤30 ml/kg RBCs, and females about 25 ml/kg. The total blood volume of males should be around 60 ml/kg and slightly less for females. (Exact values should be those obtained in your own laboratory.) Increases in red cell mass beyond the normal levels plus your accepted standard deviation should indicate a diagnosis of "polycythemia." This does not help distinguish true from secondary polycythemias but will eliminate some pseudopolycythemias such as stress polycythemia, where the problem seems to be one of a reduced plasma volume only. Tests that help distinguish between true and secondary polycythemias include:

- Erythropoietin levels: Patients with PV have normal erythropoietin levels (again these should be your own reference lab's values); 90%

of patients with secondary polycythemias for whatever reason will have ↑ erythropoietin

- Bone marrow biopsy: Bone marrow aspirate is often unhelpful in the diagnosis of PV, but a biopsy should show increased cellularity and especially increased numbers of megakaryocytes. There will also be some increase in reticulin fibers. Secondary polycythemias at best show some erythroid hyperplasia
- Bone marrow colony growth: Bone marrow cells from patients with PV will form spontaneous erythroid colonies in vitro. Normal individuals and those with the secondary polycythemias will not
- Uric acid levels: Uric acid levels are usually normal or ↑ in PV. They are rarely ↑ in secondary polycythemias
- Leukocyte alkaline phosphatase level, if reliably available, will be ↑ in PV and may be normal in other polycythemias

Management is palliative. Good management can lead to the achievement of a normal life span with good quality of life in most patients. The form of management depends on the symptoms, findings, and age of the patient.

Patients with principally an erythremic component of their polycythemia can be managed by venesection, which should be sufficient to achieve a hematocrit of ≤45. This usually requires energetic venesection initially until iron stores are depleted, but the frequency can then be reduced. The red cell numbers may be ↑ at 7 or 8 x 10^{12}/l, but it is the PCV that has the major effect on blood viscosity rather than red cell numbers, so symptomatically patients treated in this manner may avoid the complications of the disease.

Some patients need cytoreductive treatment initially, and most eventually because of pruritus, perisplenitis, or evidence of hyperviscosity (TIAs, PVD) or gout. Cytoreduction can be accomplished by oral medications such as hydroxyurea or busulphan in a dose-dependent fashion. Monitoring of WBC and platelets is necessary during the maintenance period of treatment, which may last for many years. This is probably the preferential treatment for young individuals (<55 years of age); thereafter, radiophosphorus (P32) is equally effective and more convenient. A dose of 200 mbeq initially repeated as necessary causes "remissions" (treatment-free periods) of many years. It is not recommended for younger patients because of the suspicion that it may be leukemogenic. However, the incidence of leukemia is still very low in patients treated with P32.

Individuals with PV often survive 10–20 years, but about 5% develop acute leukemia; some develop myelofibrosis.

SECONDARY POLYCYTHEMIAS

There is a pure red cell mass elevation without any evidence of myeloproliferation

- Respiratory: The relationship between the red cell mass and O_2 saturation is well established, and if Hb is relatively desaturated due, e.g., to respiratory disorders or living at high altitudes, then compensation through elevation of the red cell mass will take place. Smokers traditionally have a hematocrit which may be 5–10% higher than nonsmokers. Patients with suspected respiratory polycythemia should have their ABGs estimated; arterial saturation of <92% is abnormal
- The cyanotic Hb variants, including methemoglobinemia, usually produce mild HB elevations only, but erythrocytosis in both these and many of the high-affinity hemoglobins is relatively asymptomatic.

However, O_2 dissociation curves will show the abnormality, and in most cases the Hb variant is identifiable with structural abnormalities in both the α and β chains of the globin-suspected variant
- Cardiac erythrocytosis may occur with congenital cyanotic heart disease
- Renal erythrocytosis: Renal carcinoma, adenomas, Wilms tumors, cysts, hydronephrosis, and polycystic kidneys have been reportedly associated with secondary polycythemia
- Other tumors: Hepatocellular cancer, hepatic tumors, cerebellar haemangioblastomas, and uterine lyomyosarcomata have been associated with erythrocytosis.

OTHER MYELOPROLIFERATIVE SYNDROMES

Essential Thrombocythemia occurs in middle adult life. Patients present with thrombotic complications, but bleeding may also occur. Splenomegaly should be found, but the spleen may be atrophied due to infarction.

The differential diagnosis is from reactive thrombocytosis. In each, the platelet count may be abnormally high (>700 x 10°/l), but patients with counts of, e.g., 2000 x 10°/l are almost invariably myeloproliferative, and clusters of megakaryocytes in the bone marrow confirm the diagnosis.

Management of the disease is based on cytoreduction. Anticoagulants or aspirin should not be regarded as adequate. Alkylating agents such as Busulphan, antimetabolites such as Hydroxyurea, or Radiophosphorus are all effective. The latter is somewhat slower than, e.g., Hydroxyurea or Cyclophosphamide. If there are no treatment complications, many years' survival can be achieved, although, like PV, some patients die of associated acute leukemia or bone marrow failure due to myelofibrosis.

Myelofibrosis. In elderly patients, malignant fibrosis of the bone marrow accompanied by myeloid metaplasia (myelofibrosis) may be found. In this form the marrow stroma is taken over by reticulin and then collagen fibers, and hematopoiesis is found in the spleen and liver, both of which become enlarged. The disease is accompanied by severe wasting, anemia, thrombocytopenia, perisplenitis, and cachexia.

Management is difficult: Splenectomy is useful in prolonging good quality of life if carried out early in the disease, but often is of little value in later stages. Blood transfusion and supportive therapy are probably as effective. α Interferon may be of value in some instances, but its use has not yet been established. Erythropoietin may help with the anemia (androgen therapy had traditionally been used but response was poor). A more aggressive form of this disease may be seen in young women, where it behaves like acute myeloid leukemia.

PARAPROTEINEMIAS

Myeloma

- Myeloma is a disorder characterized by overgrowth of monoclonal plasma cells in the bone marrow and the presence of an abnormal M protein in the plasma of 80–90% of myeloma patients and the urine in 50–80%. (Techniques for identifying abnormal urinary proteins continue to improve.)

- >5% of myeloma patients have no detectable paraproteins in the plasma or urine

CLINICAL PRESENTATION

Myeloma may present with bone pain with (or without) associated fractures, anemia, infection, neurologic problems (either associated with cord compression or polyneuropathy), renal failure, hypercalcemia, or hyperviscosity

- The diagnosis is confirmed by bone marrow aspirate showing increased numbers of plasma cells that must show monoclonality by their surface light chain typing
- The peripheral blood findings are variable, but a normocytic normochromic anemia with rouleaux formation is commonly observed, and there may be leucopenia and thrombocytopenia in advanced cases. Only in the rare plasma cell leukemia are the characteristic cells actually seen in the peripheral blood
- There may be signs of bone destruction in the blood chemistry assessment (hypercalcemia), but the alkaline phosphatase is often normal or marginally ↑
- A monoclonal immunoglobulin of any class may be found, sometimes in very high concentrations in the plasma, and there may be a reduction in the normal immunoglobulin levels
- The urine shows Bence Jones protein in >1/2 of cases, representing synthesis of excess light chains. The urine may also contain excess albumin due to tubular damage by these same light chains. IgG "spikes" are the commonest in 1/2–2/3 of patients, with IgA in about 20%, and IgM, which is often separately classified, probably forming 10–15%. About 15% may have urine protein abnormalities only
- There is a certain degree of correlation between the paraprotein type and clinical attribute. IgM, IgA, and IgG3 myelomas are more likely to be associated with hyperviscosity syndromes, the rarer IgD myeloma (1%); is rather like a generalized lymphoma with hepatosplenomegaly and extramedullary disease
- Light-chain disease is associated with a poorer-than-average prognosis, as may be nonsecretory myelomas. A few patients will have double paraproteins: the so-called biclonal gammopathies

The differential diagnosis is between myelomatosis and other monoclonal gammopathies such as MGUS (see later); polyclonal elevations of immunoglobulins are frequently seen in, e.g., collagen vascular disorders or chronic infections and an increase in plasma cells in the bone marrow may also be seen in these conditions. Occasionally, myeloma presents with generalized osteopenia, especially in elderly females, and this is difficult to distinguish from the osteoporosis commonly seen in such individuals.

ASSESSMENT AND PROGNOSIS

Assessment and treatment may need to be undertaken on an emergency basis but, if not, a clinical staging system based on clinical and laboratory parameters is worth considering. The several systems available tend to reflect the total tumor burden. Older prognostic features such as the Hb level and BUN now appear to be of less value.

MANAGEMENT STRATEGY

Immediate management includes hydration, especially in patients with renal failure, correction of anemia (but take care in patients with hyperviscosity), reduction of hypercalcemia, if symptomatic, with doses of prednisolone, e.g., 16 mg/l^2 per day and the use of biphosphonates such as Etidronate 7.5 mg/kg qd. Mithramycin has also been used in patients resistant to all these maneuvers (25 μg/kg once or twice). The other emergency needing immediate treatment is pathologic fracture and, in the case of vertebral collapse with or without paravertebral disease, neurosurgical intervention may be indicated. Orthopedic repair of, e.g., fractured neck of femur is not contraindicated in myeloma.

Unlike many leukemias, myeloma treatment has traditionally been palliative. Only recently has allogenic bone marrow transplantation been used in a small number of patients, but it may be the only way of curing the disease, especially in younger patients. For most, the expected best result is the induction of a "remission," i.e., a period when the disease is apparently controlled, the level of paraprotein reduced, and the patient symptom free with an improved quality of life until relapse.

In younger patients previously untreated, a typical treatment program would consist of 6 courses of ABCM (Adriamycin, BCNU, cyclophosphamide, and prednisone at approximately monthly intervals. The alternative is probably single-agent treatment with an alkylating agent such as melphalan or cyclophosphamide. Typically, with the former, a dose of 0.25 mg/kg/day is given for 4 days. (There is some doubt as to whether adding prednisone is helpful at this time.) The treatment can be repeated every month until plateau has occurred, as measured by no further fall in the serum paraprotein. Cyclophosphamide can be used in a similar way, either IV or po, at doses of 2–250 mg/l^2 qd for 4 days. MESNA and extra fluids need to be given at this time to reduce the risk of hemorrhagic cystitis.

For relapsed patients, if they have not received combination chemotherapy, it is worth trying programs of high-dose Melphalan; Hemi body radiation is also worth considering. The role of Interferons in the treatment of myeloma, especially in maintenance regimens, is currently uncertain. Interferons do have some suppressive effect on myeloma cells. Palliative radiotherapy to painful bone lesions is also useful. Elderly patients are probably best treated with oral Mephalan as described. Plasmapheresis is temporarily effective in reducing the paraprotein level, but should be reserved for patients with acute hyperviscosity syndromes.

Other Paraproteinemias

MGUS

A relatively benign condition of Benign Monoclonal Gammopathy of Unknown Significance has been described, especially in elderly patients where it may reach an incidence of 3–4% in patients of 80 years of age. This must be distinguished from malignant paraproteinemias through a period of observation, and needs no treatment. A few patients with apparently benign disease will develop frank myeloma after many years.

SOLITARY PLASMACYTOMA

This condition is self-explanatory and should be treated like a local tumor, usually with radiotherapy. Most such patients will develop myeloma eventually, but there is no proof that treating them systemically following the appearance and management of the solitary lesion prevents the onset of frank myeloma.

WALDENSTROM'S DISEASE (MACROGLOBULINEMIA)

This disease, which is characterized by an elevation of monoclonal IgM, behaves differently to myeloma. It is almost exclusively a disease of the elderly and, again, may be often relatively benign. Presentation is most commonly that of anemia or bleeding or bruising. Bony fractures or renal disease are relatively uncommon, but occasionally neurologic symptoms can be found. Physical findings show hepatosplenomegaly in about 1/2 the patients, and adenopathy may also occur. Diagnosis is made through detecting the abnormal paraprotein and by the presence of the Waldenstrom cells (lymphoplasmacytoid cells) in the bone marrow. They are also found in lymph nodes and spleen. Bone marrow biopsy is essential to confirm the nature of the disease.

Management Treatment. When treatment is necessary because of anemia or increasing organ size, oral alkylating agents are the treatment of choice, and chlorambucil or Melphalan are of value. Typically, Melphalan 6 mg/l^2/day for 7 days at monthly intervals should suffice. Occasional patients can benefit from plasmapheresis, as hyperviscosity syndromes are sometimes life threatening. A few younger patients with more aggressive disease can be treated in the same way as myeloma.

HEAVY CHAIN DISEASE

Resembles the other paraproteinemias in that there is an abnormal serum protein that reacts to one of the heavy chains (α, γ, μ, or δ) but not with the K and n light chains. It is seen in younger patients, mostly 10–35 years old, and presents with lymphadenopathy, and GI and bone marrow involvement. A few circulating lymphoplasmacytoid cells may be seen in many cases. Prognosis is poor, and often, especially in tropical cases, there are associated diseases.

Treatment with alkylating agents, as in myeloma, may help in the short term, but this disorder is rare, and therapeutic trials of combination chemotherapy have not been conclusively carried out.

Suggested Reading

Barrett AJ, et al.: Marrow transplantation for acute lymphoblastic leukemia. Factors affecting relapse and survival. Blood, 74: 862–871, 1989.

Bithell TC: The diagnostic approach to the bleeding disorders. In Wintrobe's Clinical Haematology, pp. 1301–1324. Philadelphia, Lea & Febiger, 1993.

Gale RP, et al.: Transplantation or chemotherapy in acute myelogenous leukemia. Lancet, 1: 1119–1122, 1989.

Geller RB, et al.: Cure of acute myelocytic leukemia in adults: a reality. Leukemia, 4: 313–315, 1990.

Greer IA, Turpic AGC, Forbes CD (eds.): Haemostasis and Thrombosis in Obstetrics and Gynaecology. London, Chapman & Hall, 1992.

Lee, GR, et al., In Wintrobe Clinical Hematology. Philadelphia, Lea & Febiger, 1993.
Murphy MF, et al.: Guidelines for platelet transfusions. In Transfusion in Medicine 2: 311–18, 1992.
Roath S and Francis J: Coagulation and its inhibitors. In Int. Anaesth. Clinics 23 (2), pp. 22–35. Boston, Little & Brown, 1985.

Rheumatic Disorders

30

Robert P. Sheon

OVERVIEW AND ART OF DIAGNOSIS

Differential diagnosis of a musculoskeletal problem can be developed in 2 ways. First, however, decide whether the problem is regional and noninflammatory, such as osteoarthritis, or localized, as a bursitis.

- Is it part of a systemic disorder? Table 30–1 provides the differential diagnosis in this manner. Tables 30–2, 30–3, and 30–4 provide a differential diagnosis based upon the number of joints involved. These tables present the major diagnostic considerations if the presentation is a single swollen joint (at times the most difficult task for a rheumatologist); when the presentation consists of ≤4 swollen joints, often in an asymmetric pattern; or when onset presents with a symmetrical polyarthritis affecting >5 joints (hands and feet are considered as 1 joint for counting purposes, respectively.
- Inflammation is suspected when joints are either visibly inflamed or accompanied by morning stiffness or gelling of ≥30 min duration; fever, weight loss and fatigue may occur.
- Nonarticular rheumatic pain disorders include myofascial pain, bursitis and tendinitis, structural disorders, nerve entrapment disorders, and fibromyalgia. Table 30–5 provides features that distinguish these from the inflammatory or systemic rheumatic diseases.
- Often, osteoarthritis is a silent accompaniment to a nonarticular rheumatic pain disorder. Whereas osteoarthritis would cause pain during use or weight bearing, a superimposed nonarticular disorder such as bursitis would cause pain at night. Night pain that is worse than daytime pain is unlikely due to an arthritis.

Syndrome Analysis

Most connective tissue diseases lack any pathognomonic feature. The examiner must know the elements of each disease syndrome and then elicit those features during the examination. Table 30–6 provides a checklist for features important in a rheumatic history and physical examination.

- Is swelling visible or only a sensation? Morning stiffness/gelling duration and location will differentiate inflammatory disease from noninflammatory disease or gout. Gout seldom causes stiffness. Make certain stiffness is in true joint areas, not "all over," and not episodic, but present daily. Fibromyalgia and Parkinson's disease can cause "all over" stiffness.
- Constitutional features of fever, chills, sweats, and weight loss indicate urgent diagnosis and treatment. Chills are rarely present in connective tissue diseases. Chills indicate infection.

Table 30–1
Six Major Disease Groups

CONNECTIVE TISSUE DISEASES				
B-CELL MEDIATED	*T-CELL MEDIATED*	HEMATOLOGIC	METABOLIC	NEOPLASTIC
Rheumatoid arth	Dermatomyositis	Hemophilia	Gout	Hypertrophic pulmonary osteoarthropathy
Juvenile arth	Polymyositis	Sickle cell anemia	Pseudogout	Cancer arthropathy
Acute rheum F	Giant cell arter.	Thalassemia	Hyperparathy.	Metastasis to joint
Lupus eryrthem.	Wegener's gran.	Hemochromatosis	Hyperthyroid	Osteochondromat.
Mixed conn. tiss.	Churg/Strauss vasc	Gaucher's dis	Pancreatitis	Villonodular synov.
Felty's synd	Kawasaki's disease	Weber christian	Acromegaly	
Sjogren's synd	Takayasu's arteritis	Amyloidosis	Ochronosis	
Systemic sclerosis	Ankylosing spondylitis	Myeloma	Hyperlipidemia	
Mixed cryoglobulinemia	Reiter's syndrome	Leukemia	Diabetes	
	Psoriatic arthritis	Lymphoma		
	Chronic ulcerative colitis		ALLERGIC	
	Crohn's disease	INFECTIOUS	Henoch Schoenlein purpura	
	Granulomatous colitis	Gonococcal arth	Stevens-Johnson syndrome	
	Whipple's disease	Tuberculous arth	Drug lupus	
	Behçet's disease	Bacterial endocarditis	Serum sickness	
		Hepatitis arth	Hypersensitivity vasculitis	
		Lyme arthritis	? Sarcoid	
		Rickettsial inf.		
		Sporotrichosis		
		Fungal arthritis		
		Bacterial arthritis		
		Viral arthritis		
		Reactive arthritis		

Table 30–2
Differential Diagnosis of Monoarticular Arthritis

NONINFLAMMATORY	INFLAMMATORY	SEPTIC
Trauma/osteoarthritis	Rheumatoid monoarthritis	Bacterial
Internal derangements	Gout/pseudogout	Tuberculous
Osteonecrosis	Juvenile monoarthritis	Gonococcus
Reflex dystrophy	Spondyloarthropathy	Fungal
Hemarthrosis	Pigmented villonodular synovitis	Sporotrichosis
Neuropathic/Charcot		Viral
Paget's disease		AIDS
Joint tumors		Rickettsia

Table 30–3
Differential Diagnosis of Pauciarticular Polyarthritis (≤4 joints)

Spondyloarthropathies (HLA-B27 positive)
Reactive arthritis
- Reiter's syndrome
- Psoriatic arthritis
- Acute rheumatic fever
- Enteric arthropathies

Metabolic and crystal-induced arthropathies
Paraneoplastic syndromes
Septic arthritis
- AIDS-related arthritis
- Parvovirus
- Lyme arthritis

Seronegative rheumatoid arthritis

Table 30–4
Differential Diagnosis of Polyarticular Arthritis (≥6 joints)

Rheumatoid diseases
- Seronegative RA
- Seropositive RA
- Sjogren's syndrome
- Felty's syndrome

Other connective tissue diseases
- Systemic lupus erythematosus
- Mixed connective tissue disease
- Dermatomyositis
- Mixed cryoglobulinemia
- Adult Still's disease

Reactive arthritis
- Acute rheumatic fever
- Reiter's syndrome
- Psoriatic arthritis
- Spondyloarthritis

Hematologic
- Leukemia
- Hemochromatosis

Metabolic
- Polyarticular gout
- Pseudogout
- Dialysis arthropathy

Vasculitis
- Giant cell arteritis
- Wegener's granulomatosis

Infectious
- Endocarditis
- Lyme disease
- Parvovirus B19
- Rocky Mountain spotted fever

Miscellaneous
- Serum sickness
- Henoch-Schonlein purpura
- Enteric arthropathy
- Paraneoplastic syndrome
- Sarcoidosis

Table 30–5
Features of Nonarticular Rheumatic Pain Disorders

INFLAMMATORY RHEUMATIC DISEASES	NONARTICULAR DISORDERS
• Pain during movement • Palpable joint swelling • Abnormal tests • Aggravating factors possible • Diagnosis based on clinical examination and test results	• Pain after rest • Swelling is sensation only • All laboratory tests normal • Aggravating factors likely • Diagnosis based on physical examination maneuvers and outcome

From: Sheon RP: Nonarticular rheumatism and nerve entrapment disorders. Resident & Staff Physician, *35*(12):65–70), 1989.

- Weakness is a common complaint but must be objectively quantified. Can patient arise unassisted from a chair, lift head from bed, raise arms above head, etc.?
- If the onset followed trauma, elicit information regarding the extent of trauma (e.g., amount of damage to car); presence of abrasion, laceration, or fracture at time of injury; availability of x rays. Is litigation pending? Has patient been able to perform usual daily routine at work or at home? Specify the disabilities (e.g., can't dress, grasp, climb).
- If an ominous feature or objective signs are not evident, include a misery index: "If you were so bad that you could not get out of bed, and if that was like being in the bottom of a pit, and being restored to perfect is like being out of the pit, and there are 100 steps down into the bottom of the pit, with step #1 being terrible, where is your level of misery this week?" This version of a pain scale can discriminate irrational pain concern or alert you to search more closely for evidence of ominous disease.
- The history taking will vary with the mode of presentation and age of the patient, but should quickly eliminate ominous features. Look early and quickly for ominous features (see Table 30–6) that should be assessed at the outset of the patient encounter.
- It is not rare for patients to have overlapping features, such as sicca complex, with another disease, or the pain of a nonarticular rheumatic disorder laid upon another rheumatic disease.
- Facial asymmetry can suggest temporomandibular joint pain and dysfunction with resulting neck pain and headache; or it may be associated with other skeletal deformities such as a short leg and scoliosis.
- Observe patient arising from a chair. Then, with legs bare, have patient walk away and then toward you. Note gait, leg alignment or torsion, and balance.
- Swelling can be determined by palpating small joints with the examiner's 2 index fingers at the sides of the joint. Is the synovium normal, palpable, or boggy (like soft dough) thick? Always examine the feet; often they are deformed by a previous unrecognized attack of rheumatoid arthritis.
- Trigger points should be located when pain and symptoms occur beyond the joint boundary. See Figures 30-1 and 30-2 for common trigger point locations. Palpation should approximate 4 lb pressure. You can use the stylomastoid process as a control point. Palpation of the trigger point should reproduce the distant pain and paresthesia.

Table 30–6
History and Physical Checklist

	HISTORY		PHYSICAL
Current illness:	Onset, pattern of spread	General:	Appearance, movement
	Was swelling visible?		Body symmetry, limb length
	Duration of swelling		Flexibility, strength
	*Chills, fever, rash	Skin:	Hair loss; rashes, psoriasis
	*Weight loss?/gain?		Nailfold infarctions; leg ulc
	Stiffness duration/location	HEENT:	Temporal arteries palpable?
	Results of medications tried		Conjunctiva, mucous membranes
Family history:	Inflammatory bowel diseases		Dentition, fundoscopy
	Other rheumatic diseases	Neck:	Thyroid abnormalities; pulses
	Migraine headaches	Cardiac/pulmonary:	Rubs, murmurs, wheezes
	Joint laxity		Chest expanse
Social:	Stairs at home; location of bathrooms	Abdomen:	Organs, masses, bruit
	Tic exposure	Lymph nodes:	Cervical, groin
	Smoking/drinking	Extremities:	Deformity, color, temperature
Past history:	Allergies/operations		Pulses; Range of motion, active
	Current medical diseases		Passive; muscle symmetry
	Past medical disease	Joints:	Crepitus, tenderness
Current RX:	Prescription and non-prescription drugs		Synovitis: boggy or not?

Review of systems:	Skin rashes; psoriasis
	Raynaud's phenomenon
	Sun sensitivity & rash
	*Alopecia
	Jaw/fist clenching
	Headache, convulsions
	*Jaw claudication
	Depression, stressful event
	Dryness eyes & mouth
	Stomatitis
	*Pleuropericarditis
	Dyspnea, cough, wheeze
	*Edema, discoloration limbs
	Dysphagia, acid reflux
	Liver diseases, peptic ulcers
	Change in bowel habit
	Kidney stones, hematuria
	Dysuria, frequency
	Nocturia, balanitis
	Genital discharge
	Cervicitis
	Paresthesias, weakness
	Effusions?
	Periarticular tenderness
	Inflammation?
Spine:	Appearance bending & extending
	Effect on pain
Neurologic:	Appearance, reflexes
	Pathologic reflexes
	Gait, ability to arise unassisted

* = May be ominous sign

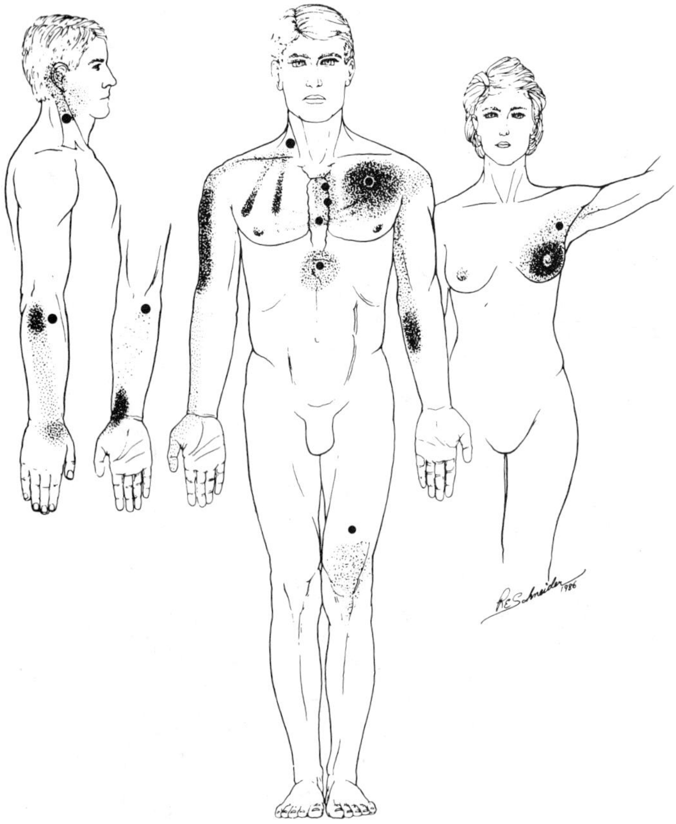

Figure 30–1. Trigger point location: front view. From: Sheon, Robert P, Moskowitz, Roland W, Goldberg, Victor M: Soft Tissue Rheumatic Pain: Recognition, Management, Prevention. 2nd Ed. Philadelphia, Lea & Febiger, 1987.

Cost-Effective Use of the Laboratory and Roentgenography

Order tests individually with thoughtful consideration of the disease presentation. For example, don't order a rheumatoid factor in young children: The various types of juvenile arthritis are usually seronegative; if ≥3 features of lupus are not present, the ANA is more likely to confuse than to help.

Complement determination and anti-DNA testing should be reserved for patients with active and diagnosed systemic LE.

Measurement of the complement component, C1q, is an inexpensive way to detect circulating immune complexes in patients suspected of having vasculitis, lupus, or systemic rheumatoid vasculitis.

The Westergren method for sedimentation rate discriminates better between normal and abnormal than other methods.

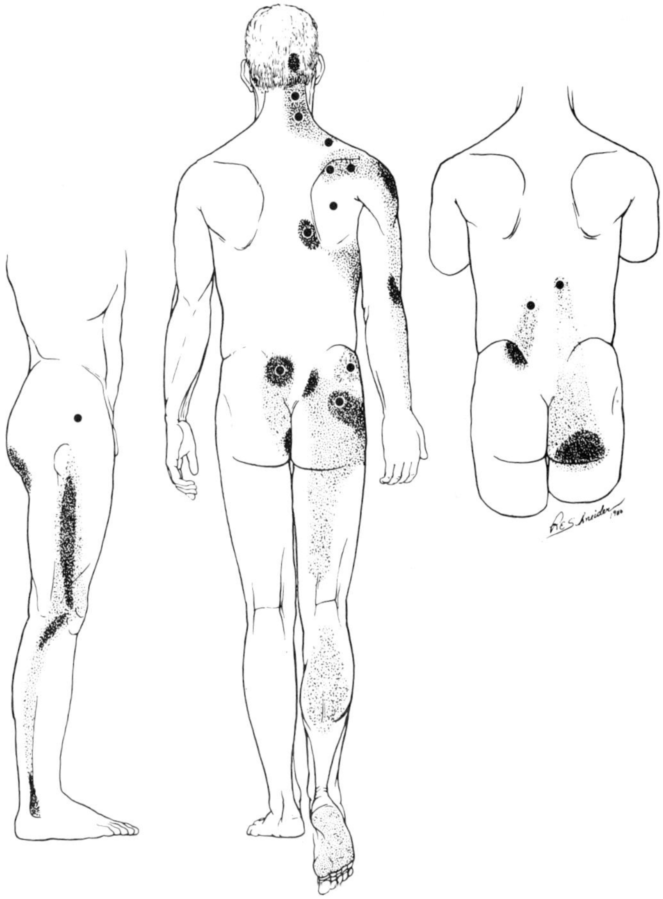

Figure 30–2. Trigger point location: lower body. From: Sheon, Robert P, Moskowitz, Roland W, Goldberg, Victor M: Soft Tissue Rheumatic Pain: Recognition, Management, Prevention. 2nd Ed. Philadelphia, Lea & Febiger, 1987.

Roentgenographic findings must be correlated to the age of the patient. Degenerative changes may be normal at advanced age and unrelated to the presenting problem.

Imaging procedures of the cervical and lumbar spine have high sensitivity but low specificity: Findings in control groups reveal significant abnormality in 20% of normal 20–year-olds, in 40% of normal 40– to 50–year-olds, and in >1/2 of those normal persons >60 years of age. Don't order these scans if you have no evidence for an ominous disease process or if you lack criteria for surgical intervention, and be certain the patient would be willing to undergo surgery if findings indicated the need for a surgical procedure. Too often the physician presents the MRI finding of disc herniation only to be told by the patient, "Oh no, I'm not that bad!" Do not waste this resource.

- If the initial patient encounter has no danger signs, begin symptomatic treatment, provide an expected outcome and advise the patient to return within a reasonable time and proceed with laboratory or radiographic procedures if symptoms persist.

PHARMACOLOGY AND THE RHEUMATIC DISEASES

NSAIDs

Patients at ↑ risk for major NSAID complications include those with hypertension, diabetes, poor renal function, liver disease, asthma or nasal polyps, peptic ulcer history, aspirin sensitivity, or advanced age.

Before initiating an NSAID, screen patient with appropriate history, CBC, chemistry panel.

Once selection of NSAID proves satisfactory, follow up with repeat laboratory tests at 2 months and then less frequently (annually or semiannually).

Adults with risks can be given nonacetylated salicylates such as choline salicylate (Arthropan), magnesium salicylate (Mobidin), or salsalate (Disalcid; Salflex; Monogesic), or combination (Trilisate).

- Patients >75 years often get as much benefit with 1000 mg acetaminophen as with NSAID. Table 30–7 reviews NSAID toxicity (after Amadio).

Steroids

Oral steroids are not indicated unless systemic inflammation is evident and less hazardous treatment has failed, or life- and limb-threatening features are evident. Why add to the patient's problems? Don't use a shortterm benefit when it carries a longterm catastrophic side effect. Steroid side effects include osteoporosis, diabetes, cataracts, glaucoma, and atherosclerosis. High doses may cause avascular necrosis of the shoulders or hips.

Ca supplements, vitamin D, avoidance of simple carbohydrates, and excess salt are helpful when longterm steroid treatment is prescribed.

Intra-articular corticosteroid injection after joint aspiration is safer, provides more symptomatic benefit, and may retard loss of cartilage. Do not repeat injection in same joint >4–6 times a year. Tables 30–8 and 30–9 provide principles for joint and soft tissue injection. See Figure 30–3.

Synovial fluid analysis is essential if acute inflammation is evident. See Table 30–10.

Get help early rather than too late! If disease is complex, or if treatment will involve costly and potentially hazardous medication, consult a rheumatologist.

If pain is persistent or if the disease is potentially deforming, consult occupational and physical therapy. See Tables 30–11 and 30–12 and Figure 30–4. Table 30–13 presents some helpful hints for providing care to patients with rheumatic complaints.

OSTEOARTHRITIS

Osteoarthritis should be considered as either compensated or decompensated. When accompanied by ligamentous instability or adjacent muscle

Table 30–7
NSAID Toxicity (After Amadio)

NSAID CLASS	GI IRRITATION	PEPTIC ULCER	CNS	TINNITUS	HEPATITIS	RENAL
Salicylates						
Aspirin	+ + + +	+ +	+	+ + +	+ +	+
Diflunisal	+	+	+	+	+	+
Propionic acid derivatives						
Carprofen	+ +	+	+	+	+	+
Fenoprofen	+ +	+	+ +	+ + +	+	+
Flurbiprofen	+ +	+	+	+	+	+
Ibuprofen	+ +	+	+	+	+	+
Ketoprofen	+ +	+	+	+	+	+
Naproxen	+ +	+ +	+ +	+ +	+	+
Naproxen sodium	+ +	+	+	+	+	+
Pyrroleacetic acid derivatives						
Indomethacin	+ + + +	+ + +	+ + + +	+	+	+ +
Sulindac	+	+	+	+	+	+
Tolmetin	+ + +	+ +	+ +	+ +	NA	+ +
Fenamates						
Mefenamic acid	+	+	+	NA	NA	+ +
Meclofenamate	+ + + (*)	+	+	+	+	+
Oxicams						
Piroxicam	+ + +	+ + +	+	+	+	+
Phenylacetic acid						
Diclofenac	+ +	+ +	+	+	+ +	+
Pyranocarboxylic acid						
Etodolac	±	±	+	+	+	+
Pyrazole derivatives						
Oxyphenbutazone	+ + + +	+ + + +	+	+	+ + + +	+
Phenylbutazone	+ + + +	+ + + +	+	+	+ + + +	+

GENERIC NAME	DOSAGE (mg)	STARTING DOSE (mg)	MAXIMUM DOSE
Salicylates	325,	650–1300 q4–6 hr	Determine by
Acetyl salicylic acid	500,	1000 q6–8 hr	serum
Zorphin	800,	1600 q 12 hr	salicylate level
Salsalate	500, 750	1000–1500 q6hr	
Magnesium salicylate	600	1200 q4–6 hr	
Choline salicylate	600	1200 q4–6 hr	
Choline magnesium	500, 750, 1000	single nightly dose 2000–4000 mg	
Diclofenac	25, 50, 75	25–75 bid–qid	200
Etodolac	200, 300	200–300 qid	1200
Ibuprofen	400, 600, 800	400–800 bid, tid, qid	3200
Indomethacin	25, 50, 75	25–75 bid, tid	225
Ketoprofen	50, 75	50–75 bid, tid	300
Meclofenamate	50, 100	50 qid	400
Nabumetone	500	500 bid	2000
Naproxen	250, 375, 500	250–500 bid	1500
Piroxicam	10, 20	20 qd	20
Sulindac	150–200	150–200 bid	450
Tolmetin	200, 400, 600	200–600 qid	1600

+ + + + highest level of toxicity among NSAIDs listed.
± negligible toxicity.
NA data not available or inconclusive.
(*) diarrhea.
Pediatric doses:
ASA: <25 kg body wt: 80–100 mg/kg/day divided 4 times/day
>25 kg body wt: 2400–3600 mg/day divided 4 times/day
Naproxen (2 yrs and older): 10–15 mg/kg divided 2 or 3 times/day
Tolmetin (2 yrs and older): 20 mg/kg/day in 3–4 divided doses/day up to 30 mg/kg/day.

Table 30–8
Principles for Soft-Tissue Injection

1. Mark site of injection with circular end of ball point pen.
2. Prepare a sterile field; use gloves or sterile technique.
3. Use the shortest needle that will reach the lesion.
4. For injecting tender points, use the needle as a probe.
5. For injecting tendon sheaths, insert the needle parallel to the tendon.
6. At site of nerve entrapment, wait a moment after needle is inserted; be certain the needle has not penetrated a nerve or vessel.
7. Use 1 or 2% local anesthetic *without epinephrine*.
   Universal precautions apply

weakness, decompensation occurs and a vicious cycle of pain, weakness, disuse and, finally, swelling occurs. Roentgenographic findings do not correlate with outcome.

When decompensated, treatment should be directed not only to pain relief but, more importantly, to restoration of muscle strength, joint protection, and elimination of bad habits and obesity.

Types include

- Primary osteoarthritis: Nodal, generalized, inflammatory (erosive), or spinal
- Secondary osteoarthritis: Following trauma, inflammation, metabolic endocrine, or neuropathic diseases

Nodal Osteoarthritis

Features include bulbous enlargement of the terminal finger joints (Heberden nodes) or proximal interphalangeal joints (Bouchard nodes); enlargement (bossing) of the great toe metatarsophalangeal joint, often with bunion formation; enlargement and limitation of movement of the first carpometacarpal joint.

Table 30–9
Principles for Joint Aspiration and Injection

1. Prepare a sterile field. Use gloves
2. Use local anesthetic without epinephrine. Make skin wheal with #25 needle tip bevel flat to skin.
3. Inject local anesthetic into synovium; withdraw needle.
4. Use #16 needle for joint aspiration. Any smaller needle may get plugged by synovium or rice bodies.
5. Use 30-cc syringe to aspirate larger joints. Aspirate slowly to avoid sucking synovium into needle tip and getting a dry tap.
6. Transfer aliquote or synovial fluid to heparinized tube for synovianalysis.
7. If crystalline steroid (methylprednisolone or triamcinolone hexacetonide) are mixed with xylocaine or procaine, a flocculant will occur with a likely prolongation of local effect.
8. Use 20–40 mg of corticosteroid and 1 cc 1% lidocaine for larger joints, and as little as 5–10 mg for smaller joints.
9. Have patient apply ice locally to prevent a painful crystal reaction.
10. Have patient avoid strenuous activity to the involved joint for two weeks.
11. Universal precautions apply.

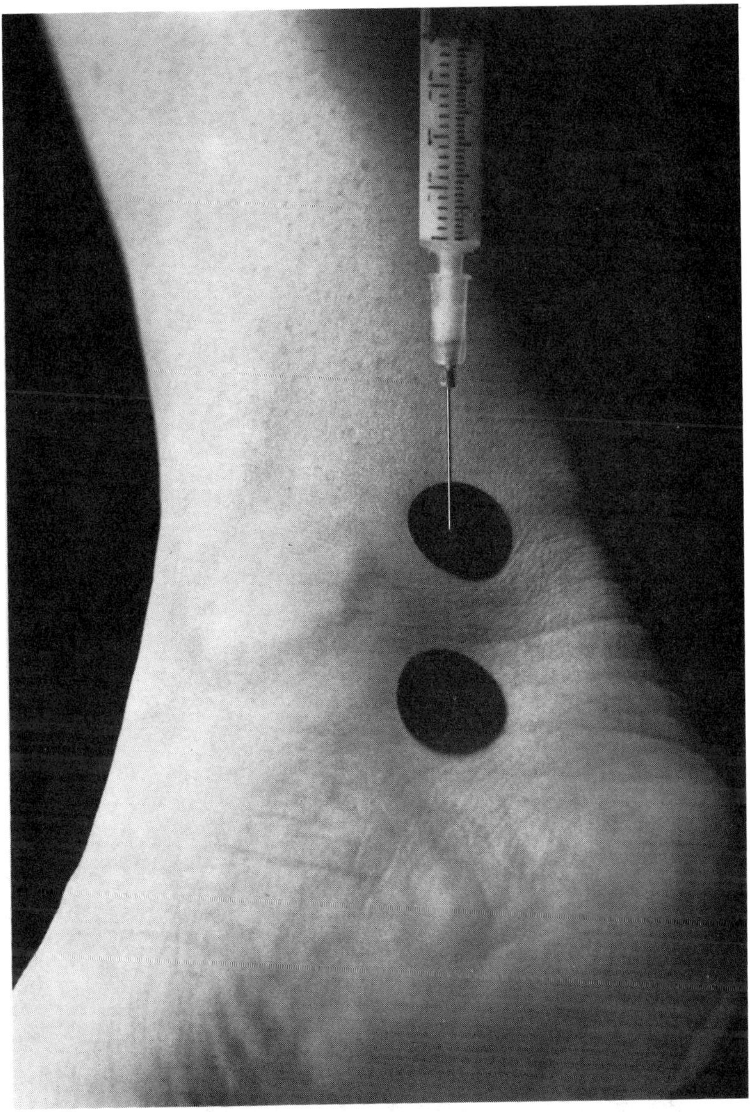

Figure 30–3. Injection sites (composite). From: Sheon, Robert P, Moskowitz, Roland W, Goldberg, Victor M: Soft Tissue Rheumatic Pain: Recognition, Management, Prevention. 2nd Ed. Philadelphia, Lea & Febiger, 1987.

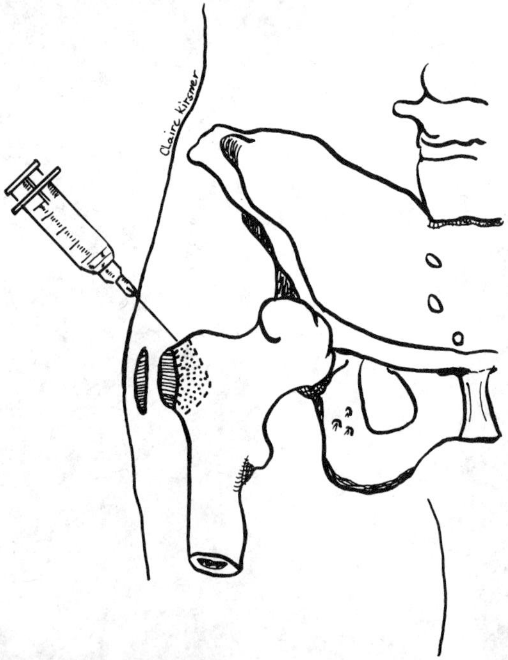

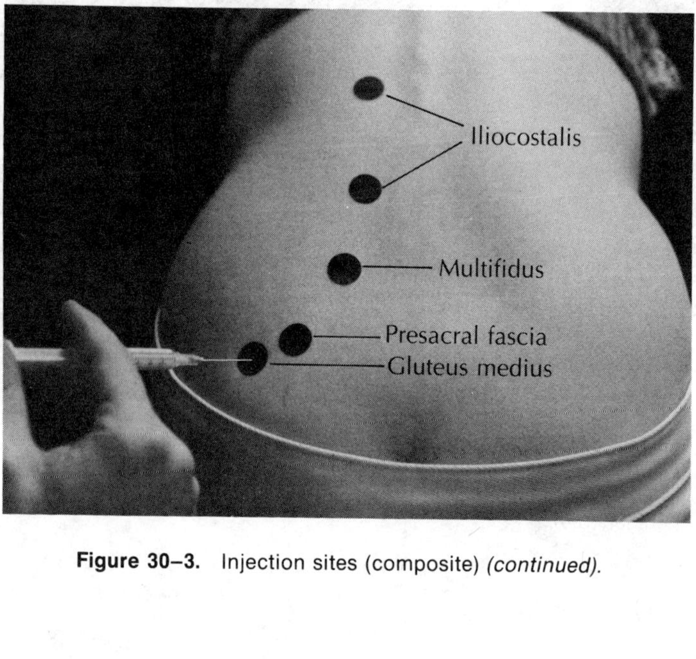

Figure 30–3. Injection sites (composite) *(continued).*

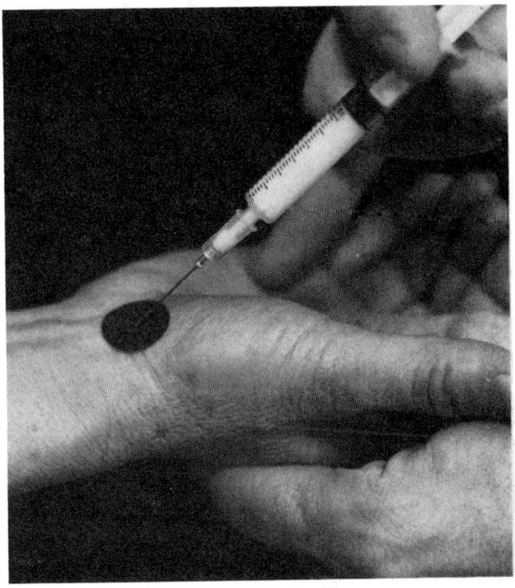

Figure 30–3. Injection sites (composite) *(continued).*

Pathogenesis: Often genetically transmitted, pathology includes fibrillation, fragmentation, thinning, and eventual loss of cartilage; formation of osteophytes; and sclerosis of subchondral bone.

Differential diagnosis: Distal finger nodes might be similar to psoriatic arthritis, tophaceous gout, or a benign tumor of bone.

- Cost-effective workup: Order x ray only when trauma has occurred, if asymmetric, or if accompanied by warmth or redness.

Initial Treatment: Pain management with oral analgesics, salicylates, NSAIDs, in that order. Joints with effusions: Aspiration and injection. If synovial fluid is turbid, do synovianalysis. See Tables 30–9 and 30–10.

Teach patient longterm behavior modification applying joint protection for each affected area (see Table 30–11). Refer to an occupational therapist for joint protection and finger exercises; splinting ad lib. Longterm behavior modification is more important than medication.

For patient education, call the Arthritis Foundation for pamphlets on Osteoarthritis and Joint Protection.

Osteoarthritis of the Hip, Knee, Spine

Often is asymptomatic; if pain awakens patient, or is worse at rest, suspect other causes for pain, particularly bursitis, tendinitis, myofascial pain disorder, gout, rheumatoid arthritis.

Features: Weight-bearing or use-related pain accompanied by ↓ or painful passive range of joint motion. Knee buckling, locking, or giving way suggests an internal derangement such as a meniscus tear.

Initial Treatment: Pain management with either salicylates or NSAIDs. Joints with effusions of >10 days' duration, when pain limits essential activity, or if persistent despite quadriceps strengthening: Aspiration and corticosteroid injection. If synovial fluid is turbid, do synovianalysis. See Tables 30–9 and 30–10.

Referral to physical therapist for exercises and home program, dietitian for weight reduction, and occupational therapist for joint protection advice. This is as important as oral medication. See Tables 30–11 & 12.

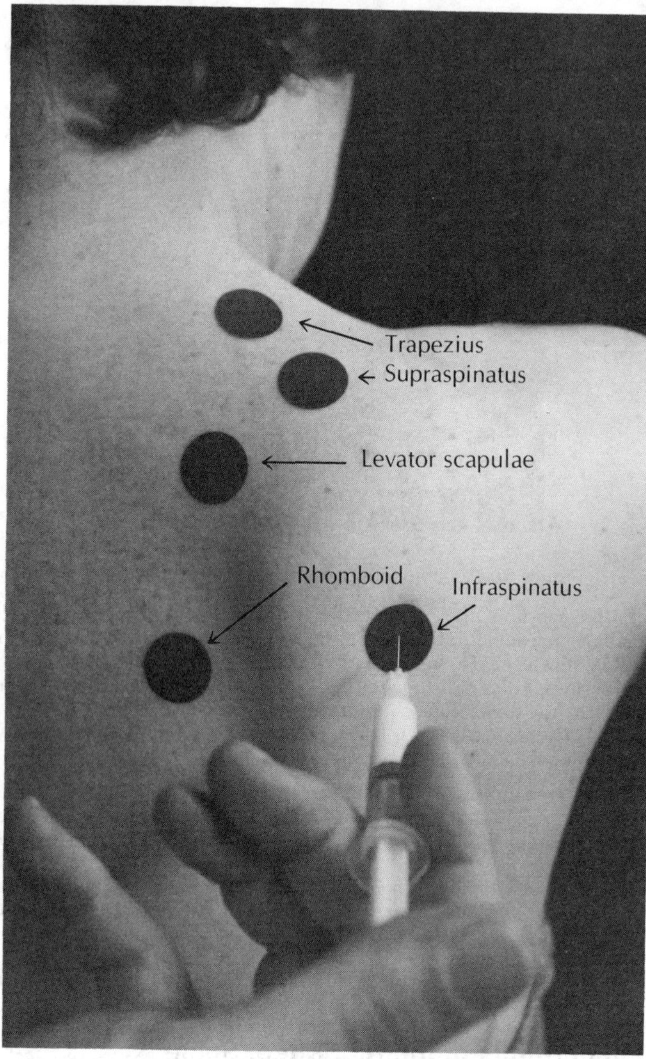

Figure 30–3. Injection sites (composite) *(continued).*

Surgical referral for osteoarthritis of the hip or knee should be restricted to patients with avascular necrosis; or patients who, after a trial of physical therapy and directed home exercises, cannot perform an essential function such as dressing, getting through a grocery store, having sex, or getting to the bathroom.

The symptomatic osteoarthritic joint will often improve with rest and modified behavior. Use NSAIDs cautiously.

- Strengthening exercises reduce pain, particularly at the wrist, hand, and knee. Elderly patients should be encouraged to use exercise therapy, rub-on medications, and acetaminophen.

Unless patient has features suggesting need for surgery and agrees to surgery, x rays are not necessary.

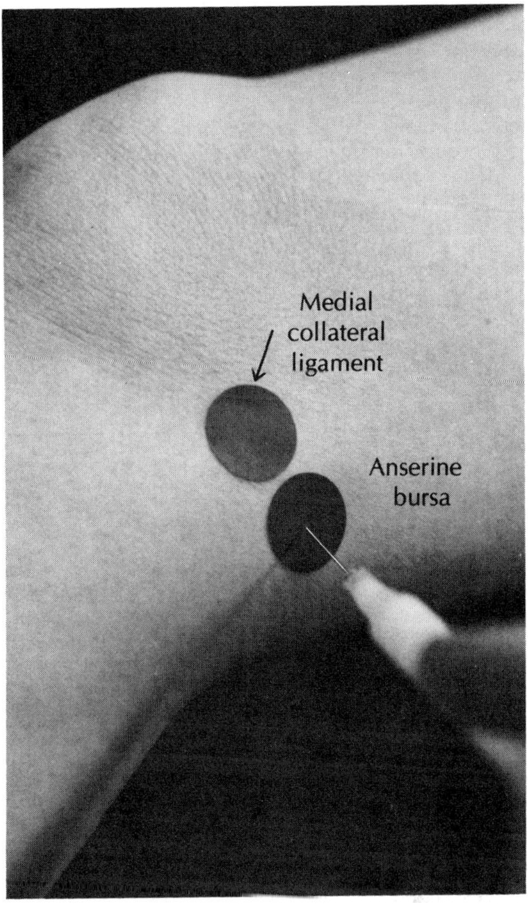

Figure 30–3. Injection sites (composite) *(continued).*

NONARTICULAR RHEUMATIC DISORDERS

These very common symptom disorders include bursitis, tendinitis, myofascial pain syndromes, structural disorders such as joint laxity (hypermobility syndrome) or body asymmetry, and fibromyalgia. They lack objective measurement and may overlay other rheumatic disorders, creating significant disability. Reserve expensive imaging for patients who have objective abnormality or who fail conservative treatment.

Diagnosis is often based on subjective features and physical examination techniques that reproduce symptoms (see Tables 30–5 and 30–6).

Nonarticular rheumatic disorders are common and easily treated without invasive procedures and with a minimum of diagnostic study. A 6-step management plan should be followed:

- Exclude other diseases through careful history, physical examination, and appropriate tests.
- Identify habits and aggravations that will cause persistence or recurrence.

Table 30–10
Synovianalysis

Basic information:
Volume, color, turbidity grade*, string sign for mucin content (one drop fluid on gloved finger, touch with thumb, and separate. A 3-inch or longer string is normal; length varies inversely with inflammation.)
Suspected problem:
Infection:
WBC, Differential; gram stain; culture
Sugar (and concomitant serum glucose)
Gout:
WBC, Differential
Crystal study with polarizing microscopy and red compensator
Rheumatoid arthritis, lupus, rheumatic fever, etc.
WBC, Differential
Latex RA titer; crystals

* Infected synovial fluid is a dirty or muddy brown (staph), green (gonococcus), and all color grades in between. If in doubt, do gram stain, sugar, culture.

- Provide an explanation for the pain and disability.
- Provide pain relief, so that exercise will be performed.
- Provide exercises to restore muscle flexibility and tone.
- Provide an expected outcome.

Regional Soft Tissue Disorders

Features include local pain and tenderness; swelling is variable; ominous findings are not present (see Table 30–6). Pain at rest often is more severe than pain during movement. Numbness and tingling may occur if the local process is adjacent to a major nerve.

Passive movement and palpation, tests, and maneuvers (e.g., the Finkelstein maneuver, trigger point palpation) can reproduce the pain. Symptom relief should follow treatment, and this corroborates diagnosis.

Etiology is usually traumatic and often subtle, such as inappropriate body position, or habits. See Table 30–11. Some common but often vague entities are

- **Carotidynia.** Throbbing pain may occur over the side of the face, head, or neck. Marked tenderness, and sometimes swelling at the carotid bifurcation, may be palpated. The condition is probably related to migraine. No diagnostic studies are available. Treatment includes drugs useful in migraine
- **Temporomandibular myofascial pain.** Pain is often referred to the neck and face, and often without jaw complaint. Palpation of the internal pterygoid muscles within the anterior pillars (with gloved finger) will elicit severe pain or tenderness. Malocclusion should be excluded with dental examination. Treatment includes use of a bite splint, behavior modification, and muscle relaxants such as cyclobenzaprine, or tricyclics, prescribed particularly at bedtime. Some patients have caffeine and theophylline sensitivity; a trial of abstaining from dark beverages may be helpful
- **Scapulothoracic syndromes,** Aching discomfort throughout the shoulder girdle, usually unilateral, with nighttime aggravation and often with diffuse arm paresthesia, may result from a trigger point

Table 30–11
Joint Protection Guide

Head and Neck

Principle: keep head aligned with trunk.
Avoid jutting head forward ("Birdwatcher's Neck," as if looking through field glasses); hold head up when reading; use large lap pillow for holding handwork higher; lower adjustable chair if work-table or desk is too low for long-waisted person. Avoid propping head forward when resting. Use proper chair for support.

Shoulder

Principle: Avoid repetitive movements or prolonged overhead use.
Vacuuming, performing pushups, or sports in which the arm moves like a piston can lead to overuse injury. Such activities should be moderated. Women with heavy breasts may benefit from use of a support brassiere. When writing, keep the involved shoulder held backward and upward.

Elbow

Principle: Repetitive and rotating motions should be moderated.
Fist clenching, using tools with a tight grip, and using the hands to push off of chairs may lead to tennis elbow. Reduce grip pressure by using pipe insulation on tool handles.

Wrist and Hand

Principle: Use larger muscles when possible; moderate repetitive activities.
Grasp with flat open palms when possible. Repetitive movements and handwork should be interrupted with other activities. Never say "I'm going to finish this even if it kills me!" Use a plastic pencil holder during prolonged writing. Use foamy pipe insulation on tool handles. Avoid clenched fists at night (a tension state); using nylon stretch gloves during sleep may help.

Low Back

Principle: Avoid prolonged standing, prolonged sitting, and improper lifting.
Bend at the knee, not at the waist. Lift with the thighs. Avoid bending over with straight knees. When prolonged standing is necessary, use a 2 × 4 × 8 inch wood block and step up on it with one foot for a few minutes, then change it to the other foot (while working in the kitchen, or if working at a machine, or as a cashier). When carrying heavy objects, carry the object out in front, turn with the feet, not by twisting the trunk. Use cushion-soled shoes when standing or working on concrete.

Knee

Principle: Maintain good alignment and quadriceps (thigh muscle) strength.
When arising from a chair, avoid using hands to push off of chair; use thigh muscles to push off. Avoid prolonged sitting. Avoid twisting the trunk; turn with the feet. Avoid stair climbing. If the home lacks a first floor toilet facility, place a portable toilet on the first floor. Avoid kneeling on hard floors; use a pad.

Foot

Principle: Shoes were meant to cover and protect the feet, not to compress them.
Aging feet sometimes enlarge or toes spread. Have shoe size measured while standing. Prolonged standing or squatting may result in foot strain. If you have flat feet, leg cramp may result from wearing flat shoes or slippers.

From: Sheon RP: Nonarticular rheumatism and nerve entrapment disorders. Resident & Staff Physician, *35*(12):65–70, 1989.

in the infraspinatus muscle, located midway between the spine of the scapula and the lower scapular pole. Palpation of the indurated firm muscle bundle reproduces the pain. An important clue is painless passive arm rotation in any plane. Injecting the trigger point is helpful and diagnostic. Other parascapular muscles may be involved. See Figures 30–1 and 30–2 for location of trigger points. (See Table 30–8 for injection technique and Table 30–11 for joint protection for the shoul-

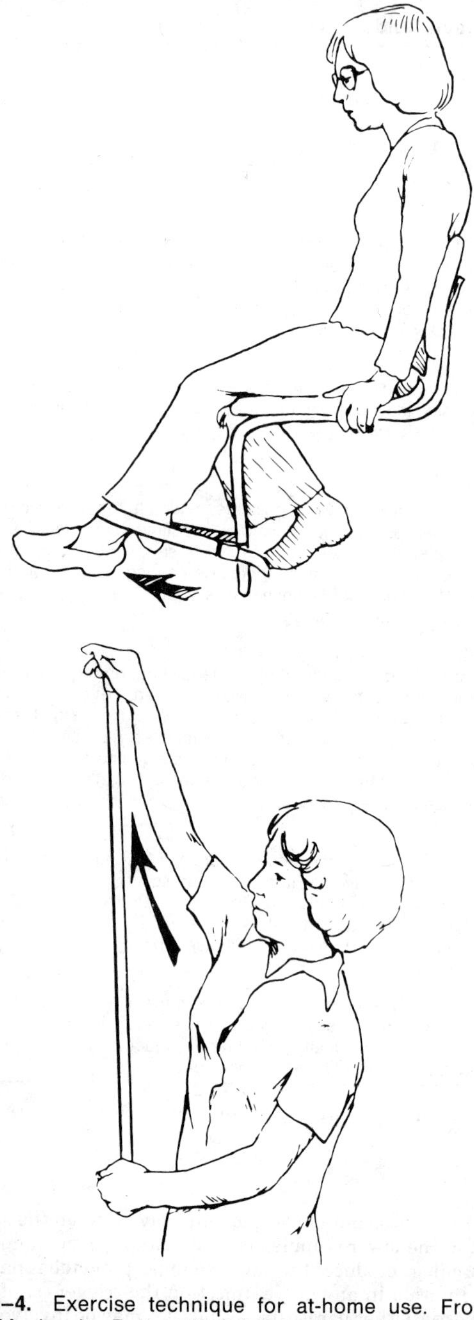

Figure 30–4. Exercise technique for at-home use. From: Sheon, Robert P, Moskowitz, Roland W, Goldberg, Victor M: Soft Tissue Rheumatic Pain: Recognition, Management, Prevention. 2nd Ed. Philadelphia, Lea & Febiger, 1987, and McCarty, Daniel J, Koopman, William J, (eds.): Arthritis and Allied Conditions. 12th Ed. Philadelphia, Lea & Febiger, 1992.

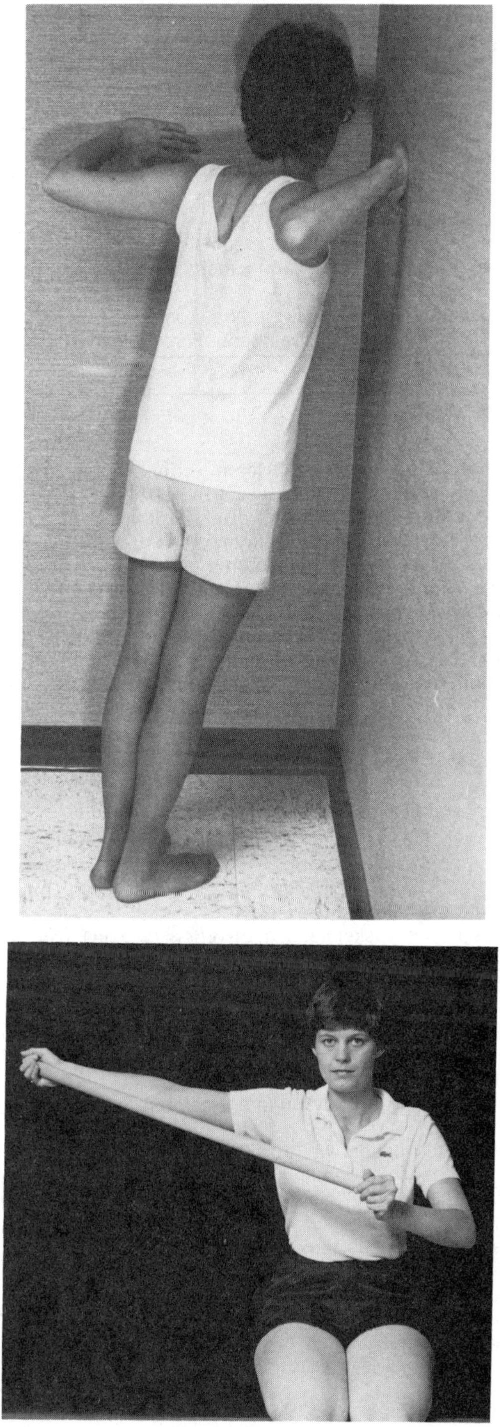

Figure 30–4. Exercise technique for at-home use *(continued).*

Table 30–12
Writing a Prescription for OT/PT

Therapist needs to know patient's name and age, diagnosis, major problems, goals, and risks.

Sample prescription for occupational therapy and/or physical therapy:

Date: April 12, 1992 Jane Doe, age 57 Diagnosis: Osteoarthritis and rheumatoid Problem: Painful swollen hands, toes, shoulders Other: Has diabetes RX: Evaluate, manage, provide home program Goals: Joint preservation, pain reduction, education about disease

der region). See Figure 30–3 for injection site. A common cause is repetitively reaching backward: For a seatbelt, into the back seat of the car, or when in the kitchen or at work

- **Shoulder impingement syndrome.** Pain during arm abduction, elevation, often with paresthesias, may result from shoulder cuff impingement under the acromion. Tenderness occurs in the vicinity of the subcoracoid bursa, below the acromioclavicular joint, and medial to the insertion of the biceps tendon. See Figure 30–5. Impingement is reproduced by grasping the patient's elbow while the arm is abducted and externally rotated, then pressing arm into acromion and

Table 30–13
Helpful Hints

1. Laying on of the examiner's hands often provides more useful information than do roentgenograms.
2. Osteoarthritis seen on roentgenograms is often unrelated to the pain syndrome.
3. Localized musculoskeletal pain disorders may be layered over another established disease process.
4. When morning stiffness does not *mainly* involve the hands and feet, rheumatoid arthritis is an unlikely diagnosis.
5. Pain so severe that the limbs cannot be touched (the touch-me-not syndrome), and with no discernible spasm, is usually of psychogenic origin.
6. Pain localized to a body quadrant seldom is due to a psychogenic cause.
7. Observing the patient while seated, while rising from a chair, while standing, and while bending forward can lead to recognition of basic *structural* alterations. "Misuse" of the musculoskeletal system may also be observed.
8. Drugs may be the least important part of treatment. Stretching exercises and avoiding aggravating factors often provide more sustained benefit than pills.

From: Sheon, Robert P, Moskowitz, Roland W, Goldberg, Victor M: Soft Tissue Rheumatic Pain: Recognition, Management, Prevention. 2nd Ed. Philadelphia, Lea & Febiger, 1987.

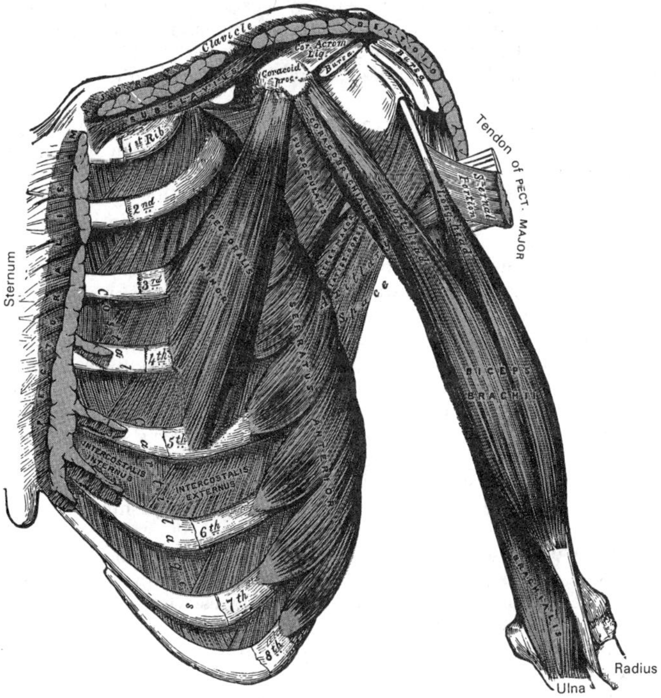

Figure 30–5. Anatomy of the shoulder, anterior view. From: Sheon, Robert P, Moskowitz, Roland W, Goldberg, Victor M: Soft Tissue Rheumatic Pain: Recognition, Management, Prevention. 2nd Ed. Philadelphia, Lea & Febiger, 1987.

rotating slightly to reproduce symptoms. The best test is instillation of xylocaine (1 cc 1%) mixed with methylprednisolone (20–40 mg) into the subcoracoid space and adjacent tissues, after careful prep. Then, active movement should be pain free. Treatment includes avoiding repetitious arm motion with elbow abducted. When necessary to perform repetitious movement, the patient should position the body so the arm can perform task out in front of the ipsilateral breast. In this manner the biceps and supraspinatus muscles avoid impingement. Physical therapy consultation is appropriate before undertaking further evaluation or orthopedic consultation

- **Carpal tunnel syndrome.** Pain, weakness, and paresthesias in median nerve distribution is suggestive. Physical examination findings include positive Tinel test, wrist compression test, or wrist tourniquet test. Electrodiagnostic study is recommended only if conservative treatment fails. If swelling is evident, or features include prolonged symmetrical morning stiffness, tests for rheumatoid arthritis should be obtained.

Patients with suggestive symptoms but without weakness or atrophy should have such conservative measures as resting wrist splints, ↓ in repetitious motion, occupational and physical therapy consultation, and avoidance of excessive gripping of the steering wheel, tools, or nocturnal hand clenching (can be treated with nylon stretch gloves worn at night with the seams to the outside). NSAIDs or injection of the volar wrist area with methylprednisolone-xylocaine mixture (see Table 30–8 and Figure 30–3) can be helpful. If conservative measures fail, then surgery is indicated

- **Trigger Finger, trigger thumb.** Complaints include snapping or locking sensation of 1 or several digits, particularly upon arising. Usually follows unusual or repetitive hand tasks. Treatment is highly satisfactory with injection of the flexor tendon sheath with steroid-xylocaine mixture (see Table 30–8 and Fig. 30–3). Splinting the digit is helpful. Provide joint protection advice (see Table 30–11)
- **Myofascial chest wall pain syndrome (costochondritis).** Inflammatory disease of the costochondral joints can occur in rheumatoid arthritis and ankylosing spondylitis (costochondritis). Much more commonly, the disorder is not inflammatory, and the term myofascial chest wall pain syndrome is preferred. What distinguishes this syndrome from other causes of chest pain is pain at rest relative to effort and exquisite costochondral tenderness. Causes include such repetitive effort as coughing, or transferring heavy objects such as moving log pile. Treatment includes behavior modification and chest wall stretching exercises. 1 simple exercise is for the patient to stand 2 feet out from the corner of a room and perform a pushup slowly into the corner for 1 or 2 min several times a day
- **Myofascial low back pain.** Perhaps as many as 90% of patients with persistent back pain lack objective causality determinants. If ominous features are not present, avoid labels suggestive of skeletal origin. Radiographic changes of disc degeneration or narrowing, spurs, unusual angulation, or congenital lumbosacral changes often have no relation to symptoms or outcome.

Much of the history and examination methods of the past have been proven unreliable.

Ominous features include a history of progressive pain that is worse with walking; paresthesia felt below the knee; leg pain that has become worse than back pain; weakness with giving way of leg; and/or physical findings of listing, flattening of the spine when patient bends forward, limitation of hip movement, diminished reflexes on 1 side, and weakness consistent with nerve root involvement.

If buttock claudication has occurred, spinal stenosis should be considered.

Roentgenographic examination should be limited to those patients whose symptoms followed significant trauma, are older, have important objective features, or have a past history suggesting possible ominous disease (e.g. osteomyelitis, tumor, family history of ankylosing spondylitis, iritis, or other systemic features, including weight loss, fever, prolonged morning stiffness, or use of corticosteroids for extended periods of time).

When ordering roentgenography, be sure to order a pelvis examination along with lumbar spine roentgenographs.

Imaging studies should likewise be reserved for the patient who has ominous features and would be willing to have surgery if the findings warrant it. Severity of pain alone is not an indication for imaging.

Conservative care includes assessment of trunk strength with corrective exercise prescription, proper shoes, and job and hobby activity modification, if necessary. Smoking and diet should be addressed. Smoking reduces O_2 content of disc and soft tissues, thus impairing natural healing. Physical therapy should be ordered early. Bed rest is of value only if an acute herniation is suspected, and then not for > a few days.

Use of NSAIDs, muscle relaxants, and trigger point injections with steroid-xylocaine mixture are a means to provide pain relief and compliance with physical therapy. See Figure 30–3.

Patients improve in direct proportion to the number of treatment modalities tried. In one study 91% of patients with proved herniated nucleus pulposis improved without surgery if cord impingement was not severe and if the patient failing one therapy was provided several alternatives in sequence.

- **Bursitis of the hip or knee.** Pain in the hip or knee that is more disturbing during rest than when walking should suggest a regional bursitis, even when significant osteoarthritis is evident. Night pain may be severe, is uncommon in osteoarthritis, and suggestive of bursitis.

Trochanteric bursitis with either superficial or deep tenderness at or posterior to the greater trochanter can be treated with either an NSAID or, if persistent, a corticosteroid-xylocaine injection (see Fig. 30–3). Relief is usual within a few days. Patient should be instructed in proper bending (with knees bent and back straight).

Anserine bursitis along the inner aspect of the knee joint commonly occurs in elderly women with thick knee panniculae. Have the knees separated with a cushion between the thighs during sleep. Night pain is common and relieved by local steroid-xylocaine injection (see Fig. 30–3).

Prepatellar bursitis may result from repeated kneeling or from foreign body penetration; septic bursitis can occur. If the bursa is swollen, do aspiration and synovial fluid examination for sugar, WBC, gram stain, and culture. Leukocyte count may not be impressive; even as low as 1,000 cells/ml may be found in septic bursitis. Many rheumatologists prefer to use oral NSAIDs and not inject this bursa after aspiration. Many would similarly treat olecranon bursitis. Surgical excision may be necessary for persistent swelling

- **Tarsal tunnel syndrome.** Foot pain that awakens the patient from sleep is characteristic. Nerve entrapment is common following ankle trauma, but may also occur from an adjacent tenosynovitis brought on by stretching the posterior tibial tendon by walking barefoot or in flat slippers. The Tinel test is best performed by rolling the examiner's thumb across the tarsal tunnel inferior to the medial malleolus. Pain reproduction is suggestive. Use of a local steroid-xylocaine injection (see Fig. 30–3) and proper footgear should provide relief

Generalized Soft Tissue Rheumatic Pain

When patients complain of diffuse stiffness and aching, or widespread arthralgia, and the sensation of joint swelling ("My rings feel tight") but without evidence of illness or synovitis, 2 entities deserve consideration: Fibromyalgia and the hypermobility syndrome. A tender point count and examination for joint laxity should be performed. (Figures 30–6 and 30–7.) Only in the absence of other diseases can these entities be considered a primary disorder.

A lengthy workup is not needed. A chemistry panel, including CPK, TSH, CBC, and Westergren sedimentation rate, may suffice. Unless objective features of connective tissue disease are in evidence, it is not necessary to order antinuclear antibodies or rheumatoid factor: Since 5% of normal persons may have low titers of these tests, and only 6% of patients with the tender point count have underlying connective tissue disease, these tests are not cost effective.

FIBROMYALGIA

Features include widespread aching and stiffness (aggravated following rest), nonrestful sleep, weather sensitivity, and fatigue. Other com-

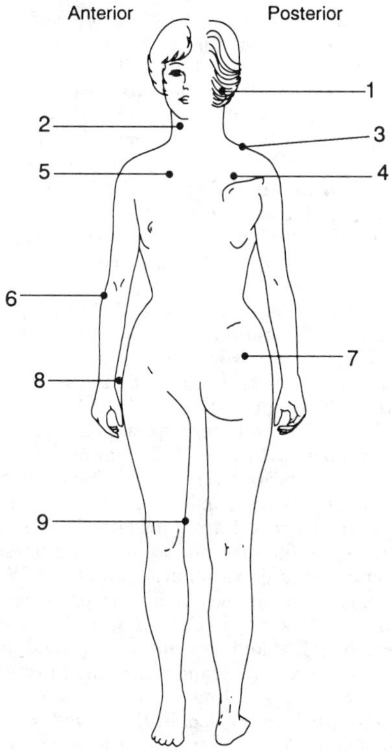

Figure 30–6. Fibromyalgia tender points. From McCarty, Daniel J, Koopman, William J: Arthritis and Allied Conditions. 12 Ed. Philadelphia, Lea & Febiger, 1992.

mon features include migraine headache, Raynaud's phenomenon, irritable bowel syndrome, paresthesia, and weakness. Figure 30–6 presents location of tender points. Diagnosis requires 11 of 18 points and few control points. Use the mid-thigh region as a control for tenderness: The sensation that occurs when the examiner presses with about 4 lb pressure is called tenderness, whereas more than that is pain, particularly when the patient grimaces or withdraws. Other control points include the forehead, mid-dorsal forearm, thumbnail compression, and midway down the third metatarsal bone. The test points should be palpated and interspersed with the control points, and they should elicit a pain response rather than a tender-only response.

Laboratory features are normal unless fibromyalgia coexists with another disease. Most patients blame a stressful event for the symptoms. Many believe alteration in Substance P and endorphins are involved.

Treatment begins by eliminating serious underlying disease with a comprehensive history and physical examination and judicious testing. When the control points are normal, the patient will be relieved to know that the examination demonstrates a non-psychological disorder; the pain is not imagined.

Medication that improves mood and sleep is helpful, including tricyclics, trazodone, meprobamate, cyclobenzaprine, or carisoprodol. These

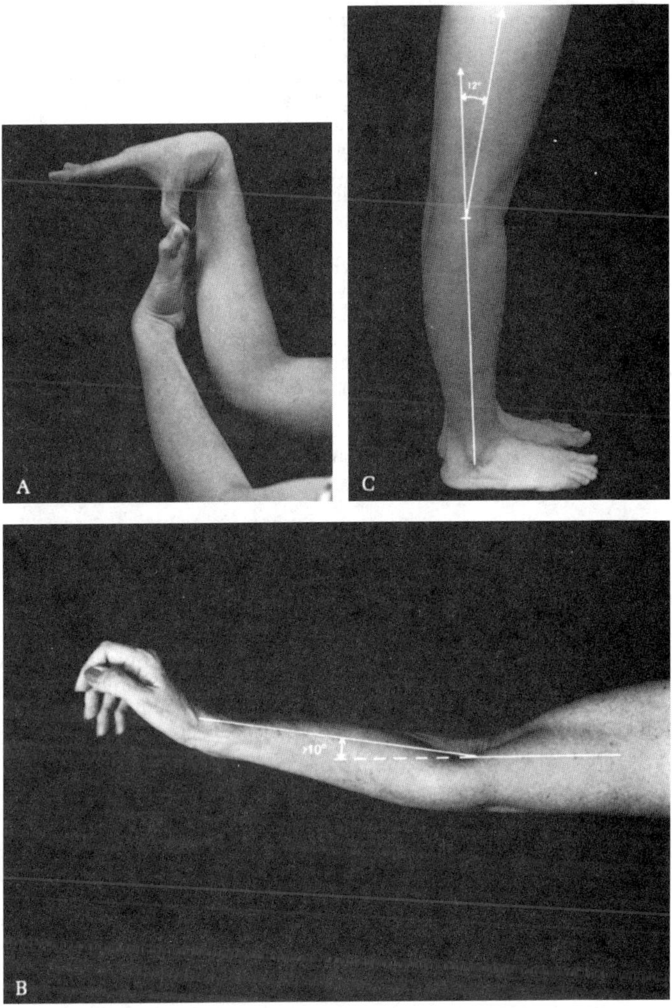

Figure 30–7. Joint laxity findings at the elbow, wrist, knee. From: Sheon, Robert P, Moskowitz, Roland W, Goldberg, Victor M: Soft Tissue Rheumatic Pain: Recognition, Management, Prevention. 2nd Ed. Philadelphia, Lea & Febiger, 1987.

agents also boost endorphins. Most important is a gradual and progressive fitness exercise program. Aquatic exercises, very light aerobic exercises, walking, and cycling can result in more prolonged pain relief than that which occurs with medication.

Severe incapacitation from fibromyalgia is rare; additional measures may include tender point injections or an ice rub and stretch routine. Behavior modification, biofeedback, and psychosocial counseling can be helpful.

HYPERMOBILITY SYNDROME

Symmetrical joint pain and back or neck pain, stiffness, and a sensation of joint swelling that is of so short duration (hours) that inflammation is unlikely, may result from loss of muscle tone in persons with diffuse joint laxity. Such patients may not be aware of joint laxity, yet they can do the following: Bend over and touch palms to floor with knees straight, extend elbows and knees >10°, draw thumb into apposition with ipsilateral forearm, draw finger back and parallel to forearm, and/or invert or evert ankle excessively.

Patients with hypermobility syndrome show joint laxity in ≥3 locations (see Fig. 30–7). Since 5% of the population have joint laxity, another factor is needed before symptoms occur. Most patients have onset after a period of inactivity, such as following pregnancy, illness, study, or a career change to a sedentary state. Then, upon attempting a physically taxing chore or sport, symptoms occur. Treatment consists of exercises that emphasize extensor muscle strengthening for the involved joints. Symptoms usually improve after several months of exercise. For patients with spinal complaints, pool aerobics may be helpful.

MONOARTICULAR ARTHRITIS

Age at onset, personal and family history, lifestyle, and personal habits history, palpation for synovial thickness, and synovial fluid analysis are essential elements for diagnosis. See Table 30–2 for differential diagnosis and Table 30–6 for important elements in a rheumatologic history and physical. Reaching the diagnosis in monoarticular arthritis is often a taxing rheumatologic exercise.

Noninflammatory Monoarthritides

- **Osteoarthritis.** Discussed earlier
- **Internal derangement** occurs in the knee, wrist, and temporomandibular joint, often without a history of trauma. The term implies a mechanical derangement that interferes with normal joint motion. Cartilage defects, ligamentous disruption, and intra-articular loose bodies are the more common disorders. Locking or buckling of the joint are usual symptoms.

When the knee is affected to the point the patient is unable to bear weight on it, refer to orthopedist. If less severe, prescribe a trial of conservative treatment. Most patients do not need surgery. Initiate use of crutches until swelling has subsided. Aspirate synovial fluid fully; do synovial fluid analysis if fluid has turbidity. Pain can be alleviated with instillation of corticosteroid and local anesthetic. See Tables 30–9 and 30–10.

Treatment for all noninflammatory degenerative monoarthropathies should include physical therapy and extensor muscle strengthening exercises (see Fig. 30–4). Pain relief often follows return of strength, irrespective of cause. Most patients with features of a meniscus tear or internal derangement improve with conservative measures. At this writing, an MRI of the knee costs $1,500; conservative treatment costs much less. Treat first, test later

- **Osteonecrosis, reflex dystrophy, Charcot joint, and hemarthro-**

sis have specific features of pain quality and severity and weight-bearing aggravation or buckling, and require management by those expert in their care

- **Paget's disease** of the spine, knee, or hip often presents with articular pain that results from secondary osteoarthritis of the involved joints. Pain often responds to joint aspiration, corticosteroid injection, ASA, and physical therapy. Serum alkaline phosphatase and urine hydroxyproline reflect disease activity. Drug treatment is usually reserved for those with elevated test results and with bone pain or in preparation for joint replacement. Treatment: Salicylates are often helpful. Active Paget's disease can be treated with etidronate 5–10 mg/kg daily for ≤6 months. If joint destruction is severe, arthroplasty should be considered. Calcitonin and mithramycin are used in special circumstances
- **Intra-articular tumors** are rare. Benign tumors present with swelling and moderate pain, and often cause locking. Malignant tumors generally cause much more pain both during movement and at rest; joint fluid is bloody and thin. MRI is helpful to diagnosis. Orthopedic consultation should be obtained for management

Inflammatory Monoarthritides

Inflammatory features of local or systemic fever, redness, and visible swelling require efficient and prompt diagnosis. Synovial fluid examination should be performed at the first visit (see Tables 30–9 and 30–10). Simply noting the mucin string sign and degree of turbidity (cloudiness) is of more value than roentgenography or scans.

RHEUMATOID ARTHRITIS

If synovium is thick and boggy, rheumatoid arthritis is most likely. The joint fluid turbidity signifies the erosiveness of the inflammatory process. Joint fluid tests for rheumatoid factor would likely be positive in high titer in adults and negative in children <16 yrs. Treatment should be aggressive

Treatment: Installation of a corticosteroid after aspiration can be performed if features of infection are not present. The injected joint should be protected from overuse for 2 weeks. NSAID in doses that parallel the degree of turbidity are prescribed (see Table 30–7). If recurrent synovitis is a problem, treatment with either hydroxychloroquine or sulfasalazine can be added (see Table 30–14). See next section's coverage of rheumatoid for comprehensive treatment.

GOUT AND PSEUDOGOUT

These conditions must be given top consideration if onset was abrupt and joint tenderness severe. Primary gout, of genetic origin, occurs in the absence of any causative factor (diuretics, alcohol, renal disease, occult hematologic or other malignancy, lead poisoning, etc.).

Synovial fluid should be examined by experienced staff; red compensation and polarized microscopy are usually necessary for crystal identification. Gout should be worked up, including tests for renal function, liver function, CBC, and uric acid determination in serum and in a 24–h urine specimen. A 24–h urine uric acid should be obtained before institution of specific therapy but after the acute attack has subsided and nonsteroidals can be replaced with colchicine.

Table 30–14
Disease-Modifying Antirheumatic Drugs (DMARDs)

DRUG BRANDS	DOSAGE	MONITOR REQUIREMENTS	SIDE EFFECTS
Methotrexate Rheumatrex	2.5-mg tabs; 5 to 20 mg single	CBC, SGPT q 2–4 weeks Chem panel q 3–6 mo	Cytopenias, hepatic fibrosis; CNS disturbances

Use with caution in patients with azotemia; avoid using with trimethoprim-sulfamethoxazole, phenylbutazone, retinoids, NSAIDs, probenecid, ethanol, cephalothin, penicillin

DRUG BRANDS	DOSAGE	MONITOR REQUIREMENTS	SIDE EFFECTS
Gold Salts	1st dose 10 mg	CBC, Platelet ct	Rash, stomatitis
Myochrysine reaction	2nd dose 25 mg	Urinalysis with each dose	Nitritoid
Solganol	then 50 mg/wk to 1200 mg, then every 2–4 weeks	Chem panel semi-annually	Nephritis, marrow toxicity
Ridaura	3–9 mg	Monthy CBC/UA	As above

(Less effective than injectible salts; useful for patients unable to travel, or for those who develop allergic reactions to injectibles)

DRUG BRANDS	DOSAGE	MONITOR REQUIREMENTS	SIDE EFFECTS
D Penicillamine Depen Cupramine	250 mg/d 1st month 500 mg bid 2nd mo	CBC/UA weekly at first, then	Rash, headache, GI upset, nephritis

then may increase q2–4 weeks; protein pneumonitis slowly to 3000 mg/d dipstick weekly

DRUG BRANDS	DOSAGE	MONITOR REQUIREMENTS	SIDE EFFECTS
Sulfasalazine AzulfidineENT	500 mg/d 1st month 500 mg/d 2nd month then if need up to 3000 mg/d	CBC/UA weekly at first than q2–4 wks albustix weekly	Rash, headache, GI upset, nephritis pneumonitis

Avoid in patients with positive ANA; past sulfa sensitivity; azotemia; hepatitis

DRUG BRANDS	DOSAGE	MONITOR REQUIREMENTS	SIDE EFFECTS
Antimalarials			
Chloroquine	250 mg/d	Eye exam with slit lamp, central fields, fundoscopy	Phototoxicity
Plaquenil	200 mg/bid		Ocular, neuro- and cardiac toxicity
Immunosuppressors			
Azathioprine (Imuran)	1 mg/kg/d up to 200 mg/day	CBC q2–4 weeks chem panel q6–12 mo	cytopenias, nausea, hepatitis
Cyclophos-phamide	1–2 mg/kg/d or 750–1000 mg bolus	CBC, Urinalysis chem panel q3–6 wks	cytopenias, hemorrhagic cystitis
Chlorambucil	2–8 mg/d	CBC q1–4 weeks chem panel q6–12 mo	cytopenias, late onset leukemias

>Cyclophosphamide and chlorambucil should be administered by those with experience. They are reserved for only life threatening disease because of their association with late onset malignancies.

Colchicine does not affect urate metabolism and can be used while waiting for urine uric acid test results. In primary gout, urine uric acid is usually normal (500–900 mg/24 h). When urine uric acid is greatly elevated, consider tumor or Lesch Nyhan syndrome.

Serum uric acid or joint fluid uric acid content, although usually elevated, may not always be so. Use of NSAIDs or aspirin may reduce the uric acid level to normal levels even though the patient is in the middle of an attack.

Treatment: Treatment of the acute attack includes NSAID treatment (indomethacin, if not contraindicated, 50 mg q 8 h) until attack subsides, usually not >48 h, or ACTH 40 U/24 h. If a diuretic is used for hypertension, try to change to other forms of antihypertensive treatment. If the diuretic is necessary, then, after the acute attack is over, and under cover of an NSAID or colchicine (0.5 or 0.6 mg bid), begin allopurinol 300 mg qd.

If renal function is good and several attacks have occurred, longterm treatment with probenecid is preferred. Again, this agent also requires cover of an NSAID or colchicine. Allopurinol is used if urine uric acid is high or if patient requires continued diuretic use or has hematologic or renal diseases.

The goal in using drugs that lower uric acid is to keep the serum uric acid level <6 mg/dl. Patients taking probenecid should not take ASA; rather, an NSAID or acetaminophen is preferred. Use maintenance NSAID or colchicine until patient is symptom free for several months and serum uric acid is normalized.

Examine all gouty patients for tophi. When present, the patient should be on life-long treatment with either allopurinol or probenecid as described above. 85% of patients with primary gout can be treated successfully with probenecid longterm; it is preferred because of less severe side effects.

Allopurinol should be used with caution in patients on coumadin, antineoplastic agents, ampicillin, amoxicillin, or ACE inhibitors, and in low dose if patient is azotemic.

- Hyperuricemia in the absence of gout is not an indication for longterm treatment with agents that lower the uric acid.

PSEUDOGOUT

May be monoarticular or polyarticular in onset. Fever can occur. Most common joints affected are the knee, ankle, and foot; rarely the great toe. The joint fluid is turbid but not "dirty"; synovial fluid microscopy with red compensator lens is important for identifying the weakly birefringent calcium pyrophosphate dihydrate crystals.

Treatment: Management of the attack is identical to treatment described for gouty arthritis attacks. Colchicine (0.5–0.6 mg bid) should be tried for intercritical treatment.

MILWAUKEE SHOULDER AND KNEE

A highly destructive basic calcium phosphate (hydroxyapatite, octacalcium phosphate, or tricalcium phosphate) arthropathy due to massive synovitis of a shoulder or knee in the elderly should be recognized early. Joint calcification and a creamy joint fluid or bloody effusion of large quantity are clues. Treat with frequent aspiration and NSAIDs.

JUVENILE MONOARTHRITIS

Without other diagnostic features, this condition may be extremely difficult to categorize. If family history is suggestive (arthritis, iritis, spondylitis, IBD), an HLA-B27 test determination is appropriate. Teenagers should have rheumatoid factor test determination, but this is not necessary for younger children.

All children with monoarticular arthritis should have ophthalmologic study with slit lamp for iritis, and ANA test determination (if positive, anterior uveitis will be more likely to occur).

Young adults should be screened carefully for sexually transmitted disease. Females may require cervical smear for gonococcus if sexually active. Joint fluid analysis is imperative on the initial visit (see Tables 30–9 and 30–10).

Complete examination is essential for signs of related diseases (see Table 30–6). Particularly examine the skin and genitalia for psoriasis and Reiter's syndrome, erythema nodosum, and erythema migrans. Perform the ENT exam for signs of mucous membrane changes and streptococcal infection, and, of course, a systematic examination as determined by the presentation.

Treatment: If joint fluid is turbid but not purulent, begin with NSAID and joint injection with corticosteroid. Lower-limb joints should be protected from weight bearing with use of crutches until joint swelling and tenderness have subsided. Defer roentgenographic examination except in patients with sepsis or trauma.

Oral anti-inflammatory treatment for children can be instituted if signs of inflammation are present: Fever, turbid joint fluid, abnormal Westergren sedimentation rate, or C-reactive protein. Preschoolers can be given non-acetylated salicylate either liquid (Arthropan; Trilisate liquid) or tablets; begin with 70–80 mg/kg in divided dosage.

Periodic determination of serum salicylate level taken 2 h after first morning dose is important in proper dosing of young children. Try to maintain salicylate level within 20–25 mg%. Reye's syndrome is rare, but during influenza or chicken pox outbreaks, salicylate therapy should be replaced with an NSAID. Naproxen (15 mg/kg/day) or tolmetin sodium (25–30 mg/kg/day) may be used.

Physical therapy home instruction is important and should begin as soon as the acute inflammation subsides.

JUVENILE SPONDYLOARTHROPATHIES

Often affect the lower extremity joints and only occasionally begin as a monoarthritis. Look for signs of sacroiliac tenderness, limited chest expanse with tape measure, family history, genital lesions of Reiter's syndrome, and nail changes. Treatment: See under Pauciarticular Polyarthritis, below.

PIGMENTED VILLONODULAR SYNOVITIS

Usually involves the hip or knee. Synovial fluid is sanguinous. Consult orthopedics.

Septic Arthritis

Bacterial infections often attack a single joint abruptly. The organism is usually spread hematologically. Older patients may not have systemic manifestations; often they suffer other debilitating diseases that lower their resistance to infection. Steroids and chemotherapy provide ↑ risk for infection.

- In younger individuals, septic arthritis is common among drug abusers, alcoholics, or those who are sexually promiscuous. The organism varies with the patient's risk factors. When the inflamed joint is associated with a tenosynovitis, look for gonococcus and tuberculosis. When the onset began with a migratory arthritis, consider bacterial endocarditis and hepatitis. If the patient works in soil (gardeners, tree surgeons), consider sporotrichosis and fungal pathogens.
- The most important treatment is early recognition. Septic arthritis can be classified as late or too late! If treatment is delayed >72 h, consider open drainage. Joint fluid should be removed daily in any event. Parenteral antibiotics are necessary in debilitated patients and those with compromised immune systems.

AIDS presents most commonly with a secondarily infected joint; the organism varies with risk factors. Those who are drug abusers tend to get staphylococcal or pseudomonas infections whereas prostitutes are more likely to have gonococcus, syphilis, or Chlamydia organisms. Other organisms associated with AIDS include mycobacterium avium intracellulare and Candida albicans. Other AIDS patients may present with features of Reiter's syndrome. See next section.

Viral arthritis and Lyme arthritis rarely present as a monoarthritis and will be discussed later.

PAUCIARTICULAR ARTHRITIS

Arthritis presentation with ≤4 swollen joints usually signifies a diagnosis other than rheumatoid arthritis and is often called a rheumatoid-variant arthritis. When the spine is affected, the term spondyloarthropathy is often used, and the HLA-B27 gene is usually present. Other rheumatic diseases without spinal involvement and in the absence of HLA-B27, and with onset following infection, are known as reactive arthritis. See Table 30–3. Treatment for the group is similar.

Diagnosis is based on extra-articular features combined with the joint findings. Extra-articular features may include involvement of the eye, heart, intestine, skin, and nails. Often the sites of tendon attachment become inflamed (enthesitis).

Spondyloarthropathies: Ankylosing Spondylitis

Onset varies with sex. Males most often start with low back stiffness and pain; the disease then slowly ascends; the neck is usually involved later. Lower extremity joints may be affected in adolescent males. Females more often present with lower limb symmetrical arthritis without spinal complaint. Chest expanse is restricted in most patients at first visit. Iritis is common.

Diagnosis should be based on the presence of ≥3 features: Back pain and stiffness not relieved by rest, sacroiliitis on x ray or bone scan, limited chest expanse (<3 inches male, 2 inches female), history of iritis (anterior uveitis), positive HLA-B27, or symmetrical inflammatory arthritis of lower limb joints. In practice, it is not necessary to test both roentgenography and HLA-B27 positivity.

Exclusions include roentgenographic findings of diffuse idiopathic skeletal hyperostosis; IBD; features of Reiter's syndrome; or psoriasis. Juvenile onset can occur, but rarely with simultaneous onset of rheumatoid arthritis; these patients then have spondylitis features and small upper limb joint involvement.

Differential diagnosis of sacroiliitis includes tuberculous spondylitis and other bacterial infections, amyloidosis, Whipple's disease, intestinal shunt-related arthritis, gout, hyperparathyroidism, Paget's disease, and neoplasia. Treatment is discussed below.

Reactive Arthritis

Inflammatory nonseptic arthritis in response to bacterial cell wall antigens has come to be known as reactive arthritis. Beginning with such well-established diseases as rheumatic fever and Reiter's syndrome, the group includes the arthritis associated with enteric pathogens and psoriatic arthritis, and the arthritis associated with IBDs.

Diagnosis is based on: Lower limb inflammatory arthritis, often involving articular and periarticular tissues; mucocutaneous lesions; urogenital lesions; and, rarely, aortitis and other cardiac lesions.

REITER'S SYNDROME

Classical features are conjunctivitis and painless stomatitis; nonseptic urethritis; lower limb arthritis (knee, ankle, feet) of ≥1 month duration; nail changes and a papular hyperkeratotic skin rash (keratodermia blennorrhagica). Circinate balanitis of the glans penis is common (see Figs. 30–8 and 30–9). Cervicitis is common in female patients. Unilateral sacroiliitis is also common.

The history must include sexual activity, risk factors for AIDS, and previous ocular, urogenital, or cutaneous involvement. Patients rarely volunteer the information.

If a joint effusion is present, synovial fluid analysis should be undertaken at the first visit to exclude infection. Joint fluid findings include moderate turbidity, ↓ mucin content, WBC range 5,000–30,000/mm^3, often with inclusion cells. If very turbid, the joint fluid should be submitted for gram stain, culture, and comparison of sugar content to simultaneous blood sugar result.

Sedimentation rate usually reflects the level of systemic disease. Leukocytosis may occur. HLA-B27 is not necessary for diagnosis and is often negative if the spine is not symptomatic.

Roentgenography of symptomatic joints may reveal sacroiliitis or a "fluffy" periostitis along the area of the plantar fascia attachment (see Fig. 30–10).

Pathogenesis: Prodromal sexually acquired or enteric infections are thought to be important in setting off the syndrome. Bacterial cell wall antigens can be found in some joint fluids. Presumably the host immune system is defective, allowing persistence of these antigens; these in turn lead to local immune-related tissue injury. Organisms that have been involved include Chlamydia, ureaplasmas, and Neisseria gonorrhoeae, Shigella flexneri and S. sonnei, Campylobacter jejuni, many salmonella and Yersinia strains; Brucella, Blastocystis hominis, Clostridium difficile, and Borrelia burgdorferi.

Differential diagnosis from rheumatoid arthritis usually is not difficult, but if onset includes symmetrical arthritis, the history is important. Urogenital or mucocutaneous lesions are required for the diagnosis of Reiter's syndrome. Erythema nodosum arthritis and sarcoidosis lack the

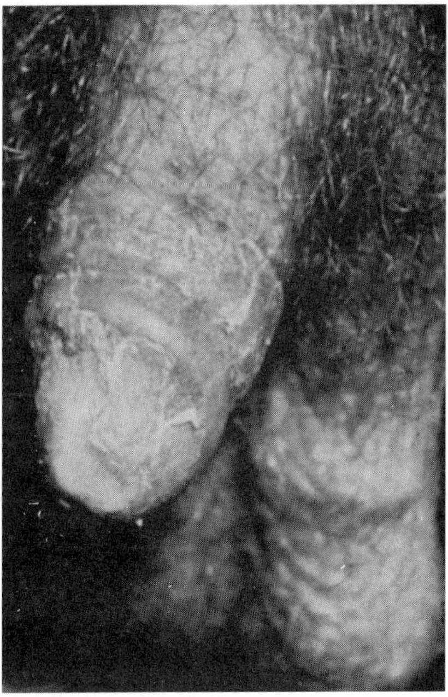

Figure 30–8. Circinate balanitis (Reiter's syndrome). Small red macules 1–2 mm in diameter coalesce into larger lesions. From Moskowitz, Roland W: Clinical Rheumatology. 2nd Ed. Philadelphia, Lea & Febiger, 1982.

stomatitis and urogenital feature. Sexually acquired infection, septicemias, and AIDS must be excluded.

The inflammatory process rarely may destroy ocular tissue, cause aortic insufficiency, and may rarely lead to articular bony erosions. The usual course of inflammation lasts several months to several years.

Treatment: For general management, see below. Patients with severe and prolonged disease may benefit from longterm antibiotic treatment as well as the measures described below.

PSORIATIC ARTHRITIS

Usually begins with an acute dactylitis: A sausage-like swelling of a single digit. The digit is painful, red, cool to touch, and diffusely swollen. Or, it may present as a symmetrical polyarthritis, however, rheumatoid factor would be negative.

Bulbous terminal finger joint with oncholysis or nail pitting is a characteristic finding. Search carefully for psoriatic involvement of the scalp, umbilicus, and gluteal cleft.

Hyperuricemia is common in patients with psoriasis, but gout is not a consideration. Gout is much more abrupt in onset and much more painful; joint fluid urate crystals are not present in psoriatic arthritis.

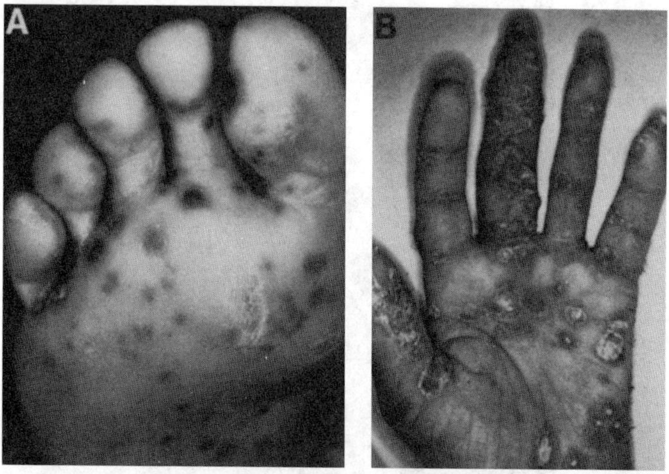

Figure 30–9. Keratoderma blennorrhagica (Reiter's syndrome). Begin as small macules, become pustular; then hyperkeratinized. Can be found on trunk and extremities also. From: McCarty, Daniel J, Koopman, William J (eds.): Arthritis and Allied Conditions. 12th Ed. Philadelphia, Lea & Febiger, 1992.

ACUTE RHEUMATIC FEVER

In recent years, young adults have been seen with rheumatic fever presenting as an acute migratory polyarthritis or sometimes a rheumatoid-like symmetrical polyarthritis. The more classical involvement of children ages 5–9 is less common. Each joint swelling is painful, often red and warm, and classically completely resolves within 1 week while another joint lights up.

A preceding sore throat may have been so inconsequential that it is not recalled. Because ↑ of streptococcal antibodies is common in carriers without disease, the diagnosis should be based on evidence of multisystem involvement and the presence of a very rapid Westergren erythrocyte sedimentation rate.

Jones Criteria for diagnosis include 2 major criteria (carditis-valvulitis or heart block; polyarthritis; chorea; erythema marginatum; subcutaneous nodules). A throat culture should be obtained for definitive evidence of a streptococcal infection, but a positive culture need not be present. Streptococcal antibodies should be elevated to several times normal levels.

Treatment in young children: Aspirin is still preferred. Begin with 75 mg/kg in divided dose. Arthropan (brand) or Trilisate (brand) liquid, a liquid choline and choline-magnesium salicylate, respectively, is easy to give to small children. A salicylate level can be obtained 2 h after a first morning dose. Try to keep the level within 20–25 mg%. The response to aspirin treatment is rapid and complete compared to that in other forms of juvenile arthritis.

If Reye's syndrome is a concern, or in teenagers and young adults, NSAIDs may be preferred. If serious carditis is present with features of pericarditis, tachycardia, heart block, or CHF, begin steroids at once, 1 mg/kg/day in divided dose.

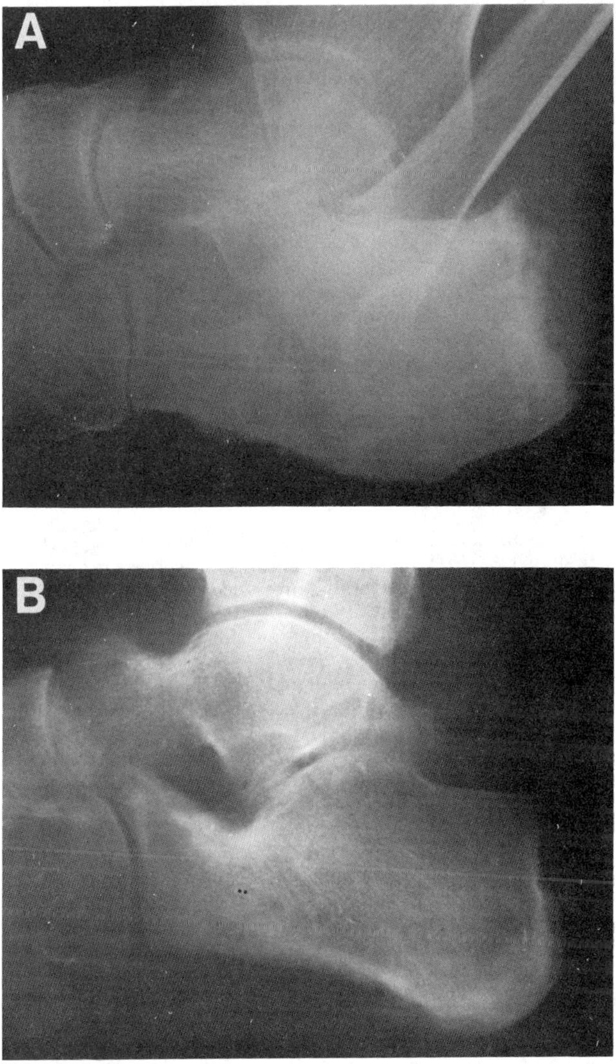

Figure 30–10. Fluffy periostitis in Reiter's syndrome. From: McCarty, Daniel J, Koopman, William J (eds.): Arthritis and Allied Conditions. 12th Ed. Philadelphia, Lea & Febiger, 1992.

Be certain to test all family members for occult streptococcal infection, and treat those infected. Patients should be followed closely for signs of carditis with weekly ECG and auscultation.

Prevention: Penicillin or similar antistreptococcal agent should be administered in order to prevent recurrences. Most reliable prophylaxis is benzathine penicillin, 1.2 million U I.M. monthly. Most experts recommend continued prophylaxis until age 40.

ENTEROPATHIC ARTHRITIS

These include IBDs such as ulcerative colitis, Crohn's disease, granulomatous colitis, and collagenous colitis. Perhaps related are the arthritis associated with intestinal bypass procedures, and with diverticulitis.

Features include lower extremity joint synovitis, skin lesions of erythema nodosum, pyoderma gangrenosum, erythema multiforme, and a painful stomatitis. Iritis is common when sacroiliitis has developed.

The arthritis may precede bowel disease, but most commonly arthritis onset coincides with the bowel disease. Small hand joints are more commonly involved with regional enteritis.

Laboratory tests are nondiagnostic. Anemia, rapid sedimentation rate, and synovial fluid findings of nonspecific inflammation are usual findings. HLA-B27 is positive if sacroiliitis occurs. Endoscopy and small bowel biopsy may be necessary for diagnosis. Synovial biopsy is usually nonspecific, but granulomas characteristic of Crohn's disease can be found.

Treatment of Ankylosing Spondylitis and Reactive Arthritis

Large joint aspiration and corticosteroid injection should be performed on the first visit. NSAIDs are helpful. The pyrroleacetic acid derivatives, particularly tolmetin, are preferable first. Indomethacin should be considered only when milder NSAIDs fail. Gastric cytoprotection with misoprostol is indicated in patients with a past history of ulcer or if using concomitant steroids.

Antibiotic therapy is controversial, but in patients with Reiter's syndrome a 2–week course of a broad-spectrum tetracycline (doxycycline or minocycline 100 mg bid) has little downside risk. Patients with onset following sexually transmitted infection should be treated with an antibiotic (doxycycline 100 mg bid for 2 weeks, or azithromycin 250 mg/day for 5 days). Sex partners should also be treated.

Persistent disease or very severe onset are indications for use of sulfasalazine. The mechanism of action is unknown, but the sulfa moiety appears to be the active ingredient. It is contraindicated in patients known to be allergic to sulfa. Begin with 500 mg enteric coated tablets bid po and followed with a full glass of water. Every few days ↑ dose until 1,000 mg tid po is achieved. Headache may occur at higher doses; lower doses may be used. Rash, hepatitis, diarrhea, leukopenia, rarely pancytopenia, and hematuria demand termination of this treatment. See Table 30–14.

Benefit should be noticeable within 8 weeks. CBCs, including platelet count, and urinalysis should be done at 3–week intervals. Periodic chemistry analysis is recommended.

The course of psoriatic arthritis and IBD is often chronic and prolonged, with unpredictable remissions. Methotrexate is useful for severe or prolonged arthritis but should be left to those expert in its use. Gold salt therapy can be used in patients with persistent ankylosing spondylitis or psoriatic arthritis.

When spondylitis is present, physical therapy and home exercise instruction help breathing and prevent a stooped posture.

Metabolic and Crystal-Induced Arthropathies

Gout and pseudogout can occur in multiple joints all at the same time. When this occurs and gout is the disease, look for underlying causes, including use of diuretics, severe calorie restriction, alcohol, renal disease, and occult neoplasm. See the previous discussion for management.

Pseudogout occurring in multiple joints may result from hemochromatosis or hyperparathyroidism. Rarely, chondrocalcinosis may occur in association with acromegaly, hypomagnesemia, hypophosphatasia, ochronosis, and oxalosis. When calcific tendinitis has also occurred, calcium apatite deposition disease is likely. Synovial fluid may show weakly birefringent clumps of amorphous material. See the previous discussion for management.

Paraneoplastic Syndromes

Cancer Arthropathy. A rheumatoid factor-negative (seronegative) asymmetric polyarthritis involving mostly the lower limb joints. Cancer presentation may occur within 3 months and can arise in any organ. If considered and searched for, the malignancy may be curable. Unfortunately, the arthritis does not always remit upon treatment of the malignancy.

Hypertrophic Pulmonary Osteoarthropathy (HOA). A triad of clubbing of the digits, periostitis of long bones, and synovitis usually of the knees. Cancer of the lung occurs in about 10% of patients.

Septic Arthritis

Two infectious arthritides that can cause a chronic pauciarticular or even a symmetrical polyarticular arthritis are Lyme disease and Parvovirus infections.

LYME DISEASE

Just as syphilis can cause a multisystem chronic illness, this Borrelia bergdorferi spirochete-caused illness can lead to perplexing disease.

Diagnosis. Features necessary for diagnosis are erythema migrans and ≥1 of the following: Arthralgias, arthritis, myalgias, headache, palpitations, heart block, visual changes, paresthesias, cognitive problems, depression, Bell's palsy, radiculopathies, fevers, lymphadenopathy, and fatigue. Without erythema migrans, the diagnosis is tenuous. At present, serologic diagnosis is not reliable. Synovial biopsy may be unrewarding. Diagnosis will be enhanced when DNA probes or other techniques are available.

Treatment of Lyme disease before cardiac or neurologic involvement can be effected with doxycycline 100 mg bid for 2 weeks. For more severe cases or late treatment, a 2–week course of ceftriaxone 2 gm/day IV may be necessary.

PARVOVIRUS B19 INFECTION

This agent has caused diverse disease ranging from erythema infectiosum to an acute symmetrical arthritis indistinguishable from rheumatoid arthritis. Serologic identification is useful only if performed within 8 weeks of onset. The arthritis is nonerosive, and patients sometimes have symptoms for up to 15 months. Laboratory findings are nonspecific; joint fluid is less inflammatory than in Reiter's syndrome. NSAIDs are helpful.

Seronegative Rheumatoid Arthritis

Approximately 10% of patients with typical rheumatoid pannus and bone erosions have a seronegative pauciarticular arthritis. Sometimes the synovitis is barely palpable. Upper-extremity joints are usually affected. Occasionally the sheep cell agglutination test will be abnormal in the presence of a normal latex rheumatoid test. The absence of other non-RA disease features, and persistence >3 months, suggests rheumatoid.

Treatment: If NSAIDs are not helpful, sulfasalazine or hydroxychloroquine should be added. Most patients with this form of rheumatoid have long remissions, but attacks may last several years.

AIDS

Approximately 5% of patients with AIDS will develop a reactive arthritis with features of Reiter's syndrome or psoriatic arthritis. Certainly if risk factors are present, HIV testing should be done. Sulfasalazine, NSAIDs, and brief steroid use is tolerated. Methotrexate should be avoided.

RHEUMATOID DISEASES

This is a diverse group of immunologically mediated diseases that lead to a deforming polyarthritis chiefly involving the hands and feet, often with multisystem involvement and damage. Monoarticular rheumatoid has been discussed.

Rheumatoid Arthritis

Diagnosis is based on the presence of 4 of the following 7 criteria:

1. Morning stiffness in joint areas of ≥1 h duration
2. Synovial swelling of ≥3 joint areas (excluding the spine) observed by a physician
3. ≥1 of the joints must include the wrist, MCP, or PIP joints
4. Simultaneous symmetrical joint swelling

(The above features must have been present for ≥6 weeks.)

5. Presence of rheumatoid nodules observed by a physician
6. Positive test for rheumatoid factor in high titer
7. Typical roentgenographic changes

Features of psoriasis, spondylitis, giant cell arteritis, or other connective tissue disorders are relative exclusions for the diagnosis.

If joint destruction is to be prevented, diagnosis must be early and vigorously treated. Early diagnosis depends on the examiner's ability to palpate joint synovium (the technique was discussed in the first section). Boggy or doughy synovitis involving the metacarpophalangeal joints and the ulnar styloid bursa are very good evidence for rheumatoid arthritis.

Systemic features include episcleritis, carditis, pleuroparenchymal lung disease, neuropathy, leg ulcers, and digital infarcts (nail fold le-

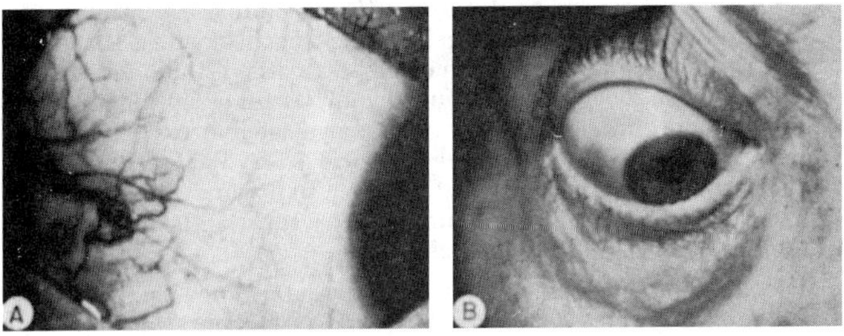

Figure 30–11. Episcleritis. From: McCarty, Daniel J, Koopman, William J (eds.): Arthritis and Allied Conditions. 12th Ed. Philadelphia, Lea & Febiger, 1992.

sions). See Figures 30–11 and 30–12. Persons with limited education tend to have more severe disease.

Ominous laboratory features include thrombocytosis, extreme ↑ of the Westergren sedimentation rate, marked ↑ of C1q or cryoglobulin, and depressed serum albumin.

Onset may occur at any age, usually insidiously, with variability from day to day. Acute onset often follows stress, trauma, or infection. Although spontaneous remission is frequent in the early years, for most patients the disease recurs, and in later life remissions are rare while relentless destructive polyarthritis is common.

Pathogenesis: Increasing evidence points to the short arm of chromosome 6; the α helix of certain DR β chains within the class II region of the major histocompatibility complex has a strong relation to rheumatoid arthritis. These genes may respond to a superantigen, possibly a bacterial heat shock protein. Then T cells invade the synovium and release cytokines, and the inflammatory pathways become activated.

Differential Diagnosis: Inflammatory polyarthritis can result from >100 diseases (see Table 30–1). Although Raynaud's phenomenon can occur in RA, other features would suggest SLE or mixed connective tissue disease. Rheumatic fever can be a difficult differential; look for extra-articular features and note the prompt response to therapeutic doses of salicylates. Polyarticular gout and pseudogout rarely affect the small

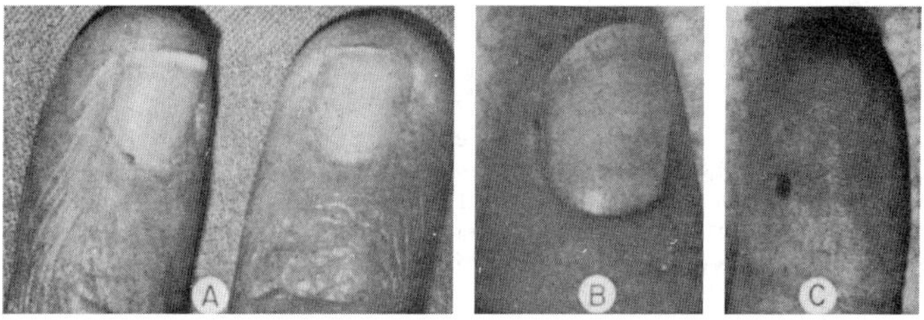

Figure 30–12. Nail fold lesion, at edge of nail, often a finding in rheumatoid vasculitis. From McCarty, Daniel J, Koopman, William J (eds.): Arthritis and Allied Conditions. 12th Ed. Philadelphia, Lea & Febiger, 1992.

hand joints; synovial fluid analysis from larger joints is essential. Lyme disease should be considered in areas that harbor the deer tic. In elderly patients with a seronegative symmetrical arthritis of the hands, giant cell arteritis should be considered, particularly with a significantly elevated sedimentation rate. A therapeutic trial of hydroxychloroquine may help avoid use of steroids if the temporal artery biopsy is negative. Reactive arthritis usually affects the lower limbs and has cutaneous features. Diseases that infiltrate joints include sarcoidosis, amyloid, hypothyroidism, and hemochromatosis.

Workup: Rheumatoid factor titer should be determined using an experienced lab. CBCs, platelet count, Westergren sedimentation rate, and baseline chemistries are necessary for assessing systemic disease severity as well as excluding other diagnoses. ANF is also helpful at baseline; some think that it is a poor prognostic finding. A baseline chest x ray for identifying rheumatoid lung disease is important. Joint changes on roentgenography are rare before 6 months of disease duration. Most rheumatologists no longer obtain a baseline joint roentgenographic survey. Characteristic erosions are a late finding, perhaps too late. If nodules, or other features of systemic disease, are evident, a quantitative cryoglobulin, fibrinogen, and sedimentation rate can be used to monitor treatment.

If synovial effusion is present, the effusion should be aspirated fully and synovial analysis carried out (Tables 30–9 and 30–10). If not purulent, a local steroid injection will be greatly helpful and can be instilled through the same needle following aspiration.

Treatment: Age, mode of presentation, serologic status, past medical history, and past drug history are all important for individualizing treatment.

Goals of treatment are to reduce pain and inflammation and prevent deformities. Absence of morning stiffness is an objective. This often requires max doses of salicylates or NSAIDs. If not, move on to methotrexate.

All patients with established rheumatoid arthritis benefit from detailed instructions in physical and occupational therapy if provided early in the course of disease. Only a few visits for home education are needed in most instances. Because of soft tissue inflammation and damage, these measures can greatly reduce pain and disability (see Table 30–12).

Mild disease, with morning stiffness of ≤1 h, moderate joint swelling without effusions, no nodules, and no constitutional features, can be treated with nonacetyl salicylates or NSAIDs. But, if the disease does not improve within a few weeks, begin either hydroxychloroquine or sulfasalazine and continue the NSAID or salsalate. See introduction and Tables 30–7 and 30–14.

Moderate disease: Patients with boggy synovium and recurrent effusion should be strongly considered for gold salt therapy, methotrexate, or both. Most rheumatologists do not like oral corticosteroids in any schedule. The osteoporosis and poor resistance to infection due to the arthritis are often compounded by steroids.

These problems are avoided by joint aspiration and steroid injections at 8– to 12–week intervals until remission occurs.

Long-acting drugs are often used sequentially: Gold salts or antimalarials are tried first, always in conjunction with salicylates or NSAIDs.

- Gold salt therapy by injection is preferred; save auranofin for patients who have remitted with gold salts but then develop side effects. If patient is a late failure on gold, try pumping the gold back to weekly doses for 6 doses; if successful, resume a q 3–week schedule. See Table 30–14.

If gold and chloroquine fail, move on to sulfasalazine, then d-penicillamine, and lastly azathioprine.

Never use sulfasalazine and methotrexate together. Similarly, sulfa-based antibiotics should be avoided with methotrexate. Severe bone marrow depression can result.

Methotrexate should be considered early in older patients. It is safer than an NSAID in the very old.

Severe disease: Patients with episcleritis or vasculitis should be considered for d-penicillamine treatment. Because the drug may take several months to work, most rheumatologists would use oral prednisone beginning with 1 mg/kg in divided dose. If this fails, nitrogen mustard, bolus cyclophosphamide, or high-dose steroid or bolus steroid therapy can be considered, but should be undertaken only by an experienced physician.

Synovectomy is a consideration if joint effusion of a single joint is resistant to repeated aspiration/injection treatment. Arthroscopic synovectomy of a knee or shoulder can be helpful.

Arthroplasty of a major joint should be considered if intensive therapy both with adequate medication and physical therapy have failed. Indications for elbow or shoulder arthroplasty include inability to feed, dress, or perform toilet activity. Indications for lower extremity joints are inability to dress, walk from car through grocery store, inability to perform sexually if desired, or intractable night pain.

When patients have had severe GI or pulmonary side effects with salicylates and NSAIDs, then gold salt therapy and intra-articular steroid injections should be tried and oral medication avoided. Never inject the same joint more often than every 6 weeks.

- Patients with sinusitis, nasal polyps, or marked GI sensitivity can be tried on nonacetylated salicylates, including choline salicylate, salsalate, or magnesium salicylate. Gold salt therapy may be very helpful for such patients. Methotrexate can also aggravate pulmonary problems but can be cautiously tried.

If laryngeal involvement is a problem, particularly with hoarseness, ACTH can be helpful. Give 40 U 3 times a week for 2–3 weeks.

When C1–C2 subluxation occurs, with paresthesias to scalp and arms, prescribe a hard cervical collar and get prompt orthopedic consultation. Patients with severe hand deformities are likely to have moderate but silent C1–2 subluxation. They are at risk during intubation for a general anesthetic. Such patients should have high cervical CT beforehand, and the anesthesiologist should be apprised.

Novel therapies unavailable at this time are provided in Table 30–15.

Sjogren's Syndrome

Diagnosis is based on occurrence of keratoconjunctivitis sicca, xerostomia, and an autoimmune disease. Most patients can be screened with fluorescein or Rose Bengal staining. The Schirmer test is easily performed and can be used to follow the course of the disease. Sialogram, scintigraphy, and lip biopsy are only occasionally necessary. Antinuclear antibodies, rheumatoid factors, anti-Ro (SS-A), and Anti-La (SS-B) antibodies occur in the majority of patients; thyroglobulin antibodies, cryoglobulins, and anti-DNA may be found even in the absence of any evident connective tissue disease.

These patients are subject to focal neurologic and neuropsychiatric sequelae. Cerebral vasculitis may be seen on MRI.

These patients also may develop lymphoproliferative diseases with pseudolymphoma and malignant lymphomas. Diffuse interstitial pneu-

Table 30–15
Newer, Novel Drugs Under Investigation

AGENT	MECHANISM	SIDE EFFECTS
Cyclosporin	Reduces IL-2 production	Nephrotoxic
Levamisole		
Minocycline	Inhibits collagenase	Vertigo, rash, phototoxicity; nausea
Amiprilose hydrochloride	Anti-inflammatory; reduces IL-2	Visual, nausea, headache
Superoxide dismutase	Reduces free radical	??
Tenidap	Anti IL-1; antioxidation	
Gamma Interferon		Fever, headache, GI upset
N-(fluorenyl-9-methoxy-carbonyl amino acids (Leumedins)	Stimulates leukotriene B4	
2-cyanoaziridine	T- and B-cell inhibitor	Rash, liver enzymes incr.
Anti-CD4 or 5	T-cell modulation	Rash, fever
Monoclonal antibodies	Anti CD-4 and CD-7	Anaphylaxis risk
Antithymocyte globulin	Deletion of T-cell clones	Fever, urticaria, vasculitis

monitis, and renal diseases with glomerulosclerosis and renal tubular acidosis, can occur.

Treatment: This includes that of the underlying rheumatic disease. Shohl's citrate solution can help. Mix 1 ounce in 32 ounces of water. Ingest in divided dose daily. Prescribe 1 g ascorbic acid qd. Used for 30 days, patients claim to experience relief. Oral symptoms may be helped by sipping a glass of water containing a few drops of oil of peppermint. Sour candy also may help.

Felty's Syndrome

Consists of a triad of rheumatoid arthritis, leukopenia, and splenomegaly. Also, anemia, lymphadenopathy, and leg ulcers are common. The bone marrow is usually hyperplastic. Hypersplenism is common. Splenectomy is of variable benefit and should be considered if 2 serious infections have occurred. Most patients can be treated with gold salts or penicillamine. In this condition, the baseline WBC is used and the drug withheld if the WBC falls to 50% of the baseline, or the absolute neutrophil count drops to lower levels.

OTHER CONNECTIVE TISSUE DISEASE

With rare exception, diagnosis is based on syndrome identification. Too many patients are seen with minimal evidence of disease but with significant laboratory features. About 1/2 of these patients will develop fully developed syndromes, most commonly rheumatoid arthritis.

The history must be done with care. Patients don't volunteer information. They are often focused on fatigue and disability from arthritis. Ask each patient to carefully review systems (see Table 30–6). Include a drug history for those drugs that can induce drug lupus; ask about breast augmentation and occupational exposure to agents that can cause scleroderma-like features when they are present.

Pathogenesis: As in rheumatoid arthritis, these diseases are likely to result from the individual's genetic susceptibility and environmental factors, including ultraviolet light exposure and infectious agents.

Systemic Lupus Erythematosus

Features include

- Skin and mucous membrane changes, including malar rash, discoid rash, photosensitivity, alopecia, and oral ulcers
- Arthritis (often of fingers, and intermittent)
- Serositis, including pleuritis, pericarditis, and mesenteritis
- Nephritis with persistent proteinuria or casts
- Hematologic disease, including thrombocytopenia, hemolytic anemia; often with leukopenia of <4,000 cells and a positive direct Coomb's test
- Evident immunologic disorder with positive LE prep, positive test for syphilis, anti-DNA, or anti-Sm antigens
- ANA in significant titer

≥4 positive features are needed for diagnosis. Patients with <4 criteria can be designated as having "undifferentiated connective tissue disease.".

Patients tend to have certain patterns of disease, and new flares usually follow the initial pattern

- **Skin-joint disease:** Mild disease with any or all of the skin manifestations and significant symmetrical polyarthritis. No major organ involvement
- **Hematologic disease:** This can occur as an isolated idiopathic thrombocytopenia or as an autoimmune hemolytic anemia
- **Brain, heart, kidney disease:** Convulsions, psychosis, depression, transverse myelitis, endocarditis with Libman-Sachs valvulitis, or nephrotic syndrome.

Drug lupus can present as any of the above, rarely with nephritis. Such patients may require steroids. The offending drugs include procainamide, hydralazine, anticonvulsants, isoniazid, levodopa, propylthiouracil, penicillamine, sulfasalazine, and lithium. Each year adds more to the list. Although antihistone antibodies are common in drug lupus, they are neither diagnostic nor specific. Although the clinical features ultimately clear when the offending drug has been removed, the ANA remains positive and in high titer for years.

Differential diagnosis depends on mode of presentation and duration. Consider other photosensitizing diseases, such as porphyria, bacterial endocarditis, syphilis, Lyme disease, AIDS, histoplasmosis, other systemic infections, paraneoplastic syndromes, sarcoidosis, and hematologic diseases.

Workup should initially include CBC with differential, ANA, chemistry panel, urinalysis, and chest x ray. Then, in addition, depending on features, echocardiogram, further immunologic tests, including anti-double stranded DNA, C3, C1q, and creatinine clearance and 24–h urine protein.

Treatment and follow-up

- **Skin-joint disease:** NSAIDs, nonacetylated salicylates, and hydroxychloroquine are often effective. Stubborn joint swelling can be treated with intra-articular injections of corticosteroids. Try to avoid steroids at this level of disease, but follow the patient closely for evidence of more systemic disease. Anti-DNA is not of value unless serositis or nephritis have appeared. If the patient is planning pregnancy, anticardiolipin lupus anticoagulant, SS-A and SS-B antibody tests should be obtained.
- **Hematologic disease:** Low-dose prednisone (0.5 mg/kg/day) with slow taper is necessary. These patients should be monitored as above.
- **Brain and transverse myelitis:** These patients should be treated with parenteral bolus corticosteroids as soon as symptoms suggest diagnosis. Don't wait for test results. As soon as the emergency spinal tap has been obtained, use ≥250 mg solumedrol q 6 h. MRI of the spinal cord can be helpful for assessing transverse myelitis. Anticardiolipin antibodies and the lupus anticoagulant should be tested.
- **Carditis** usually responds to prednisone (beginning with 1 mg/kg/day in divided dose). Glomerulonephritis and nephrotic syndrome should have nephrology consultation, with renal biopsy to guide treatment. Evidence of proliferative glomerulonephritis is currently treated with bolus cyclophosphamide or nitrogen mustard and corticosteroids. This process is seen more commonly in noncaucasians. Be more alert to nephritis in them.

Antiphospholipid Syndrome

Features include arterial and venous thrombosis, stroke, transverse myelitis, fetal loss, and thrombocytopenia. Assessment should include both anticardiolipin and lupus anticoagulant. Patients may or may not have any connective tissue disease, but features for SLE should be sought.

At the present time, patients with CNS disease, or venous and arterial thrombosis, are treated with longterm anticoagulation; those also with SLE are treated additionally with steroids. Patients who have had miscarriages can often be carried to term using daily prednisone (0.5–1.0 mg/kg/day) and aspirin.

Mixed Connective Tissue Disease

Similar to SLE but with 3 distinguishing features

- Sausage-like swelling of fingers with evolution of features of rheumatoid arthritis, scleroderma, myositis, and lupus
- Presence of anti-U1 RNP in high titer ribonucleoprotein
- Low incidence of cardiac or renal disease

May have ↑ incidence of pulmonary fibrosis, pulmonary hypertension, Sjogren's syndrome, and Hashimoto's thyroiditis.

Treatment for most patients is corticosteroids in moderate to high doses. Those patients with a predominant arthritis manifestation can be treated with antimalarials and NSAIDs. Those patients with scleroderma features are least likely to improve. No prospective studies are available. No data is available on use of d-penicillamine for this group.

SYSTEMIC SCLEROSIS

A group of local or generalized connective tissue diseases with the major manifestation of fibrosis and degeneration of skin (scleroderma), synovium, muscles; less commonly the internal organs.

CLASSIFICATION OF SCLERODERMA

Systemic Sclerosis. Diffuse cutaneous scleroderma: With early appearance of pulmonary, cardiac, GI, and renal disease. Limited cutaneous scleroderma: With skin limited to face and distal limbs; late onset of pulmonary arterial hypertension, biliary cirrhosis. Commonly known as CREST Syndrome (with Calcinosis; Raynaud's phenomenon; Esophageal dysfunction; Sclerodactyly; and Telangiectasia).

Localized Scleroderma. Morphea: Single or multiple plaques of leathery skin with pigmentation.

Linear Scleroderma. Deep cutaneous fibrosis, with or without melorheostosis.

FEATURES

Raynaud's phenomenon may precede disease by months or years. The diffuse type may begin with generalized edema; widespread dysesthesia may be very uncomfortable and last for many months.

Speckled antinuclear antibodies are common but of no significance. Anti-topoisomerase I antibodies (Scl-70) tend to occur in the diffuse type of scleroderma, and pulmonary interstitial fibrosis is linked.

Anticentromere antibodies have remarkable specificity for limited cutaneous scleroderma. These patients can present with a malignant form of Raynaud's with digital gangrene as the first manifestation of disease.

DIFFERENTIAL DIAGNOSIS

Environmental agents that can trigger scleroderma-like changes include silica dust, silicone, vinyl chloride, trichlorethylene, bleomycin, cisplatin, benzene, phenylenediamines, epoxy resins, carbidopa, hydroxytryptophan, toxic oil syndrome, and the graft vs. host disease.

TREATMENT

No controlled data exist supporting a specific form of treatment. Dermatologists like penicillin for localized scleroderma. Anecdotal data suggest a positive outcome. For diffuse disease, most rheumatologists use d-penicillamine for ≥3 years. See Table 30–14. Treatment of Raynaud's phenomenon includes local cold protection with gloves, face mask, and nifedipine (30–90 mg/day); reserpine 0.5 mg bid, dibenzyline 10 mg tid, or biofeedback training, can be tried sequentially. Asymptomatic proteinuria may herald renal scleroderma and malignant hypertension. A nephrologist should be involved as soon as the condition is recognized.

Patients with systemic sclerosis should be followed with monitoring of BP and DLCO, and with attention to joint range of motion, nutrition, dentition, and renal function.

Polymyositis/Dermatomyositis

Features include

- Symmetric weakness of neck and girdle muscles
- Elevated serum skeletal muscle enzymes (e.g., CPK, SGOT (AST))
- Electromyographic changes consistent with an inflammatory myopathy
- Muscle biopsy findings of fiber necrosis, inflammation, phagocytosis, and regeneration, and variation in fiber size

Electron microscopy should be part of a routine workup.. Diagnosis requires 3 of the above.

Skin changes for dermatomyositis include the characteristic heliotrope eyelid, Gottron's patches (red scaly patches over the metacarpophalangeal joints), and rose-red rash on face, trunk, or limbs. Dermatomyositis is more common in children and in patients who have an occult neoplasm.

Synovitis of hands, pulmonary interstitial infiltration, myocardiopathy, vasculitis of the intestinal tract, dysphagia, or dysphonia can occur.

Ominous features are dysphonia (aspiration pneumonia can occur), CPK ↑ >10,000, lack of response to prednisone within 1 month, and extensive rash (occult neoplasm).

PATHOGENESIS

HLA-DR3, HLA-DR52, and HLA-B8 are frequently related. Anti-Jo-1 antibodies and anti-synthetase autoantibodies may be found also. Picornaviruses, Coxsackievirus, and Toxoplasma gondii have been implicated.

DIFFERENTIAL DIAGNOSIS

The list of causes for dysfunction of muscle is extensive. Most are noninflammatory. Toxic myopathies from alcohol, cocaine, colchicine, clofibrate, and penicillamine may be difficult to differentiate and need to be excluded. Muscular dystrophies have a helpful family history. Polymyalgia and fibromyalgia do not cause weakness.

TREATMENT

Corticosteroid therapy is still the cornerstone of treatment. Depending upon severity at onset, prednisone dosage of 1–2 mg/kg is given with slow taper for 6 months. Divided doses at tid is necessary in the beginning. If vasculitis is present, IV delivery is necessary. Single morning maintenance dosages are determined by enzyme levels. Steroid myopathy is an insidious lower-extremity problem that requires trial-and-error care. Use of urine creatine ratios may be helpful in this situation.

Use bedrest along with passive range of motion until enzymes ↓. Then progress with graded exercises.

When more aggressive treatment is needed, methotrexate, azathioprine, or cyclophosphamide have had variable success. Cyclophosphamide 1–4 mg/kg should be seriously considered in childhood resistant myositis. IV Immune serum globulin has been reported helpful in a 15–year-old resistant to all other forms of treatment. Dosage reported was 1 gm/kg/day for 2 consecutive days each month.

Necrotizing Vasculitis

A protean group of diseases that affect many organ systems, with ischemia resulting from inflammation and swelling of the vascular tree. Table 30–16 summarizes the histopathology and some demographic features.

Constitutional features of fever, weight loss, myalgia, and anemia are common at presentation. Limited forms are not uncommon, with less illness and greater difficulty in diagnosis. Progress has been made in identifying serologic markers specific for vasculitis.

Antineutrophil cytoplasmic antibodies can be found in systemic necrotizing vasculitis, particularly Wegener's granulomatosis. The specificity and sensitivity are not yet known.

PATHOGENESIS

Because of the sporadic occurrence of vasculitis, lack of familial involvement, lack of association with any specific infectious agent, and marked variability of case presentation, these diseases likely represent an immunopathogenic response to infection. Indeed, the finding of hepatitis virus in association with cryoglobulinemia and polyarteritis nodosum is suggestive of this mechanism.

Systemic vasculitis should be considered if 3 organ systems appear affected by a systemic inflammatory process. Electromyography for denervation may prove neurologic system involvement if needed. Most of these patients will have either articular swelling (giant cell arteritis, Wegener's granulomatosis), skin lesions, pulmonary lesions, or evidence of renal involvement as well.

WORKUP

Sedimentation rate, sinus and chest x ray, sinus biopsy if the sinus walls appear involved; abdominal visceral angiography if renal or neurologic systems appear involved; skin and muscle biopsy if arteriogram is negative or inconclusive.

In patients with predominant CNS involvement, cerebral arteriography is often necessary; in many cases MRI is inconclusive.

DIFFERENTIAL DIAGNOSIS

Other conditions to consider include cardiac myxoma, multiple cholesterol embolization syndrome, subacute bacterial endocarditis and other systemic infections, lues, leukemia and paraneoplastic syndromes, hypersensitivity reactions, carcinoid, and porphyria.

TREATMENT

Wegener's granulomatosis should be treated with cyclophosphamide and prednisone as soon as diagnosis is evident. Oliguric renal failure may occur within days of onset.

Polyarteritis nodosum may respond to corticosteroid given in daily (1–2 mg/kg) divided dose, but if not quickly responsive, cyclophosphamide is added, even when hepatitis virus is evident. Most rheumatologists would initiate treatment with combination therapy (prednisone and cyclophosphamide) because late sequelae are less likely and pro-

Table 30–16
Features of Vasculitis Syndromes

	POLYARTERITIS NODOSA	CHURG-STRAUSS SYNDROME	WEGENER'S GRANULOMATOSIS	HYPERSENSITIVITY VASCULITIS	HENOCH-SCHÖNLEIN PURPURA	GIANT CELL (TEMPORAL) ARTERITIS	TAKAYASU ARTERITIS
Type of vessels involved	Medium and small muscular arteries, and sometimes arterioles	Small arteries and veins, often arterioles and venules	Usually small arteries and veins, sometimes larger vessels	Arterioles and venules, often small arteries and veins	Arterioles and venules, often small arteries and veins	Vessels of all sizes	Elastic arteries and selected muscular arteries
Distribution and localization	Visceral, cutaneous, and, infrequently cerebral vessels and lung	Upper and lower respiratory tract, viscera, heart, and skin	Upper and lower respiratory tract, often kidney, and infrequently skin, heart, viscera, and brain	Predominantly skin and less commonly viscera, heart, and synovium	Predominantly skin, gastrointestinal, kidney, and synovian	Predominantly temporal arteries, and less often any other large, medium, and small vessels	Aorta, arch vessels, and other major branches (coronary, renal, visceral), and pulmonary arteries
Type of vasculitis and inflammatory cell infiltrate	Necrotizing, with mixed cells and few eosinophils, rarely granulomatous	Necrotizing or granulomatous, with mixed cells and prominent eosinophils	Necrotizing or granulomatous, with mixed cells and occasional eosinophils	Leukocytoclastic or lymphocytic, with variable number of eosinophils, occasionally granulomatous	Leukocytoclastic, mixed-cell, or lymphocytic, with variable number of eosinophils	Granulomatous, with variable number of giant cells, sometimes only lymphoplasmacytic	Granulomatous, with few giant cells in active phase, and sclerosing fibrosis in chronic stage, with scanty infiltrate

Special features	Focal segmental involvement of vessels; coexisting acute and healed vascular lesions, or normal and affected vessels; microaneurysms	Extravascular necrotizing granulomas with prominent eosinophils; may manifest as "limited form"	Geographic pattern of tissue necrosis and positive antineutrophil cytoplasmic antibodies; may manifest as "limited form"	May be associated with myocarditis, interstitial nephritis, or hepatitis	IgA immune deposits in affected tissue	Affected extracranial large vessels indistinguishable from Takayasu arteritis; may form aneurysm or cause dissection	Aneurysmal in 20%; may be segmental, and cause rupture or dissection
Demographic and environmental predisposition	Vascular lesion of infantile polyarteritis is indistinguishable from fatal cases of Kawasaki disease	Most patients have asthma or history of allergy	Occurs in all ages, with a slight male preponderance; associated with HLA-DR2; may respond to antimicrobial agents	Patients may have history of drug or chemical allergy, vaccination, or occult malignancy	Predominantly children and young adults	Virtually all patients with temporal arteritis are over age 50; may be clinically asymptomatic	Most commonly in women of childbearing age; more prevalent in the Orient; an important cause of renovascular hypertension in adolescents

From: Hunder GG, Arend WP, Bloch DA, et al.: The American College of Rheumatology 1990 criteria for the classification of vasculitis. Arthritis Rheum, *33*:1065–1144, 1990.

longed high-dose steroid therapy can be avoided. Late occurrence of malignancy, particularly of bladder cancer, is common. Hopefully other effective nonsteroidal treatment will be found.

Giant cell arteritis usually responds to corticosteroids, beginning with prednisone 60–80 mg/day as a single dose. After several weeks, this dose may be ↓ by 10 mg every 2 weeks, then from 20 mg the taper can be ↓ 1 mg/week. Symptomatic stability is more important than sedimentation rate. If steroids are ineffective, or causing great distress, methotrexate can be substituted. Add the methotrexate (10–20 mg/week in a single dose each week) and slowly taper the steroid after the fourth week. Visual symptoms are present in about 1/3 of patients.

NSAIDs have no role in these diseases, may cover up important symptoms and add to the renal injury, and should not be used.

See the previous section on use of corticosteroids and Table 30–14 for use of immunosuppressive medication.

Suggested Reading

Baker DG, Schumacher HR: Acute monoarthritis. N Engl J Med 329: 1013, 1993.

McCarty Daniel J, Koopman William J (eds.): Arthritis and Allied Conditions. 12th Edition. Philadelphia, Lea & Febiger, 1992.

Sheon RP, Pinals RS: Bursitis, Tendinitis, Myofascial Pain. 3rd Edition. Atlanta, The Arthritis Foundation, 1991.

Sheon Robert P, Moskowitz Roland W, Goldberg Victor M: Soft Tissue Rheumatic Pain: Recognition, Management, Prevention. 2nd Edition. Philadelphia, Lea & Febiger, 1987.

Amadio P Jr, Cummings DM, Amadio P: Nonsteroidal anti-inflammatory drugs. Tailoring therapy to achieve results and avoid toxicity. Postg Med 93(4):73–88, 1993.

Sodium, Potassium, and Calcium Disturbances

31

M. Gabriel Khan

HYPONATREMIA

Definition: A serum Na <135 mEq (mmol)/l, after exclusion of pseudohyponatremia, usually due to severe hyperlipidemia and hyperproteinemia, or hyperglycemia, causing a shift of water from cells. Every 100 mg/dl (5.6 mmol/l) ↑ in glucose above normal causes a ↓ in serum Na of 1.5 mEq (mmol/l). **Note:** 1 mEq/l Na or K = 1 mmol/l Na or K.

Causes

All causes are due to Na loss or water gain (Fig. 31–1).

Na LOSS

- Renal loss: Diuretics, renal salt-wasting diseases, and primary adrenal insufficiency. (Secondary adrenal insufficiency is not a cause since the renin angiotensin aldosterone system is intact and controls Na-K balance; ACTH has little effect.)
- GI loss: Vomiting, diarrhea, fistulas
- Third-space loss: Ascites, burns

These conditions are readily identifiable clinical problems that can be spotted without resort to serum and urine osmolality, urine electrolytes, or complicated algorithms that describe tonicity and volume of compartments.

WATER GAIN DUE TO INCREASED ADH SECRETION

↑ secretion of ADH causes a ↓ in renal free-H_2O excretion, thus a ↓ in serum Na, ↓ serum osmolality, ↑ urine osmolality, and a urinary Na >25 mEq/l. In contrast a low effective circulating plasma volume as with CHF produces urinary Na <15 mEq/l and Cl <15 mEq/l in the absence of diuretic use. Serum osmolality = 2 (Na) + (glucose ± 18) + (BUN ÷ 2.8); normal range: 275–295 mOsm/l.

Causes of water gain include

1. Increased ADH From the Pituitary or Hypothalamus (see Fig. 31–1)

- Decreased circulating plasma volume as seen in CHF, liver failure, nephrotic syndrome, other hypoproteinemias, and severe hypothyroidism
- Drugs (especially narcotics), tricyclics, phenothiazines, vincristine
- Pain, vomiting, psychosis

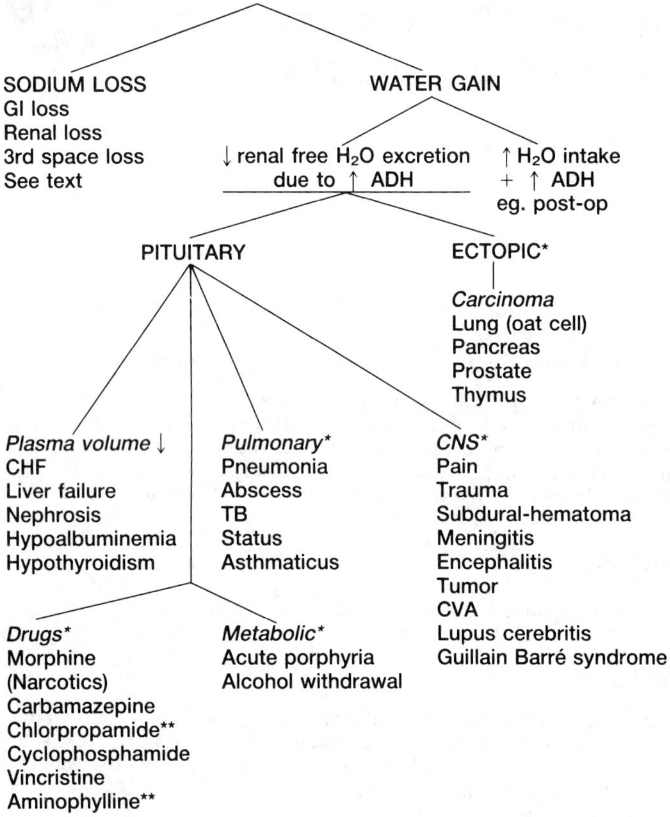

* So-called SIADH
** Potentiate ADH action

Figure 31–1. Causes of true hyponatremia.

- CNS lesions: Trauma, subdural hematoma, meningitis, encephalitis, tumor, CVA, lupus cerebritis, Guillain-Barré syndrome
- Pulmonary infections, pneumonias, abscess, TB
- Metabolic: Acute intermittent porphyria, alcohol withdrawal

2.–Ectopic ADH production

- From tumors: Carcinomas, especially oat cell of lung, pancreas, prostate, and thymus

3.–ADH potentiating drugs

- Chlorpropamide (adenylate cyclase activation)
- Aminophylline, caffeine (phosphodiesterase inhibition)

In some of the above-mentioned conditions (1–3), hypothalamic or posterior pituitary ADH is ↑, there is ectopic production regardless of serum osmolality, or there is enhancement of ADH action on renal tubules as with chlorpropamide. Thus, the listing of these conditions in most textbooks as the syndrome of inappropriate (SI)ADH secretion is questionable. The so-called syndrome confuses the facts and relegates clinical medicine to complicated algorithms that require determination of serum and urine osmolality and volume status.

A relevant history and physical examination usually reveal volume status and most causes listed in Figure 31–1. including the above-mentioned causes of ↑ ADH production or enhancement. Serum electrolytes, creatinine, if needed, and chest x ray arc assessed. At this point, if a cause is not readily identifiable, assessment of serum and urine osmolality and urine Na is advisable. If the hyponatremia is due to conditions causing ↑ ADH secretion (Fig. 31–1), then serum osmolality is low, urine osmolality relatively higher, urine Na >25 mEq/l; serum uric acid and urea are low and the hyponatremia responds to fluid restriction.

Clinical Manifestations

Acute hyponatremia, especially if associated with ↓ serum osmolality, may cause confusion, weakness, lethargy, nausea and vomiting, seizures, respiratory arrest, and coma. Chronic hyponatremia causes mild symptoms: Headache, lethargy, muscle cramps, agitation, and confusion.

Treatment

- **Hyponatremia due to Na loss:** Correct with IV infusion of isotonic (0.9%) saline. When urine output is adequate, KCl is added to the infusion to maintain a normal serum Na and K
- **Severe hyponatremia with seizures:** The hypotonic state with reduced serum osmolality causes H_2O to pass into cells, producing dangerous cerebral edema. This is a life-threatening situation and is usually seen with serum Na in the range of 95–115 mEq/l, especially where an acute ↓ in Na has occurred: e.g., a ↓ from 140 to 120 in 24–48 h. Seizures may be unresponsive to diazepam or phenytoin. Table 31–1 gives guidelines for the administration of hypertonic saline. There is no advantage in calculating the deficit and trying to restore this in 12–24 h since it is not advisable to ↑ the serum Na from the baseline beyond 10 mEq (mmol)/l in the first 24 h, and cer-

Table 31–1
Guidelines for Correction of Serum Sodium < 114 mEq (mmol)L with Hypertonic Saline

PRESENCE OF	SALINE 1 L CONTAINS mEq/L	INFUSE VOLUME	TOTAL mEq = mmol	EXPECTED ↑ SERUM Na AND mEq/L/h
CNS symptoms or signs; no seizures	3% = 500	500 ml over 5 h then	250 50/h	7 ± 1 1.4 mEq/L/h
Seizures	5% = 850	300 ml over 3 h then* slow infusion if needed**	250	7 ± 1 2.3 mEq/l /h

* Furosemide 20–40 mg; K replacement and fluid restriction
** Do not increase serum Na to above 120 mEq (mmol)/L in first 24 h. Measure serum Na 2 hourly for 6 h, then as needed.

tainly not advisable to ↑ the total serum Na to >120 mEq/l in the first 24 h

- **Acute hyponatremia with CNS symptoms and/or signs in the absence of seizures:** If the serum Na has fallen quickly over a period of days to <115 mEq/l, give 300–500 ml 3% saline over 5 h, then 40 mg furosemide. 3% saline, 0.5–1.4 mEq/l/h infused over a few hours should suffice to raise the serum Na 10 to max 14 mEq from baseline over the first 24 h. Thereafter, water restriction should suffice to ↑ serum Na about 5 mEq (mmol)/l daily
- **Patients without seizures and CNS signs** should be treated with fluid restriction 750 ml/day for 2 days, 1 l/day for 3 days, then 1.2 l/day until the serum Na reaches >130 mEq/l

It is important not to correct the Na deficit too rapidly to normal levels because this may cause central pontine myelinolysis, albeit rarely. The possible role of the rate and extent of correction of hyponatremia in the development of pontine myelinolysis remains uncertain; malnutrition and alcoholism ↑ the risk of this complication. Concentrations as high as 29.2% saline have been used to ↑ serum Na 10–20 mmol from baseline in 24 h in patients with seizures unresponsive to diazepam and phenytoin without adverse effects. This approach is not recommended, however. A formula can be used to estimate the Na deficit, volume of 3% NaCl, and duration of infusion. However, such calculations often result in the use of too large an amount of Na infused. Use 120 mEq/l as a goal. Na deficit = 0.6 (or 0.5 for women; 50% lean wt = total body H_2O) x wt (kg) x (120 – measured Na). The suggested number of hours for correction by NaCl infusion = (120 – measured Na).

Give half the above-calculated deficit in the first 24 h. See Table 31–1 for a more practical and prudent approach to the correction of severe acute hyponatremia.

Demeclocycline impedes the effect of ADH on the distal and convoluted tubules of the kidney, resulting in free H_2O excretion. Its effect may not be apparent for >1 week. Dosage: 300–600 mg bid in patients with chronic hyponatremia. Caution: The drug is metabolized in the liver and a ↓ in dosage is required in the presence of hepatic failure to avoid nephrotoxicity.

HYPOKALEMIA

Definition: Intracellular K concentration is approximately 30 times higher than extracellular. Fall of serum K 1 mEq represents approximately a 300-mEq deficit. The serum K level dictates an alteration of the K gradient across myocardial cell membranes that can result in severe electrical changes and cardiac arrhythmias. Serum K levels <3 mEq/l can produce premature atrial or ventricular beats, junctional tachycardias, ventricular tachycardia, or fibrillation. A low serum K reduces VF threshold and ↑ the risk of sudden death.

Causes

- of serum K <3.5 mEq (mmol)/l include
- Renal loss: Diuretics, renal diseases including renal tubular acidosis, and hyperaldosteronism

- GI loss: Vomiting, nasogastric suction, diarrhea, laxative abuse, and villous adenoma
- Shift into cells: (a) alkalosis: Every 0.1 ↑ in pH causes a ↓ of 0.5 mEq K/l; (b) insulin and glucose infusion, β agonists, and hypokalemic periodic paralysis

Treatment

- Mild K depletion 3–3.5 mEq/l: This is usually asymptomatic but requires correction in patients on digoxin or diuretics, or in the presence of IHD, hepatic encephalopathy, or metabolic acidosis, where serum K <3.5 reflects severe K depletion. Give KCl orally
- Moderate K depletion 2.5–2.9 mEq/l: Correction can be with oral therapy. IV is used if a line already exists or if symptoms such as weakness, confusion, or arrhythmias and/or digitalis toxicity are present
- Severe depletion, K <2.5 mEq/l or metabolic acidosis with K <3.5: IV KCl is necessary, given in 0.9% saline. In some cardiac patients, where Na load may be hazardous, the first liter given in 0.9% saline can alternate with 5% dextrose/H_2O (D5W). However, severe K depletion must not be corrected with K in dextrose solution because this ↑ the K shift into cells under the activity of insulin
- Liquid and oral preparations containing adequate K, 20 mEq, and Cl, 20 mEq, include: K-Lor in liquid or packets, Kaochlor 10%, Kay Ciel and Kay-Ciel; K-Lyte Cl contains 25 mEq K, 25 Cl
- K tablets. K-Dur 20 and K Contin contain 20 mEq KCl. Micro-K = 8 mEq, Micro-K = 10 mEq; Slow-K = 8 mEq
- IV KCl: IV for serum K 2.5–3 mEq/l: 40 mEq KCl added to 1 l 0.9% saline given q 8 h = 125 ml q h = 5 mEq K/h (for cardiacs with CHF, dilute in 1 l 5% dextrose/H_2O) IV KCl always should be given in saline. May need to add oral KCl to prevent fluid overload: e.g., K-Dur-20 or K-Contin 20 mEq tid. Max rate without cardiac monitor 10 mEq K/h. Above solution 250 ml/h (note the large volume required). Max K dosage: 20 mEq/h.
- In life-threatening situations with serum K <2 mEq/l or <3 mEq/l with metabolic acidosis. Put 60 mEq KCl/l in 0.9% saline, infuse through a large vein, run at 333 ml/h, but not in a central vein, because cardiac toxicity may result if a bolus >20 mEq/h is infused directly into the heart. Only extremely rarely is 30 mEq/h needed. K concentration/h and volume of fluid/h that can be tolerated are important considerations.

HYPERKALEMIA

Causes

Serum K >5 mEq (mmol)l: Quickly exclude pseudohyperkalemia (poor phlebotomy techniques, hemolysed specimen, severe thrombocytosis, leukocytosis), then approach systematically. See Fig. 31–2

Manifestations

Alteration in cardiac excitability is the most important sequelae, with typical ECG changes

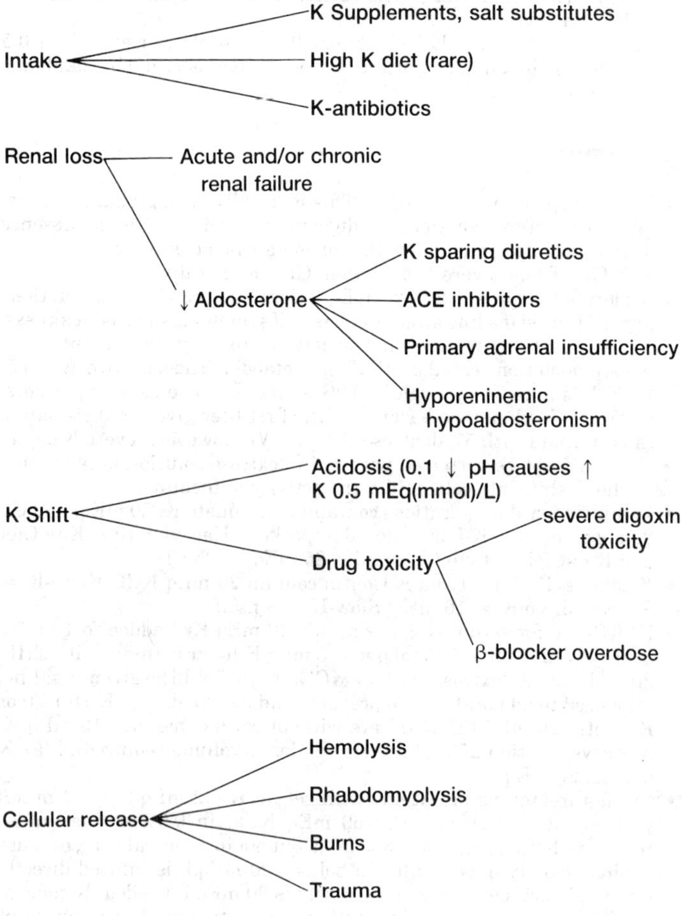

Figure 31–2. Hyperkalemia.

- Narrow-based peaked T ("tented") waves occur mainly in V2-V4 when serum K is >6 mEq/l (Fig. 31–3), PR interval may be prolonged
- K >7 mEq/l: QRS widens. The S wave moves steeply into the T wave: There is no longer a normal isoelectric ST segment. P waves flattened or absent
- K >8 mEq/l, absent P, wide QRS, peaked T (sine wave)
- VF or asystole; VT may occur with K >6 mEq/l without the above ECG changes

Treatment

Serum K >6 mEq/l and/or ECG manifestations dictate rapid correction of hyperkalemia.

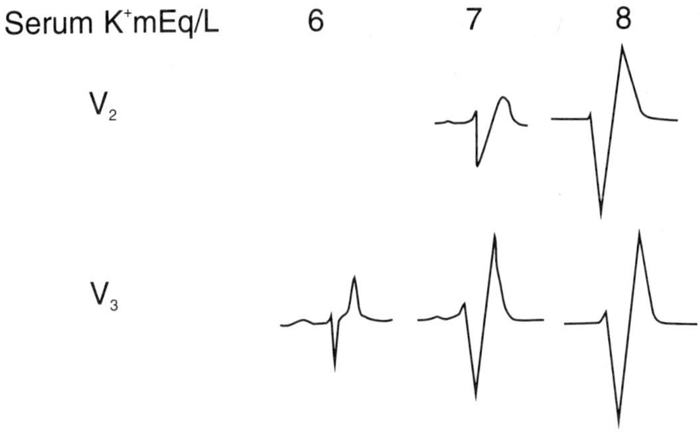

Figure 31–3. Electrocardiographic Signs of Hyperkalemia.

K^+ > 5.7 mEq (mmol)/L: Earliest signs; T wave peaked, narrow base ("tented"); PR interval may be prolonged.
> 7 mEq/L: P wave flat or absent; QRS widens, prominent S wave.
> 8 mEq/L: S wave becomes wider and deeper, and moves steeply into the T wave; there is virtually no isoelectric ST segment; occasionally ST segment elevation.

RESTRICT INTAKE OF K

Curtail dietary K, salt substitutes, K supplements, and/or K-retaining medications (K-sparing diuretics and ACE inhibitors).

PROMOTE SHIFT INTO CELLS

Sodium bicarbonate IV, 2 ampules 88 mEq (mmol) over 15 min produces immediate K shift into cells. Effect lasts 1–2 h. Repeat in 2 h if no effect and ECG signs persist. Caution: Can precipitate CHF, tetany, or intracellular acidosis.

Insulin (Regular) 10 U in 50 ml 50% dextrose, IV bolus, or 10 U in 500 ml 20% D/W over 1 h; effect is immediate, lasts about 2 h, and should ↓ serum K 1 mEq/l after 2 h.

Albuterol (salbutamol) IV or **fenoterol** (β_2 agonists) aerosol have an immediate effect but short duration. This approach should be considered where $NaHCO_3$ is contraindicated or has had little effect.

STABILIZE CARDIAC CELL MEMBRANE

For serum K >6.5 or ECG signs of hyperkalemia: CaCl or Ca gluconate 10–20 ml, 10% IV bolus over 3 min; action within min and lasts about 30–60 min. If no salutary response in 5 min, repeat dose.

PROMOTE RENAL LOSS OF K

Furosemide 80–160 mg IV plus isotonic saline, depending on cause of ↑ K.

Fludrocortisone 0.5–2 mg po if hypoaldosteronism is suspected.

PROMOTE GI LOSS

Na or Ca polystyrene sulphonate bind K and release Na or Ca in the colon. Enemas have a quicker onset of colonic action (within 1 h).

Sodium polystyrene sulfonate (Kayexalate, Resonium A): 50 g powder in 200 ml of 20% sorbitol solution retained for about 1 h and given q 4–6 h. Orally 15–30 g powder in H_2O, then sorbitol 50 ml 20% solution to facilitate quick transit to the colon and elimination; repeat q 4–6 h.

Calcium polystyrene sulphonate (Resonium Calcium) exchanges Ca for K and is preferable in patients with CHF and severe renal failure where Na load may be hazardous. Caution: Conditions prone to hypercalcemia. Dosage is the same for both resins.

Dialysis. Failure to maintain K <7 mEq/l with the above measures, rapidly increasing K, increasing ECG signs (especially if due to renal failure or rhabdomyolysis) often require hemodialysis; peritoneal dialysis is less efficient.

HYPERCALCEMIA

Normally, serum Ca is controlled primarily by the action of PTH, Vitamin D, and to a lesser extent calcitonin, on bone, kidneys, and intestine. Normal serum Ca range: 8.8–10.4 mg/dl (2.2–2.6 mmol/l).

Causes

Bone Pathology Increased bone resorption: Increased osteoclastic activity; ↑ PGE2 or PTH-like chemicals and mechanical erosion

- Carcinomas: Breast, lung, kidney, ovary, prostate, pancreas
- Hematologic: Myeloma, lymphomas
- Hyperparathyroidism
- Paget's disease

Kidney Increased reabsorption of Ca in the proximal tubule and ↓ Ca excretory capacity

- Hyperparathyroidism
- Thiazide diuretics
- Familial hypocalciuric hypercalcemia

Intestine Increased absorption

- Excessive intake of Ca, Vitamin D
- Milk alkali syndrome
- Vitamin D effect, as with sarcoidosis

Bone and Intestine

- Hyperparathyroidism
- Vitamin D intoxication
- Sarcoidosis: Increased level and sensitivity to Vitamin D

Others Vitamin A intoxication, prolonged immobilization, thyrotoxicosis, Addison's disease, lithium therapy

Symptoms and Signs

- GI: Anorexia, vomiting, constipation, ileus, peptic ulcer or pancreatic abdominal pain, stones, bones and groans of hyperparathyroidism
- Renal: Hypercalcemia interferes with renal mechanisms for the reabsorption of Na and H_2O: Polyuria caused by osmotic diuresis and impaired concentrating ability results in volume depletion, hemodynamic deterioration, and renal insufficiency, which further ↑ serum Ca. Pain due to nephrolithiasis may occur
- CNS: Change in mental status: Confusion, lethargy, agitation, hyporeflexia, psychosis, coma
- CVS: Shortened QT interval, arrhythmias

Acute Management

Medical therapy is indicated in patients with serum Ca levels >12 mg/dl (3 mmol/l) and/or if symptoms are present and when the patient's underlying disease warrants treatment. Serum Ca levels are adjusted if serum albumin is low: A ↓ of 1 g/dl of albumin causes a 0.8 mg/dl ↓ in serum Ca (a ↓ of 10 g/l of albumin causes a 0.2 mmol/l ↓ in serum CA). In patients with Ca levels >14 mg/dl (3.5 mmol/l), urgent treatment is required. Suggested steps in how to manage this clinical situation are given in Figure 31–4. For details of drugs, see Table 31–2.

Acute management always requires rapid volume expansion. Give 500 ml 0.9% NaCl rapidly, then 2–4 l q 24 h.

Furosemide IV 20 mg q 6–12 h is commenced only after volume repletion with 2–4 l isotonic saline IV. The effect of furosemide depends on the delivery of Ca to the ascending limb. Higher doses, (80–100 mg) furosemide are not usually necessary and may cause volume depletion with hemodynamic deterioration. A dose of 10–20 mg IV q 6 h is preferable in the elderly or in patients at risk for CHF. The urinary output is measured hourly and should be replaced with IV saline, rate adjusted to match urine output.

Calcitonin is the most rapid-acting osteoclast inhibitor and is indicated for the rapid lowering of life-threatening serum Ca levels >16 mg/dl (4 mmol/l). However, the drug has a mild effect and should not be used as sole drug therapy.

Dosage: 2–8 IU/kg IV over 24 h or 4–8 IU/kg SC q 6 h. Caution: Do allergy test in patients with history of allergy: 1 IU intradermal prior to therapy; use plastic IV bag, not glass.

Corticosteroids enhance the activity of calcitonin and should be added, especially in patients with sarcoidosis, Vitamin D intoxication, myeloma, or breast carcinoma. Alternatively, plicamycin should follow the administration of calcitonin if no contraindications exist.

Plicamycin (Mithramycin) may cause significant nephrotoxicity, hepatotoxicity, and thrombocytopenia. Usually given as 1 dose, max 2 doses. Reduce dose 50% with renal failure.

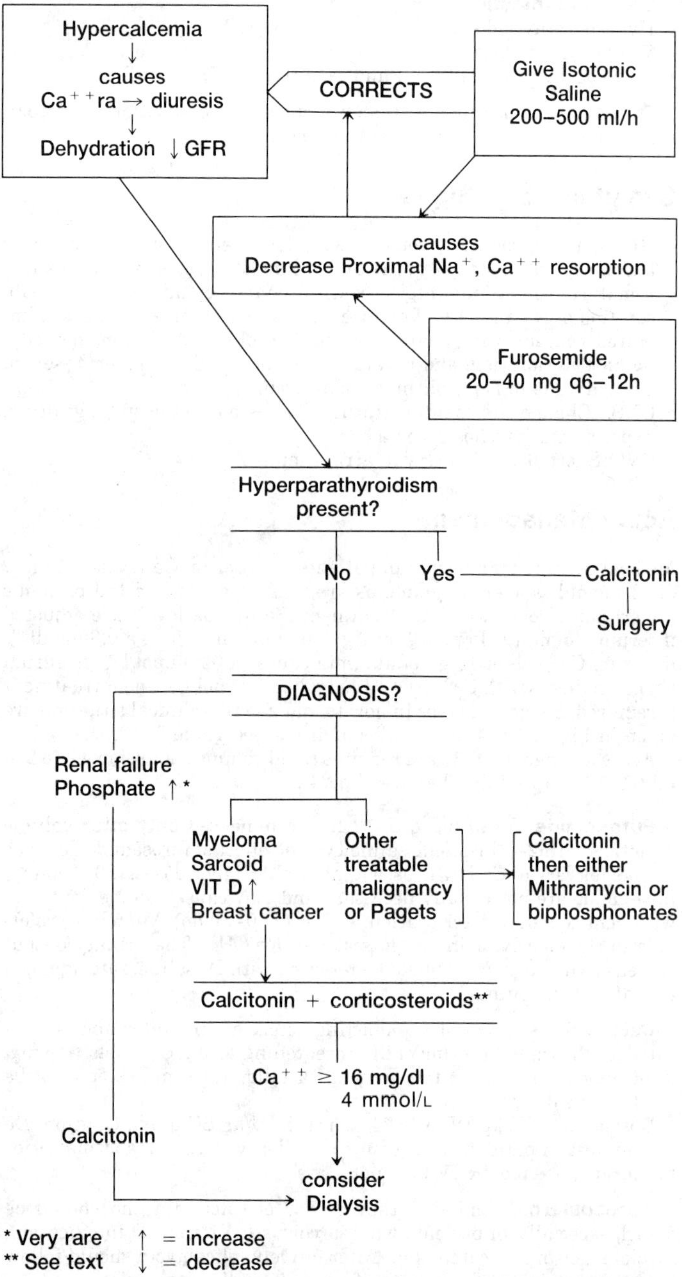

Figure 31–4. Acute Management of Hypercalcemia.

Table 31–2
Drugs Used in the Management of Hypercalcemia

DRUG	MECHANISM	ONSET OF ACTION	INDICATIONS—ADVICE	C/I	DOSAGE
Phosphate	Ca^{++} ↑ deposition to bone and soft tissue ↓ GI absorption ↓ Bone breakdown	2–3 days (chronic management)	Chronic hypercalcemia. Keep serum phosphate in normal range.	Serum phosphate elevated, renal failure	Oral: 250–500 mg q 6 h. IV not recommended.
Glucocorticoids	↑ Ca^{++} excretion ↓ GI absorption ↓ Osteolytic activity	36–72 h	Sarcoidosis, breast carcinoma, myeloma, vitamin D intoxication	—	Prednisone 30–40 mg twice daily
Calcitonin (salmon; Salcatonin)	↑ Renal excretion of Ca^{++} ↓ Release of Ca^{++} from bone ↑ Phosphate excretion in urine	Immediate but mild ↓ Ca^{++}	Hypercalcemia unresponsive to saline & furosemide hyperparathyroidism vitamin D malignancy: with ↑ phosphate levels	Allergy +ve skin test	4 8U/kg q 6 or 12 h SC or IM for 1–2 days
Plicamycin (Mithramycin)	Osteoclast toxin, ↓ bone resorption	12–24 h	Symptomatic serum $Ca^{++} > 3.5$ mmol/L (15 mg/dL)	Hepatic & renal failure, ↓ platelets	10–25 μg/kg IV infusion over 6 hours. Repeat in 3 days only if absolutely necessary
Biphosphonates	↓ bone resorption by osteoclasts	2–5 days	Malignancy, Paget's	Severe renal failure	See text.

Chronic Management

- Low Ca/high Na diet
- High fluid intake: 2–4 l/day
- Prednisone 30–40 mg bid for 3 days, then decreasing doses
- Oral phosphate, where the serum phosphate is normal and in the absence of renal failure
- The combination of phosphate and corticosteroids
- Indomethacin: 75–150 mg qd for PGE_2-associated hypercalcemia
- Biphosphonates inhibit bone resorption and have a role along with saline infusion in stable patients with only moderate symptoms. These agents are more potent and have a longer duration of action than calcitonin and are far less toxic than plicamycin. Disodium etidronate or pamidronate is available.

Disodium etidronate (Didronel). Dosage: For Paget's or malignancy: 5 mg/kg po once daily for ≤6 months, or 10 mg/kg for 3 months. For severe hypercalcemia of malignancy: 7.5 mg/kg in 250 ml 0.9% saline IV over 4 h qd for 3–7 days. On day of last IV dose, commence oral dose 20 mg/kg once daily for 1 month.

Pamidronate 60–90 mg in 1 l saline or 5% D/W IV over 24 h.

Caution: Avoid food, especially Ca products, for 2 h before and after biphosphonates. Discontinue treatment if fractures occur. Reduce dose in renal impairment. CI with severe renal failure.

Gallium nitrate inhibits bone resorption by absorbing and reducing solubility of hydroxy-apatite crystals. Lowering of serum Ca occurs in 3–5 days, i.e., a slower action than calcitonin, but causes a higher response rate. Adverse effects include nephrotoxicity. Avoid in patients with renal insufficiency. Dosage: 200 mg/m^2 in 1 l 0.9% saline IV over 24 h qd for 5 days. Maintain adequate hydration with ≥2 l saline IV daily.

Suggested Reading

Bilezikian John P: Review article: Drug therapy: Management of acute hypercalcemia. New Eng J Med, *326*: 1996, 1992.

Diabetes Mellitus

32

Richard Beaser and Robyn L. Houlden

Diagnosis. The recommended screening test for diabetes is a fasting plasma glucose level. A fasting plasma glucose >115 mg/dl (6.4 mmol/l) indicates a need for further testing (Fig. 32–1). According to criteria developed by the National Diabetes Data Group, any of the following are considered diagnostic of diabetes

- Presence of classic symptoms—polyuria, polydipsia, ketonuria, and rapid weight loss—together with a random venous plasma glucose level ≥ 200 mg/dl (11.1 mmol/l)
- Fasting venous plasma glucose ≥ 140 mg/dl (7.8 mmol/l) on >1 occasion
- Fasting plasma glucose <140 mg/dl (7.8 mmol/l) and a 2–h plasma

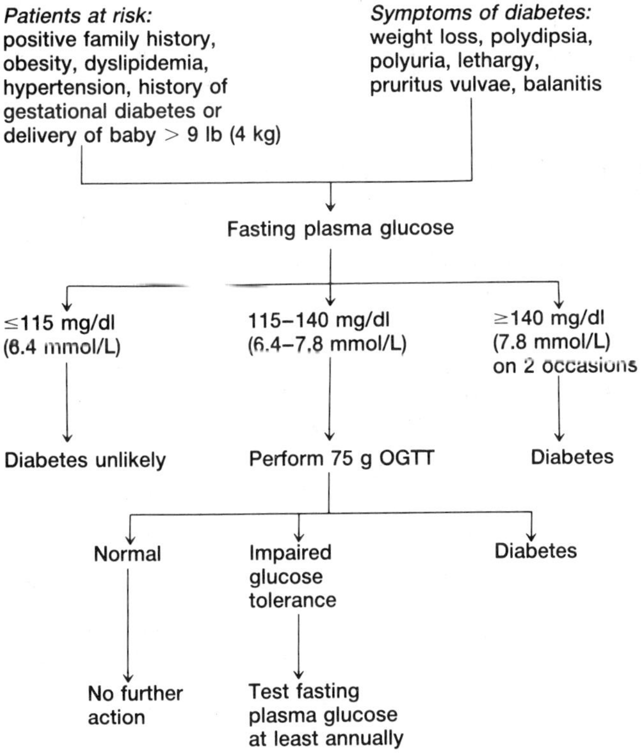

Figure 32–1. Screening for Diabetes.

Table 32–1
Definition of Diabetes

	FASTING GLUCOSE [mg/dl (mmol/L)]	PEAK GLUCOSE [mg/dl (mmol/L)]	2 HOUR GLUCOSE [mg/dl (mmol/L)]
Normal	≤115 (6.4)	<200 (11.1)	<140 (7.8)
Impaired glucose tolerance	<140 (7.8)	>200 (11.1)	140–200 (7.8–11.1)
Diabetes mellitus	≥140 (7.8)	OGTT not needed	
Diabetes mellitus	<140 (7.8)	≥200 (11.1)	≥200 (11.1)

OGTT = oral glucose tolerance test
The test should be done:
- after 3 days of a diet supplying more than 150 g of carbohydrates per day
- in the morning after a 10–14 hour fast
- with the patient lying down or sitting in a quiet room, without smoking

glucose >200 mg/dl (11.1 mmol/l) with 1 intervening value >200 mg/dl (11.1 mmol/l) following a 75–g glucose load on >1 occasion (Table 32–1)

Types. Table 32–2 outlines the differences in the 2 major types of diabetes mellitus.

Impaired Glucose Tolerance. Individuals with IGT have plasma glucose levels that are higher than normal but lower than those consid-

Table 32–2
Characteristic Features of the 2 Main Types of Diabetes Mellitus

	TYPE I: INSULIN-DEPENDENT DIABETES MELLITUS (IDDM)	TYPE II: NONINSULIN-DEPENDENT DIABETES MELLITUS (NIDDM)
Prevalence	10%	90%
Age of onset	typically onset <30 years but any age possible	onset usually >40 years
Body weight	usually thin	>80% obese
Presentation	acute onset, with polyuria, polydipsia, weight loss, lethargy, pruritus vulvae, balanitis	insidious onset, micro- and macrovascular complications may be present at diagnosis
Etiology	inadequate insulin secretion due to autoimmune destruction of the pancreatic β-cells	impaired insulin secretion, increased hepatic glucose production and peripheral insulin resistance
Ketosis	prone	not prone
Genetics	HLA-DR3 and DR4 common; 50% concordance in identical twins	HLA unrelated; 100% concordance in identical twins

ered diagnostic for diabetes mellitus. Of all patients with IGT, 1–5% a year develop overt diabetes mellitus. Individuals with IGT have a greater than normal risk for macrovascular complications but do not appear to have a ↑ risk for the microvascular complications of diabetes.

ACUTE COMPLICATIONS OF DIABETES

Diabetic Ketoacidosis

DEFINITION

- Hyperglycemia: Glucose usually >250 mg/dl (14 mmol/l)
- Hyperketonemia: Ketones present in the blood and urine
- Acidosis: pH <7.2 or bicarbonate <15 mEq (mmol)/l

CAUSES

DKA is always caused by insulin deficiency, either absolute (e.g., a previously undiagnosed patient or one who omitted insulin) or relative (e.g., too little insulin injected or antagonism by stress hormones) (Fig. 32–2).

SIGNS AND SYMPTOMS

DKA is characterized by nausea, vomiting, dehydration, fruity breath, Kussmaul (rapid and deep) respirations, abdominal pain, and CNS depression, with drowsiness progressing to coma.

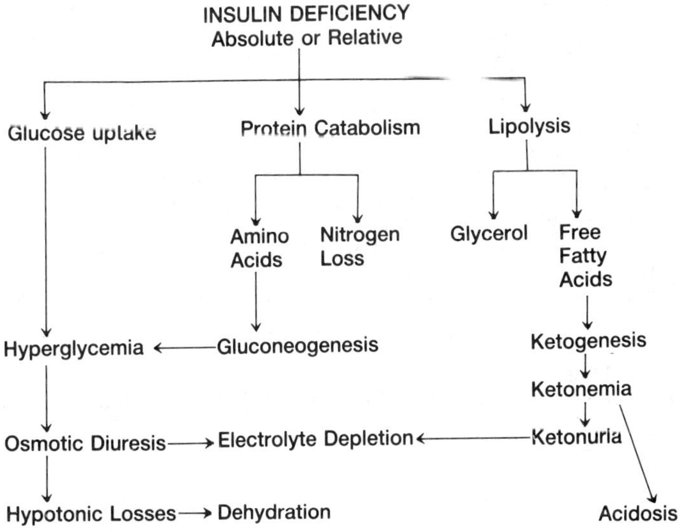

Figure 32–2. Pathogenesis of Diabetic Ketoacidosis.

TYPICAL LABORATORY ABNORMALITIES

- Plasma glucose >300 mg/dl (17 mmol/l)
- Urinary and plasma ketones
- Bicarbonate <15 mEq (mmol)/l
- Arterial pH <7.2
- ↑ anion gap—usually >16 mEq (mmol)/l
- Low plasma Na: Hyperglycemia lowers Na level by 1.6 mEq (mmol)/l for every 100 mg/dl (5.5 mmol/l) ↑ in blood glucose >100 mg/dl (5.5 mmol/l)
- ↑ urea and creatinine
- Elevated WBC: May occur in the absence of infection

OTHER LABORATORY ABNORMALITIES

- Elevated amylase: May be ↑ in >50% of patients without evidence of pancreatitis. Salivary isoenzyme is usually responsible for the ↑
- Mild to moderate ↑ in creatinine kinase (CPK): May occur in 25–40% of patients without ECG or clinical evidence of MI
- Mild to moderate ↑ of hepatic transaminases (AST and ALT) in 25–50% of patients without clinical evidence of hepatic disease

MANAGEMENT

- The initial goal of therapy is to treat life-threatening emergencies, including dehydration, insulin deficiency, and K deficiency
- Monitor vital signs, blood glucose, Na, K, chloride, bicarbonate, and urea q 2 h until stable. Typical fluid and electrolyte deficits are shown in Table 32–3
- Fluid replacement: Initial goals are to restore circulating volume, reverse hypotension, and maintain cerebral, coronary, and renal perfusion. Isotonic saline (0.98% NaCl) is usually the initial choice of rehydrating fluid. For patients who are hypernatremic or at risk for CHF, a solution containing half (0.45%) isotonic saline may be preferred. The rates and volumes of administration will depend on the patient's clinical status. As a guide, give 1 liter/h x 1 h, 500 ml/h x 2 h, 250 ml/h x 4 h, then 150 ml/h. Reduce fluid administration in the elderly and in patients with cardiac disease, and check cardiopulmonary status regularly. Fluid replacement should normally be completed over 12–24 h. However, with mild cases of DKA, fluid replacement may be completed in the emergency room over 6–8 h
- K replacement: Hypokalemia is a significant cause of mortality. K levels may be normal or ↑ initially due to the metabolic acidosis. However, total body K levels are always depleted. Administer K replacement from the outset unless the initial K level is >6.0 mEq

Table 32–3
Typical Fluid and Electrolyte Deficits in Diabetic Ketoacidosis

FLUID OR ELECTROLYTE	DEFICIT
Water	60–100 ml/kg
Sodium	6–12 mEq (mmol)/kg
Potassium	4–6 mEq (mmol)/kg
Phosphate	2–5 mEq (mmol)/kg

Table 32–4
Potassium Replacement for Diabetic Ketoacidosis

PLASMA POTASSIUM LEVEL [mEq (mmol)/L]	POTASSIUM INFUSION [mEq (mmol)/kg/hr]
<3.0	>0.5
3.0–4.0	0.4
4.0–5.0	0.3
5.0–6.0	0.1–0.2
>6.0	0 (until K^+ <6.0)

(mmol)/l or oliguria is demonstrated by bladder catherization. Guidelines for K replacement are shown in Table 32–4. ECG monitoring may be helpful in assessing K status (see Fig. 31–3).

- Insulin: If the blood glucose is >270 mg/dl (15 mmol/l), give a bolus of short-acting insulin 0.15 U/kg IV. Then start a continuous infusion of short-acting insulin of 0.1 U/kg/h. The blood glucose level should ↓ at an average rate of 75 mg/dl (4.0 mmol/l/h). If no response has occurred after 2–4 h, double the infusion rate of short-acting insulin. Once the blood glucose has reached 250 mg/dl (<14 mmol/l), start 5% dextrose/H_2O at 100 ml/h in addition to the insulin infusion. This permits continued administration of insulin to abolish ketosis while protecting the patient from hypoglycemia. In addition, ↓ the insulin infusion rate to 1–2 U/h to maintain the plasma glucose at 150–250 mg/dl (8–14 mmol/l). When the acidosis is corrected and the patient able to drink and eat, give the patient's usual dose of SQ insulin and discontinue the insulin infusion 2 h later
- Bicarbonate: Its use in DKA is controversial. It may precipitate or worsen hypokalemia, leading to cardiac arrhythmias; cause a paradoxical ↓ of CSF pH, leading to worsening of the CNS depression; and cause a shift in the Hb O_2 disassociation curve (Bohr effect), leading to tissue hypoxia. Indications for bicarbonate therapy include: Severe acidosis (pH <7.0); serum HCO_3- <10 mEq (mmol)/l; acidosis accompanied by hypotension, shock, or arrhythmias; and hyperkalemia (serum K >6.5 mEq (mmol)/l). Administer 1–2 mEq (mmol)/kg of sodium bicarbonate in 500 ml of 0.9% NaCl over 2 h. Check the arterial pH 30 min after the bicarbonate infusion finishes and give further doses of bicarbonate until the pH is >7.0. The amount of bicarbonate administered should generally not be >3 mEq (mmol)/kg over 12 h
- Identify and correct the precipitating cause. It is important to teach patients proper management of sick days at home

Hyperglycemic Hyperosmolar Coma

HHC usually occurs in older patients with Type II diabetes who cannot recognize thirst or express their need for H_2O. A precipitating factor is usually present (e.g., MI, CVA, infection, diuretics, total parenteral nutrition, glucocorticoids, or phenytoin). The pathogenesis of hyperosmolar coma is shown in Figure 32–3. Hyperglycemia results in a chronic osmotic diuresis that causes dehydration and loss of K and Na. Renal impairment from dehydration and declining creatinine clearance with aging is usually present and contributes to the hyperglycemia and hyperosmolality. Ketosis is absent, which is probably due to several reasons: A critical amount of insulin is still present and capable of suppressing lipolysis; there is less ↑ of counterregulatory hormones than in DKA;

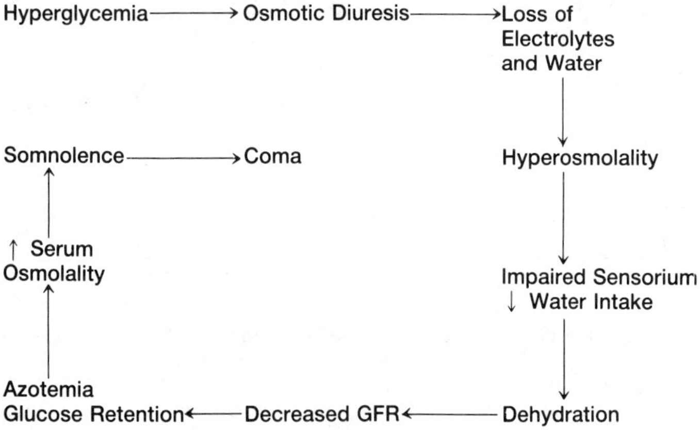

Figure 32–3. Pathogenesis of Hyperosmolar State.

and the hyperosmolality itself may suppress lipolysis. Patients present with dehydration, often with shock, and disorientation progressing to coma.

LABORATORY FINDINGS

- Severe hyperglycemia (blood glucose >600 mg/dl [30 mmol/l])
- Absence of, or slight, ketosis
- Calculated or measured serum hyperosmolality >330 mOsm (mmol)/kg H_2O
- Profound dehydration with ↑ urea and creatinine
- Serum Na may be normal or high due to dehydration

MANAGEMENT

- Rehydration should be done more slowly than in DKA. Monitoring of central venous pressure or PCWP is often necessary to aid in the management of fluids in elderly patients with renal and cardiac failure. Serum Na <150 mEq (mmol)/l: Use 0.9% NaCl. Serum Na >150 mEq (mmol)/l and *normotensive,* use 0.45% NaCl
- K replacement should be administered as in the management of DKA
- Insulin should be given as outlined for DKA. Most patients are quite sensitive to insulin. Rehydration alone may produce a substantial ↓ in blood glucose by improving renal plasma flow and glomerular filtration
- Identify and treat the precipitating cause

Hypoglycemia

Most common cause of visits to the emergency room among patients with diabetes. The incidence ↑ as patients strive for tighter glycemic control. Adrenergic symptoms are caused by activation of the sympathetic nervous system and include diaphoresis, palpitations, tremor, anxiety, and pallor. Neuroglycopenic symptoms include cognitive impairment, visual changes, hunger, seizures, and loss of consciousness. They are produced by neuronal dysfunction secondary to glucose deprivation. Glucose is the only fuel the brain can use as an energy source. The brain cannot synthesize or store glucose and is dependent on a continuous supply from the circulation.

MANAGEMENT

- Conscious patient: Give 10 g rapidly absorbable glucose, i.e., 1 of the following: 4 oz (125 ml) juice or regular soft drink, sugar (2 cubes, 2 packets, or 2 tsp), several small candies. Wait 5–10 min. If the patient does not improve, repeat the treatment. After the patient recovers, give a snack equivalent to 1 starch and 1 protein exchange if the next regularly scheduled meal or snack is >1 h away. Chocolate and ice cream should be avoided due to their fat content
- Unconscious patient: Give 25 ml of 50% dextrose/H_2O IV bolus or 1 mg of glucagon SQ or I.M. every 5–10 min until the patient awakens, then feed orally
- Identify the precipitating cause. Patients should be taught how to adjust food and insulin for changes in diet and activity. Hypoglycemia induced by the longer-acting sulphonylureas or long-acting insulins can be prolonged. Glucose levels should be followed for 24 h. The patient may need to be admitted to hospital for a continuous glucose infusion

Differential Diagnosis of Coma in Patients with Diabetes

See Table 32–5.

Table 32–5
Differential Diagnosis of Coma in Patients with Diabetes

SIGNS AND SYMPTOMS

DIAGNOSIS	VENTILATION	DEHYDRATION	PRESSURE	SKIN
DKA	+ + +	+ + +	Normal/Low	Warm
HONC	+ + + +	Normal/Low	Normal	
Hypoglycemia	0	0	Normal	Cool, Clammy
Lactic Acidosis	+ + +	0	Low	Warm
Nonmetabolic	0 to +	0 to +	Variable	Normal

LABORATORY TESTS

DIAGNOSIS	GLUCOSE	KETONES
DKA	>300 mg/dl (17 mmol/L)	+ + to + + + +
HONC	>800 mg/dl (44 mmol/L)	0 to +
Hypoglycemia	<50 mg/dl (3.0 mmol/L)	0
Lactic Acidosis	Variable	0 to +
Nonmetabolic	Variable	0 to +

CHRONIC COMPLICATIONS OF DIABETES

Macrovascular Disease

- Cardiovascular disease is the leading cause of death in patients with diabetes, particularly in women who lose their premenopausal protection against CHD. Atherosclerotic lesions tend to occur at an earlier age and to be more diffuse. Peripheral vascular disease is a major factor for the increased risk of amputation in patients with diabetes
- Modifiable risk factors should be changed. Smoking must be stopped. Dyslipidemia should be treated, initially with nonpharmacologic therapy: Weight ↓, a ↓ in total fat intake to <30% of calories with <10% of these coming from saturated fatty acids, and a ↓ in dietary cholesterol. Lipid-lowering agents should be added if nonpharmacologic therapy is not successful (see Chap. 9)

Retinopathy

- Nonproliferative (background) retinopathy (dot and blot hemorrhages, hard and soft exudates, microaneurysms) is present in 50% of patients with Type I diabetes 10 years after onset of symptoms. Proliferative retinopathy (growth of new capillaries and fibrous tissue within the retina and into the vitreous chamber) is present in 50% of patients after 15 years
- Refer to an ophthalmologist: All patients with Type I diabetes who are >10 years old and have had the disease for >5 years; all patients with diabetes who at diagnosis are >30 years old; and all female patients planning a pregnancy in the near future. Pregnant women should be reassessed early in the first trimester and seen each trimester thereafter unless more frequent visits are indicated for retinal disease
- Laser therapy can halt the progression of retinal disease. Vitrectomy (surgical removal of the vitreous) may help restore vision in severely diseased eyes with a significant retinal bleed

Nephropathy

- End stage renal disease occurs in 30–40% of patients with Type I diabetes. Renal disease manifests itself by the appearance of persistent proteinuria, usually after 10–15 years
- Urinalysis and serum creatinine should be checked at least annually
- After the patient has had diabetes for >5 years, total urinary protein excretion (in the patient with proteinuria on urine dipstick) or microalbuminuria (in the patient with no detectable proteinuria on routine urinalysis) should be measured annually
- BP should be measured at every follow-up visit
- When persistent proteinuria or declining renal function is confirmed, the patient should be referred to a nephrologist for medical treatment and to a dietician for instruction in low-protein diets
- Aggressive treatment of hypertension is the only therapy that slows progression of established diabetic nephropathy. Antihypertensive agents that may be used include ACE inhibitors, Ca antagonists, and cardioselective β-blockers (may mask symptoms of hypoglycemia)

Neuropathy

- The most common chronic complication of diabetes. Affects 50% of patients with long-standing diabetes
- Distal symmetrical sensory-motor polyneuropathy: Glove and stocking loss of sensation for pin prick and light touch. Vibration sense and reflexes are diminished. Pain is typically nocturnal. May be relieved by amitriptyline 10–150 mg/day at hs or capsaicin cream applied 3–4 times a day to the affected area

Autonomic Neuropathy

- Orthostatic hypotension: May respond to salt supplementation, fludrocortisone acetate (Florinef) 0.05–0.2 mg/day, or midodrine hydrochloride (Amatine) 2.5 mg tid. (See Chapter 15)
- Gastroparesis: May present with nausea and vomiting secondary to delayed gastric emptying. Cisapride 5–10 mg bid to qid, metoclopramide 5–10 mg tid or qid, or domperidone 10 mg tid or qid may help. All of these agents are taken 15–30 min before meals
- Diabetic diarrhea: May respond to tetracycline 250 mg qid for 7 days, loperamide hydrochloride (Imodium) 2 mg with each bowel movement up to 16 mg/day, or diphenoxylate hydrochloride (Lomotil) 5 mg tid or qid
- Diabetic cystopathy (neurogenic bladder): Results in chronic urine retention. May respond to bethanechol 10–20 mg tid to stimulate detrusor function or intermittent self-catherization
- Impotence: May be managed with penile implant, intrapenile injections of papaverine and phentolamine, or an external suction device

Focal Neuropathies

- Cranial mononeuropathy: Unilateral 3rd nerve paresis is the most common. Presents with abrupt onset of diplopia, typically accompanied by orbital or retro-orbital pain. Ptosis may occur, but pupillary function is spared. Usually resolves in 6 weeks–6 months
- Mononeuropathy/mononeuropathy multiplex: May involve ≥1 nerves of the extremities or trunk. Results from ischemic infarction of the nerve and is heralded by the acute onset of muscle weakness and pain in the area supplied. Spontaneous recovery occurs in 3–6 months

Foot Care

- In patients with neuropathy or peripheral vascular disease, a minor trauma to the foot can often lead to skin ulceration, infection, and ultimately gangrene. Feet should be examined at each follow-up visit. Patients must be taught preventive foot care.

MANAGEMENT OF DIABETES MELLITUS

Diabetic Way of Eating

- All patients should be referred to a dietitian for instruction on appropriate meal plans. In the obese patient with Type II diabetes, weight

Table 32–6
Estimation of Desirable Body Weight

BUILD	WOMEN	MEN
Small	−10%	−10%
Medium	100 lb (45 kg) for 1st 5 ft (150 cm); 5 lb/inch for each inch >5 ft (0.9 kg/cm) for each cm >60 cm)	106 lb (48 kg) for 1st 5 ft (150 cm) of height; 6 lb/inch for each inch >5 ft (1.1 kg/cm) for each cm >60 cm)
Large	+10%	40 kcal (170 kJ)/kg

CALORIE REQUIREMENTS

ACTIVITY LEVEL	ADULTS
Sedentary	10–12 cal/lb (22–26 kcal/kg) (90–110 kJ/kg) DBW
Moderate activity	12–14 cal/lb (26–31 kcal/kg) (110–130 kJ/kg) DBW
High activity	14–16 cal/lb (31–35 kcal/kg) (130–140 kJ/kg) DBW

DBW = desired body weight

↓ is the most important goal. In the patient with Type I diabetes, proper timing of meals and snacks, and consistency of food quantities, are important to good glycemic control

- Energy: Individual energy needs are difficult to predict accurately. An approximation can be obtained with Table 32–6
- Carbohydrates: 55–60% of total calories. Unrefined, high-fiber, complex carbohydrates are preferred
- Protein: ≤15% of total calories (0.8 g/kg desirable body weight)
- Fat: <35% of total calories. Fat should be reduced through restriction of saturated fat to <10% of total calories. Polyunsaturated fat should contribute <10% of calories, with monounsaturated fat supplying the remainder of energy needs
- Alcohol: Consumption should be restricted in patients with obesity, hypertension, or hypertriglyceridemia. Alcohol may also impair recognition and recovery from hypoglycemia
- Noncaloric sweeteners (e.g., aspartame, sucralose) may be used in moderation. Nutritive sweeteners (e.g., sorbitol, fructose, and sucrose) may be included as a free food when the total serving provides ≤60 kJ (15 kcal)
- Na: Intake should be restricted to <90 mEq (mmol)/day in hypertensive patients

Exercise

- A physical activity plan should be developed for each patient. Aerobic exercise is preferred
- Capillary blood glucose should be checked before and after exercise so that the patient can learn to adjust diet and/or hypoglycemic medications to activity. Mild exercise of short duration may require little change other than extra carbohydrates. More prolonged exercise may require a ↓ in the insulin dose. Patients should avoid injecting into an exercising limb, as exercise may ↑ the rate of absorption

Table 32–7
Insulin Preparations

INSULIN	ONSET (h)	PEAK (h)	DURATION (h)
Animal			
Regular	0.5	2–4	6–8
Semilente	1–2	3–8	10–16
NPH	1–2	6–12	18–26
Lente	1–3	6–12	18–26
Ultralente	4–6	minimal at 8–20	28–36
Protamine Zinc	4–6	14–24	26–36
Human			
Regular	0.5	2–4	6–8
NPH	1–2	6–12	18–24
Lente	1–3	6–12	18–24
Ultralente	4–6	minimal at 8–20	28–36

- The major risk of exercise in patients taking insulin or oral hypoglycemic agents is hypoglycemia. This may occur during or ≤20 h after exercise
- Exercise should be prescribed with caution in patients with cardiovascular disease, neuropathy, proliferative retinopathy, or hypoglycemia unawareness. An exercise stress test may be indicated in certain patients before starting an exercise program

Hypoglycemic Medication

The need for oral hypoglycemic agents or insulin in addition to nonpharmacologic therapy depends on the type of diabetes, the severity of symptoms, and the degree of metabolic control desired. All patients with Type I diabetes must be treated with insulin. With Type II diabetes, insulin is used in patients who fail to respond to oral hypoglycemic agents or who have persistent symptoms of hyperglycemia. Insulin may also be required in patients with Type II diabetes during surgery or intercurrent illness. Insulin Preparations are shown in Table 32–7.

HUMAN VS. ANIMAL INSULIN

The onset, peak, and duration of action of human insulin is faster and shorter than animal insulins. Human insulin is preferred for patients initiating insulin therapy, pregnant women, individuals with allergies or immune resistance to animal-derived insulins, and those who may use insulin only intermittently (i.e., patients with Type II diabetes) because the reintroduction of insulin may create an anamnestic antibody response. The Diabetes Control and Complications Trial (DCCT) demonstrated that Intensive Diabetes Therapy (IDT) of Type I diabetes, and, by implication, the lowest glycosylated hemoglobin (see monitoring section) safely achievable, reduce the risk of developing diabetes-related complications. Therefore, many patients, including those with Type II diabetes using insulin, may elect to use intensive therapy, or at least intensify their conventional therapy program.

INSULIN REGIMENS

With conventional insulin therapy, the same dose of insulin is given each day, varying only for marked deviations from the usual routine (e.g., large meals, ↑ activity). The approach is based on the assumption that each day is metabolically similar to the previous day and that a fixed dose adequately anticipates the quantity of insulin needed. Conventional fixed-dose insulin therapy may be useful for some patients with Type I diabetes and for many patients with Type II diabetes who require insulin. Conventional insulin therapy regimens include

- Single dose of intermediate-acting insulin before breakfast may be sufficient for some patients early in Type I diabetes (anywhere from the first few months to years) or Type II diabetes as the pancreas can still secrete endogenous insulin in response to meal stimulation. The starting dose of SQ insulin in adults with newly diagnosed Type I diabetes should be 10–15 U intermediate-acting insulin. A single dose of intermediate-acting insulin is usually inadequate to manage Type I diabetes optimally longterm
- Single dose of intermediate- and short-acting insulin 30 min before breakfast is useful if the fasting blood glucose level is acceptable but prelunch hyperglycemia is present
- Split dose of intermediate-acting insulin before breakfast and supper (or bedtime): The evening injection provides basal insulin during the night
- Split dose of mixed intermediate- and short-acting insulin before breakfast and supper: Adding short-acting insulin to the pre-supper dose of insulin can minimize post-supper hyperglycemia
- Mixed intermediate- and short-acting insulin before breakfast, short-acting insulin before supper, and intermediate-acting insulin at bedtime: Giving the evening intermediate-acting insulin at bedtime is often effective in normalizing fasting hyperglycemia without producing nocturnal hypoglycemia. This regimen is the recommended "conventional" insulin treatment pattern for both Type I and Type II patients using conventional therapy. This program may be "intensified" by providing guidelines for adjusting the dose of regular insulin given before breakfast and before supper.

Many patients are now choosing intensive diabetes therapy, using either multiple (≥3) daily injections (MDI) of insulin, or an insulin infusion pump (subcutaneous insulin infusion, or CSII). The dose of regular insulin is based on results of self-monitoring of blood glucose levels and is designed to achieve glucose levels that are within or close to the normal range. Changes in dosage are also made to accommodate variations in food intake and activity level. Indications for starting intensive insulin therapy include

- Less than ideal control with conventional insulin therapy
- Pregnancy (start before conception)
- Variable lifestyles (shift work, athletes, etc.)

Contraindications for intensive diabetes therapy include:

- Patients with far advanced complications such as renal failure
- Patients with coronary artery or cerebrovascular disease
- Children younger than 13
- Patient unwilling or unable to participate actively in their treatment or to perform frequent self-monitoring of blood glucose levels

Caution should be used in:

- Patients with hypoglycemic unawareness or having frequent, severe hypoglycemia using intensive diabetes therapy

- The elderly

Intensive insulin therapy using multiple daily injections includes

- Short-acting insulin before each meal and intermediate-acting insulin at bedtime. The dose of short-acting insulin is adjusted based on the capillary blood glucose, meal size, and planned activity
- Short-acting insulin before each meal and long-acting insulin before breakfast or supper: Ultralente provides a relatively peakless basal insulin, and the short-acting insulin controls postprandial hyperglycemia. Generally, about half of the total daily dose of insulin is given as ultralente, with the remainder initially divided equally before each meal and then adjusted as necessary
- Insulin pump to infuse short-acting insulin SQ continuously: Approximately 40–60% of the total daily dose is given as a basal insulin infusion over 24 h to mimic basal insulin secretion. The remainder is given as 3 premeal insulin boluses.

ORAL HYPOGLYCEMIC AGENTS

Oral hypoglycemic agents should be used in patients with Type II diabetes when diet and exercise have failed to achieve individual treatment goals. Sulphonylureas are the first-line drugs. The biguanide, metformin, may be a useful first-line drug in the very obese. Combination therapy with metformin and a sulphonylurea may be tried when target glycemic control is not achieved with either agent alone.

Tolbutamide (orinase, Rastinon). Supplied: Tablets 500 mg, 1 g. Dosage: 0.5 g bid or tid, max 2 g/day. Metabolized by the liver. Has the shortest duration of action and may be less likely to cause hypoglycemia in erratic eaters or the elderly. Duration of action: 6–12 h.

Acetohexamide (Dimelor). Supplied: Tablets 500 mg. Dosage: 0.25–0.5 g once daily, max 0.5 g tid. Metabolized by the liver. Duration of action: 12–18 h.

Chlorpropamide (Diabinese). Supplied: Tablets 100, 250 mg. Dosage: 100–250 mg once daily with breakfast, max 500 mg once daily (elderly 100 mg once daily). 70% metabolized by the liver; 30% excreted intact by the kidneys. Can cause hypoatremia due to potentiation of vasopressin action. Duration of action: 36+ h.

Glyburide (Diabeta, Micronase), **Glibenclamide** (Euglucon). Supplied: Tablets 2.5, 5 mg. Dosage: 2.5–5 mg qd or bid, max 20 mg/day (elderly 1.25 mg qd bid, max. 10 mg/day). Metabolized by the liver. Duration of action: 12–24 h.

Glipizide (Glucotrol). Supplied: Tablets 5, 10 mg. Dosage: 5 mg once daily, max 20 mg bid. Metabolized by the liver. Duration of action: 10–24 h.

Gliclazide (Diamicron). Supplied: 80 mg. Dosage: 80 mg bid, max 160 mg/day. (Elderly 40 mg bid). Duration of action: 10–24 h.

Metformin (Glucophage). A biguanide. Supplied: Tablets 500 mg. Dosage: 500 mg bid or tid with meals to minimize GI upset. Excreted by the kidney. Avoid with renal or liver impairment, or illness that may lead to hypoxia. Duration of action: 7–19 h.

Monitoring

- Second voided urine glucose testing: Easy and inexpensive; however, there is poor correlation between simultaneous blood and urine glucose measurements. In addition, the renal threshold for glucose varies greatly from patient to patient, and in the same patient from time to time

- Self-monitoring of blood glucose: Mandatory for patients on insulin therapy and desirable for patients on oral hypoglycemic agents. More frequent tests are performed on sick days, with changes in exercise or meal patterns, on travel days, or when hypoglycemia is suspected. Allows daily glucose patterns to be visualized and correlated with insulin, food, and activity
- Urine ketone testing: Should be performed during illness or when blood glucose >360 mg/dl (20 mmol/l)
- Glycated Hb (glycosylated Hb, HbAlc), nonfasting: Created by glycation of the amino-terminal valine of the β subunit of Hb. Reflects blood glucose control over the preceding 3 months (the life span of RBCs). The normal value depends on the method used and the laboratory. May be ↓ with hemolytic and chronic anemias, and with renal failure. Alternating episodes of hyperglycemia and hypoglycemia may give a pseudo-normal result
- Fructosamine: Measures glycated albumin and reflects glucose control over the previous 2–3 weeks. May be useful in pregnancy and other states when changes in glycemic control over weeks rather than months is important. Test may be interfered by hypoproteinemia, hemolysis of the blood sample, hypertriglyceridemia, and hyperbilirubinemia.

Education

Patient education is essential for compliance with a management regimen. All patients should be offered an education program covering the important aspects of self-care, knowledge, and skills. Ongoing counseling is necessary to achieve longterm compliance. Table 32–8 outlines guidelines for the goals of therapy in diabetes.

Surgery

Patients with diabetes who require surgery must be adequately controlled to avoid hypoglycemia, hyperglycemia, and ketosis during surgery. With elective surgery, the patient should be under as good metabolic control as possible and free of ketosis. With emergency surgery, any acidosis and dehydration should be corrected before the procedure.

Minor Procedure Without a General Anesthetic

Patients treated with oral hypoglycemic agents

- Hold morning dose of oral hypoglycemic agents
- Monitor blood glucose before, during, and after surgery
- Give IV fluids to provide hydration and prevent hypoglycemia
- Give supplemental short-acting insulin SC if blood glucose >250 mg/dl (14 mmol/l)

Patients treated with insulin

- Administer 1/2 to 2/3rd of the usual morning dose of intermediate-acting insulin SQ

Table 32–8
Targets for Control of Diabetes

	OPTIMAL	ACCEPTABLE	COMPROMISED
Blood glucose			
• fasting	80–120 mg/dl (4–7 mmol/l)	<180 mg/dl (10 mmol/L)	>180 mg/dl (10 mmol/L)
• after eating	90–180 mg/dl (5–10 mmol/L)	<220 mg/dl (12 mmol/L)	>220 mg/dl (12 mmol/L)
Glycated hemoglobin (% of upper limit)	<110	<140	>140
Total cholesterol	<200 mg/dl (5.2 mmol/L)*	<240 mg/dl (6.2 mmol/L)*	>240 mg/dl (6.2 mmol/L)
LDL-cholesterol	<130 mg/dl (3.4 mmol/L)*	<160 mg/dl (4.1 mmol/L)*	>160 mg/dl (4.1 mmol/L)
HDL-cholesterol	>45 mg/dl (1.1 mmol/L)*	>35 mg/dl (0.9 mmol/L)	<35 mg/dl (0.9 mmol/L)
Triglycerides	<150 mg/dl (1.7 mmol/L)*	<220 mg/dl (2.5 mmol/L)	>220 mg/dl (2.5 mmol/L)
Body mass index			
• male <65 years	<25	<27	>27
• female <65 years	<24	<26	>26
Blood pressure (mm Hg)**	<140/90	<160/95	>160/95

* Should be adjusted for other risk factors. Less strict targets may be appropriate for older patients with limited life expectancy.
** For patients with diabetic nephropathy, it has been suggested that optimal blood pressure should be 130/80 to 135/85 mmHg; however, conclusive evidence is lacking.
Reprinted with permission. Expert Committee of the Canadian Diabetes Advisory Board. Clinical practice guidelines for treatment of diabetes mellitus. CMAJ, *147:* 697–712, 1992.

- Hold the usual morning dose of short-acting insulin
- Infuse 5% dextrose/water at 100 ml/h while the patient is NPO
- Monitor the blood glucose immediately after the operation and q 4 h thereafter
- Give extra short-acting insulin SC in small amounts for blood glucoses >200 mg/dl (12 mmol/l)
- If the patient is drinking and eating well, give the usual evening dose of insulin

Major Procedure with a General Anesthetic

Patients not well controlled on oral hypoglycemic agents

- Discontinue oral hypoglycemic agents the night before surgery
- On the morning of surgery, start an infusion of 5% dextrose/water at 100 ml/h
- Also, start an insulin drip by diluting 100 units of short-acting insulin in 500 ml of 0.9% NaCl
- Check the blood glucose q 2 h preoperatively, q 1 h during surgery, and q 2 h postoperatively, and adjust each infusion as outlined in Table 32–9
- When patient is eating and drinking well, resume oral hypoglycemic

Table 32–9
Insulin-Glucose Infusion for Surgery

BLOOD GLUCOSE (mg/dl) (mmol/L)	INSULIN INFUSION (ml/hr)	INSULIN INFUSION (units/hr)	D_5W INFUSION (ml/hr)
<70 (4)	2	0.4	150
71–100 (4–6)	5	1.0	125
101–150 (6.1–8)	7	1.4	100
151–200 (8.1–10)	10	2.0	100
201–250 (10.1–14)	15	3.0	100
251–300 (14–16)	20	4.0	75
>300 (16)	25	6.0	50

agents if changes will be made to the patient's meal plan and exercise program; otherwise switch the patient to a SQ insulin regimen

Patients well controlled on insulin

- Hold the usual SQ insulin on the morning of surgery
- Start an infusion of 5% dextrose/water at 100 ml/h
- Also, start an insulin drip by diluting 100 U of short-acting insulin in 500 ml of 0.9% NaCl
- Check the blood glucose q 2 h preoperatively, q 1 h during surgery, and q 2 h postoperatively and adjust each infusion as outlined in Table 32–9
- Continue the insulin and glucose infusions until the patient is able to take food, and then restart the usual dose of SQ insulin
- Continue both the insulin and glucose infusions for 1–2 h after the SQ insulin has been given to prevent the blood glucose level from rising before the SQ insulin has begun to work

Patients not well controlled on insulin

- Start insulin drip and glucose infusion as outlined above the day before surgery

Suggested Reading

American Diabetes Association: Clinical practice guidelines recommendations 1991–1992. Diabetes Care, *15* (suppl 2):1, 1992.

Endocrine Diseases

33

Robyn L. Houlden

THYROID DISEASES

Thyroid Tests

Serum total thyroxine T_4 reflects the total T_4 concentration (both free and bound). Used for screening and follow-up of hyper- and hypothyroidism. The disadvantage of TT_4 as a screening test is that it is affected by changes in the concentration of thyroxine binding globulin (TBG).

Serum Total T_3 is used for diagnosis and follow-up hyperthyroidism. May be useful in certain hyperthyroid states where the serum T_4 is normal ("T_3 toxicosis"). Like total T_4, it is affected by changes in TBG.

T_3 resin uptake is used to distinguish hyper- and hypothyroidism from ↑ and ↓ TBG concentrations. The test measures indirectly the unoccupied binding sites for T_4 and T_3 on TBG. It is performed by mixing radiolabeled T_3 with the patient's serum, adding a resin, and then determining the amount of radiolabeled T_3 bound to the resin.

Causes of a high T_3RU include

- Hyperthyroidism (more binding sites occupied with T_4)
- Salicylates, dilantin, and clofibrate (compete with T_4 for binding to TBG)
- Decreased TBG production secondary to androgen therapy, severe hypoproteinemia, glucocorticoid excess, or hereditary TBG deficiency

Causes of a low T_3RU include

- Hypothyroidism (fewer binding sites occupied with T_4)
- Increased TBG production secondary to estrogen therapy, pregnancy, acute hepatitis, acute intermittent porphyria, or hereditary TBG excess

Free thyroxine index (FT_4I) is used to correct changes in TBG by normalizing discordant serum T_4 and T_3RU values. It is calculated by multiplying T_4 by the T_3 ratio (T_3RU of patient ÷ T_3RU for normal subjects).

Free T_4 and Free T_3 are currently used to diagnose thyroid disease because the serum total T_4 and T_3 may be altered by changes in protein binding.

TSH is the screening test of choice for hypo- and hyperthyroidism (Fig. 33–1). Also used to evaluate thyroid hormone replacement for hypothyroidism and suppression therapy for thyroid cancer. Conventional TSH assays were not sensitive enough to differentiate between hyperthyroid and euthyroid individuals at the lower range. The newer third-generation immunometric assays ("sensitive" TSH) are able to distinguish normal from hyperthyroid patients.

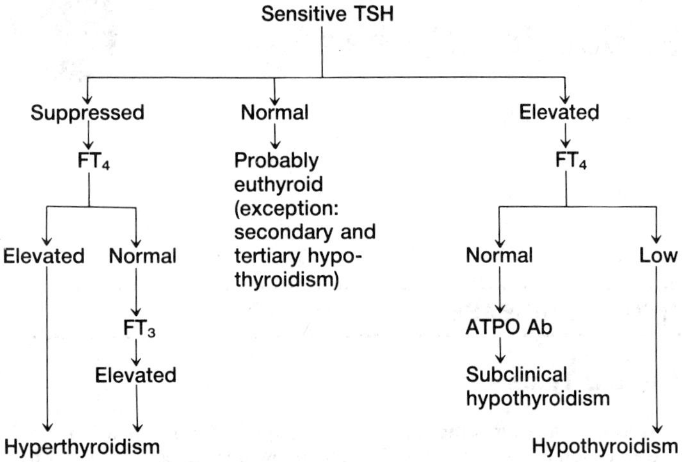

FT_4 = Free T_4
FT_3 = Free T_3
ATPO Ab = antithyroid peroxidase antibodies

Figure 33–1. Screening for thyroid disease.

TRH Stimulation Test is used in patients with suspected hyperthyroidism in whom thyroid function tests are equivocal. TRH 200 μg is injected IV over 15–30 sec. Serum TSH levels are drawn at 0, 30 and 60 min. Side effects are brief (1–2 min) and include nausea, facial flushing, metallic taste, and the urge to micturate. The normal response is a tenfold ↑ relative to the basal level. Blunted or absent responses are seen in hyperthyroidism, pituitary hypothyroidism, acromegaly, glucocorticoid therapy, chronic renal failure, severe systemic illness, depression, and normal elderly subjects. This test has become less useful since the availability of "sensitive" TSH assays.

Antithyroid peroxidase (microsomal) and Antithyroglobulin antibodies are used primarily in making a diagnosis of Hashimoto's thyroiditis. Antithyroid peroxidase antibodies are more sensitive than antithyroglobulin antibodies.

Thyroglobulin indicates the presence of functioning thyroid tissue. Used primarily in thyroid cancer for follow-up of patients who have had thyroid gland ablation. Best measured off thyroid hormone suppression therapy. Levels ↑ with the occurrence of metastases. May also be useful in distinguishing factitious hyperthyroidism from thyroiditis.

Thyroidal RAIU: Radioactive iodine is administered po and the uptake is measured over the thyroid with a scintillation counter. The count is usually done at 24 h, when the uptake plateaus. A measurement is frequently done at 6 h as well, as the RAIU may reach a max earlier with severe hyperthyroidism. The RAIU is useful in the differential diagnosis of hyperthyroidism and in calculating the dose of ^{131}I needed for radioactive iodine therapy (Table 33–1).

Table 33–1
Thyroid Scanning and RAIU Findings in Hyperthyroidism

DISEASE	THYROID SCAN	RADIOACTIVE IODINE UPTAKE (RAIU)
Graves' disease	diffuse goiter	increased
Toxic multinodular goiter	patchy uptake	high normal to elevated
Thyroiditis	little uptake	low

Euthyroid Sick Syndrome

Refers to patients with nonthyroidal illness and abnormal thyroid tests. Primary thyroid disease is not present. The abnormal thyroid function tests are the result of abnormalities in serum thyroid hormone binding and extrathyroidal thyroid hormone metabolism. The syndrome can be classified into the following categories

- Low T_3 syndrome is most common. Characterized by normal or slightly ↑ total T_4, low T_3, ↑ reverse T_3 (rT_3), and normal TSH levels. Due to ↓ extrathyroidal conversion of T_4 to T_3. Occurs with severe systemic illnesses and following the administration of some drugs (dexamethasone, cholecystographic dyes, amiodarone, high doses of propranolol)
- Low T_3 and Low TT_4 syndrome is characterized by low total T_4, low T_3, high rT_3, normal or slightly ↓ TSH, and an impaired TSH response to TRH stimulation. Postulated to be due to a circulating inhibitor of T_4 binding to thyroid-binding proteins. The normal or low TSH may reflect hypothalamic adaptation to severe illness. Occurs in severely ill patients. There is no evidence that treatment with levothyroxine helps. The low T_4 and T_3 may be an adaptive mechanism to spare protein catabolism
- High total T_4 syndrome is characterized by a high total T_4 and normal T_3. Causes include TBG excess inherited or secondary to liver disease (acute viral hepatitis, chronic active hepatitis, primary biliary cirrhosis), estrogen therapy, or acute intermittent porphyria; familial dysalbuminemic hyperthyroxinemia (abnormal binding of T_4 by albumin); ↑ TBPA; drug-related from amiodarone, oral cholecystographic contrast agents (iopanoic acid [Telepaque] or ipodate [Oragrafin]), and high doses of propranolol

Hypothyroidism

CAUSES

- Primary (intrinsic thyroid disease): Hashimoto's thyroiditis (chronic lymphocytic thyroiditis); recovery phase of subacute or silent thyroiditis; thyroid gland ablation (thyroidectomy, postradioactive iodine treatment, external radiation); drugs (excess iodine, antithyroid agents, lithium carbonate)
- Secondary (TSH deficiency): Disease of the pituitary gland
- Tertiary (TRH deficiency): Disease of the hypothalamus

CLINICAL MANIFESTATIONS

The onset may be slow and unnoticed. The most important symptoms diagnostically are generalized weakness, tiredness, and lethargy; cold intolerance; dry skin and hair loss; memory impairment. Other symptoms and signs include weight gain; constipation; muscle cramps, aching and stiffness; facial and peripheral edema; heavy, prolonged menstrual periods; deepening of the voice; hearing loss; bradycardia; pseudomyotonia (delay in the relaxation phase of the deep tendon reflexes); and carpal tunnel syndrome

TREATMENT

Sodium L-thyroxine (Eltroxin, Synthroid). Supplied: Tablets 25, 50, 75, 88, 100, 112, 125, 150, 175, 200, 300 μg. Dosage: <60 years with no cardiac disease start with 100 μg/day. Assess adequacy of dose with sensitive TSH in 6–8 weeks. (Elderly start with 25 μg/day and ↑ every 6-8 weeks. Warn the patient that initiation of thyroid hormone replacement may precipitate angina or palpitations.)

MYXEDEMA COMA

- Severe hypothyroidism with unresponsiveness, hypothermia, hypotension, hypoventilation, hyponatremia, bradycardia
- Precipitating illness or event is usually present
- Treat promptly without waiting for laboratory confirmation

MANAGEMENT

- Thyroid hormone replacement: 500 μg of sodium levothyroxine IV bolus, then 50–100 μg IV bolus qd until oral therapy can be substituted
- Respiratory support: Hypoventilation may lead to CO_2 retention and CNS unresponsiveness. Monitor ABGs and provide intubation and mechanical ventilation if indicated
- Hypotension may respond poorly to pressor agents until thyroid hormone is replaced. Carry out volume replacement cautiously with isotonic fluids
- Hypothermia: Warm passively with blankets
- Hyponatremia is caused by impaired free water clearance. Usually corrected by L-thyroxine therapy and fluid restriction. If severe, may require partial correction with hypertonic saline (See Chap. 31)
- Hypoglycemia is rare. Correct with 5% dextrose/water IV
- Glucocorticoids are given to cover the possibility of concomitant ACTH or adrenal insufficiency. Give hydrocortisone sodium succinate (Solu-Cortef) 100 mg IV q 8 h
- Identify and treat any precipitating illnesses

Hyperthyroidism

CAUSES

- Graves' disease
- Thyroiditis: Subacute (pseudogranulomatous, de Quervain's); silent (painless); radiation-induced
- Toxic multinodular goiter
- Toxic solitary thyroid adenoma (Plummer's disease)
- Exogenous thyroid hormone ingestion: iatrogenic, factitious
- Excess TSH production: Pituitary adenoma, trophoblastic tumors

- Ectopic T_4 production: Struma ovarii, metastatic follicular thyroid cancer

SYMPTOMS

- Heat intolerance, excessive sweating
- Nervousness, irritability
- Weight loss with normal or ↑ appetite
- Palpitations
- Tiredness, tremulousness
- Proximal muscle weakness
- Diarrhea
- Scanty or absent periods
- Dyspnea on exertion
- Elderly patients often present differently with lethargy, atrial fibrillation, CHF, weight loss with anorexia, muscle weakness, and wasting. The absence of adrenergic and hyperkinetic symptoms is sometimes called apathetic or masked hyperthyroidism

SIGNS

- Tachycardia, hyperkinesis, agitation, goiter, fine tremor, brisk reflexes, warm moist skin, proximal muscle wasting, onycholysis (separation of the nail from its bed distally)
- Noninfiltrative eye signs: Lid lag, lid retraction, and stare can occur in all hyperthyroid patients. Infiltrative signs: Periorbital edema, chemosis, conjunctivitis, exophthalmos, and ophthalmoplegia usually occur only in Graves' disease
- Pretibial myxedema is a less common feature of Graves' disease; the skin appears brown and indurated

MANAGEMENT OF GRAVES' DISEASE

Graves' disease is the most common cause of hyperthyroidism, with a female to male ratio of 8 to 1. It is distinguished from other forms of hyperthyroidism by the presence of diffuse thyroid enlargement, ophthalmopathy, and occasionally pretibial myxedema. Ophthalmopathy is present in 20–40% of patients with recent onset Graves' disease and may develop before hyperthyroidism, at the onset of hyperthyroidism, or years later, after the patent's hyperthyroidism has been treated. Graves' disease is an autoimmune disease mediated by thyroid-stimulating immunoglobulins (TSAb or TSI). These antibodies recognize the TSH receptor as antigen, attach to the receptor, and activate the thyroid follicular cell. At present the treatment of Graves' disease is directed at the thyroid gland rather than at the basic immunologic process.

RAI is the treatment of choice for most adults with Graves' disease. The most commonly used isotope is ^{131}I in a dose of 4–10 mCi (150–370 megaBq). The dose is determined by the size of the thyroid and the RAIU. The response to RAI is slow and patients may remain hyperthyroid for 3 months. Occasionally patients require a second or third treatment if they are still hyperthyroid 6–12 months after RAI. Patients with severe hyperthyroidism, a cardiac condition, or an elderly age should be rendered euthyroid with antithyroid drugs and β blockers before treatment with RAI, as radiation thyroiditis may occur with leakage of stored hormone and exacerbation of the hyperthyroidism. Antithyroid drugs should be stopped 4–7 days before RAI and may be restarted 3 days afterward.

There is no ↑ incidence of thyroid cancer, leukemia, or birth defects after doses of RAI used to treat hyperthyroidism. The most common complication of RAI is the development of hypothyroidism. Patients must be monitored lifelong and started on thyroid hormone replacement as soon as they become biochemically hypothyroid.

PTU and methimazole (Tapazole) block thyroid peroxidase and inhibit thyroid hormone synthesis. Both agents have weak immunosuppressive effects. PTU also inhibits the extrathyroidal conversion of T_4 to T_3. The half-life of PTU is 1–2 h whereas methimazole is 6–8 h. The major reason to choose antithyroid drug therapy is that a spontaneous remission of Graves' may occur, allowing drug therapy to be discontinued and leaving the patient with normal thyroid function. Remissions occur in 30–50% of patients treated for 1 year. Factors believed to favor the probability of a remission include female sex, recent onset of symptoms, mild or moderate severity of symptoms, and modest thyroid enlargement.

PTU. Supplied: Tablet 50, 100, 250 mg. Dosage: Initial dose is 100–200 mg 3–4 times a day. The larger doses are given to patient with more severe clinical hyperthyroidism and/or a large goiter. After the patient becomes euthyroid (usually 6–8 weeks), taper dose by 1/3 every 4–6 weeks to a maintenance dose of 50 mg once daily.

Methimazole (Tapazole). Supplied: Tablets 5, 10 mg. Dosage: Initial dose is 5–10 mg tid. Maintenance dose is 5–15 mg once daily.

Carbimazole (Neo-mercazole) (UK). Supplied: Tablets 5 mg. Dosage: Initial dose is 30–60 mg once daily. Maintenance dose is 5–15 mg once daily.

Continue therapy for 12–18 months, then discontinue. The vast majority of relapses occur with 3–6 months of cessation of therapy, at which time alternative treatment is recommended.

Adverse Effects: Most common complications are dermatologic (pruritus, urticaria). May subside with no treatment. Generally do not require discontinuation of drug therapy. Agranulocytosis is the most serious side effect. Occurs in 0.2% of patients, usually within the first 3 months. It is an idiosyncratic reaction and not dose related. Patients should be instructed to report immediately any symptoms suggestive of agranulocytosis, such as fever or sore throat. The drug should be stopped immediately and the WBC checked. Routine blood counts are not helpful.

Surgery: Subtotal thyroidectomy is reserved for children who are noncompliant or cannot be controlled with antithyroid drugs, and patients with large goiters with pressure symptoms. The patient should be made euthyroid pre-operatively with an antithyroid drug. Iodide (SSKI 1–2 drops po tid) is usually added for 2 weeks before surgery. This ensures that the patient is euthyroid and also reduces the vascularity of the gland. Patients who cannot tolerate antithyroid drugs can be managed pre-operatively with high doses of propranolol.

Beta blockers are useful in controlling the adrenergic manifestations of hyperthyroidism such as tachycardia.

Dosage: propranolol 20–40 mg qid. The dose should be titrated to produce the desired symptoms. If blockers are contraindicated, verapamil has a role.

MANAGEMENT OF TOXIC MULTINODULAR GOITER

Antithyroid drugs have no role in the longterm treatment of a multinodular goiter, as spontaneous remissions rarely occur. The treatment of choice is RAI. As with Graves' disease, elderly patients and patients with heart disease should be rendered euthyroid with antithyroid drugs before RAI. Large doses of RAI 10–30 mCi (370–1110 megaBq) are given because the thyroid uptake of ^{131}I is usually only moderately ↑. Occasionally, with a large gland causing tracheal compression, surgery is the treatment of choice.

MANAGEMENT OF TOXIC SOLITARY ADENOMA

Lobectomy is the treatment of choice in a younger patient. In an older person, RAI may be indicated. The dose used should be large (20–30 mCi [740–1110 megaBq]) to destroy the nodule.

Thyroid Storm

- Severe, life-threatening hyperthyroidism
- Usually develops in an undiagnosed hyperthyroid patient who has another major stress or illness (i.e., infection, injury, or surgery)
- Clinical manifestations include fever, tachycardia, nausea, vomiting, abdominal pain, and cardiac failure
- Features of the precipitating illness (i.e., fever, tachycardia) may be difficult to distinguish from thyroid storm
- Free T_4 and T_3 are ↑, but no more so than in "ordinary" hyperthyroidism

Management includes general supportive measures (IV fluids, glucose for hypoglycemia, acetaminophen and cooling blanket for fever—avoid aspirin as it displaces thyroid hormones from their binding proteins) and antithyroid drugs, which may be given po or by nasogastric tube. PTU is theoretically preferable to methimazole as it also inhibits extrathyroidal production of T_3.

PTU. Dosage: 300–400 mg po initially followed by 250 mg q 6 h.

Methimazole. Dosage: 30–40 mg po initially followed by 20–30 mg po q 8 h. After stabilization, the dosages of either preparation should be ↓ to the usual ones used for treatment of hyperthyroidism.

Iodide is the most effective agent for lowering serum T_4 acutely. It inhibits release of thyroid hormones. Iodide therapy should be initiated 1–2 h after starting antithyroid medications as the iodide could theoretically be used to synthesize additional thyroid hormone, thereby worsening the clinical state. If the patient is unable to take oral medications, 1 g of sodium iodide can be administered as a continuous infusion over 12 h q 12 h.

Lugol's solution 10 drops po q 8 h or SSKI 5 drops po q 8 h can also be used.

Propranolol 40–80 mg po q 6 h can be used to block the catecholamine effects. If the patient is nauseated, may give 1–2 mg IV over 5 min q 4–6 h with cardiac monitoring.

Dexamethasone 2 mg IV q 6 h is recommended for 24–48 h as high doses of glucocorticoids block the peripheral conversion of T_4 to T_3.

Sodium ipodate is an iodide-containing oral cholecystographic agent that impairs the conversion of T_4 to T_3. May be given instead of iodide in a dosage of 1 g po once daily.

Subacute Thyroiditis

Also called pseudogranulomatous, de Quervain's or giant-cell thyroiditis. The most common cause of thyroid pain. Believed to be viral in etiology although the exact causative agent is unknown. A history of preceding upper respiratory infection is common. Presents with abrupt onset of neck pain, malaise, myalgias, and fever. Clinical manifestations of hyperthyroidism occur in 50% of patients. Serum T_4 and T_3 levels may be ↑ due to release of preformed hormone. The ESR is usually ↑. RAIU is low in the acute stage due to follicular cell destruction. In most patients symptoms subside over 2–6 weeks. Transient hypothyroidism occurs in 15–25% of cases. Permanent hypothyroidism occurs in <10%.

TREATMENT

Salicylates (650 mg qid) or other nonsteroidal agents can be used for pain relief. Prednisone (30–40 mg once daily) can be used for severe pain in patients unresponsive to salicylates. Treatment should be continued for 2–3 weeks and then tapered. Propranolol (20–40 mg tid to qid) may be used for relief of symptoms of hyperthyroidism. Antithyroid drugs are not indicated and do not work. Transient hypothyroidism may be treated with temporary thyroid hormone replacement.

Silent Thyroiditis (Painless Thyroiditis)

Inflammatory disorder characterized by abrupt onset of hyperthyroid symptoms and a painless, nontender goiter. The etiology is uncertain but is probably a form of autoimmune thyroid disease. Treatment is the same as subacute thyroiditis except that salicylates are omitted. Silent thyroiditis occurs in 3–5% of women in the postpartum period and may recur with subsequent pregnancies.

Solitary Thyroid Nodules

Most thyroid nodules are benign. The goal is to select for surgery those patients whose nodules are at risk for malignancy, and to avoid unnecessary operations on nodules that are likely to be benign. In some clinical situations carcinoma is more likely to be present and a more aggressive approach is justified. These include

- History of therapeutic irradiation to the head, neck, or chest
- Age <40 years
- Male sex
- Family history of thyroid carcinoma (i.e., medullary thyroid carcinoma with MEN Type II)
- Compression of adjacent structures (i.e., trachea, esophagus, vocal cord or sympathetic nerves, superior vena cava)
- Palpable regional lymph nodes and/or abnormalities in distant sites (i.e., lung, bone)

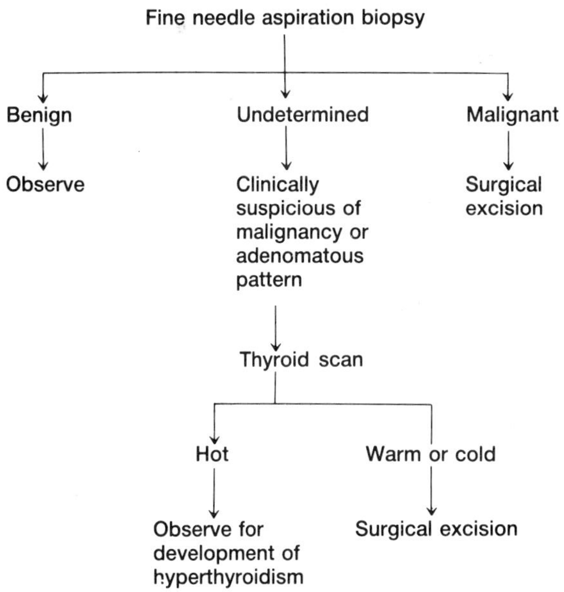

Figure 33–2. Investigation of the solitary thyroid nodule.

INVESTIGATION

- FNA biopsy is the initial procedure in the evaluation of thyroid nodules in many centers. Requires persons skilled in the technique and in cytopathology. Follicular lesions pose a problem as it is difficult to distinguish benign from malignant ones. Figure 33–2 outlines management of the solitary thyroid nodule based on FNA biopsy as the initial diagnostic test
- Thyroid radioisotope scan: The most commonly used isotopes are ^{123}I, ^{131}I , and ^{99m}Technetium. Nodules appear hypofunctioning ("cold" or "cool"), isofunctioning ("warm"), or hyperfunctioning ("hot") Thyroid cancer cells do not trap radionuclides as well as normal thyroid cells and appear hypofunctioning on scanning. However, most cold nodules are still benign (only 10–15% are malignant)
- Thyroid ultrasound: Nodules are classified as solid, cystic, or mixed solid/cystic. Malignancy is three- to fourfold more frequent in solid compared to cystic nodules.

ADRENAL DISEASES

Adrenal Insufficiency

CAUSES

- Primary (Addison's disease): Autoimmune (most common cause); infectious (tuberculosis, fungal, cytomegalovirus, AIDS); infiltrative (amyloidosis, sarcoidosis, metastatic carcinoma, hemochromatosis); hemorrhage (anticoagulants, DIC); iatrogenic: Drugs that block steroid hormone synthesis (ketoconazole, mitotane, metyrapone, aminoglutethimide)

- Secondary: Hypothalamic-pituitary-adrenal axis suppression following exogenous glucocorticoids; pituitary and hypothalamic lesions

CLINICAL MANIFESTATIONS

- Weight loss, fatigue, anorexia, nausea, vomiting, postural hypotension
- Hyperpigmentation with primary adrenal insufficiency (particularly in the creases of the hand, over the knuckles, in the axillae, over the gingival and buccal mucosa, in the areola of the breasts, and in the perineum. Scars formed after the onset of adrenal insufficiency may also be pigmented.)
- Autoimmune Addison's disease may be associated with other autoimmune diseases such as Hashimoto's thyroiditis, pernicious anemia, vitiligo, hypoparathyroidism, premature ovarian or testicular failure, and diabetes mellitus
- Symptoms and signs of other pituitary hormone deficiencies may be present (e.g., LH, FSH, GH, TSH) with secondary adrenal insufficiency

LABORATORY FINDINGS

- Hyponatremia, hyperkalemia (usually in the range of 5.4–5.9 mEq [mmol]/l), mild metabolic acidosis
- Increased blood urea or BUN
- Low or normal blood glucose
- Normocytic-normochromic anemia, lymphocytosis, eosinophilia
- Hypercalcemia (infrequently)

DIAGNOSTIC PROCEDURES

- Treatment should not be delayed in the seriously ill patient with acute adrenal insufficiency. A plasma cortisol and ACTH level should be drawn for future interpretation. A low plasma cortisol and a ↑ plasma ACTH level is diagnostic of primary adrenal insufficiency
- Short ACTH Test is a useful screening test if the index of suspicion is low (i.e., weak, tired, normally pigmented subject in whom one wishes to rule out Addison's disease). Administer 250 μg of synthetic ACTH (Cosyntropin, Cortrosyn) IV and draw plasma cortisol levels at 0, 30, and 60 min. The normal increment in plasma cortisol is >7 μg/dl (200 nmol/l), and the absolute level achieved should be >20 ≤μg/dl (500 nmol/l). A normal response rules out primary adrenal insufficiency. Most patients with secondary adrenal insufficiency do not respond normally because of secondary atrophy of the adrenal cortex
- Plasma ACTH levels, if available, are an easy way to differentiate primary and secondary adrenal insufficiency. Levels are ↑ in primary and low in secondary adrenal insufficiency
- Prolonged ACTH stimulation test is useful for differentiating primary and secondary adrenal insufficiency when an assay for plasma ACTH is not available or cause is uncertain. Collect a baseline 24-h urine free cortisol and creatinine. Infuse synthetic ACTH 250 μg in 500 ml

of 0.9% NaCl over 8 h (8 A.M. to 4 P.M.) on 3 consecutive days with concomitant 24–h urine collections for free cortisol and creatinine. Also draw serum cortisol levels at 8 A.M. and 8 P.M. daily. When adrenal insufficiency is strongly suspected, the patient should receive coverage with dexamethasone 0.5 mg bid during the test. Patients with primary adrenal insufficiency have no ↑ in their serum and urinary cortisol levels. Patients with secondary adrenal insufficiency exhibit a gradual, usually stepwise, ↑ in their plasma and urinary cortisol levels due to reactivation of their anatomically intact adrenal glands. Levels ↑ 2–3 times baseline by the third day. The daily urinary creatinine should be ±10% to ensure complete and consistent urine collections

- Insulin Tolerance Test is useful for: Confirming the diagnosis of suspected secondary adrenal insufficiency; assessing the functioning of the hypothalamic-pituitary-adrenal axis following longterm glucocorticoid therapy to determine whether glucocorticoids can be stopped safely (glucocorticoid therapy should be held for 36 h prior to the insulin tolerance test). After overnight fasting, the patient is injected with 0.15 U of short-acting insulin/kg IV bolus. Plasma cortisol levels are collected at 0, 30, 60, and 90 min. A physician should be in attendance and glucose must be available for IV administration if severe symptoms of hypoglycemia occur. An adequate degree of hypoglycemia must be obtained (blood glucose ≤40 mg/dl [2.2 mmol/l]). A normal cortisol response is an ↑ of ≥7 μg/dl (200 nmol/l) with a peak level of >20 μg/dl (550 nmol/l). An inadequate response is seen with primary and secondary adrenal insufficiency
- Adrenal calcifications may be seen on plain films of the abdomen in patients with primary adrenal insufficiency from tuberculosis

TREATMENT OF ACUTE ADRENAL INSUFFICIENCY

- Therapy should be instituted immediately. Diagnostic investigations, with the exception of a serum cortisol and plasma ACTH, should be postponed until the patient is completely well
- Volume repletion: Give 1–2 l 0.9% NaCl over the first 2 h, followed by 3–5 l over the following 24 h
- Glucocorticoid therapy: 100 mg hydrocortisone sodium succinate (Solu-Cortef) IV bolus followed by 100 mg IV q 8 h. The dosage should be ↓ by 50% each day thereafter until the maintenance dosage is achieved, assuming the patient's course is uncomplicated
- Mineralocorticoid therapy is not required initially since cortisol in large doses (>100 mg/day) has enough salt-retaining activity. However, when the dose is ↓ below this level, treatment with fludrocortisone (Florinef) should be started in patients with primary adrenal insufficiency
- Precipitating factors should be corrected, such as infection, trauma, surgery, myocardial infarction, or noncompliance with glucocorticoid therapy
- General supportive measures should be provided, such as treatment of persistent electrolyte abnormalities, hypoglycemia, hypothermia, and hypotension refractory to IV fluids and glucocorticoids

MANAGEMENT OF CHRONIC ADRENAL INSUFFICIENCY

- Maintenance of glucocorticoid replacement may be given with 1 of the following:

1. Hydrocortisone 20 mg on waking and 10 mg at 4–6 P.M.
2. Prednisone 5 mg on waking and 2.5 mg at 4–6 P.M.
3. Cortisone acetate 25 mg on waking and 12.5 mg at 4–6 P.M.

Patients should be told to double their dose of glucocorticoid with a mild illness. If they cannot take their steroid by mouth, it should be given parenterally. Patients should wear a medical identification bracelet or necklace giving details of their condition

- Maintenance mineralocorticoid replacement is usually given with fludrocortisone acetate (Florinef) in doses of 0.05–0.2 mg qd in patient with primary adrenal insufficiency. If the dose is excessive, edema, hypokalemia, and hypertension may result
- Minor surgery: 100 mg of hydrocortisone hemisuccinate I.M. or 100 mg of hydrocortisone sodium succinate IV should be given with the premedication
- Major surgery: The steroid regimen outlined for acute adrenal crisis should be adopted

Cushing's Syndrome

CAUSES

- ACTH dependent: Pituitary adenoma (Cushing's disease) (70%); ectopic ACTH syndrome (10%); ectopic corticotropin releasing hormone (rare)
- ACTH independent: Adrenal adenoma (10%); adrenal carcinoma (10%); micronodular adrenal disease (rare); iatrogenic (exogenous glucocorticoids)

CLINICAL MANIFESTATIONS

- Truncal obesity, facial rounding (moon facies)
- Proximal muscle weakness
- Thin skin with purple striae, ecchymoses, facial plethora
- Osteoporosis
- Hypertension
- Glucose intolerance or diabetes mellitus
- Nephrolithiasis
- Oligomenorrhea, acne, hirsutism, loss of libido
- Psychologic disturbances (depression, emotional lability)

DIAGNOSTIC PROCEDURES

Figure 33–3 outlines the investigation of Cushing's syndrome

- Overnight dexamethasone suppression test is used as a screening test. Administer dexamethasone 1.0 mg po at 11 P.M. and draw a plasma cortisol at 8 A.M. the following morning. A normal response is suppression of plasma cortisol to <5 μg/dl (140 nmol/l). False positive responses (failure of suppression in the absence of Cushing's syndrome) are common and may be due to stress, obesity, high estrogen states (pregnancy, estrogen therapy, and oral contraceptives), various drugs (phenobarbital, dilantin, primidone, and phenothiazines), alcoholism, and depression
- 24–h urine free cortisol provides a useful screen when combined with the overnight dexamethasone suppression test. Values are ↑ in hypercortisolism and in some patients with uncontrolled diabetes
- Low-dose dexamethasone suppression test is used to confirm suspected

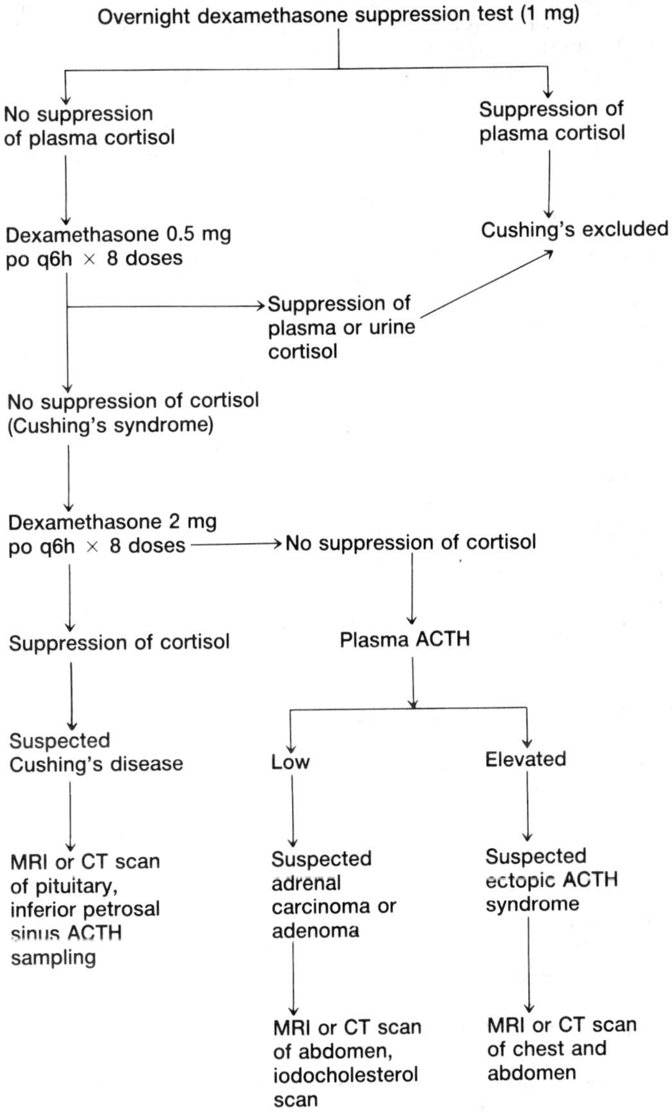

Figure 33–3. Investigation of Cushing's Syndrome.

Cushing's syndrome if screening tests are abnormal. Administer dexamethasone 0.5 mg po q 6 h for 48 h. Measure plasma cortisol qd at 8 A.M. Also collect daily 24–h urine collections for free cortisol and creatinine excretion. A normal response is suppression of urine free cortisol to <25 μg/24 h or a ↓ in plasma cortisol to <5 μg/dl (140 nmol/l)

- High-dose dexamethasone suppression test is used to differentiate

Cushing's disease from ectopic ACTH production or adrenal cortisol-secreting tumors. Administer dexamethasone 2.0 mg po q 6 h for 48 h. Measure morning plasma cortisol and 24–h urine free cortisol levels as in the low-dose dexamethasone suppression test.

1. Cushing's disease: Suppression of urinary cortisol to <50% of baseline and suppression of plasma cortisol to <5 μg/dl (140 nmol/l) (rarely, a bronchial carcinoid or an ACTH-secreting thymoma may give the same result).
2. Ectopic ACTH syndrome and adrenal tumors: Lack of adequate suppression

- Plasma ACTH levels are also useful to differentiate the various causes of Cushing's syndrome: Cushing's disease (high normal to moderately ↑); ectopic ACTH syndrome (usually very high [>200 pg/ml (44 pmol/l)]; adrenal tumors (low)
- Radiographic procedures: Cushing's disease (CT scan or MRI of the pituitary); ectopic ACTH syndrome (CT scan or tomograms of the chest); adrenal tumors (CT scan or MRI of the abdomen, iodocholesterol scanning)

TREATMENT

- Cushing's disease: Transsphenoidal surgery
- Ectopic ACTH syndrome: Treatment of the underlying tumor if possible; correction of hypokalemia with K replacement and spironolactone; drugs that block steroid synthesis: Ketoconazole, metyrapone, aminoglutethimide, and o,p'-DDD (Mitotane)
- Adrenal tumors: Adrenalectomy

Primary Hyperaldosteronism

Autonomous overproduction of aldosterone occurs in about 2% of patients with hypertension

CAUSES

- Aldosterone-producing adenoma (85%)
- Bilateral adrenocortical hyperplasia (15%)
- Dexamethasone-suppressible hyperaldosteronism (rare)
- Adrenocortical carcinoma (rare)

CLINICAL MANIFESTATIONS

- Hypertension may be resistant to usual antihypertensive medications. It is rarely malignant
- K depletion may produce muscle weakness, easy fatigability, polyuria, and polydipsia

INVESTIGATIONS

- Serum K <3.5 mEq (mmol)/l after the patient has remained off diuretics for 3 weeks and adhered to a high Na diet (>120 mEq [mmol]/day) for ≥3 days merits further investigation
- 24–h urinary aldosterone excretion is usually ↑ in primary hyperaldosteronism

- Captopril suppression test: 25 mg of captopril is given po. The patient remains seated, and PRA and plasma aldosterone are drawn 2 h later. Plasma aldosterone does not suppress <15 ng/dl (415 pmol/l) in patients with primary hyperaldosteronism
- Saline suppression test: 2 liters of 0.9% NaCl are infused over 4 h with the patient recumbent. Plasma aldosterone does not suppress <8.5–10 ng/dl (235–275 pmol/l) with primary hyperaldosteronism
- Furosemide stimulation test: 40 mg of furosemide is given IV and the patient lies down for 1 h to promote diuresis, followed by standing for 2 h. PRA fails to rise and remains <1.7 ng/ml/hr (0.47 ng/l/s)

Differentiating Adrenal Adenoma from Bilateral Hyperplasia

- 8 A.M. plasma 18–hydroxycorticosterone levels on a high-Na diet: >100 ng/dl are usually found with an adenoma and <100 ng/dl with hyperplasia
- Plasma aldosterone levels after 4 h of upright posture: ↓ with an aldosterone-producing adenoma and ↑ with bilateral hyperplasia

PROCEDURES TO LOCALIZE AN ADRENAL ADENOMA

- CT or MRI scan of the adrenals
- Adrenal vein catherization with aldosterone and cortisol sampling
- ^{131}I iodocholesterol scanning

TREATMENT

- Bilateral adrenal hyperplasia: Spironolactone (Aldactone) 100–400 mg qd or amiloride 10–20 mg qd restores K balance. Hypertension may be treated with Ca channel-blocking agents or angiotensin-converting enzyme inhibitors
- Aldosterone-producing adenoma: Unilateral adrenalectomy

Pheochromocytoma

Tumor of chromaffin tissue that produces excessive catecholamines. 90% are found in the adrenals. 10% are extra-adrenal, usually in the organ of Zuckerkandl, located at the bifurcation of the abdominal aorta. 10% are familial and may be part of Type II MEN syndrome. 10% are bilateral and 10% are malignant (see Chap. 1).

ANTERIOR PITUITARY DISEASES

Hyperprolactinemia

CLINICAL MANIFESTATIONS

- Women: Amenorrhea, galactorrhea, infertility
- Men: Decreased libido, impotence, infertility

DIFFERENTIAL DIAGNOSIS

- Physiologic: Pregnancy, postpartum, newborn, stress
- Pituitary disorders: Prolactin-secreting pituitary tumor; acromegaly; empty sella syndrome
- Hypothalamic disorders: Craniopharyngioma; metastatic disease; pituitary stalk section or compression
- Hypothyroidism
- Chronic renal failure
- Liver disease
- Chest wall or spinal cord lesions
- Drugs: Phenothiazines, tricyclic antidepressants, reserpine, α-methyldopa, estrogen therapy, oral contraceptives, metoclopramide, H_2 blockers, opiates, verapamil

WORKUP

- Serum prolactin: Values >150 ng/ml (μg/l) suggest a pituitary tumor. Modest elevations (30–100 ng/ml [μg/l]) often present a diagnostic challenge
- Exclude pregnancy, estrogen administration, hypothyroidism, and drug-induced hyperprolactinemia
- CT or MRI scan: Perform if no cause is identified. Indicated even with mild hyperprolactinemia since tumors may be poorly functioning
- Assess estrogen status in amenorrheic women with serum estradiol or response to medroxyprogesterone acetate (Provera) 10 mg qd for 5 days. Assess gonadal status in men by clinical history and serum testosterone

THERAPY OF PROLACTINOMAS

- Women with hyperprolactinemia without evidence of an adenoma, or with a microprolactinoma (<10 mm) and not desiring pregnancy: <10% of microadenomas grow the size of macroadenomas; ≤30% disappear spontaneously. Close follow-up with no drug treatment is an option. Many patients are started on bromocriptine to reduce the risk of osteoporosis associated with estrogen deficiency
- Women with hyperprolactinemia or a microprolactinoma desiring pregnancy or restoration of menstruation: Bromocriptine (Parlodel), a dopamine agonist, restores prolactin to normal in 80–85% of patients with microadenomas. Galactorrhea usually ceases in a few weeks, and ovulatory menses are established within the first 2 months of treatment. Supplied: Tablets 2.5, 5 mg. Dosage: Start with 1.25 mg given with food at bedtime to minimize the side effects of nausea, vomiting, and postural hypotension. Gradually ↑ the dose until milk secretion has ceased or, in the case of menstrual dysfunction, until the menstrual cycle has returned to normal. Transsphenoidal surgery: Initial cure rate of 70–80% with a late recurrence rate of ≤20–30%
- Pregnant women with a microprolactinoma: Discontinue bromocriptine once pregnancy is confirmed. Follow patient clinically throughout pregnancy. Complications occur in <5% of patients and may be safely treated by reinstitution of bromocriptine
- Women with a macroprolactinoma (>10 mm): Bromocriptine reduces prolactin to normal in 70–80% and causes tumor ↓ to <1/2 the original size in 50%. Surgery cure rate <50% with a late recurrence rate of 20–50%. Generally reserved for patients unresponsive to bromocrip-

tine or needing tumor debulking. Radiotherapy or proton beam therapy is usually reserved for bromocriptine nonresponders not cured by surgery
- Pregnant women with a macroprolactinoma have a 15% risk of tumor enlargement. Monitor visual fields monthly. Reinstitute bromocriptine if tumor enlarges. Surgery may be used for nonresponders
- Men with a microprolactinoma or a macroprolactinoma: Management is similar to that for women. With bromocriptine therapy, testosterone levels ↑ as prolactin ↓. It may take 3–6 months for restoration of normal sexual function.

Acromegaly

The clinical syndrome caused by excess secretion of growth hormone GH.

CLINICAL MANIFESTATIONS

- Headache, visual field defects (bitemporal hemianopsia)
- Growth of hands, feet, and head. Increase in ring, glove, or shoe size. Ask for old photographs for comparison
- Coarsening of facial features, skin tags (fibroma moluscum), ↑ perspiration
- Hepatomegaly, cardiomegaly, thyromegaly
- Arthralgias and arthritis, carpal tunnel syndrome
- Glucose intolerance, hypertension
- Amenorrhea, ↓ libido

DIAGNOSIS

The diagnostic workup of acromegaly is outlined in Figure 33–4
- IGF–1 (Somatomedin-C) level: ↑ in acromegaly. Acts as a mediator of some of the effects of GH and integrates GH secretion
- Glucose suppression test with GH levels: 100 g po glucose load is given, and GH levels are measured at baseline, 1, and 2 h. Normally, administration of glucose suppresses GH secretion. In acromegaly, the tumor is autonomous and does not respond to hyperglycemia. About 20–30% show no change in GH levels, 20–40% show a paradoxical ↑, and 5–7% show suppression but not to normal levels.
- TRH stimulation test: Increase in GH in response to TRH 200 μg IV bolus is seen in 80–90% of patients
- CT scan or MRI of sella turcica
- Prolactin: Excess secretion is found in 30% of patients with acromegaly
- Plasma GHRH levels: Occasionally needed to identify the very rare case of acromegaly caused by excess GHRH secretion

MANAGEMENT

- Surgery results in improvement in ≤90%. In patients whose GH levels return to normal, recurrence occurs in 5%. With incomplete tumor removal, the recurrence rate is >50%. Patients must be followed indefinitely after treatment to assess the efficacy of control of GH secretion and tumor growth. Typically, patients are evaluated 3 months postoperatively with measurement of IGF-1 levels and performance of a glucose suppression test. TRH testing may also be per-

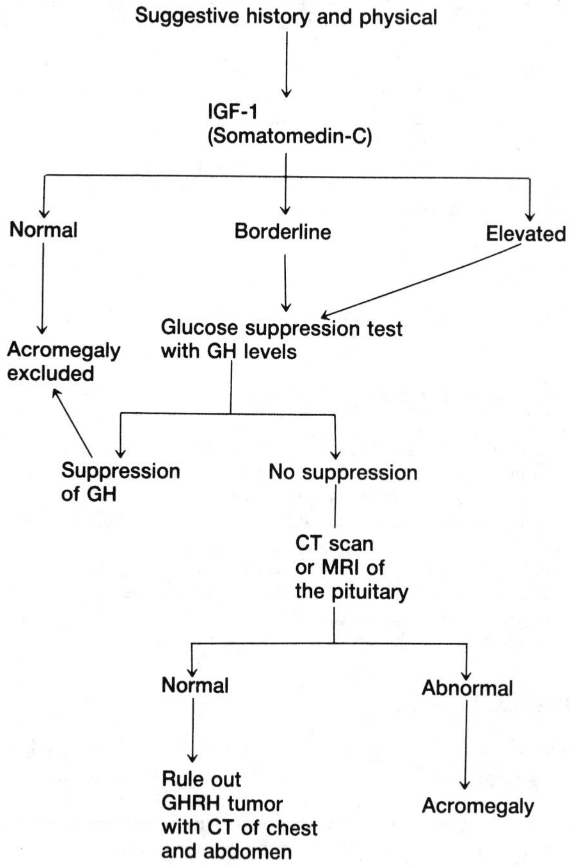

Figure 33–4. Diagnosis of Acromegaly.

formed if it was abnormal before treatment. CT scanning or MRI are used to follow tumor size. Visual field should be followed, particularly in patients who had abnormalities on baseline studies

- External irradiation is used to treat residual tumor from surgery and for inoperable patients. Annual assessment is necessary as late hypopituitarism can occur
- Bromocriptine is useful for cases resistant to surgery and radiotherapy. Used in doses of 10–20 mg qd with meals.

POSTERIOR PITUITARY DISORDERS

Polyuria

Defined as a persistent 24-h urinary volume >2.5 l.

CAUSES

- Osmotic diuresis secondary to excessive solute secretion (i.e., hyperglycemia) or other agents (i.e., mannitol, loop diuretics)

- Primary polydipsia with suppression of AVP (ADH) by excessive water intake
- Central (neurogenic) diabetes insipidus with absolute or partial deficiency of AVP

1. Idiopathic: Familial; sporadic
2. Secondary: Trauma (head injury, surgery to hypothalamic-pituitary region); neoplasms (hypothalamic, pituitary, craniopharyngioma, metastatic); granulomas (sarcoid, histiocytosis); infection (meningitis, encephalitis); external radiation

- Nephrogenic diabetes insipidus with resistance to AVP in the kidney

1. Idiopathic: Familial; sporadic
2. Secondary: Metabolic (hypercalcemia, hypokalemia); toxic (lithium, demeclocycline, methoxyflurane, colchicine, amphotericin, vinblastine, gentamicin, methicillin); vascular (sickle cell disease or trait); infectious (pyelonephritis); postobstructive; other (sarcoidosis, polycystic kidney, amyloidosis)

DIFFERENTIAL DIAGNOSIS OF POLYURIA

In principle, it should be easy to differentiate the various causes of polyuria. A comparison of urinary osmolality during dehydration and after the administration of aqueous vasopressin should reveal a rapid ↑ in osmolality only in patients with central diabetes insipidus. In patients with primary polydipsia, urinary osmolality should ↑ normally in response to dehydration. However, these distinctions are not always as clear because of a number of factors

- Chronic polyuria of any etiology interferes with the maintenance of the renal medullary concentration gradient. This washout effect diminishes the maximal concentrating ability of the kidney
- Most patients with central diabetes insipidus maintain a small capacity to secrete AVP during severe dehydration
- Many patients with acquired nephrogenic diabetes insipidus have an incomplete deficit in AVP action and will concentrate their urine during severe dehydration

INDIRECT TESTING

AVP secretion is indirectly assessed through changes in urinary osmolality during dehydration and after vasopressin administration

- The patient is maintained on complete fluid restriction. Testing is performed during the working day rather than overnight so that the patient is adequately supervised and severe dehydration is avoided. The patient is weighed every hour and the test is stopped if >3% of the initial body weight is lost
- Urinary volume and osmolality are measured every hour. When the urinary osmolality reaches a plateau, as indicated by an hourly ↑ of <30 mOsm/kg (mmol/kg) for 3 successive hours, 5 U of aqueous vasopressin are administered SQ. Urinary osmolality is measured 30 and 60 min later. The last urinary osmolality obtained before the administration of vasopressin and the highest value obtained after the injection are compared
- In subjects with normal pituitary function, urinary osmolality does not ↑ by >9% after the injection of vasopressin. In central diabetes insipidus, the ↑ in urinary osmolality after vasopressin is >9%. Patients with nephrogenic diabetes insipidus usually show little ↑ in urinary osmolality with dehydration and no further ↑ after vasopres-

sin injection. Patients with primary polydipsia often require prolonged water deprivation before a plateau in urinary osmolality is reached and urinary osmolality fails to rise by >9% after the administration of vasopressin

DIRECT TESTING

- Plasma vasopressin levels are measured at the end of the dehydration test. The results are plotted on a nomogram depicting the normal relationship between plasma Na or osmolality and plasma AVP in normal subjects (Fig. 33–5). If the relationship between plasma AVP and osmolality ↓ below the normal range, a diagnosis of central diabetes insipidus is made
- Partial nephrogenic diabetes insipidus and primary polydipsia can be differentiated by analyzing the relationship between plasma AVP and urinary osmolality at the end of the dehydration period (Fig. 33–6).

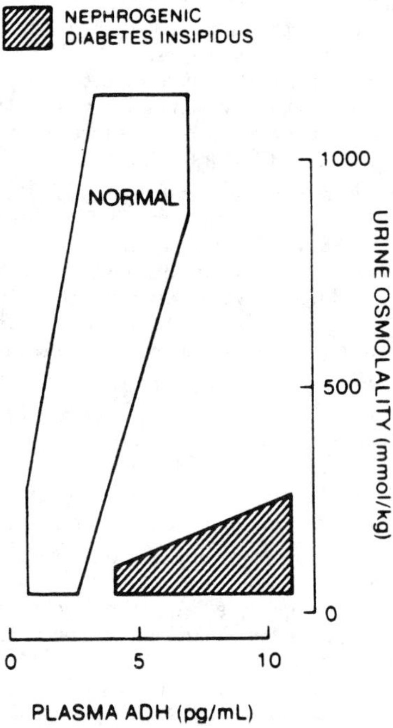

Figure 33–5. Relationship between plasma vasopressin and urine osmolality during dehydration in patients with the 3 forms of diabetes insipidus. Patients with neurogenic diabetes insipidus and primary polydipsia have values within the normal range (open area) in contrast to patients with nephrogenic diabetes insipidus, who have hypotonic urine despite high plasma ADH (cross-hatched area). From Zerbe RL, Robertson GL: Disorders of ADH. Medicine North America *13:*1570, 1984.

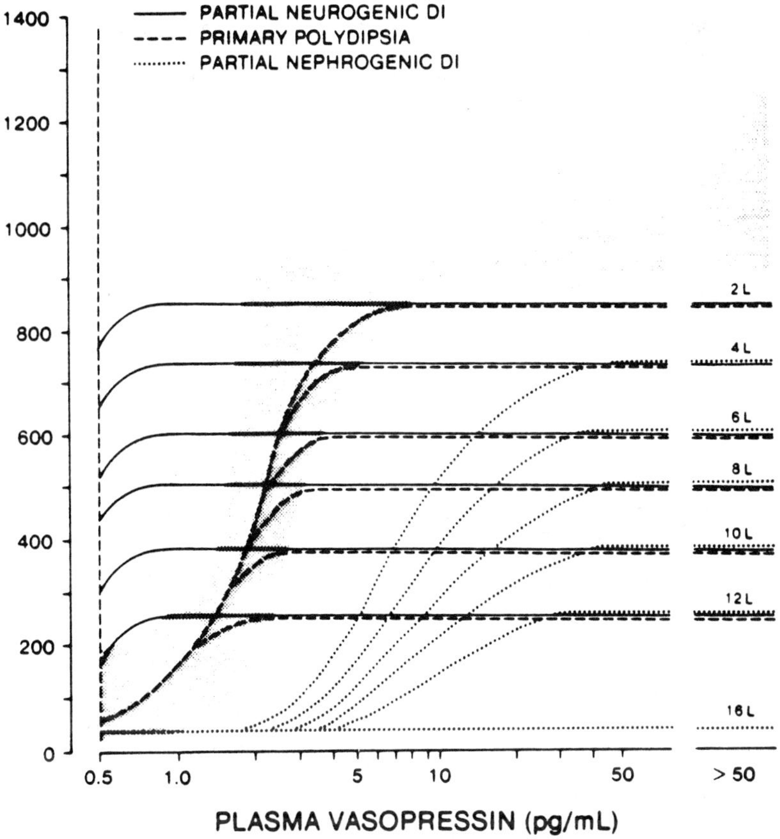

Figure 33–6. Relationship between plasma AVP and plasma osmolality in neurogenic diabetes insipidus, nephrogenic diabetes insipidus and primary polydipsia. From: Robertson GL: Diagnosis of diabetes insipidus. *In* Diabetes insipidus in man. Edited by Czernichow P, Robinson AG. Basel, S. Karger, 1985, p 176.

CHRONIC TREATMENT OF NEUROGENIC DIABETES INSIPIDUS

- Desmopressin (DDAVP) is a synthetic vasopressin analog. Supplied: Metered dose intranasal spray pump delivering 10 μg per depression. Dose: Must be individualized. Average daily dose for adults is 10–40 μg qd. Initially, start with a single evening dose to control nocturia. May add a morning dose if required to control daytime polyuria
- Chlorpropamide (Diabinese) ↑ renal tubular sensitivity to circulating endogenous AVP. Effective in ≤80% of patients. Dose: 250–500 mg bid. Adverse effects: May cause hypoglycemia.

TREATMENT OF NEPHROGENIC DIABETES INSIPIDUS

- Correct any underlying disorder
- Thiazide diuretics (i.e., hydrochlorothiazide 50 mg qd) with Na restric-

tion may ↑ urinary concentration by a vasopressin-independent mechanism
- Amiloride may be useful in patients with nephrogenic diabetes insipidus from lithium therapy as it prevents the uptake of lithium in the collecting ducts

HIRSUTISM

- Hirsutism is defined as the excessive growth of terminal hair (coarse and pigmented) in androgen-sensitive regions (e.g., beard area, trunk, and inner upper thighs).

CAUSES

- Adrenal: Cushing's syndrome; androgen-producing tumors; congenital adrenal hyperplasia (CAH)
- Ovarian: Polycystic ovarian disease (PCOD); insulin resistance; ovarian tumors
- Combined ovarian and adrenal: Idiopathic hirsutism (mostly ovarian)
- Medication: Androgens, anabolic steroids
- Most common causes are PCOD and idiopathic hirsutism

INVESTIGATIONS

- History: Inquire concerning

1. Age of onset: Prepubertal hirsutism suggests CAH; peripubertal onset is compatible with PCOD and idiopathic hirsutism
2. Mode of onset: Abrupt onset and rapid progression suggest an androgen-secreting tumor
3. Menstrual abnormalities: Common in PCOD
4. Galactorrhea: Hyperprolactinemia is a rare cause of hirsutism
5. Medications: Inquire about the use of anabolic steroids
6. Family history: Frequently positive for hirsutism with PCOD and idiopathic hirsutism

- Physical: Document

1. Amount and distribution of hair: Facial, periareolar, and lower abdominal hair is common; hair over the upper chest, upper abdomen, and upper back suggests more severe androgen excess
2. Signs of virilization (clitoromegaly, balding, deepening of voice, and ↑ muscle mass) suggest an androgen-secreting tumor
3. Features of Cushing's syndrome
4. Presence of ovarian or adrenal masses

- Serum testosterone: A level <2 ng/ml (7 nmol/l) suggests an ovarian tumor. Often mildly ↑ in PCOD
- Serum DHEA-S: A level >6630 ng/ml (18 μmol/l) suggests an adrenal tumor. May be mildly ↑ in PCOD
- Serum gonadotropins: A ↑ ratio of LH/FSH (>2.5) may be seen in the early follicular phase with PCOD
- Plasma 17–hydroxyprogesterone: ↑ suggests late-onset CAH. ACTH stimulation test may be needed to confirm this diagnosis
- Serum prolactin: Useful to rule out hyperprolactinemia
- Overnight dexamethasone suppression test: Perform if Cushing's syndrome is suspected (Fig. 33–3)

- Adrenal CT scan: Perform if adrenal tumor is suspected
- Pelvic and vaginal ultrasound: Ovaries may be enlarged with multiple cysts in PCOD

Polycystic Ovarian Disease

Exact pathophysiology is not known but is probably multifactorial, involving disorders of the adrenals, ovaries, and hypothalamus. Diagnosis is made after excluding other causes of hirsutism. The ultrasound finding of polycystic ovaries is nonspecific and can occur in a variety of hyperandrogenic anovulatory states. Clinical manifestations vary. Classic signs and symptoms consist of chronic anovulation, amenorrhea/oligomenorrhea, and slowly progressive hirsutism onsetting just after menarche. Obesity, acne, and infertility are common. Family history is often positive for similar complaints.

Idiopathic Hirsutism

Menstrual cycles are usually regular and ovulatory. The hirsutism tends to start in the late teens or early twenties. Family history is common. Most women have ↑ ovarian production and bioavailability of androgens

MANAGEMENT

- Local measures (electrolysis, shaving, bleaching, and waxing) are often useful by themselves or while awaiting the full benefits of drug therapy
- Weight loss may improve hirsutism by increasing hepatic production of sex hormone binding globulin (SHBG) and thereby reducing bioavailable testosterone
- Oral contraceptive agents ↓ ovarian androgen secretion by suppressing gonadotropin secretion and ↑ SHBG levels decreasing the levels of free testosterone. Avoid agents containing desogestrel, as this progestin has enhanced androgenic activity. Agents containing desogestrel, norethindrone or ethynodiol diacetate are generally preferred. Maximum therapeutic effect takes 9–12 months
- Anti-androgens: Spironolactone (Aldactone). Supplied: Tablets 25, 100 mg. Dosage: Usual initial dose is 50 mg bid. Max therapeutic effect takes 9–12 months. Adverse effects: Nausea, irregular menses or amenorrhea, fatigue, and headache. Spironolactone must not be given during pregnancy because it interferes with normal masculinization of a male fetus. Cyproterone acetate (Androcur) (Canada). Supplied: Tablets 50 mg. Dosage: Initial dose with severe hirsutism is 25–50 mg days 5–14 of each calendar month. In mild hirsutism or with maintenance therapy, 2 mg days 5–14 may be sufficient. An estrogen (ethinyl estradiol 25 μg days 5–25) is given to induce regular menstrual bleeding. Adverse Effects: Nausea, fatigue, and ↓ libido.

Late-Onset Congenital Adrenal Hyperplasia

May be present in 1–5% of hirsute women. Most commonly caused by a partial block in 21–hydroxylase activity, which leads to ↑ serum levels of 17–OHP. Diagnosed by ACTH stimulation: Inject ACTH 250 μg I.M. or IV and draw 17–OHP levels at 0, 30, and 60 min. Patients with a partial enzymatic defect demonstrate ↑ 17–OHP levels (>2000 ng/dl) after ACTH. Treatment consists of dexamethasone (Decadron) 0.25–0.50 mg at bedtime.

Suggested Reading

Thyroid Disorders

Caldwell G, Kellet HA, Gow SM, et al.: A new strategy for thyroid function testing. Lancet, *1*: 1117, 1985.

Adrenal Disorders

Carpenter PC: Diagnostic evaluation of Cushing's syndrome. Endocrinol Metab Clin North Am,*17*(3): 445, 1988.

Young WF Jr, Hogan MJ, Klee GG, et al.: Primary aldosteronism: Diagnosis and treatment. Mayo Clin Proc, *65*:96, 1990.

Pituitary Disorders

Melby JC: Therapy of Cushing's disease: A consensus for pituitary microsurgery (editorial). Ann Intern Med, *109*:445, 1988.

Melmed S, Braunstein GD, Chang RJ, Becker DP: Pituitary tumours secreting growth hormone and prolactin. Ann Intern Med, *105*:238, 1986.

Robertson GL: Differential diagnosis of polyuria. Annu Rev Med, *39*: 425, 1988.

Hirsutism

Rittmaster RS, Loriaux DL: Hirsutism. Ann Intern Med, *106*:95, 1987.

McKenna, TJ: Pathogenesis and treatment of polycystic ovary syndrome. N Engl J Med, *318*:558, 1988.

Massachusetts General Hospital: Normal Reference Laboratory Values

The following is a list of reference values, general methods, and conversion factors for tests commonly ordered at the Massachusetts General Hospital and recorded in the Case Records. It reflects the revision of tabular summaries previously published (Normal Laboratory Values. N Engl J Med 1946, 234:24–8; 1950, 243:748–53; 1956, 254:29–35; 1960, 262:84–91; 1963, 268:1462–9; 1967, 276:167–74; 1970, 283:1276–85; 1974, 290:39–49; 1978, 298:34–45; 1980, 302:37–48; and 1986, 314: 39–49). The present values were compiled with with the aid of Leonard Ellman, M.D., J. Larry Jameson, M.D., Ph.D., and Kurt Bloch, M.D. Values for analytes obtained in more than one laboratory are not listed since the reference ranges differ. Values are expressed in the units used at this institution (MGH units) and the units of the Système international d'Unités (SI units), with a factor to convert MGH units to SI units by multiplication.

General Chemistry

ANALYTE	FLUID*	MGH UNITS	SI UNITS	METHOD OR INSTRUMENT	FACTOR FOR CONVERSION TO SI UNITS
Acid phosphatase, prostatic	S	0–0.8 U/liter	0.0–13.0 nkat/liter	Kinetic method	16.67
Alanine aminotransferase (ALT, SGPT)	S			Kinetic method	0.01667
Female		7–30 U/liter	0.12–0.50 μkat/liter		
Male		10–55 U/liter	0.17–0.91 μkat/liter		
Albumin	S	3.1–4.3 g/dl	31–43 g/liter	Colorimetry (bromocresol purple)	10
Aldolase	S	0–7 U/liter	0–117 nkat/liter	Kinetic method	16.67
Alkaline phosphatase	S			Kinetic method	0.01667
Female		30–100 U/liter	0.5–1.67 μkat/liter		
Male		45–115 U/liter	0.75–1.92 μkat/liter		
Alkaline phosphatase, leukocyte	WB			Histochemistry	
Female (not taking oral contraceptives)		30–160	None		None
Male		33–188	None		None
Alpha$_1$-antitrypsin	S	85–213 mg/dl	0.85–2.13 g/liter	Nephelometry	0.01
Alpha-fetoprotein (nonmaternal)	S	<10 IU/ml	<7.75 μg/liter	Immunoassay	0.775
Ammonia	P	12–55 μmol/liter	12–55 μmol/liter	Enzymatic analysis	1
Amylase	S	53–123 U/liter	0.88–2.05 nkat/liter	Kinetic method	0.01667
	U	0–375 U/liter	0–6.25 μkat/liter	Kinetic method	
Angiotensin-converting enzyme (ACE)	S	10–50 U/liter	167–834 nkat/liter	Kinetic method	16.67
Aspartate aminotransferase (AST, SGOT)	S			Kinetic method	0.01667
Female		9–25 U/liter	0.15–0.42 μkat/liter		
Male		10–40 U/liter	0.17–0.67 μkat/liter		
Bicarbonate (HCO_3^-)	WB, S	22–26 meq/liter	22–26 mmol/liter	Calculation	1
Bilirubin, direct	S	0.0–0.4 mg/dl	0–7 μmol/liter	Colorimetry	17.1
Bilirubin, total	S	0.0–1.0 mg/dl	0–17 μmol/liter	Colorimetry	17.1
CA-19-9	S	<37.0 U/ml	<37.0 kU/liter	Immunoassay	1
CA-125	S	<20.0 U/ml	<20.0 kU/liter	Immunoassay	1
Calcium	S	8.5–10.5 mg/dl	2.1–2.6 mmol/liter	Colorimetry	0.25

	U	0.0–300 mg/day	0.0–7.5 mmol/day	Atomic absorption	0.025
Calcium, ionized	P	4.0–4.6 mg/dl	1.0–1.15 mmol/liter	Ion-selective electrode	1
Carbon dioxide content, total	S	24.0–30.9 l/liter	24.0–30.9 mmol/liter	Carbon dioxide electrode	1
Carbon dioxide, partial pressure, arterial ($PaCO_2$)	WB	35–45 mm Hg	4.7–6.0 kPa	Carbon dioxide electrode	0.1333
Carboxyhemoglobin	WB	<5% of total hemoglobin	<0.05 fraction of total hemoglobin saturation	Multiwavelength spectrophotometry	0.01
Carcinoembryonic antigen (CEA)	P, S	0.0–3.0 ng/ml	0.0–3.0 μg/liter	Immunoassay	1
Cerebrospinal fluid (adult)	CSF				
Albumin		11–48 mg/dl	0.11–0.48 g/liter	Nephelometry	0.01
Cell count		0–5 mononuclear cells/μl	0–5 × 10^6 cells/liter	Manual count	1 × 10^6
Chloride		120–130 mEq/liter	120–130 mmol/liter	Coulometry	1
Glucose		50–75 mg/dl	2.8–4.2 mmol/liter	Enzymatic analysis	0.05551
IgG		8.0–8.6 mg/dl	0.08–0.086 g/liter	Nephelometry	0.01
Pressure		70–180 mm of water	70–180 arbitrary units	Manual measurement	1
Protein		15–45 mg/dl	0.15–0.45 g/liter	Turbidometry	0.01
Ceruloplasmin	S	23–43 mg/dl	230–430 mg/liter	Oxidase activity	10
Chloride	P, S	100–108 mEq/liter	100–108 mmol/liter	Coulometry	1
	U	10–200 mEq/liter	10–200 mmol/liter	Coulometry	1
Cholesterol	S			Colorimetry	0.02586
Desirable		<200 mg/dl	<5.18 mmol/liter		
Borderline high		200–239 mg/dl	5.18–6.19 mmol/liter		
High		≥240 mg/dl	≥6.20 mmol/liter		
Copper	P	70–155 μg/dl	11.0–24.4 μmol/liter	Atomic absorption	0.1574
	U	0–60 μg/dl/day	0.0–0.94 μmol/day	Atomic absorption	0.01574
Creatine kinase (CK)	S			Kinetic method	0.01667
Female		40–150 U/liter	0.67–2.50 μkat/liter		
Male		40–150 U/liter	0.67–2.50 μkat/liter		
Creatine kinase iscenzymes, MB fraction	S	0–7.5 ng/ml >5% in acute MI	0–7.5 μg/liter 2>0.05	Immunoassay	1

(continued)

* S denotes serum, WB whole blood, P plasma, U urine, CSF cerebrospinal fluid, and PRP platelet-rich plasma.

General Chemistry *(continued)*

ANALYTE	FLUID*	MGH UNITS	SI UNITS	METHOD OR INSTRUMENT	FACTOR FOR CONVERSION TO SI UNITS
Creatine kinase isoenzyme index	S	0.0–3.0% relative index	None	$\frac{\text{ng/ml}}{\text{total CK(U/liter)}} \times 100$	None
Creatinine	S	0.6–1.5 mg/dl	53–133 μmol/liter	Colorimetry	88.4
	U	15–25 mg/kg/day	0.13–0.22 mmol/kg/day		0.0088
Fecal fat (as stearic acid)		1–7 g/day	3.5–25 mmol/day	Gravimetry	3.515
Gamma-glutamyl transpeptidase (GGT)	S	1.0–60.0 U/liter	0.02–1.00 μkat/liter	Kinetic method	0.01667
Globulin	S	2.6–4.1 g/dl	26–41 g/liter	Calculation: total protein – albumin	10
Glucose, fasting	P	70–110 mg/dl	3.9–6.1 mmol/liter	Enzymatic analysis	0.05551
High-density lipoprotein, cholesterol, as major risk factor	S	<35 mg/dl	<0.91 mmol/liter	Colorimetry	0.02586
Ketones	S, U	Negative	Negative	Colorimetry (nitroprusside)	
Lactic dehydrogenase (LDH)	S	110–210 U/liter	1.83–3.50 μkat/liter	Kinetic method	0.01667
Lactic dehydrogenase isoenzymes	S			Electrophoresis	0.01
LD_1		17–27%	0.17–0.27		
LD_2		28–38%	0.28–0.38		
LD_3		18–28%	0.18–0.28		
LD_4		5–15%	0.05–0.15		
LD_5		5–15%	0.05–0.15		
Total LDH (when isoenzymes determined)		110–250 U/liter	1.83–4.23 μkat/liter		
Lactic acid	P	0.5–2.2 mmol/liter	0.5–2.2 mmol/liter	Enzymatic analysis	1
Lipase	S	4–24 U/dl	0.67–4.00 μkat/liter	Kinetic method	0.1667

Low-density lipoprotein cholesterol	S			Calculation	0.02586
Desirable		<130 mg/dl	<3.36 mmol/liter		
Borderline high risk		130–159 mg/dl	3.36–4.11 mmol/liter		
High risk		≥160 mg/dl	≥4.13 mmol/liter		
Magnesium	S	1.5–2.0 mEq/liter	0.8–1.0 mmol/liter	Colorimetry	0.5
5′-Nucleotidase	S	1–11 U/liter	0.02–0.18 μkat/liter	Kinetic method	0.01667
Osmolality	S	280–296 mOsm/kg of water	280–296 mmol/kg	Freezing-point depression	1
Oxygen, partial pressure, arterial (PaO_2); room air, age dependent	WB	75–100 mm Hg	10.0–13.3 kPa	Oxygen electrode	0.1333
Oxygen saturation, arterial	WB	96–100%	0.96–1.00	Pulse oximetry	0.01
pH, arterial	WB	7.35–7.45 pH units	7.35–7.45 pH units	pH electrode	1
Phosphorus, inorganic	S	2.6–4.5 mg/dl	0.84–1.45 mmol/liter	Spectrophotometry	0.3229
	U	average, 1 g/day	average, 32 mmol/day		32.29
Potassium	S	3.5–5.0 mEq/liter	3.5–5.0 mmol/liter	Ion-selective electrode	1
	U	Diet dependent	Diet dependent	Ion-selective electrode	1
Prostate-specific antigen	S			Immunoassay	1
Female		0.0–0.5 μg/liter	0.0–0.5 μg/liter		
Male <40 yr old		0.0–2.0 μg/liter	0.0–2.0 μg/liter		
Male ≥40 yr old		0.0–4.0 μg/liter	0.0–4.0 μg/liter		
Protein, total	S	6.0–8.0 g/dl	60–80 g/liter	Colorimetry	10
	U	<165 mg/day	<0.165 g/day	Turbidometry	0.001
Sodium	S	135–145 mEq/liter	135–145 mmol/liter	Ion-selective electrode	1
	U	Diet dependent	Diet dependent	Ion-selective electrode	1
Triglycerides (fasting)	S	40–150 mg/dl	0.45–1.69 mmol/liter	Spectrophotometry	0.01129
Urea nitrogen (BUN)	S	8–25 mg/dl	2.9–8.9 mmol/liter	Conductivity	0.357
Uric acid	S			Colorimetry	59.48
Female		2.3–6.6 mg/dl	137–393 μmol/liter		
Male		3.6–8.5 mg/dl	214–506 μmol/liter		

* S denotes serum, WB whole blood, P plasma, U urine, CSF cerebrospinal fluid, and PRP platelet-rich plasma.

Endocrine Chemistry

ANALYTE	FLUID*	MGH UNITS	SI UNITS	METHOD OR INSTRUMENT	FACTOR FOR CONVERSION TO SI UNITS
Aldosterone					
Standing (normal-salt diet)	S, P	4–31 ng/dl	111–860 pmol/liter	Immunoassay	27.74
Recumbent (normal-salt diet)	S, P	<16 ng/dl	<444 pmol/liter	Immunoassay	27.74
Normal-salt diet (100–180 meq of sodium)	U	6–25 μg/day	17–69 nmol/day	Immunoassay	2.774
Low-salt diet (10 meq of sodium)	U	17–44 μg/day	47–122 nmol/day	Immunoassay	2.774
High-salt diet	U	0–6 μg/day	0–17 nmol/day	Immunoassay	2.774
Androstenedione	S	60–260 ng/dl	2.1–9.1 nmol/liter	Immunoassay	0.0349
Antidiuretic hormone (arginine vasopressin)	P	1.0–13.3 pg/ml	1.0–13.3 ng/liter	Immunoassay	1
Calcitonin	S			Immunoassay	1
Female		0–20 pg/ml	0–20 ng/liter		
Male		0–28 pg/ml	0–28 ng/liter		
Catecholamines					
Dopamine	U	65–400 μg/day	424–2612 nmol/day	Liquid chromatography	6.53
	P	0–30 pg/ml	0–196 nmol/liter	Liquid chromatography	6.53
Epinephrine	U	1.7–22.4 μg/day	9.3–122 nmol/day	Liquid chromatography	5.458
Supine	P	0–110 pg/ml	0–600 pmol/liter	Liquid chromatography	5.458
Standing	P	0–140 pg/ml	0–764 pmol/liter	Liquid chromatography	5.458
Norepinephrine	U	12.1–85.5 μg/day	72–505 nmol/day	Liquid chromatography	5.911
Supine	P	70–750 pg/ml	0.41–4.43 nmol/liter	Liquid chromatography	0.005911
Standing	P	200–1700 pg/ml	1.18–10.0	Liquid chromatography	0.005911
Chorionic gonadotropin (hCG) (non-pregnant)	S	<10 mIU/ml	<10 IU/liter	Immunoassay	1
Corticotropin (ACTH)	P	6.0–76.0 pg/ml	1.3–16.7 pmol/liter	Immunoassay	0.2202
Cortisol	P			Immunoassay	27.59
Fasting, 8 a.m.–12 noon		5.0–25.0 μg/dl	138–690 nmol/liter		
12 noon–8 p.m.		5.0–15.0 μg/dl	138–410 nmol/liter		
8 p.m.–8 a.m.		0.0–10.0 μg/dl	0–276 nmol/liter		
Cortisol, free	U	20–70 μg/day	55–193 nmol/day	Immunoassay	2.759
C peptide	S	0.30–3.70 μg/liter	0.10–1.22 nmol/liter	Immunoassay	0.33

11-Deoxycortisol (after metyrapone)	P	>7.5 μg/dl	>216 nmol/liter	Immunoassay	28.86
1.25-Dihydroxyvitamin D	S	16–42 pg/ml	38–101 pmol/liter	Immunoassay	2.4
Erythropoietin	S	<19 mU/ml	≤19 U/liter	Immunoassay	1
Estradiol	S, P			Immunoassay	3.671
Female					
Premenopausal adult		23–361 pg/ml	84–1325 pmol/liter		
Postmenopausal		<30 pg/ml	<110 pmol/liter		
Prepubertal		<20 pg/ml	<73 pmol/liter		
Male		<50 pg/ml	<184 pmol/liter		
Gastrin	P	0–200 pg/ml	0–200 ng/liter	Immunoassay	1
Growth hormone	P	2.0–6.0 ng/ml	2.0–6.0 μg/liter	Immunoassay	1
Hemoglobin A_{1c}	P	3.8–6.4%	0.038–0.064	Liquid chromatography	0.01
Homovanillic acid	U	0.0–15.0 mg/day	0–82 μmol/day	Liquid chromatography	5.489
17-Hydroxycorticosteroids	U			Colorimetry	2.759
Female		2.0–6.0 mg/day	5.5–17 μmol/day		
Male		3.0–10.0 mg/day	8–28 μmol/day		
5-Hydroxyindoleacetic acid (lower in women than in men)	U	2–9 mg/day	10–47 μmol/day	Colorimetry	5.23
17-Hydroxyprogesterone	S			Immunoassay	3.026
Female					
Prepubertal		0.20–0.54 μg/liter	0.61–1.63 nmol/liter		
Follicular		0.02–0.80 μg/liter	0.61–2.42 nmol/liter		
Luteal		0.90–3.04 μg/liter	2.72–9.20 nmol/liter		
Postmenopausal		<0.45 μg/liter	<1.36 nmol/liter		
Male					
Prepubertal		0.12–0.30 μg/liter	0.36–0.91 nmol/liter		
Adult		0.20–1.80 μg/liter	0.61–5.45 nmol/liter		
25-Hydroxyvitamin D	S	8–55 ng/ml	20–137 nmol/liter	Immunoassay	2.496
Insulin	S	0–29 μU/ml	0–208 pmol/liter	Immunoassay	7.175

(continued)

* S denotes serum, WB whole blood, P plasma, U urine, CSF cerebrospinal fluid, and PRP platelet-rich plasma.

Endocrine Chemistry *(continued)*

ANALYTE	FLUID*	MGH UNITS	SI UNITS	METHOD OR INSTRUMENT	FACTOR FOR CONVERSION TO SI UNITS
17-Ketogenic steroids	U			Colorimetry	3.467
Female		3.0–15.0 mg/day	10–52 μmol/day		
Male		5.0–23.0 mg/day	17–80 μmol/day		
17-Ketosteroids	U			Colorimetry	3.467
Female and male ≤10 yr old		0.1–3.0 mg/day	0.4–10.4 μmol/day		
Female and male 11–14 yr old		2.0–7.0 mg/day	6.9–24.2 μmol/day		
Female ≥15 yr old		5.0–15.0 mg/day	17.3–52.0 μmol/day		
Male ≥15 yr old		9.0–22.0 mg/day	31.2–76.3 μmol/day		
Metanephrines, total	U	0.0–0.90 mg/day	0.0–4.9 μmol/day	Spectrophotometry	5.458
Parathyroid hormone	P	10–60 pg/ml	10–60 ng/liter	Immunoassay	1
Parathyroid-related protein	P	<1.5 pmol/liter	<1.5 pmol/liter	Immunoassay	1
Pregnanediol	U			Gas chromatography	3.12
Female		0.2–6.0 mg/day	0.6–18.7 μmol/day		
Follicular phase		0.1–1.3 mg/day	0.3–5.3 μmol/day		
Luteal phase		1.2–9.5 mg/day	3.7–29.6 μmol/day		
Pregnancy		Gestation-period dependent	Gestation-period dependent		
Male		0.2–1.2 mg/day	0.6–3.7 μmol/day		
Pregnanetriol	U	0.5–2.0 mg/day	1.5–6.0 μmol/day	Gas chromatography	2.972
Prolactin	S			Immunoassay	1
Female		0–15 ng/ml	0–15 μg/liter		
Male		0–10 ng/ml	0–10 μg/liter		
Renin activity	P			Immunoassay	0.2778
Normal salt intake					
Recumbent 6 hr		0.5–1.6 ng/ml/hr	0.14–0.44 ng/(liter · sec)		
Upright 4 hr		1.9–3.6 ng/ml/hr	0.53–1.00 ng/(liter · sec)		

Low salt intake					
Recumbent 6 hr		2.2–4.4 ng/ml/hr	0.61–1.22 ng/(liter · sec)		
Upright 4 hr		4.0–8.1 ng/ml/hr	1.11–2.25 ng/(liter · sec)		
Upright 4 hr, with diuretic		6.8–15.0 ng/ml/hr	1.89–4.17 ng/(liter · sec)		
Somatomedin C	P			Immunoassay	1
Female					
Preadolescent		60.8–724.5 ng/ml	60.8–724.5 μg/liter		
Adolescent		112.5–450.0 ng/ml	112.5–450.0 μg/liter		
Adult		141.8–389.3 ng/ml	141.8–389.3 μg/liter		
Male					
Preadolescent		65.5–841.5 ng/ml	65.5–841.5 μg/liter		
Adolescent		83.3–378.0 ng/ml	83.3–378.0 μg/liter		
Adult		54.0–328.5 ng/ml	54.0–328.5 μg/liter		
Testosterone, total, morning sample	P			Immunoassay	0.03467
Female		20–90 ng/dl	0.7–3.1 nmol/liter		
Male, adult		300–1100 ng/dl	10.4–38.1 nmol/liter		
Testosterone, unbound, morning sample	P			Equilibrium dialysis	34.67
Female, adult		0.09–1.29 ng/dl	3–45 pmol/liter		
Male, adult		3.06–24.0 ng/dl	106–832 pmol/liter		
Thyroglobulin	S	0–60 ng/ml	0–60 μg/liter	Immunoassay	1
Thyroid-hormone-binding index		0.83–1.17	0.83–1.17	Charcoal resin	1
Thyroid-stimulating hormone	S	0.5–5.0 μU/ml	0.5–5.0 mU/liter	Immunoassay	1
Thyroxine, free	S	0.8–2.7 ng/dl	10–35 pmol/ligter	Direct equilibrium dialysis	12.87
Thyroxine-binding globulin	S	Age and sex dependent	Age and sex dependent	Immunoassay	
Thyroxine, free, index		4.6–11.2	4.6–11.2	Calculation	1
Thyroxine, total (T_4)	S	4–12 μg/dl	51–154 nmol/liter	Immunoassay	12.87
Triiodothyronine, total (T_3)	S	75–195 ng/dl	1.2–3.0 nmol/liter	Immunoassay	0.01536
Vanilmandelic acid (VMA)	U	1.4–6.5 mg/day	7.1–32.7 μmol/day	Liquid chromatography	5.046

* S denotes serum, WB whole blood, P plasma, U urine, CSF cerebrospinal fluid, and PRP platelet-rich plasma.

Immunology

ANALYTE	FLUID*	MGH UNITS	SI UNITS	METHOD OR INSTRUMENT	FACTOR FOR CONVERSION TO SI UNITS
Autoantibodies					
Adrenal gland	S	Negative at 1:10 dilution	Not applicable	Indirect immunofluorescence	
Anticentromere antibodies	S	Negative at 1:40 dilution	Not applicable	Indirect immunofluorescence	
Anti-native DNA antibodies	S	Negative at 1:10 dilution	Not applicable	Indirect immunofluorescence	
Antineutrophil antibodies, direct	WB	Negative	Not applicable	Autologous immunologic assay	
Antineutrophil antibodies, indirect	S	Negative	Not applicable	Staphylococcal conjugated immunologic assay	
Antinuclear antibodies	S	Negative at 1:8 dilution	Not applicable	Indirect immunofluorescence	
La	S	None detected	Not applicable	Indirect immunofluorescence	
Mitochondrial	S	Negative at 1:20 dilution	Not applicable	Indirect immunofluorescence	
RNP	S	None detected	Not applicable	Indirect immunofluorescence	
Ro	S	None detected	Not applicable	Indirect immunofluorescence	

Sm	S	None detected	Not applicable	Indirect immunofluorescence	
Smooth muscle	S	Negative at 1:20 dilution	Not applicable	Indirect immunofluorescence	
Thyroid colloid and microsomal antigens	S	Negative at 1:10 dilution	Not applicable	Indirect immunofluorescence or hemagglutination	
C1-esterase-inhibitor protein	S	12.6–24.6 mg/dl	0.13–0.25 g/liter	Nephelometry	0.01
Complement					
C3	S	83–177 mg/dl	0.83–1.77 g/liter	Nephelometry	0.01
C4	S	15–45 mg/dl	0.15–0.45 g/liter	Nephelometry	0.01
Total hemolytic (CH_{50})	S	150–250 U/ml	150–250 U/liter	Sheep red-cell hemolysis	1
Factor B	S	17–42 mg/dl	0.17–0.42 g/liter	Nephelometry	0.01
Immunoglobulin, quantitation	S			Nephelometry	
IgA		70–312 mg/dl	0.7–3.12 g/liter		0.01
IgG		639–1349 mg/dl	6.39–13.49 g/liter		0.01
IgM		56–352 mg/dl	0.56–3.52 g/liter		0.01
IgE		<103 IU/ml	<247 μg/liter		2.4
Rheumatoid factor (fasting sample)	S	<30 IU/ml	<30 kIU/liter	Nephelometry	1
Viscosity	S	1.4–1.8 relative viscosity units, as compared with water	1.4–1.8 relative viscosity units, as compared with water	Ostwald viscometry	1

* S denotes serum, WB whole blood, P plasma, U urine, CSF cerebrospinal fluid, and PRP platelet-rich plasma.

Hematology and Coagulation

ANALYTE	FLUID*	MGH UNITS	SI UNITS	METHOD OR INSTRUMENT	FACTOR FOR CONVERSION TO SI UNITS
Alpha$_2$-antiplasmin, functional	P	80 – 130%	0.80–1.30	Chromogenic assay	0.01
Anti-factor VIIIC titer	P	0 Bethesda units	0 Bethesda units	Automated clotting assay	1
Antiplatelet antibodies	P	Negative	Negative	Serotonin release	1
Antithrombin III	P				
Immunologic		22–39 mg/dl	220–390 mg/liter	Immunoassay	10
Functional		80–120%	0.80–1.20	Chromogenic assay	0.01
Bleeding time		2–9.5 min	2–9.5 min	Surgicutt	1
Clot retraction	P	50–100%/2 hr	0.50–1.00/2 hr	Manual	0.01
D-Dimer screen	P	<0.5 μg/ml	<0.5 mg/liter	Latex agglutination	1
Differential blood count	WB			Automated cell counter	0.01
Neutrophils		45–74%	0.45–0.74		
Bands		0–4%	0.00–0.04		
Lymphocytes		16–45%	0.16–0.45		
Monocytes		4–10%	0.04–0.10		
Eosinophils		0–7%	0.00–0.07		
Basophils		0–2%	0.00–0.02		
Erythrocyte count	WB	4.15–4.90 × 10^6/mm^3	4.15–4.90 × 10^{12}/liter	Automated cell counter	1
Erythrocyte sedimentation rate	WB			Manual (modified Westergren method)	1
Female		1–30 mm/hr	1–30 mm/hr		
Male		1–13 mm/hr	1–13 mm/hr		
Factor I, fibrinogen	P	0.15–0.35 g/dl	4.0–10.0 μmol/liter	Automated clotting assay	29.41
Factor II, prothrombin	P	60–140%	0.60–1.40	Automated clotting assay	0.01
Factor V	P	60–140%	0.60–1.40	Automated clotting assay	0.01
Factor VII	P	60–140%	0.60–1.40	Automated clotting assay	0.01
Factor VIII	P	50–200%	0.50–2.00	Automated clotting assay	0.01
Factor IX	P	60–140%	0.60–1.40	Automated clotting assay	0.01

Factor X	P	60–140%	0.60–1.40	Automated clotting assay	0.01
Factor XI	P	60–140%	0.60–1.40	Automated clotting assay	0.01
Factor XII	P	60–140%	0.60–1.40	Automated clotting assay	0.01
Factor XIII screen	P	Negative	Negative	Urea clot dissolution	1
Ferritin	S			Immunoassay	1
Normal		>20 ng/ml	>20 μg/liter		
Borderline deficient		13–20 ng/ml	13–20 μg/liter		
Deficient		0–12 ng/ml	0–12 μg/liter		
Excessive		>400 ng/ml	>400 μg/liter		
Fibrin(ogen) degradation products	S	<10 μg/ml	<100 mg/liter	Latex agglutination	10
Fletcher factor screen	P	Negative	Negative	Automated clotting assay	1
Folate (folic acid)	S			Immunoassay	2.266
Normal		≥3.3 ng/ml	>7.3 nmol/liter		
Borderline deficient		2.5–3.2 ng/ml	5.7–7.3 nmol/liter		
Deficient		<2.5 ng/ml	<5.7 nmol/liter		
Glucose-6-phosphate dehydrogenase (erythrocyte)	WB	5–15 U/g of hemoglobin	5–15 U/g of hemoglobin	Colorimetry	1
Haptoglobin	S	13–163 mg/dl	0.13–1.63 g/liter	Nephelometry	0.01
Hematocrit	WB			Automated cell counter	0.01
Female		37–48%	0.37–0.48		
Male		42–52%	0.42–0.52		
Hemoglobin	WB			Automated cell counter	10
Female		12–16 g/dl	120–160 g/liter		
Male		13–18 g/dl	130–180 g/liter		
Iron	S	50–150 μg/dl	9.0–26.9 μmol/liter	Colorimetry	0.1791
Iron-binding capacity	S	250–410 μg/dl	45–73 μmol/liter	Colorimetry	0.1791
Leukocyte count	WB	4.3–10.8 × $10^3/mm^3$	4.3–10.8 × 10^9/liter	Automated cell counter	1
Lupus inhibitor tests				Automated clotting assay	1
Tissue-thromboplastin-inhibition test	P	Negative	Negative		

(continued)

* S denotes serum, WB whole blood, P plasma, U urine, CSF cerebrospinal fluid, and PRP platelet-rich plasma.

Hematology and Coagulation *(continued)*

ANALYTE	FLUID*	MGH UNITS	SI UNITS	METHOD OR INSTRUMENT	FACTOR FOR CONVERSION TO SI UNITS
Dilute Russell's viper venom test	P	Negative	Negative		
Platelet neutralization procedure	P	Negative	Negative		
Anticardiolipin antibody	S			Immunoassay	1
IgG		0–23 Anti-IgG units	0–23 arbitrary units		
IgM		0–11 Anti-IgM units	0–11 arbitrary units		
Mean corpuscular hemoglobin (MCH)	WB	28–33 pg/cell	28–33 pg/cell	Automated cell counter	1
Mean corpuscular hemoglobin concentration (MCHC)	WB	32–36 g/dl	320–360 g/liter	Automated cell counter	10
Mean corpuscular volume (MCV)	WB	86–98 μm^3	86–98 fl	Automated cell counter	1
50:50 Mixing studies	P	Correction = factor deficiency		Automated clotting assay	1
Osmotic fragility of erythrocytes	WB	Increased if hemolysis occurs at >0.5% sodium chloride		Spectrophotometry	1
Partial-thromboplastin time, activated	P	24–37 sec	24–37 sec	Automated clotting assay	1
Peroxide hemolysis	WB	<10%	<0.10	Manual	0.01
Plasminogen, functional	P	80–130%	0.80–1.30	Chromogenic assay	0.01
Platelet aggregation	PRP	>65% aggregation in response to adenosine diphosphate, epinephrine, collagen, ristocetin, and arachidonic acid		Platelet aggregometry	Not applicable
Platelet count	WB	150–350 × $10^3/mm^3$	150–350 × 10^9/liter	Automated cell counter	1

Platelet, mean volume	WB	6.6–11.0 μm^3	6.6–11.0 fl	automated cell counter	1
Protein C	P				0.01
Immunologic		70–140%	0.70–1.40	Immunoassay	
Functional		70–140%	0.70–1.40	Automated clotting assay	
Protein S	P				0.01
Total antigen		70–140%	0.70–1.40	Immunoassay	
Functional		70–140%	0.70–1.40	Automated clotting assay	
Prothrombin time	P	8.8–11.6 sec	8.8–11.6 sec	Automated clotting assay	1
Red-cell distribution width	WB	11.5–14.5%	0.115–0.145	Automated clotting assay	0.01
Reptilase time	P	Within 5 sec of control	Within 5 sec of control	Automated clotting assay	1
Reticulocyte count	WB	0.5–2.5% red cells	0.005–0.025 red cells	Manual	0.01
Ristocetin cofactor (functional von Willebrand factor)	P	50–150%	0.50–1.50	Platelet agglutination	0.01
Thrombin time	P	Within 5 sec of control	Within 5 sec of control	Automated clotting assay	1
Vitamin B_{12}	S			Immunoassay	0.7378
Normal		205–876 pg/ml	151–646 pmol/liter		
Borderline		140–204 pg/ml	103–150 pmol/liter		
Deficient		<140 pg/ml	<103 pmol/liter		
von Willebrand factor (vWF) antigen (factor VIII:R antigen)	P	50–150%	0.50–1.50	Immunoassay	0.01
von Willebrand factor multimers	P	Normal distribution	Normal distribution	Western blotting	1

* S denotes serum, WB whole blood, P plasma, U urine, CSF cerebrospinal fluid, and PRP platelet-rich plasma.
Reprinted, with permission, from N. Engl J Med, *327*:718, 1992.

Abbreviations

Abbreviation	Meaning
-C	cholesterol
1st° . . .	first-degree . . .
<	less than; under
>	greater than; more than; in excess of; over (age); above; exceeding
A-V	atrioventricular
ABE	acute bacterial endocarditis
ABG	arterial blood gas
ACC	American College of Cardiology
ACE	angiotensin-converting enzyme
ADA	adenosine deaminase
ADH	antidiuretic hormone
ADP	adenosine 5′-diphosphate; adenosine diphosphate
AED	automated external defibrillator
AF	atrial fibrillation
AG	anion gap
AHA	American Heart Association
AIDS	acquired immunodeficiency syndrome
ALT	alanine aminotransferase
AML	acute myeloid leukemia
AMP	adenosine monophosphate
ANA	antinuclear antibody
APSAC	anisoylated plasminogen-streptokinase activator complex
ARDS	adult respiratory distress syndrome
ARF	acute respiratory failure
ASA	amino salicylate
ASD	atrial septal defect
AST	aspartate aminotransferase
ATPase	adenosinetriphosphatase
ATIII	antithrombin III
AVNRT	A-V nodal reentrant tachycardia
BAL	bronchoalveolar lavage
BASIS	Basel Antiarrhythmic Study of Infarct Survival
BHAT	Beta Blocker Heart Attack Trial
bid	twice a day; twice daily
BMT	bone marrow transplant
BP	blood pressure
BPPV	benign paroxysmal positional vertigo
BUN	blood urea nitrogen
Ca + +/Ca +/Ca	calcium
CABS	coronary artery bypass surgery
CaCl	calcium chloride
CAP	community-acquired pneumonia
CAS	coronary artery spasm
CAST	Cardiac Arrhythmia Suppression Trial
CBC	complete blood count
CCU	coronary care unit; critical care unit
CF	complement fixation
CHD	coronary heart disease; ischemic heart disease
CHF	congestive heart failure
CK	creatine kinase

Abbreviation	Meaning
CLL	chronic lymphocytic leukemia
CMV	Cytomegalovirus
CNS	central nervous system
CoA	coenzyme A
CO_2	carbon dioxide
CONSENSUS	Cooperative North Scandinavian Enalapril Survival Study
COPD	chronic obstructive pulmonary disease; obstructive lung disease
CPK	creatine phosphokinase
CPR	cardiopulmonary resuscitation
CRF	chronic renal failure
CRH	corticotropin releasing hormone
CSF	cerebrospinal fluid
CT	computed tomography; computerized tomographic
CVP	central venous pressure
CVS	cardiovascular system
D5W	5% dextrose in water
DA/TMP	Dapsone-Trimethoprim
DCM	dilated cardiomyopathy
DFA	direct fluorescent antibody
DHE 45	Dihydroergotamine
DIC	diffuse intravascular coagulation
dl (dL)	deciliter
DOPA	dihydroxyphenylalanine
DPG	diphosphoglycerate
DVT	deep venous thrombosis
D/W	dextrose in water
E.	Escherichia
ECG	electrocardiogram, electrocardiographic
EF	ejection fraction
ELISA	complement fixation
EMD	electromechanical dissociation
EMF	electromotive force
EMG	electromyogram
EP	electrophysiologic
EPO	erythropoeitin
ERCP	endoscopic retrograde cholangiopancreatography
ESR	erythrocyte sedimentation rate
EXCEL	Expanded Clinical Evaluation of Lovastatin
FB	fiberoptic bronchoscopy
FDA	Food and Drug Administration
FEV	forced expiratory volume
FIO_2	fractional concentration of inspired oxygen
FFP	fresh frozen plasma
FSH	follicle stimulating hormone
FT_4I	free thyroxine index
FUO	fever of unknown origin
FVC	forced vital capacity
g	gram
GFR	glomerular filtration rate
GI	gastrointestinal
GISSI	The Gruppo Italiano per lo Studio della Strepto chinasi Nell Infarto Miocardico
GN	glomerulonephritis
GNB	gram negative bacteria

Abbreviation	Meaning
GUSTO	Global Utilization of SK and tPA for Occluded Coronary Arteries
GVH	graft versus host
h	hour(s)
Hb	hemoglobin
HCl	hydrochloric acid
HCM	hypertrophic cardiomyopathy
HCTZ	hydrochlorothiazide
HDL	high density lipoprotein
HF	heart failure
HIV	human immunodeficiency virus
HLA	human leukocyte antigen
HMG-CoA	3-hydroxy-3-methylglutaryl coenzyme A
HOA	hypertrophic pulmonary osteopathy
HR	heart rate
HSV	Herpes Simplex Virus
HV	His to ventricular
I.M.	intramuscular(ly)
IABP	intra-aortic blood pump
IBD	inflammatory bowel disease
ICU	intensive care unit
IHD	ischemic heart disease
IF	immunofluorescence
IgG	immunoglobin g
IgM	immunoglobin M
IM	internal medicine
INR	International Normalized Ratio
IPG	Impedance plethysmography
ISA	intrinsic sympathomimetic activity
ISI	International Sensitivity Index
ISIS-2	The Second International Study of Infarct Survival
IV	intravenous(ly)
J	joule
JVP	jugular venous pressure
K	potassium
KS	Kaposi's sarcoma
KCl	potassium chloride
kg	kilogram
L	liter
L-	levo-
LAD	left anterior descending
LATE	Late Assessment of Thrombolytic Efficacy
LBBB	left bundle branch block
LDH	lactate dehydrogenase
LDL	low-density lipoprotein
LGV	lymphogranuloma venereum
LH	luteinizing hormone
LV	left ventricular; left heart
LVH	left ventricular hypertrophy
M	molar
MAT	multifocal atrial tachycardia
MCHC	mean corpuscular hemoglobin concentration
MCP	metacarpophalangeal
MDI	metered-dose inhaler
meq/mEq	milliequivalent
mCi	millicurie
MegaBq	MegaBecquerel

Abbreviation	Meaning
MESNA	mercaptoethane sulfate
MET	metabolic exercise equivalents; metabolic equivalent
mg	milligram
MI	myocardial infarction
MIAMI	Metroprolol in Acute Myocardial Infarction
MIBG	I131 meta-iodo-benzyl-guanidine
MIC	minimum inhibitory concentration
MITI	myocardial infarction triage
ml (mL)	milliliter
mmol	millimole
MPGN	membrane proliferative glomerulonephritis
MPTP	1-methyl-4-phenyl-1, 2, 3, 6-tetrahydropyridine
MR	mitral regurgitation
MRI	magnetic resonance imaging
MRSA	methicillin resistant staphylococcus aureus
MSK	musculoskeletal system
Na+/Na	sodium
NaCl	sodium chloride
NBT	nitro blue tetrazolium
NG	nasogastric
ng	nonogram
NHLBI	National Heart Lung Blood Institute
nmol	nanomole
NMS	neuroleptic malignant syndrome
NPO	nothing by mouth
NSAID	nonsteroidal anti-inflammatory drug
NTG	nitroglycerine
NYHA	New York Heart Association
O_2	oxygen
PA	pulmonary artery
$PaCO_2$	arterial carbon dioxide tension
PaO2	arterial oxygen tension
PAS	periodic acid—Schiff
PAT	paroxysmal atrial tachycardia
PB	protected brush
PCWP	pulmonary capillary wedge pressure
PEEP	positive end-expiratory pressure
PEER	peak expiratory flow rate
pg	picagram
PIOPED	Prospective Investigation of Pulmonary Embolism Diagnosis
PMN	polymorphonuclear neutrophils
pmol	picomole
PND	paroxysmal nocturnal dyspnea
po	by mouth
PPD	purified protein derivative of tuberculin
PRBC	packed red blood cells
prn	as the occasion arises
PSVT	paroxysmal supraventricular tachycardia
PT	prothrombin time
PTH	parathyroid hormone
PTU	propylthiauracil
PTT	partial thromboplastin time
PVD	peripheral vascular disease
q	every
q 4 h	every 4 hours

Abbreviation	Meaning
qd	daily
qid	four times a day
PRA	plasma renin activity
RA	receptor antagonist
RAIU	radioactive iodine uptake
RBBB	right bundle branch block
RBC	red blood cell
RCM	restrictive cardiomyopathy
RPR	rapid plasma reagin
S-A	sinoatrial
SAVE	Survival and Ventricular Enlargement
SBE	subacute bacterial endocarditis
SC	subcutaneous
SHEP	Systolic Hypertension in the Elderly Program
SHMD	specific heart muscle disease
SK	streptokinase
SLE	systemic lupus erythematosus
SO_4	sulfate
SOLVD	studies of left ventricular dysfunction
sp(p)	subspecies
ST	Sinus tachycardia
SVT	supraventricular tachycardia
TBPA	thyroid binding pre-albumin
TEE	transesophageal echocardiogram; Transesophageal echocardiography
TIA	transient ischemic attack
tid	three times a day
TIMI	Thrombolysis in Myocardial Infarction
TMP/SMX	Trimethoprim-sulfamethoxazole
TPA	tissue plasminogen activator
TPN	total parenteral nutrition
TPNH	triphosphopyridine nucleotide
TRH	thyrotropin stimulating hormone
TSH	thryroid stimulating hormone
TT	total thyroxine
TTP	thrombotic thromcytopenic purpura
T_3RU	T_3 resin uptake
U	unit
UA	urine anions
UC	urine cations
UGI	upper gastrointestinal
V	volt
V-A	ventriculoatrial
VA	Veterans' Administration
VF	ventricular fibrillation
VHeFT	Veterans Administration Cooperative Vasodilator Heart Failure Trial
VIP	vasoactive intestinal peptide
VLDL	very low-density lipoprotein
VMA	vanillylmandelic acid
$\dot{V}O_2$	oxygen consumption
VPB	ventricular premature beat
VPC	ventricular premature contraction
VQ	ventilation/perfusion (V/Q)
VSD	ventricular septal defect
VT	ventricular tachycardia
WBC	white blood cell; white blood count

Abbreviation	Meaning
WHO	World Health Organization
WPW	Wolff-Parkinson-White
≤	less than or equal to; equal to or less than; # or less; # or fewer
≥	greater than or equal to; at least; more than or equal to; # or more
μ	micro
μm	micrometer
μmg	micromilligram
β	beta
↓	decrease(d); reduction
↑	increase; rise

Index

Page numbers in *italics* indicate illustrations; numbers followed by "t" indicate tables.

ALGORITHM FOR THE MANAGEMENT OF SUSPECTED PULMONARY EMBOLISM

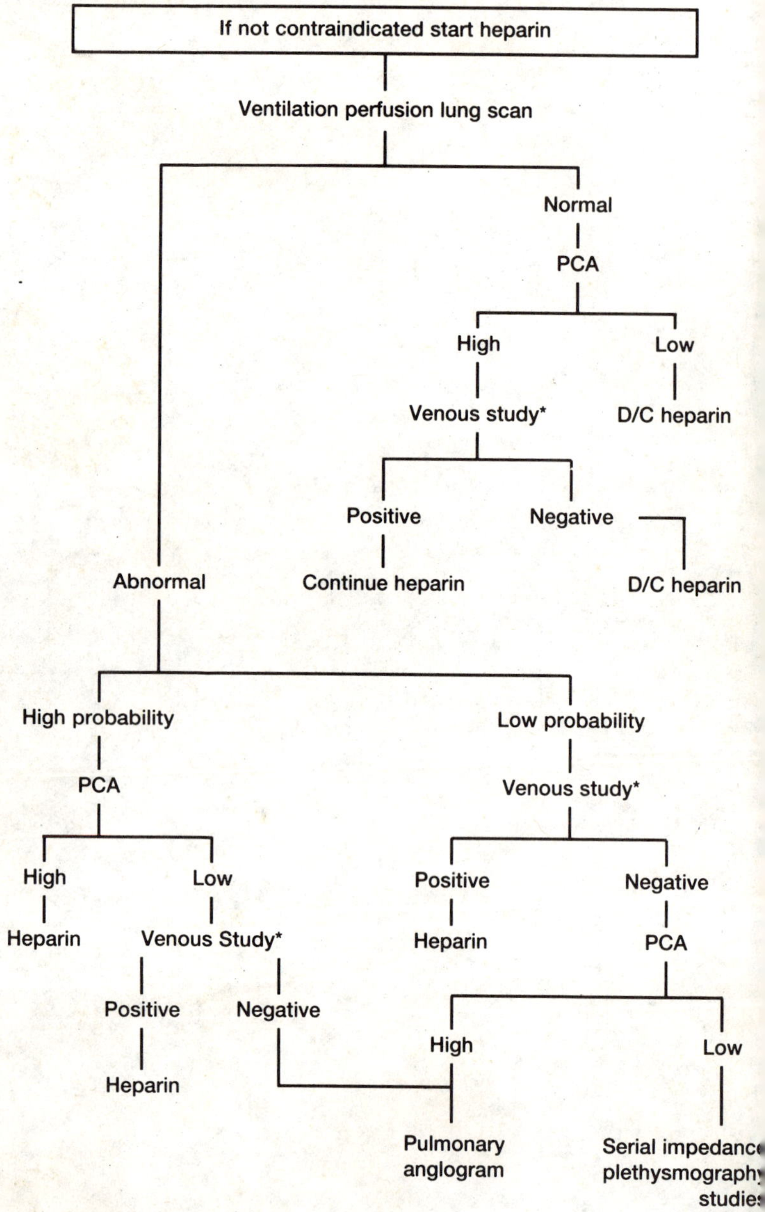

PCA = Probability from clinical assessment

D/C = Discontinue

*Venous study = Impedance plethysmography, venogram, or Duplex scanning

M. Gabriel Khan, Lucy B. Palm